The Wrist

Diagnosis and
Operative Treatment

VOLUME TWO

The Wrist
Diagnosis and Operative Treatment

Edited by

WILLIAM P. COONEY, M.D.
Chair, Division of Hand Surgery, Mayo Clinic and
Mayo Foundation; Professor of Orthopedics,
Mayo Medical School; Rochester, Minnesota

RONALD L. LINSCHEID, M.D.
Emeritus, Department of Orthopedics, Mayo Clinic and
Mayo Foundation; Emeritus Professor of Orthopedics,
Mayo Medical School; Rochester, Minnesota

JAMES H. DOBYNS, M.D.
Emeritus, Department of Orthopedics, Mayo Clinic and
Mayo Foundation; Emeritus Professor of Orthopedics,
Mayo Medical School; Rochester, Minnesota

with 2620 illustrations, 64 in color

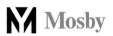

St. Louis Baltimore Boston Carlsbad Chicago Naples New York Philadelphia Portland
London Madrid Mexico City Singapore Sydney Tokyo Toronto Wiesbaden

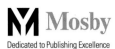
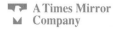

Dedicated to Publishing Excellence

A Times Mirror
Company

Vice President and Publisher: Anne S. Patterson
Editor: Robert A. Hurley
Developmental Editor: Lauranne Billus
Editorial Assistant: Jori Matison
Project Manager: Linda Clarke
Associate Production Editor: Deborah Ann Cicirello
Composition Specialist: Kevin D. Dodds
Designer: Chris Robinson
Cover Designer: Carolyn O'Brien
Manufacturing Manager: William A. Winneberger, Jr.

Printed in the United States of America
Composition by Mosby Electronic Production, Philadelphia
Printing/binding by Maple-Vail Book Manufacturing Group

Mosby–Year Book, Inc.
11830 Westline Industrial Drive
St. Louis, Missouri 63146

Library of Congress Cataloging in Publication Data
The wrist : diagnosis and operative treatment / [edited by] William P.
  Cooney, Ronald L. Linscheid, James H. Dobyns.
    p.   cm.
    Includes bibliographical references and index.
    ISBN 0-8016-6644-9
    1. Wrist.   I. Cooney, William Patrick, 1943-   II. Linscheid,
  R. L. (Ronald Lee), 1929-   .   III. Dobyns, James H.
    [DNLM: 1. Wrist Injuries. 2. Wrist. 3. Wrist Joint.   WE 830
  W95517 1998]
  RD559.W752   1998
  617.5′ 74—dc21
  DNLM/DLC
  for Library of Congress   97-14867
                                                            CIP

98 99 00 01 02 / 9 8 7 6 5 4 3 2 1

CONTRIBUTORS

Peter C. Amadio, M.D.
Consultant, Division of Hand Surgery, Mayo Clinic
and Mayo Foundation; Professor of Orthopedics,
Mayo Medical School; Rochester, Minnesota

Kai-Nan An, Ph.D.
Chair, Division of Orthopedic Research, Mayo Clinic
and Mayo Foundation; Professor of Bioengineering,
Mayo Medical School; Rochester, Minnesota

Robert D. Beckenbaugh, M.D.
Consultant, Division of Hand Surgery, Mayo Clinic
and Mayo Foundation; Professor of Orthopedics,
Mayo Medical School; Rochester, Minnesota

Keith A. Bengtson, M.D.
Consultant, Department of Physical Medicine and
Rehabilitation, Mayo Clinic and Mayo Foundation;
Instructor in Physical Medicine and Rehabilitation,
Mayo Medical School; Rochester, Minnesota

Michel Y. Benoit, M.D.
Assistant Professor, Department of Orthopedic
Surgery and Rehabilitation, University of Vermont,
Burlington, Vermont

Richard A. Berger, M.D., Ph.D.
Consultant, Division of Hand Surgery, Mayo Clinic
and Mayo Foundation; Associate Professor of
Orthopedics, Mayo Medical School; Rochester,
Minnesota

Allen T. Bishop, M.D.
Consultant, Division of Hand Surgery, Mayo Clinic
and Mayo Foundation; Assistant Professor of
Orthopedics, Mayo Medical School; Rochester,
Minnesota

Steven D. Bogard III, M.A., P.T.
Supervisor, Department of Physical Medicine and
Rehabilitation, Mayo Clinic and Mayo Foundation,
Rochester, Minnesota

Jeffrey R. Bond, M.D.
Consultant, Department of Diagnostic Radiology,
Mayo Clinic and Mayo Foundation; Assistant
Professor of Radiology, Mayo Medical School;
Rochester, Minnesota

Thomas DeBartolo, M.D.
Hand Special Fellow, Division of Hand Surgery,
Mayo Clinic and Mayo Foundation, Rochester,
Minnesota. Present address: Hand Surgeon, Mason
City Clinic, Mason City, Iowa

Joseph M. Failla, M.D.
Hand Special Fellow, Division of Hand Surgery,
Mayo Clinic and Mayo Foundation, Rochester,
Minnesota. Present address: Consultant, Hand
Surgery, Department of Orthopedics, Henry Ford
Hospital, Detroit, Michigan

Marc Garcia-Elias, M.D.
Visiting Scientist at the Division of Orthopedic
Research, Mayo Clinic and Mayo Foundation,
Rochester, Minnesota. Present address: Department
of Orthopedics, Hospital General de Catalunya,
Barcelona, Spain

Guillaume Herzberg, M.D.
Visiting Scientist at the Division of Hand Surgery,
Mayo Clinic and Mayo Foundation, Rochester,
Minnesota. Present address: Head of Hand and
Upper Extremity Orthopedic Unit, Hopital Edouard
Herriot, Lyon, France

Emiko Horii, M.D.
Visiting Clinician at the Department of
Orthopedics, Mayo Clinic and Mayo Foundation,
Rochester, Minnesota. Present address: Branch
Hospital of Nagoya University, Higashiku, Nagoya
City 461, Japan

Damien C.R. Ireland, M.D.
Resident in Orthopedics, Mayo Graduate School of
Medicine, Rochester, Minnesota. Present address:
Consultant Orthopaedic Surgeon, Royal Australian
Navy; Director, Victorian Hand Surgery &
Rehabilitation Centre, Melbourne, Australia

George B. Irons, M.D.
Emeritus, Division of Plastic Surgery, Mayo Clinic
and Mayo Foundation; Emeritus Professor of Plastic
Surgery, Mayo Medical School; Rochester,
Minnesota. Present address: Fountain Hills, Arizona

Scott H. Kozin, M.D.
Hand Special Fellow, Division of Hand Surgery, Mayo Clinic and Mayo Foundation, Rochester, Minnesota. Present address: Instructor, Department of Orthopedics, Temple University School of Medicine, Philadelphia, Pennsylvania

Jon Loftus, M.D.
Assistant Professor, Orthopedic Surgery and General Surgery, SUNY Health Science Center, Department of Orthopedic Surgery, Syracuse, New York

Mary W. Marzke, Ph.D.
Visiting Scientist at the Division of Orthopedic Research, Mayo Clinic and Mayo Foundation, Rochester, Minnesota. Present address: Associate Professor, Department of Anthropology, Arizona State University, Tempe, Arizona

Brian J. McGrory, M.D.
Senior Resident in Orthopedics, Mayo Graduate School of Medicine, Rochester, Minnesota. Present address: Private Practice, Portland, Maine

Elizabeth Mohror, O.T.R.
Occupational Therapist, Department of Physical Medicine and Rehabilitation, Mayo Clinic and Mayo Foundation, Rochester, Minnesota. Present address: Alexandria, Minnesota

Margaret A. Moutvic, M.D.
Consultant, Department of Physical Medicine and Rehabilitation, Mayo Clinic and Mayo Foundation; Instructor in Physical Medicine and Rehabilitation, Mayo Medical School; Rochester, Minnesota

Owen J. Moy, M.D.
Consultant, Department of Orthopedic Surgery, Mayo Clinic Jacksonville, Jacksonville, Florida. Present address: Consultant, Hand Center of Western New York, Upstate New York Medical College, Syracuse, New York

Michael S. Murphy, M.D.
Hand Special Fellow, Division of Hand Surgery, Mayo Clinic and Mayo Foundation, Rochester, Minnesota. Present address: Instructor, Department of Orthopedics, Johns Hopkins Medical School, Union Memorial Hospital, Baltimore, Maryland

Peter M. Murray, M.D.
Hand Special Fellow, Division of Hand Surgery, Mayo Clinic and Mayo Foundation, Rochester, Minnesota. Present address: Chief of Hand Surgery, Wilford Hall, Lackland Air Force Base, U.S. Air Force, San Antonio, Texas

Andrew K. Palmer, M.D.
Hand Special Fellow, Division of Hand Surgery, Mayo Clinic and Mayo Foundation, Rochester, Minnesota. Present address: Professor of Orthopedic Surgery, Department of Orthopedic Surgery, SUNY Health Science Center, Syracuse, New York

Hamlet A. Peterson, M.D.
Chair, Division of Pediatric Orthopedics, Mayo Clinic and Mayo Foundation; Professor of Orthopedics, Mayo Medical School; Rochester, Minnesota

John M. Rayhack, M.D.
Hand Special Fellow, Division of Hand Surgery, Mayo Clinic and Mayo Foundation, Rochester, Minnesota. Present address: Private Practice, Tampa, Florida

Douglas S. Reagan, M.D.
Hand Special Fellow, Division of Hand Surgery, Mayo Clinic and Mayo Foundation, Rochester, Minnesota. Present address: West Des Moines, Iowa

Spencer A. Rowland, M.D.
Resident in Orthopedics, Mayo Graduate School of Medicine, Rochester, Minnesota. Present address: San Antonio Orthopaedic Group, P.A., San Antonio, Texas

Leonard K. Ruby, M.D.
Visiting Scientist at the Division of Orthopedic Research, Mayo Clinic and Mayo Foundation, Rochester, Minnesota. Present address: Professor of Orthopedic Surgery, Tufts University; Chair, Division of Hand Surgery, Department of Orthopedic Surgery, Tufts University School of Medicine, New England Medical Center; Boston, Massachusetts

Frédéric A. Schuind, M.D.
Research Fellow at the Division of Orthopedic Research, Mayo Clinic and Mayo Foundation, Rochester, Minnesota. Present address: Service d'Orthopedie-Traumatologie, Cliniques Universitaires des Bruxelles, Hopital Erasme, Bruxelles, Belgium

Ann H. Schutt, M.D.
Consultant, Department of Physical Medicine and Rehabilitation, Mayo Clinic and Mayo Foundation; Associate Professor of Physical Medicine and Rehabilitation, Mayo Medical School; Rochester, Minnesota

Julio Taleisnik, M.D.
Resident in Orthopedics, Mayo Graduate School of Medicine, Rochester, Minnesota. Present address: Clinical Professor of Surgery (Orthopedics), University of California, Irvine, Irvine, California

Steven M. Topper, M.D.
Hand Special Fellow, Division of Hand Surgery, Mayo Clinic and Mayo Foundation, Rochester, Minnesota. Present address: Assistant Professor of Orthopaedic Surgery, University of Colorado Health Science Center; Clinical Assistant Professor of Surgery, Uniformed Services University of Health Sciences, F. Edward Hebert School of Medicine; Clinical Assistant Professor of Orthopaedic Surgery, University of Colorado Health Science Center; Colorado Springs, Colorado

David Vickers, M.B.B.S.
Visiting Professor at the Division of Hand Surgery, Mayo Clinic and Mayo Foundation, Rochester, Minnesota. Present address: Clinical Professor, University of Queensland, Watkins Medical Centre, Brisbane, Australia

Edward R. Weber, M.D.
Hand Special Fellow, Division of Hand Surgery, Mayo Clinic and Mayo Foundation, Rochester, Minnesota. Present address: Private Practice, Little Rock, Arkansas

Michael B. Wood, M.D.
Consultant, Department of Orthopedics, Mayo Clinic and Mayo Foundation; Professor of Orthopedics, Mayo Medical School; Rochester, Minnesota

Thomas W. Wright, M.D.
Hand Special Fellow, Division of Hand Surgery, Mayo Clinic and Mayo Foundation, Rochester, Minnesota. Present address: Assistant Professor, Department of Orthopedic Surgery, Division of Hand Surgery, University of Florida, Gainesville, Florida

The entire current staff as well as past residents and fellows within the Division of Hand Surgery at the Mayo Clinic dedicate this book to Drs. Ronald L. Linscheid and James H. Dobyns. We do so noting their effective contributions to knowledge of and treatment rendered to disorders of the wrist.

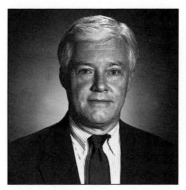 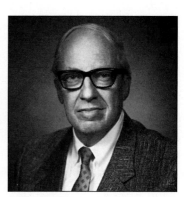

Ronald L. Linscheid, M.D.   *James H. Dobyns, M.D.*

The wrist is a complex articulation essential to the performance of many human activities. A wide range of motion, analogous to that of a swiveled universal joint, provides incremental positioning of the hand and simultaneously allows extensive alteration in the transmission of force to the hand. That the wrist-hand unit may be considered a product of advantageous evolutionary adaptations is addressed in the first chapter. The forging of morphologic changes in the carpus of our hominid precursors, as they used progressively more sophisticated tools, appears to be a significant factor in developing the capabilities that distinguish modern humans. These changes gave distinct advantages to the survival of our species.

The nomenclature of the carpus has long been the plaything of anatomists and the bane of medical students. Yet, naming structures is relatively simple compared with the task of discerning the interrelationships of the complex topology of individual carpal bones and simpler still than understanding the dynamic biomechanical functions of the bones, joints, and ligaments of the wrist. Accurate anatomic descriptions of the carpus are rather recent, and careful kinematic study of the carpus only became possible with the advent of the x-ray a scant century ago, as reviewed in Chapter 2. Application of modern techniques to study force transmission, joint contact areas, and relative displacement of individual and combinations of carpal bones has added greatly to our appreciation of the normal as well as the pathophysiologic functions of these joints. A review of the anatomy and physiology of the wrist is presented in Chapter 3.

Several prescient early works on the wrist, especially the outstanding text of E. Destot,* were largely ignored in the interval between the two World Wars. A marked resurgence of interest in the wrist began in the late 1960s and early 1970s. This is evidenced by the increasing number of published articles on wrist-related subjects as well as several recent well-written single-author or multiauthor books. This dissemination of knowledge has had a beneficial and expansive effect on the diagnosis and treatment of carpal injuries and conditions, as is apparent to anyone whose observations have spanned the last three decades.

A new comprehensive text on a subject that is already extensively covered requires some justification. That justification, we believe, is that an extensive body of work has developed and is continuing around the early core publications of the Mayo group, beginning 25 to 30 years ago. Wrist investigation became and continues to be such an integral part of the training program in which we were involved that a school of thought concerning all aspects of the wrist has evolved. The onus on this group to publish a text earlier was delayed by the publication of a superb single-author text, *The Wrist* * by Julio Taleisnik, in 1985. This and other single-author texts have the advantages of a focused point of view and this is often easier to absorb. Nevertheless, the many investigations of a school of workers in a given interest produce a ferment of productivity that spills over into the occasional text as well as often cited publication. By the time any text, including this one, is published, the fermentation flow has progressed beyond the text, but the themes of the past, present, and future are revealed and the historical support for these themes is firmly in place.

One of the delights of being part of a professional fermenting process is to enjoy spreading of the zest, particularly when many other individuals and schools become involved, leading the progress and taking the point position. Wrist enthusiasts know that the state of the art will continue to change indefinitely as we recognize increasing problems with the wrist and the effect of an increasingly active population.

The greatest verity of the ages is "this too shall pass!" and it is true of the current basic, diagnostic, and treatment thoughts in this text. The corollary is "that which passes will be replaced!" and our hope is that this book will stimulate inquisitive minds to make dynamic advances. If this is accomplished, our purpose will have been more than served and the labor of its production amply rewarded.

James H. Dobyns, M.D.
Ronald L. Linscheid, M.D.

---

* Destot E: *Injuries of the wrist: a radiological study* (translated by FRB Atkinson), New York, 1926, Paul B Hoeber.

* Taleisnik J: *The wrist,* New York, 1985, Churchill Livingstone.

In the last 10 to 15 years, the level of interest in the wrist, its injuries, and its diseases has increased exponentially. This era of the wrist may, in fact, be attributed in large part to the singular devoted interest of the coeditors of this text, Drs. Ronald L. Linscheid and James H. Dobyns. Their classic paper on post-traumatic carpal instability[*] helped to inaugurate an increasing national and international interest in the wrist. In recognition of these contributions, we dedicate this book to our mentors in wrist surgery.

With a long and dedicated record of interest in the wrist at the Mayo Clinic, it appeared quite appropriate and beneficial to place together in a single source the teachings of these mentors as well as those of the subsequent staff of the Division of Hand Surgery at our institution. We wanted, as well, to include distinguished alumni who shared, yet not infrequently disagreed with, our concepts and surgical approaches to problems involving the wrist.

We identify three significant reasons why we were motivated to undertake an extensive and comprehensive text on the wrist. First, we believe that a tremendous wealth of information based on clinical studies and basic science has originated from the talents and energies of the staff and hand fellows in training at the Mayo Clinic. Publications related to this work have been quite extensive but never compiled into a single source. Using this information as a framework, together with an exhaustive review of the literature and knowledge of the variability in surgical techniques used to treat disease and injury about the wrist, we wish to provide our readers with the preferred operative approaches for the most common problems affecting the wrist.

Second, there has been no major in-depth text regarding the wrist since the excellent publication by Dr. Julio Taleisnik and the multiauthor text on the wrist edited by Dr. David Lichtman. The field of wrist pathology and the depth of understanding of wrist disease and injury have progressed substantially since the time of those publications. Indeed, a specialized interest group identified as The Wrist Investigators Workshop Group developed to meet the need of ongoing educational discussions regarding the wrist. At present, there is not a single reference source that details the rationale, techniques, and results of operative intervention on the wrist. This book is an effort to fill that void.

Third, an in-depth presentation of the writings of the editors, the current staff of our institution, and other related investigators appeared to be a timely contribution to our knowledge on this subject.

The book starts with a short history of the wrist and its disorders by Drs. Linscheid and Dobyns, followed by anthropology and comparative anatomy, a special interest of both coeditors, but particularly of Dr. Linscheid. The book then continues with sections on anatomy, surgical approaches, pathomechanics, and diagnostic examination and imaging. The major sections deal with fractures of the wrist, carpal instability, dislocations, the distal radioulnar joint, arthritis of the wrist, developmental disorders, complications and tendinitis, and tumors of the wrist. We conclude with a section on rehabilitation and both physical and occupational therapy directed toward the wrist. The book is designed to be comprehensive in both diagnosis and treatment, with a special emphasis as indicated by the title on the operative treatment of disorders involving the wrist. We are hopeful that the textbook will serve as a continuing guide for preoperative planning and interoperative judgment in reconstructive surgery of the wrist.

"The Future," the final section, provides a look ahead. It places this textbook, in fact, back into the hands of the readers, providing them the background and opportunity to expand on the information presented. The wrist was considered a new frontier in the 1970s, and great progress has been made in solving many of its problems. However, there is still a great deal to accomplish, with many challenges ahead. The need is great to identify and critically investigate disorders and deformities that affect the wrist by applying what we have learned in research laboratories and in the clinical setting from outcome analysis and prospective reviews. Our goal is to provide our patients with a functional wrist and, as a result, useful and productive lives.

We hope that this contribution as well as our previous efforts will be rewarded by knowing that we have aided a few and that other physicians and surgeons have aided many as a result of becoming increasingly knowledgeable about the wrist.

Developing this textbook on the wrist has been a stimulating and pleasurable educational experience that was salted with hard work and represents a team effort. It would not have been possible without collaboration from my partners within the Hand Clinic; the dedicated service of Ms. Deborah Hughes, my secretary; and the excellence in manuscript preparation from our Section of Publications: Ms. Margery Lovejoy, Ms. Reneé Van Vleet, and Ms. Roberta Schwartz. That this text reads well is a reflection of the diligence and persistence of our editor from Mayo's Section of Publications, Dr. Carol Kornblith, who reviewed and corrected every chapter. Finally, the exquisite art was done by Beck Visual Communications, Inc., of Minneapolis, Minnesota, and members of Mayo's Section of Visual Information. We hope these combined efforts have given you—student, resident, fellow, physician, and surgeon—an excellent text on which to base your knowledge of disorders of the wrist.

---

[*] Linscheid RL, Dobyns JH, Beabout JW, et al.: Traumatic instability of the wrist. Diagnosis, classification, and pathomechanics, *J Bone Joint Surg Am* 54:1612-1632, 1972.

William P. Cooney, M.D.

CONTENTS

VOLUME ONE

I BACKGROUND

1   CARPAL COMPREHENSION: A SHORT LOOK AT A HISTORY OF UNDERSTANDING THE WRIST JOINT, 2
R.L. Linscheid, J.H. Dobyns

2   ANTHROPOLOGY AND COMPARATIVE ANATOMY, 14
M.W. Marzke, R.L. Linscheid

II ANATOMY

3   GENERAL ANATOMY, 32
R.A. Berger

4   BONES AND JOINTS, 61
M. Garcia-Elias, J.H. Dobyns

5   LIGAMENT ANATOMY, 73
R.A. Berger

6   VASCULAR AND NEUROLOGIC ANATOMY OF THE WRIST, 106
W.P. Cooney

III SURGICAL APPROACHES

7   ARTHROTOMY, 126
L.K. Ruby

8   ARTHROSCOPIC ANATOMY OF THE WRIST, 169
W.P. Cooney

IV PATHOMECHANICS OF WRIST INJURIES

9   FORCE TRANSMISSION THROUGH RADIOCARPAL JOINT, 190
E. Horii, M. Garcia-Elias, K-N An

10   KINEMATICS OF THE RADIOCARPAL JOINT, 205
M. Garcia-Elias, W.P. Cooney

11   MECHANICS OF THE DISTAL RADIOULNAR JOINT, 219
F.A. Schuind, R.L. Linscheid

V EXAMINATION OF THE WRIST

12   PHYSICAL EXAMINATION OF THE WRIST, 236
W.P. Cooney, A.T. Bishop, R.L. Linscheid

13   IMAGING OF THE WRIST, 262
J.R. Bond, W.P. Cooney, R.A. Berger

14   WRIST ARTHROSCOPY, 284
A.K. Palmer, J. Loftus

VI FRACTURES OF THE WRIST

15   FRACTURES OF THE DISTAL RADIUS, 310
W.P. Cooney

16   MALUNION OF THE DISTAL RADIUS, 356
B.J. McGrory, P.C. Amadio

17   SCAPHOID FRACTURES AND NONUNION, 385
R.L. Linscheid, E.R. Weber

18   LUNATE FRACTURES: KIENBÖCK'S DISEASE, 431
A.K. Palmer, M.Y. Benoit

19   ISOLATED CARPAL FRACTURES, 474
W.P. Cooney

VII CARPAL INSTABILITY

20   CLASSIFICATION OF CARPAL INSTABILITY, 490
J.H. Dobyns, W.P. Cooney

21   SCAPHOLUNATE INSTABILITY, 501
J. Taleisnik, R.L. Linscheid

22   LUNOTRIQUETRAL SPRAINS, 527
A.T. Bishop, D.S. Reagan

23   CARPAL INSTABILITY NONDISSOCIATIVE, 550
T.W. Wright, J.H. Dobyns

24   RADIOCARPAL INSTABILITY AND RADIOCARPAL DISLOCATIONS, 569
D.C.R. Ireland

25 POST-TRAUMATIC ARTHRITIS OF THE
    WRIST, 588
    W.P. Cooney, T. DeBartolo, M.B. Wood

VIII DISLOCATIONS AND FRACTURES

26 PERILUNATE DISLOCATIONS, 632
    S.H. Kozin, M.S. Murphy, W.P. Cooney

27 PERILUNATE FRACTURE DISLOCATIONS,
    651
    G. Herzberg, W.P. Cooney

28 AXIAL DISLOCATIONS AND FRACTURE
    DISLOCATIONS, 684
    M. Garcia-Elias, W.P. Cooney

29 ISOLATED CARPAL DISLOCATIONS, 696
    L.K. Ruby

VOLUME TWO

IX INJURIES OF DISTAL RADIOULNAR
    JOINT

30 TEARS OF THE TRIANGULAR
    FIBROCARTILAGE OF THE WRIST, 710
    W.P. Cooney

31 FRACTURES OF THE DISTAL RADIOULNAR
    JOINT, 743
    J.M. Rayhack, W.P. Cooney

32 DORSAL AND PALMAR DISLOCATIONS OF
    THE DISTAL RADIOULNAR JOINT, 758
    M. Garcia-Elias, J.H. Dobyns

33 ULNOCARPAL ABUTMENT, 773
    O.J. Moy, A.K. Palmer

34 ARTHRITIS DEFORMITY: RESECTION
    ARTHROPLASTY AND FUSION, 788
    J. Taleisnik, L.K. Ruby

35 DISORDERS OF THE DISTAL RADIOULNAR
    JOINT, 819
    R.L. Linscheid

X RHEUMATOID ARTHRITIS

36 CLINICAL EVALUATION OF THE ARTHRITIC
    WRIST, 870
    J.H. Dobyns

37 SOFT-TISSUE RECONSTRUCTION, 887
    M.B. Wood

38 WRIST FUSION: PARTIAL AND COMPLETE,
    899
    J.M. Rayhack, M.B. Wood

39 TOTAL WRIST ARTHROPLASTY, 924
    R.D. Beckenbaugh

40 VARIANT FORMS OF ARTHRITIS: JUVENILE
    RHEUMATOID ARTHRITIS, SYSTEMIC
    LUPUS ERYTHEMATOSUS, AND PSORIATIC
    ARTHRITIS, 945
    S.A. Rowland, J. Taleisnik

XI DEVELOPMENTAL DISORDERS

41 MADELUNG'S DEFORMITY, 966
    D. Vickers

42 GROWTH-PLATE INJURIES, 982
    D. Vickers

43 DEFORMITIES AND PROBLEMS OF THE
    WRIST IN CHILDREN WITH MULTIPLE
    HEREDITARY OSTEOCHONDROMATA, 991
    H.A. Peterson

44 THE CHILD'S WRIST: DIAGNOSTIC AND
    TREATMENT PROBLEMS, 1002
    J.H. Dobyns, W.P. Cooney

45 ATHLETIC INJURIES OF THE WRIST, 1031
    S.M. Topper, M.B. Wood, W.P. Cooney

XII COMPLICATIONS OF WRIST
     INJURIES AND TREATMENT

46 COMPLICATIONS OF INJURIES OF THE
    WRIST (AND CHRONIC PAIN
    MANAGEMENT), 1076
    W.P. Cooney, O.J. Moy, M.B. Wood

47 COMPARTMENT SYNDROMES AND
    ISCHEMIC CONTRACTURE: HAND, WRIST,
    AND FOREARM, 1107
    J.M. Failla

48 SYNOVITIS OF THE WRIST, 1137
    P.M. Murray, R.A. Berger

XIII SOFT-TISSUE PROBLEMS AND
      NEOPLASMS

49 GANGLIONS OF THE WRIST, 1166
    S.H. Kozin, A.T. Bishop

50 TENDINITIS OF THE WRIST, 1181
    S.H. Kozin, A.T. Bishop, W.P. Cooney

51 CARPAL TUNNEL SYNDROME, 1197
    R.D. Beckenbaugh

52 TUMORS OF THE WRIST, 1234
    G.B. Irons, J.H. Dobyns

XIV REHABILITATION OF THE WRIST

53   PHYSICAL THERAPY MODALITIES, 1262
      S.D. Bogard III

54   WRIST REHABILITATION AND SPLINTING:
      OCCUPATIONAL THERAPY, 1272
      A.H. Schutt

55   WORK REHABILITATION, 1287
      E. Mohror, M.A. Moutvic

56   OVERUSE SYNDROME, 1295
      K.A. Bengtson, D.C.R. Ireland

XV THE FUTURE

57   ANTICIPATIONS AND NEEDS, 1306
      J.H. Dobyns, W.P. Cooney, R.L. Linscheid

      COLOR PLATES FOLLOW PAGES 48, 80,
      304, AND 1156.

IX

INJURIES OF DISTAL RADIOULNAR JOINT

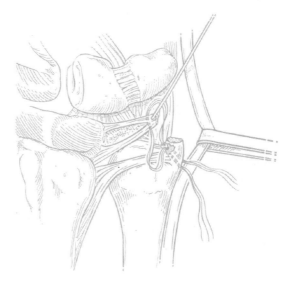

TEARS OF THE TRIANGULAR FIBROCARTILAGE OF THE WRIST

William P. Cooney, M.D.

ANATOMY AND BIOMECHANICS
CLINICAL PRESENTATION
DIAGNOSTIC EXAMINATIONS
WRIST ARTHROSCOPY
CLASSIFICATION
TREATMENT
   ACUTE TRAUMATIC TEARS OF THE TFC
   ISOLATED TFC TEARS: ACUTE REPAIR
   OPEN REPAIR OF THE TFC
   OPEN REPAIR OF TFC TYPE IA (RADIAL
      LESIONS)
   TECHNIQUE OF RADIAL REPAIR

OPEN REPAIR OF ULNAR TFC TEARS
   (AVULSIONS)
REATTACHMENT OF THE ULNAR STYLOID (BONE
   AVULSION INJURY)
OPEN REPAIR OF PALMAR TFC TEARS
OPEN REPAIR OF THE RADIAL AVULSION TFC
   TEAR
ARTHROSCOPIC REPAIR OF THE TFC
ARTHROSCOPIC TREATMENT OF DEGENERATIVE
   TEARS
AUTHOR'S PREFERRED TREATMENT

With increasing interest in the problems of injury to the ulnar side of the wrist, the importance of the triangular fibrocartilage (TFC) as a key element in the stability and force transmission across the wrist has been recognized.[2,3,11,12,19] Some have considered the TFC complex as the "new frontier" of wrist surgery, and it is true that the TFC and distal radioulnar joint (DRUJ) have received less attention than more common wrist fractures and ligament injuries. New clinical,[10,11,13,39] biomechanical,[3,67,76,77] and anatomic studies[*] are addressing the importance of this structure (see Chapter 11).

My colleagues and I have recognized injury to the TFC as from acute traumatic events or as attritional problems associated with aging.[24,51,65,66,68] Patients present with complaints of pain and instability related to the wrist itself or, more commonly, to rotation stress (pronation and supination) discomfort of the forearm.

When faced with instability and pain on the ulnar side of the wrist, most surgeons have excised the TFC[21,30,42,51] or the entire DRUJ.[14,26,42] Not until 1989, following an article by Palmer,[63] was appropriate attention paid to the importance of the TFC and an understanding developed of its role in stability and function of the wrist and forearm. Bowers,[11,12] in descriptions of problems of the DRUJ, further emphasized the functional potential of this tough internal ligament that appears to bear both compression and tensile loads, depending on loading directions and forces involved. Bowers and others[*] improved knowledge of the TFC as the prime structural support of the ulnar side of the wrist. Retention rather than resection became a guiding principle, and operative interventions of limited resection, repair, and reconstruction of the TFC have emerged.[24,39] This chapter examines briefly the anatomy and force-bearing constraints of

---

[*] References 2,4,6,13,20,45,47,48.

[*] References 4,12,19,20,36,76.

the TFC, the clinical presentation of patients with acute and chronic injuries, the classification of TFC injuries, and the principal recommendations for treatment and their alternatives. Our preferred treatment program is presented.

ANATOMY AND BIOMECHANICS

The TFC itself is a fibrocartilaginous disk that has its origin on the distal radius and insertion at the base of the ulnar styloid (Fig. 30-1). The radial origin is strongly attached by sharp fibers to the entire rim of the junction of the lunate fossa of the distal radius and the sigmoid notch of the DRUJ. The palmar edge of the TFC serves as the origin of the palmar ulnolunate and ulnotriquetral ligaments.[79,80] These ligaments do not, in fact, have a direct origin from the distal ulna, as commonly described and depicted.[3,12] The ulnar insertion is described as at the base of the ulnar styloid, but in fact, there are fibers that wrap around the styloid and that do not always connect to the base. The dorsal edge of the TFC can blend imperceptibly with the dorsal radioulnar ligament. Bowers preferred not to name specific ligaments because identification can be difficult. He noted peripheral thickening of the TFC that becomes the fibrous rim of dorsal and palmar attachments from the distal radius to the ulna (Fig. 30-2). Because there is confusion regarding the separation of these structures, Palmer[63] named the entity the triangular fibrocartilage complex (TFCC).

The central third of the TFC is a cartilaginous weightbearing area and, as such, does not have or require a vascular supply.[6,81] Recent work by Chidgey[18-20] and by Adams and Holley[2] has clarified the microstructure of the central and peripheral portions of the TFC complex. They noted that certain areas take up compression or contact loads (Fig. 30-3) and other more peripheral areas resist not only lateral displacement (Fig. 30-4) but distal to proximal directed loads from the wrist to the forearm.[76] The vascular supply of the TFC has also been studied, and it has been confirmed that its blood supply is greatest at the periphery (Fig. 30-5).[6,53,81] Tension loads are noted in these same areas and therefore tensile forces and vascular supply appear to be related. With aging, the central portion of the TFC is affected. In a classic study, Mikic[54] demonstrated the age-related changes of degeneration of the TFC. From his work it is recognized that after age 40 years, degenerative perforations (tears?) of the TFC may be quite routine and are not necessarily pathologic; a linear deterioration of tears can be appreciated. Mikic[54] further demonstrated that congenital perforations of the TFC did not occur. From a historic point of view, Kauer[45] and others[48] pointed out the cartilaginous nature of the central portion of the TFC. These authors as well as af Ekenstam and

Hagert[4] separated the central from the peripheral ligamentous attachment and identified dorsal and palmar radioulnar ligaments.

My colleagues and I have adopted the concept of a single nonhomogeneous structure for the TFC with a central cartilaginous and peripheral fibrous portion with multiple interactive areas of support. We believe that the TFC functions as a buffer or cushion between the distal end of the ulna and the radioulnar carpal joint and that it is the primary ligament of support for the radius to the ulnar side of the carpus. Others share this concept of function, noting that the TFC carries about 20% of the axial load from the wrist to the forearm and that it is a major stabilizer of the DRUJ[67] and the ulnar carpus.

What is unclear is the precise role of the TFC in maintaining support for the DRUJ compared with other associated structures such as the interosseous membrane, pronator quadratus, extensor carpi ulnaris (ECU) tendon sheath,[16] ulnar collateral ligaments, and superficial and deep forearm fascia.[4,67,76] Differences in ulna variance[26,28] (positive or negative) are also important and appear to determine, in part, the thickness of the compression loading aspect of the TFC in different positions of forearm pronation-supination.[62] Greater ulna variance in pronation assumes greater load to the TFC and to the distal ulna, but with supination the compressive load would be less.[28,43] Most TFC injuries occur with forearm pronation. Tightening of the dorsal and palmar aspects of the TFC (or dorsal and palmar radioulnar ligaments) is a final factor in determining how tears of the TFC occur because ligament instability of the DRUJ depends on the position of forearm pronation or supination.

CLINICAL PRESENTATION

Patients who have tears of the TFC present with a history of recurrent wrist pain, loss of strength, and painful rotation of the DRUJ. These may occur alone or in association with other wrist injuries.[5] Clinically, tears of the TFC may be difficult to distinguish from other causes of ulnar wrist pain, particularly ulnacarpal abutment,[25] lunotriquetral dissociation, ECU tendinitis, and degenerative changes within the DRUJ.[7,15,31,83,84] A careful clinical history and examination are essential to place injury to the TFC within the differential diagnosis of ulnar wrist pain.[5,11] The history should establish that a rotational injury or stress occurred to the DRUJ or that there has been chronic and persistent discomfort with activities related to the DRUJ. Most injuries have a component of hyperextension of the wrist with a rotation load. The history of injury may include fractures of the distal radius such as Colles'[15,31] or Galeazzi's fracture; sudden rotational stress to the forearm; a twisting fall onto the hand and

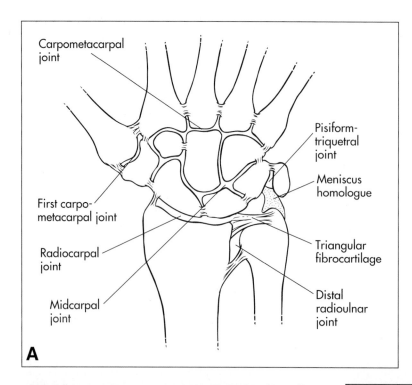

Carpometacarpal joint

Pisiform-triquetral joint

Meniscus homologue

First carpo-metacarpal joint

Radiocarpal joint

Triangular fibrocartilage

Midcarpal joint

Distal radioulnar joint

A

FIGURE 30-1

Triangular fibrocartilage (*TFC*). **A,** The TFC is a portion of the ulnar carpal ligament complex that includes the meniscus homologue and ulnar collateral ligaments. **B,** Cross-sectional anatomy of wrist demonstrates TFC relationship to scapholunate (*large arrowhead*) and lunotriquetral ligaments. **C,** Cross-sectional anatomy of distal radioulnar joint (*DRUJ*) (*small arrowhead in* **B**) and radiocarpal joint shows tight ligamentous attachments of the TFC to the distal radius (*Rad*), ulnar styloid, and ulnar collateral ligaments. (Carpal scaphoid and lunate bones removed.) **D,** Fetal anatomy demonstrates firm attachment of TFC to the ulnar border of the distal radius and to the base of the ulnar styloid. *C,* capitate; *H,* hamate; *Lun,* lunate; *RC,* radiocarpal; *Scap,* scaphoid; *T, Triq,* triquetrum.

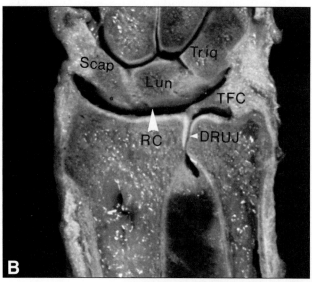

B

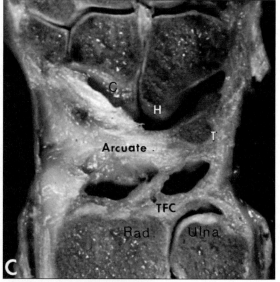

C

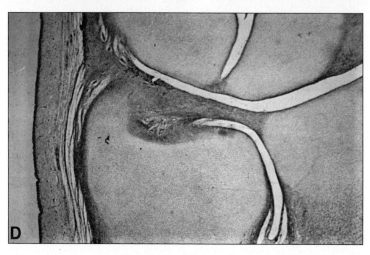

D

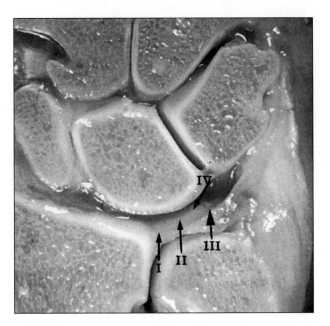

FIGURE 30-2

Zones of the triangular fibrocartilage. The triangular fibrocartilage has four separate functional zones. Zone I is the radial attachment. Zone II is the central cartilaginous area. Zone III is the area of ulnar attachment near the base of the ulnar styloid. Zone IV is the palmar attachment. (See Color Plate 58.)

wrist associated with a radial head fracture (the Essex-Lopresti lesion)[27,29]; or "wrist sprain" in which a significant rotation load was involved.[21,23,70] Aching discomfort with extremes of rotation is present and often associated with decreased strength, particularly in activities such as twisting a jar lid, doorknob, or steering wheel. The patient may experience a sensation of catching or snapping of the wrist, but there is no true subluxation or dislocation of the DRUJ.

The physical examination is important for a correct diagnosis of injury to the TFC. By careful palpation, one can identify tenderness and pain directly over the TFC and distinct from the lunotriquetral joint[70] or ECU sheath.[16] Stress loading the DRUJ at the extremes of pronation and supination is often critical to diagnosis because pain expressed at these positions is pathognomonic of a TFC injury. Dorsal-palmar ballottement of the distal ulna (the piano key sign) is a second important stress test (Fig. 30-6). Tenderness at the base of the ulnar styloid or along the ulnar collateral ligament complex may suggest injury to the TFC. Direct compression of the ulnar head against the seat of the sigmoid fossa does not produce pain. Tenderness and painful motion vary with the type of TFC tear. The tear from the base of

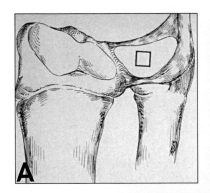
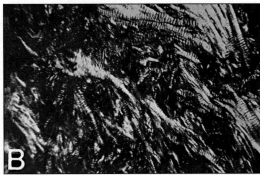
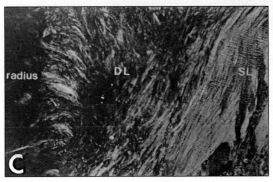

FIGURE 30-3

Microstructure of the triangular fibrocartilage, central area. **A,** Origin of biopsy specimen from central portion of the articular disk. **B,** Transverse histologic section of central region shows short collagen fibers in multiple directions, suggesting compression loads. **C,** Transverse histologic section through articular disk shows superficial layer (*SL*) and deep layer (*DL*). The superficial layer of fibers has a more oriented pattern than the deep layer. (Polarized light; ×6.) (*From Chidgey.[18] By permission of WB Saunders.*)

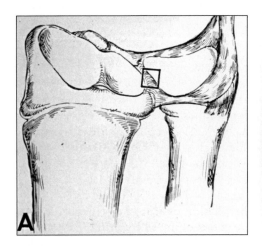
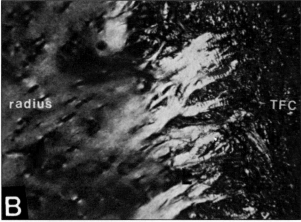

FIGURE 30-4

Microstructure of the triangular fibrocartilage (TFC). Radial border area of biopsy specimen. **A,** Origin of the radial attachment of the TFC (articular disk) from the distal radius. **B,** Transverse histologic section of radial origin. Note short thick fibers that extend from the radius into the articular disk. (Polarized light; ×16.) *(From Chidgey.[18] By permission of WB Saunders.)*

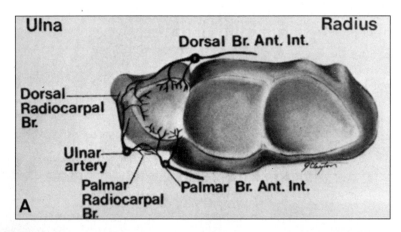

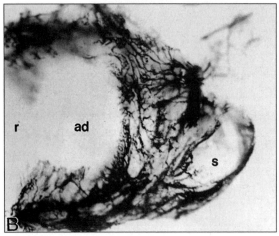

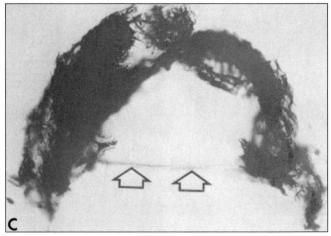

FIGURE 30-5

Vascular supply to the triangular fibrocartilage (TFC). **A,** Arterial anatomy of the TFC shows extrinsic blood supply from dorsal and palmar branches (*Br.*) of the anterior (*Ant.*) interosseous (*Int.*) artery as well as dorsal and palmar branches of the ulnar artery. *(From Thiru et al.[81] Copyright, American Society for Surgery of the Hand, by permission of Churchill Livingstone.)* **B,** Microvascular articular disk demonstrates that the vascular ring around the disk is incomplete because the radial border is avascular. The radial edge or attachment of the vascular plexus extends between the radius (*r*) and the disk (*ad*). A rich vascular supply is noted at the base styloid area between the disk and the styloid (*s*) process. *(From Mikic.[53] By permission of JB Lippincott.)* **C,** Axial view of TFC after vascular perfusion and tissue clearing. The inner portion of the TFC is devoid of vessels and no vessels enter the TFC from its radial attachment (*arrows*). *(From Bednar et al.[6] Copyright, American Society for Surgery of the Hand, by permission of Churchill Livingstone.)*

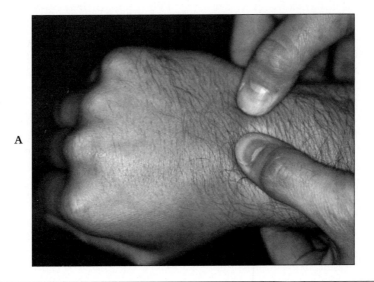

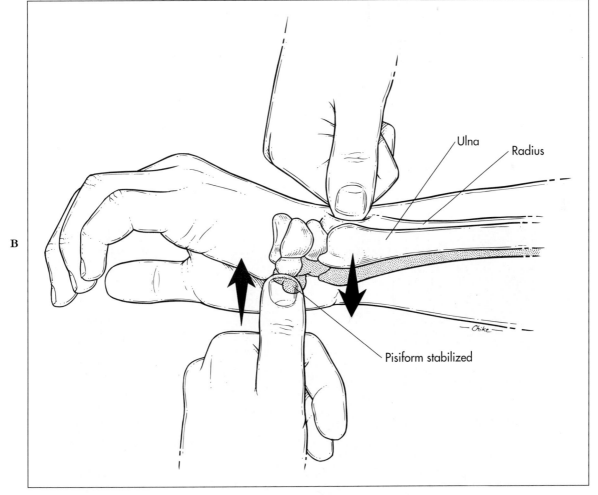

FIGURE 30-6

Physical examination of the triangular fibrocartilage. **A,** Positive ballottement by dorsal to palmar pressure demonstrates pain or instability or both. **B,** Diagrammatic demonstration of piano key sign of dorsal radioulnar joint instability.

the ulnar styloid has tenderness and pain with stress referred to the ulnar aspect of the wrist, whereas a palmar avulsion tear of the TFC has pain and tenderness along the palmar ulnar side of the wrist just proximal to the pisiform. We have found that diagnostic injections into the DRUJ can separate TFC or other primary DRUJ injuries from other causes of ulnocarpal wrist pain. Part of the difficulty in diagnosis of TFC tears in patients with ulnar wrist pain is that many patients have more than one pathologic area[80] and that TFC tears, in particular, are associated with other conditions affecting the wrist. The isolated TFC tear can be difficult to diagnose solely from the clinical examination. Carefully planned ancillary examinations provide the background for further tests and an appropriate diagnosis.

DIAGNOSTIC EXAMINATIONS

In the evaluation of ulnar wrist pain, in particular TFC tears, routine radiographs of the wrist may not be helpful. In tears from the ulnar styloid, a fleck of bone from the distal ulna can be seen on plain films (Fig. 30-7). The presence of positive ulna variance, ulna-carpal abutment, arthritis of the DRUJ, ulnar styloid avulsion fracture, or other findings may suggest that the TFC is not the specific cause of the presenting wrist pain. Otherwise the radiographs of the wrist are usually normal and serve only to eliminate other sources of pain. The arthrogram of the wrist[8,34,72,73]

(radiocarpal and distal radioulnar joints) is probably the first and most important examination to detect TFC injuries (Fig. 30-8). It is true that in patients older than age 40 years, the arthrogram becomes less reliable[55]; yet in most patients it is the first test that is specific and reliable for pathologic features related to the TFC.[38] Video arthrography, arthrotomography,[8] and stress arthrography[6] have also been suggested but are generally not helpful in determining the specific diagnosis. This is especially true for peripheral TFC tears. Arthrography of the DRUJ is often positive for a peripheral TFC tear when the radiocarpal examination is negative (Figs. 30-8, *E* and *F*).[49,72,73] The suggestion of multiple joint arthrography is particularly helpful in evaluating TFC tears.[34,38] An ulnar tear at the base of the TFC may not be observed on a radiocarpal arthrogram, but irregularity or pooling of dye at the periphery of the TFC can be picked up on DRUJ arthrography (Fig. 30-8, *G*).[34]

The second examination that has increased in popularity is the magnetic resonance image of the ulnar side of the wrist (Fig. 30-9).[17,35,69,88] Alone or enhanced with gadolinium or saline, the magnetic resonance image can show the TFC quite well in profile with the joint articular fluid and can demonstrate various levels and locations of tears of the TFC. Other tests such as bone scan scintigraphy or computed tomography are too nonspecific or inconclusive to be of great value in examination for TFC lesions, unless there is joint instability, in which case the computed tomography study may be diagnostic.[46] Previous concern that

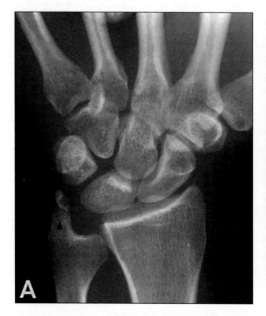
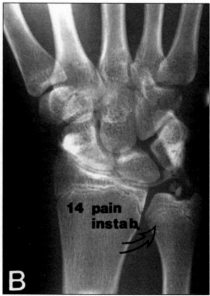

FIGURE 30-7

Radiographs of wrist, peripheral tears. **A,** Ulnar styloid avulsion fracture associated with triangular fibrocartilage tear. **B,** Avulsion of ulnar styloid base, yet negative result of arthrogram associated with instability (*instab.*) of the distal radioulnar joint.

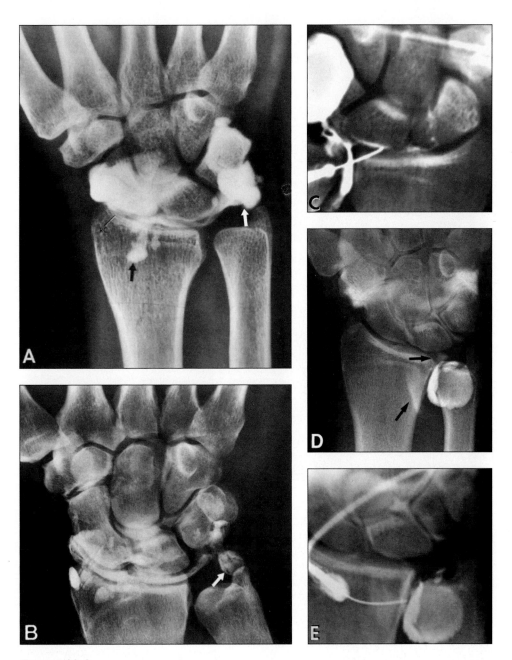

FIGURE 30-8

Arthrography of wrist. **A,** Normal posteroanterior arthrogram of the radiocarpal joint (*RC*) shows a well-filled radiocarpal joint, a small ulna prestyloid recess (*arrow, right*) and palmar radiocarpal recess (*arrow, left*). Smooth border of the triangular fibrocartilage (*TFC*) is noted. **B,** Filling a large prestyloid recess (*arrow*) should not be confused by a peripheral (ulnar insertion) TFC tear. Posteroanterior arthrogram shows the large prestyloid recess. (*A and B, From Resnick D:* Medical Radiology and Pathology, *Eastman Kodak Co., Rochester, New York, vol 52, number 3, 1976, p 57.*) **C,** Radiocarpal arthrogram shows a radial border tear of the TFC. **D,** Radiocarpal arthrogram shows a large central tear of the TFC (*top arrow*). Communication noted into the midcarpal joint extending to the capsule of the dorsal radioulnar joint (*arrow, bottom*). **E,** Radioulnar joint arthrogram (series 1): no dye leakage.

Continued.

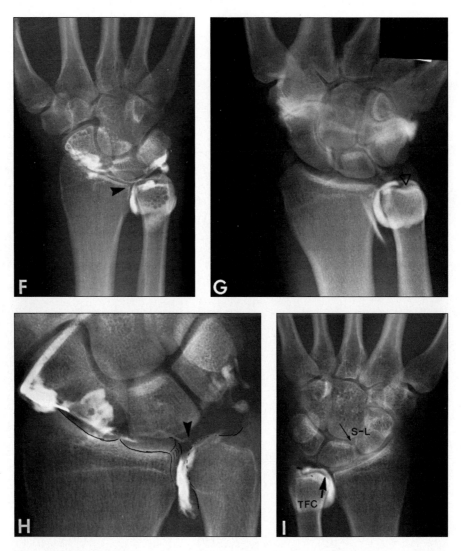

FIGURE 30-8, CONT'D.

F, Radioulnar joint arthrogram (series 3): dye communication with radiocarpal joint; radial border tear of the TFC (*arrowhead*). **G,** Radioulnar joint arthrogram shows peripheral tear (*arrowhead*) at the base of the ulnar styloid; dye in radiocarpal joint. **H,** Palmar tear (*arrowhead*) with dye from radiocarpal joint entering through a palmar ulnocarpal ligament tear into the radioulnar joint. **I,** Two-phase arthrogram. Positive midcarpal arthrogram (faint dye) (*small arrow*) through scapholunate (*S-L*) ligament and negative distal radioulnar joint arthrogram (*large arrow*).

the magnetic resonance image cannot show traumatic tears may be negated by the increased sophistication of the technique.

WRIST ARTHROSCOPY

The advent of wrist arthroscopy as a diagnostic test has specifically improved the diagnosis of injuries of the TFC.[9,13,22,37] With triangulation, the location and extent of TFC injury can be assessed quite accurately. For tears in the radial central or palmar aspects of the TFC, the degree of tearing and loss of resilience of the

TFC should be noted. With the ulnar peripheral tear, the loss of ballottement or trampoline of the TFC will be a specific sign of injury that should always be tested (see Fig. 30-18). A normal TFC is quite firm to probing, whereas peripheral tears produce a laxity or loss of resilience that is difficult to miss. The arthroscopic procedure also provides an excellent view of other internal derangements of the wrist that emphasizes the need for a complete examination before making the definitive diagnosis or initiating treatment.

My colleagues and I perform wrist arthroscopy during distraction with the tourniquet elevated (see Chapters 8 and 14).[9] The arthroscope is inserted first in

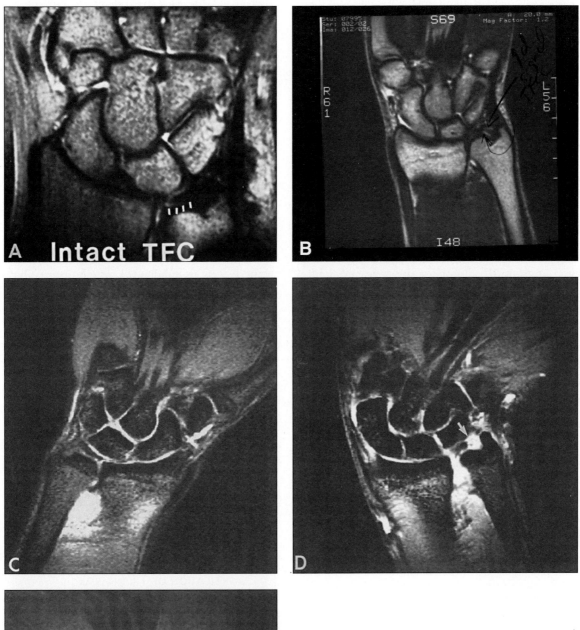

Figure 30-9

Magnetic resonance image (MRI) of the triangular fibrocartilage (*TFC*). **A,** T2-weighted, saline contrast MRI shows intact outline of the TFC between radius and ulnar styloid. **B,** Complete tear of central portion of the TFC. **C,** Normal articular disk (T2-weighted). **D,** Peripheral TFC tear (*arrow*) (T2-weighted). **E,** Degenerative central tear (*arrow*) of TFC. *(C, D, and E, From Diagnostic des ulno Karpalen Komplexes in MR Movie,* Handchir Microchir Plast Chir *26:115-119, 1994. By permission of Hippokrates Verlag GmbH.)*

the dorsal 3-4 portal with the triangulation probe in the dorsal 4-5 or 6 radial portal. Switching the scope to the 4-5 portal and probing from radial to ulnar should be performed as a routine part of examination. Rotation of the DRUJ helps to determine TFC tightness and DRUJ stability. If there is a central TFC tear, degenerative changes on the head of the ulna can be assessed.

CLASSIFICATION

The work by Bowers[11,12] has been important in our overall examination and understanding of derangements of the DRUJ (see box below). In his classification, the present chapter discusses group II and group IV, acute joint disruptions, specifically subgroup C, the isolated TFC disruptions without instability. We are also interested in group III, chronic or late-appearing joint disruptions—without radiographic arthritis (see box below). Bowers and others proposed specific treatment

alternatives for each of the five groups or types of derangement of the DRUJ.* For the isolated TFC injury, the specific treatment may be best directed at the type of TFC abnormality as classified by Palmer and by my colleagues and me. In the Palmer classification (see box below), there are two broad categories: class I, traumatic tears, and class II, degenerative tears. Depending on the location of tear within the class of traumatic or degenerative lesions and the presence or absence of associated chondromalacia changes, different treatment modalities are considered. The Mayo classification (see box on p. 721) of the traumatic TFC tears is based on the zones of the triangular fibrocartilage (Fig. 30-2) and consists of a different recognition of peripheral tears, with different emphasis given to the location of the tears.

In the Palmer classification (Fig. 30-10), the traumatic lesions are subdivided into four types. Type I is a central tear within the cartilaginous substance of the TFC. It may be horizontal, vertical, or stellate in shape. It differs from the vertical tear that is juxtaposed to the sigmoid notch and lunate fossa of the distal radius. Type II is an avulsion tear from the base of the ulnar styloid. It is the soft-tissue equivalent of an ulnar styloid avulsion fracture. Type III is a tear of the palmar third of the TFC, usually involving the ulnocarpal ligaments. Type IV is a radial avulsion of TFC, with or without bone from the distal radius and usually associated with fractures of the distal radius.

Degenerative tears of the TFC appear to result from the normal aging process, yet some individuals are

---

* References 12,42,44,49,59,62,64.

CLASSIFICATION OF DISORDERS OF THE DISTAL RADIOULNAR JOINT AND TRIANGULAR FIBROCARTILAGE COMPLEX (BOWERS)

I. Fractures—acute
   A. Radioulnar joint surface fracture
      1. Sigmoid cavity of radius
      2. Ulnar head
   B. Styloid fracture—isolated
      1. Tip
      2. Base (see II, A and C)
II. Joint Disruption—acute
   A. Isolated dislocations
   B. Triangular fibrocartilage injuries—partial (see IV, C)
   C. Disruptions associated with other injuries
III. Joint Disruption—chronic
IV. Joint Disorders
   A. Length discrepancies
      1. Ulna too long
      2. Ulna too short
   B. Arthritis
      1. Post-traumatic arthritis and osteoarthritis
      2. Rheumatoid arthritis
      3. Ulnar head chondromalacia
   C. Triangular fibrocartilage tears, perforations, and attritional changes
V. Joint Area Problems
   A. Extensor carpi ulnaris subluxation or dislocation
   B. Ulnocarpal problems
      1. Pisotriquetral arthrosis
      2. Lunotriquetral ligament tears
      3. Midcarpal instability
   C. The Darrach solution as a problem

CLASSIFICATION OF TRIANGULAR FIBROCARTILAGE COMPLEX INJURY (PALMER)

I. Traumatic Tear (types)
   I   Central
   II   Medial (± styloid fracture)
   III   Distal (ulnocarpal)
   IV   Lateral (radial attachment, distal radius fracture)
II. Degenerative Tear (stages)
   I   TFC wear
   II   TFC wear and chondromalacia
   III   TFC perforation and chondromalacia
   IV   TFC perforation
      + chondromalacia
      + lunotriquetral ligament tear
   V   TFC perforation
      + ulnocarpal arthritis

TFC, triangular fibrocartilage complex.
Modified from Palmer AK.[63] Copyright, American Society for Surgery of the Hand, by permission of Churchill Livingstone.

clinically symptomatic. The degenerative tears are divided into five different types based on arthroscopic and radiographic pathologic features (see box on p. 720). The first type (stage I) is simple TFC wear without a central perforation. The second type (stage II) involves TFC wear but with lunate and ulnar head chondromalacia. The third type (stage III) involves perforation of the articular disk with lunate or ulna chondromalacia. The fourth type (stage IV) includes perforation of the TFC, chondromalacia, and a lunotriquetral ligament tear. The fifth type (stage V) includes all of the above plus ulnocarpal arthritis. Positive ulna variance is associated with many of these stages leading to ulnacarpal abutment. All of the degenerative tears are central rather than peripheral and they are stellate, cleavage-type tears, not the linear tears seen with trauma.

The Mayo classification of traumatic tears identifies the radial rim tear as the most common in our experience (Fig. 30-11). This is the type I traumatic tear. It is a vertical tear from dorsal to palmar within 1 to 2 mm of the radial border of the lunate fossa of the distal radius. It is a tear capable of repair. The type II traumatic tear is a central tear of the TFC within the cartilaginous central portion of the TFC. It varies in direction and shape and is accessible to arthroscopic excision. The type III tear is an ulnar insertion tear of the TFC. It is assumed to be an avulsion of the TFC from the base of the ulnar styloid. The type IV tear is a palmar tear of the TFC from the ulnocarpal ligaments that can occur alone or in association with injury to the lunotriquetral ligaments.

The Mayo classification of degenerative tears is based on treatment options and is similar to the classification above. The type I tear is a central degenerative

stellate tear that requires open or arthroscopic excision. The type II tear is central and associated with ulnocarpal impingement. Central excision of the TFC and either ulna recession (shortening) or distal ulna excision (Feldon procedure)[30,86] should be considered. The

---

MAYO CLASSIFICATION OF TRIANGULAR FIBROCARTILAGE TEAR (TREATMENT AND LOCATION BASED)

Traumatic Tear (types)
  I Radial rim (detachment)
  II Central
  III Ulnar (equivalent ulnar styloid fracture)
  IV Palmar

Degenerative Tear (types)
  I Central (stellate) tear
  II Central tear, ulnocarpal impingement
  III Central tear, impingement, lunotriquetral ligament tear
  IV Central tear, impingement, lunotriquetral arthritis (radioulnar arthritis?)

Treatment
  Traumatic Tear
    I, III, IV Surgical repair
    II Excision
  Degenerative Tear
    I Excision
    II Excision and ulna recession
    III Excision, lunotriquetral reconstruction, ulna recession
    IV Ulna excision (Darrach) versus ulna recession only

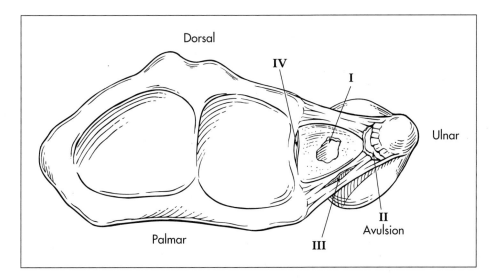

FIGURE 30-10

Classification of triangular fibrocartilage (TFC) tears (Palmer). I = Central tear (perforation). II = Peripheral, ulnar styloid tear. III = Peripheral, palmar tear (TFC and ulnocarpal ligaments). IV = Peripheral tear, radial border.

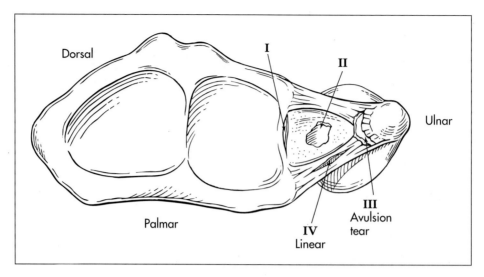

FIGURE 30-11

Classification of traumatic triangular fibrocartilage (TFC) tears (Mayo). I = Peripheral radial rim tear. II = Central tear. III = Peripheral tear, ulnar insertion. IV = Peripheral tear, palmar attachments.

type III tear includes impingement and lunotriquetral ligament disruption. The latter involves lunotriquetral instability and not simply a lunotriquetral central perforation. The treatment of stage III includes TFC tear excision, ulnar recession, and either lunotriquetral ligament reconstruction or lunotriquetral fusion (see Chapter 22). The type IV tear includes a central tear, ulnocarpal impingement, and lunotriquetral and often distal radioulnar joint arthritis. Treatment considerations are ulna recession only or excision of the distal ulna.

TREATMENT

ACUTE TRAUMATIC TEARS OF THE TFC

Traumatic injuries of the TFC and ulnar styloid are controversial with respect to surgical repair.* With fractures of the distal radius, the majority opinion is that the ulnar styloid fracture or TFC tear does not need open treatment.[3] My colleagues and I do not necessarily support that concept. That is not to say that the forearm should not be immobilized in supination after distal radius fractures or that pinning of the DRUJ in some Colles-type and nearly all Galeazzi's fractures of the radius is not reasonable considering the level of DRUJ instability. Rather, we agree with Mikic[54] that the DRUJ is the forgotten joint of the wrist when associated with most fractures. It appears to "play second fiddle" to the fracture of the distal radius or both bone forearm fractures. Many surgeons recognize and accept that if there is displacement of

the ulnar styloid of 3 to 4 mm or more (particularly with a fracture of the base of the ulnar styloid) then closed reduction and pinning or open reduction of the joint is required. Few experienced wrist surgeons, however, consider the ulnar styloid fracture a problem. Most agree that Colles' fractures with a TFC tear or ulnar styloid fracture do quite well without open treatment. We believe that a more careful examination of the TFC and associated DRUJ is essential before making a decision regarding conservative or operative treatment of the TFC tear (or ulnar styloid fracture).

In general, we prefer open treatment of TFC tears with or without ulnar styloid fractures. Our preference and technique for open repair of the ulnar styloid are reported below. Our results suggest that we may need to look at early repair of these injuries more frequently than in the past.

Acute instability of the DRUJ not associated with fracture but with other soft-tissue injuries may be a more important reason for open treatment of TFC injuries. Examples of this instability are discussed in other chapters. They include TFC or ulnar styloid injury associated with perilunate dislocations of the wrist; acute, complete ulnocarpal ligament tears that may include the ECU sheath, TFC, lunotriquetral joint, and palmar ulnocarpal ligaments; the Essex-Lopresti injury that produces instability at proximal and distal radioulnar joints; and finally, cases of ulnar translation of the wrist in which carpal ligaments are torn palmarly along with a lateral (ulnar) displacement injury of the DRUJ. These injuries, although infrequent, demand stabilization of the DRUJ by TFC repair or reattachment of an ulnar styloid fracture displacement.[27,39,40,62]

_____

* References 1,10,11,21,24,25,30,37,39,42,49,51,52,58,60,61,68.

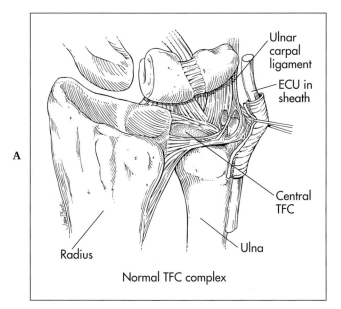

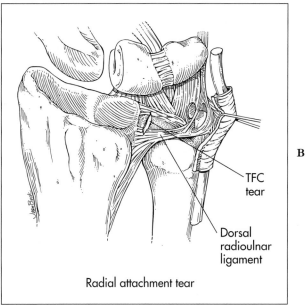

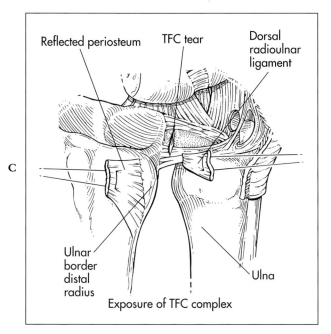

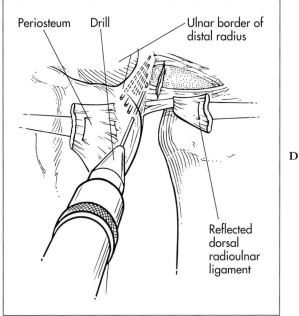

FIGURE 30–14

Diagrammatic presentation of repair of a radial rim tear of the triangular fibrocartilage (*TFC*). **A,** TFC complex shows the broad origin of the TFC and dorsal radioulnar ligament from the edge of the lunate fossa of the distal radius; the insertion of the TFC is at the base of the ulnar styloid; note origin and interconnections of palmar ulnocarpal ligaments with the TFC and ulnar styloid. **B,** Location of typical radial attachment tear within 1 to 2 mm of the ulnar border of the distal radius. **C,** Operative approach to the radial tear is performed by detaching the dorsal radioulnar ligament from the distal radius as well as reflecting periosteum for exposure of the dorsal ulnar aspect of the distal radius. **D,** Drill holes are placed from dorsal ulnar aspect of the distal radius in a palmar ulnar direction to exit along the ulnar rim of the distal radius (radial attachment of TFC).

Continued.

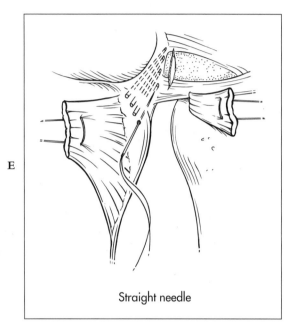

E

Straight needle

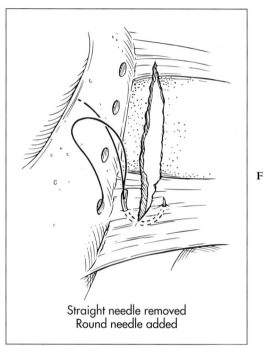

F

Straight needle removed
Round needle added

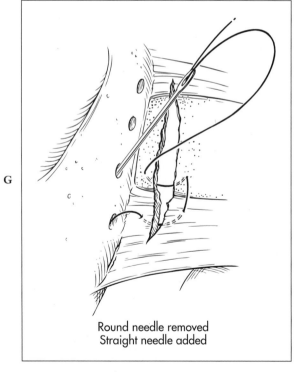

G

Round needle removed
Straight needle added

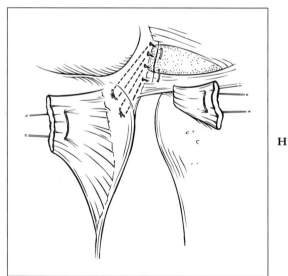

H

FIGURE 30-14, CONT'D.

E, Suture placement (3-0, resorbable preferred) by mattress suture through the radial edge of the TFC through drill holes placed in the ulnar border of the distal radius. The bony edge is freshened for a new radial attachment. **F,** Suture placement through free ulnar edge of the TFC and edge brought radially to the ulnar border of the radius. **G,** Retrieval of suture with retrograde or reversed Keith needle. **H,** Tightening of sutures over dorsal aspect of the radius pulling the TFC snugly against the ulnar border of the distal radius.

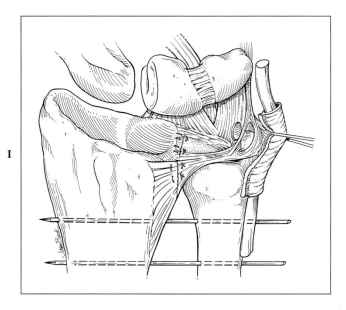

I

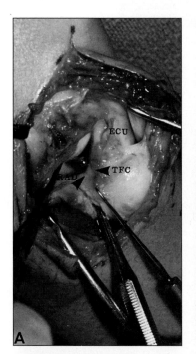

A

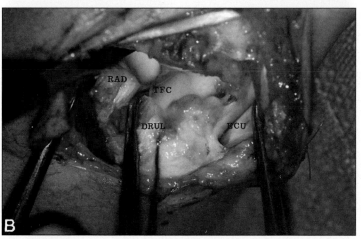

B

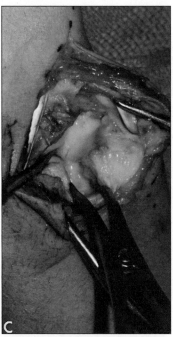

C

FIGURE 30-14, CONT'D.

I, Closure of dorsal radioulnar ligaments over repaired TFC. Stabilization of distal radioulnar joint in midrotation with two Kirschner wires (0.045-0.625 in.) to prevent breakage. *ECU,* extensor carpi ulnaris.

FIGURE 30-15

Surgical exposure and repair of the triangular fibrocartilage (*TFC*). **A,** Dental probe inserted through the radial border of the TFC demonstrates a 4-mm tear (*arrowheads*) (right wrist). **B,** Dental probe into the edge of radial tear. The dorsal radioulnar ligament (*DRUL*) has been reflected (under neck of probe) to provide exposure of the TFC. **C,** Lamina spreader is placed proximal to the distal radioulnar joint to aid exposure of the TFC.

Continued.

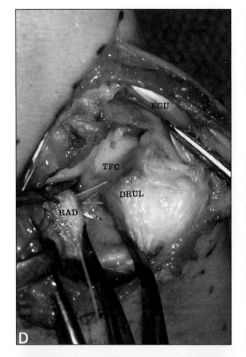

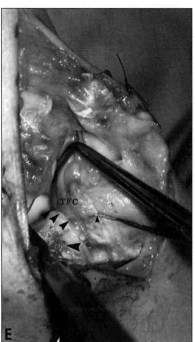

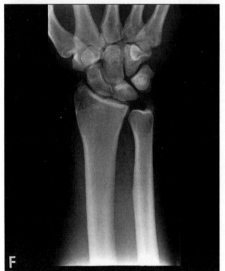

FIGURE 30-15, CONT'D.

D, Suture placement (mattress suture) from ulnar border of the distal radius into the radial edge of the TFC. **E,** Completed repair of TFC with suture knots placed over the dorsal ulnar aspect of the distal radius (*arrowheads*). **F,** Stable distal radioulnar joint after repair. *ECU,* extensor carpi ulnaris; *RAD,* radius.

retinacular flap tagged for later repair. The ECU is mobilized ulnarly and the ulnar styloid region is exposed. The ulnocarpal joint is entered with a transverse incision parallel to the TFC. Small needles placed into the radioulnar carpal joint and the DRUJ help to demonstrate the precise location of these narrow joint openings. Once exposed, the TFC is mobilized from a radial to ulnar direction with a blunt elevator used within the radiocarpal joint. Any granulation tissue or hypervascular connective tissue is débrided to the base or fovea of the ulnar styloid near the head of the ulna.

For reinsertion, most authors suggest creating a small trough for reattachment of the TFC to the ulna. A reasonable alternative is to pull the TFC dorsally

and ulnarly over the base of the ulnar styloid, which duplicates normal direction of insertion. At least three mattress sutures of 2-0 or 3-0 absorbable or nonabsorbable material are required for a strong repair. If the TFC does not reach far to the ulna fovea, it can be attached to the base of the ulnar styloid or ulnar distal aspect of the ulnar head. The most important principle is that the TFC is attached to well-vascularized strong tissue ulnarly and not to granulation tissue to restore normal tension. Attachment to ligament or bone is equally advantageous.

Normal TFC tension (trampoline test) can be used to judge the tautness of the repair. We recommend placement of the forearm in neutral rotation to slight supination and pinning the DRUJ extra-articularly in

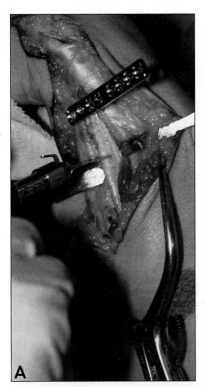

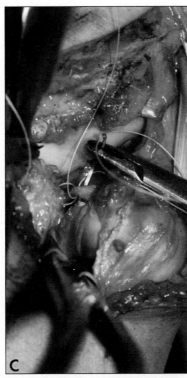

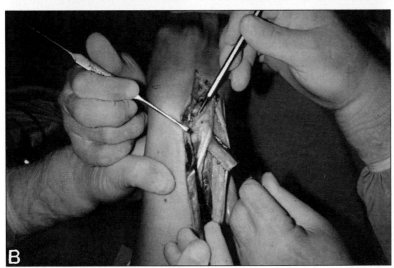

FIGURE 30-16

A, Ulnar osteotomy for more extensive exposure of the distal radioulnar joint; ulnar recession after triangular fibrocartilage (TFC) repair. **B,** Retraction of distal ulna and exploration of the TFC tear site. **C,** Direct suture repair of the TFC to the free ulnar border of the distal radius.

this position before tightening the repair sutures. Tension on the TFC can then be assessed. Dorsal capsule repair and imbrication of the extensor retinaculum about the ECU tendon completes the procedure. Unless there are abnormalities related to the ECU sheath,[16] a retinacular stabilization of the ECU sheath is probably not necessary.

Immobilization in a long arm cast for 6 weeks is recommended, followed by 3 to 4 weeks in a Munster or ulnar gutter splint to protect the repair during the mobilization period.

From previous series[39] and our experience with peripheral detachment of the TFC from the ulnar styloid, one should expect that other carpal injuries such as

scaphoid fractures, distal radius fractures, or perilunate carpal instabilities may also be present. These conditions should be considered and treated on their own merits.

REATTACHMENT OF THE ULNAR STYLOID (BONE AVULSION INJURY)

In the cases in which the ulnar styloid is fractured or avulsed from the distal ulna and in which there is displacement of more than 2 to 3 mm from its normal position, open repair of the ulnar styloid is recommended.[5,77,80] The technique involves an ulnar incision 2 cm long centered over the distal ulna. The dorsal branch of the ulnar nerve is protected. With sharp dissection onto bone, the periosteum is raised and reflected to expose the ulnar avulsion site proximally and to grasp the ulnar styloid distally. The ends of bones may need to be freshened with a rongeur. For internal fixation, two Kirschner wires are inserted retrogradely and drilled through the ulnar styloid.

A tension band wire is inserted through the TFC attachment and bone distally and passed proximally into a drill hole in the proximal ulna at the head-neck junction (Fig. 30-17). The two Kirschner wires within the ulnar styloid are then drilled distal to proximal with the ulnar styloid held and reduced with a bone-holding clamp or small Kocher forceps. The tension band wire is tightened. The forearm should be in midrotation to slight supination during the realignment of the styloid. The Kirschner wires can be retained for 3 to 4 weeks or removed, if the tension band wire provides a firm reduction.

Bowers[12] prefers a different technique that uses a dorsal approach to visualize the entire TFC, because the lesions may extend along the ulnolunate and ulnotriquetral ligaments. He performs a direct repair of the ulnar styloid with an interosseous wire from the tip of the styloid proximally through the fracture site and exiting radially along the ulnar shaft. Both techniques can provide firm reattachment of the ulnar styloid and TFC to the ulna.

OPEN REPAIR OF PALMAR TFC TEARS

Of the four types of traumatic TFC tears, the palmar tear is probably the least common (or least recognized). The palmar aspect of the TFC does not have a strongly organized "palmar radioulnar ligament" compared with the dorsal radioulnar ligament. Tears of the palmar TFC are related to injuries of the ulnolunate and ulnotriquetral ligaments and can have related ulnocarpal complex multiplane disruptions.

My colleagues and I[24] have recognized five palmar TFC ligament injuries and have proceeded with open repair of the palmar aspect of the TFC, lunotriquetral ligaments, and ECU tendon sheaths when that complex of injuries occurs. For maximum exposure, an ulnar osteotomy is performed, derotating the ulna and releasing the ECU sheath (Fig. 30-16). Examination of the ulnar attachment of the TFC by ulnar rotation and distraction of the wrist for exposure are often required. With this surgical approach, the ulnopalmar ligaments and palmar aspect of the TFC are reached and directly sutured. The repair is performed with a mattress suture of 2-0 Vicryl if a dorsal approach is used because the knot would remain within the radiocarpal joint. The repair may include the palmar lunotriquetral ligaments, ulnar collateral complex, and the ECU tendon sheath.

The palmar TFC tear may also appear to be a chronic subluxation of the DRUJ at presentation, suggesting that more than a TFC tear is involved in the instability.[11,33,75,78] Stress testing demonstrates palmar instability of the head of the ulna. Plain radiographs are usually normal, but axial tomography[4,47,56] of the DRUJs comparing injured and uninjured sides demonstrates palmar displacement of the ulna with respect to the distal radius (actually, the radius is displaced dorsally to the stable ulna). In this circumstance, direct repair of the TFC and associated ulnocarpal ligaments may not be feasible. A palmar approach to the DRUJ is recommended to evaluate the abnormality and to repair or reconstruct the ulnocarpal ligaments. We have used a variation of the Hui-Linscheid procedure[33,41] to reinforce the palmar aspect of the TFC and to provide a rim of fibrous tissue to repair and tighten the ulnocarpal ligaments. This repair technique is described in greater detail in Chapter 42.

OPEN REPAIR OF THE RADIAL AVULSION TFC TEAR

The lateral avulsion tear from the radial attachment is an injury most commonly associated with fractures of the distal radius.[15,31] The injury typically involves the sigmoid fossa and the lunate fossa of the distal radius. Radiographs show the ulnar spread of the distal ulna away from the radius, with attached bone from the lunate fossa of the distal radius. An arthrogram demonstrates communication between the radiocarpal and the distal radioulnar joints. Closed reduction of the distal radius fracture with supination of the forearm may provide adequate alignment of the fracture fragments such that cast immobilization of the injury is often sufficient. However, if reduction cannot be achieved by closed means, then open reduction of the lunate fossa (or sigmoid fossa) of the distal radius is recommended, with appropriate reduction and Kirschner-wire fixation of the displaced fracture fragments that are attached to the TFC. If all distal radius fractures were analyzed by tomography and arthrography, this particular injury of the TFC would probably be the most common. The vast majority heal bone to bone as part of the treatment of the distal radius fracture and do not present late problems of pain, weakness, or carpal instability.

ARTHROSCOPIC REPAIR OF THE TFC

Poehling and several other authors[37,61,71,85,87] have demonstrated that arthroscopy is accurate in the diagnosis of abnormalities involving the TFC and has the potential for arthroscopic reconstructive repair of the TFC. For this procedure of arthroscopic repair, the operative approach is to place the scope in the dorsal 3-4 portal and the examining probe in the dorsal 4-5 portal. With the triangulation probe, the location and extent of the TFC tear can be determined. If there is a tear in the central region of the TFC, simple excision of the loose edge of the TFC

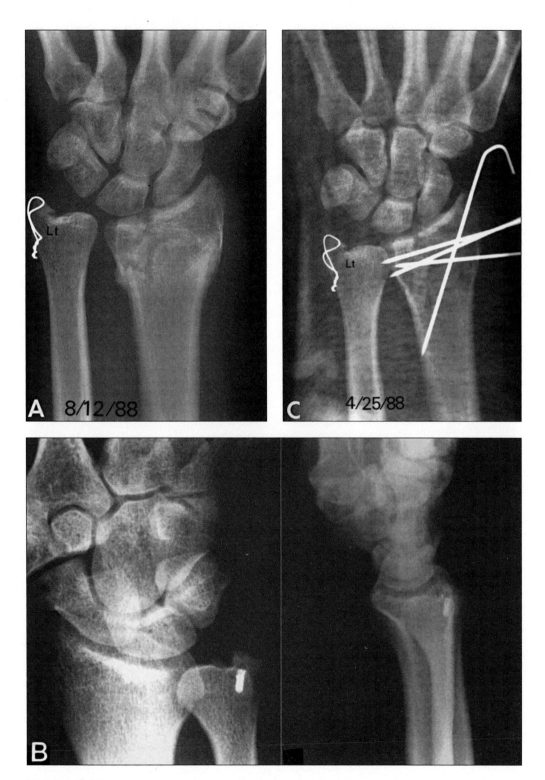

FIGURE 30-17

A, Tension band repair technique for avulsion of ulnar styloid associated with intra-articular distal radius fracture. **B,** Mitek anchor. Posteroanterior (*left*) and lateral (*right*) radiographs depict placement of the Mitek anchor in the distal ulna. *(From Walker LG: Stabilization of the distal radioulnar joint after ulnar styloid nonunion using Mitek anchors, Orthop Rev 23:769-772, 1994. By permission of Excerpta Medica, Inc.)* **C,** Radial avulsion tear associated with distal radius fracture and ulnar styloid fracture through its base; both repaired by open reduction and internal fixation. *Lt,* left.

with a suction punch and radial side cutting shaver may be sufficient.[37] If there is a radial horizontal tear, the proximity to the distal radius and ability to repair or resect the tear can be assessed. With palpation, the resilience (trampoline effect) of the TFC can be observed to help determine if resection, or repair is preferable (Fig. 30-18). Also, the head of the ulna can be palpated and positive ulna variance can be assessed.

For excision of the TFC, one needs instruments for cutting and then removing and débriding the TFC (Fig. 30-19, *A*).[71] These include a banana or hook knife, suction punch, radial side cutting shaver, and grasping forceps. With the scope in the dorsal 3-4 portal, observing the TFC from a radial perspective, the 4-5 portal is the working entrance to the wrist (Fig. 30-19, *A*). First, the tear is elevated with a probe. Second, the free edge is excised with the banana knife. Third, the free fragment is removed

with the grasping forceps. Fourth, the suction punch is used to clean up the edges of the TFC, which is then further trimmed with the motorized radial side cutting shaver (Figs. 30-19, *C* and *D*). In some cases, it is first necessary to débride the joint with the radial side cutting shaver to improve visualization of the entire wrist. In most cases, it is also necessary to switch the scope from the 3-4 to the 4-5 portal and approach the ulnar side of the TFC from the 3-4 portal.

For treatment of the avulsion tear on the ulnar aspect of the TFC, arthroscopic repair techniques have evolved (Fig. 30-20).[61,74,85] First, it is necessary to confirm the lesion by noting the loss of resilience in the TFC and noting vascular granulation tissue response at the base of the ulnar styloid. The steps involved in TFC avulsion repair include placement of a Tuohy needle from radial to ulnar into the joint. The needle should pierce the free edge of the TFC, and a

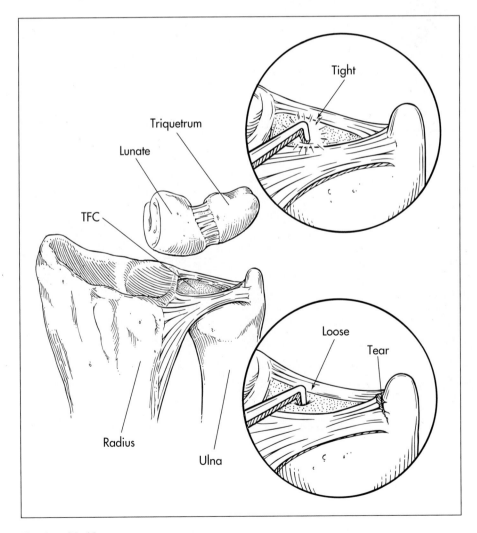

FIGURE 30-18

Trampoline effect to test resilience (tightness) of the triangular fibrocartilage (*TFC*) before and after peripheral repair.

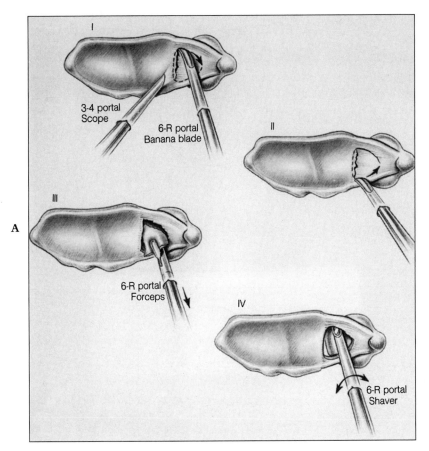

A

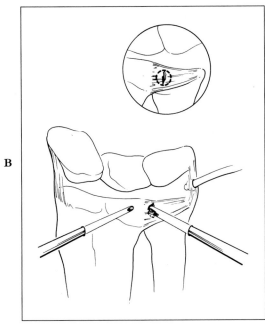

FIGURE 30-19

A, Illustration of the triangular fibrocartilage complex articular disk resection by using a curved banana blade (right wrist). The blade is oriented with the concave surface facing radially and proximally to begin the dorsal cut. Viewed from the 3-4 portal with the blade in the 6-R portal. *(From Whipple TL, editor: Arthroscopic surgery: the wrist, Philadelphia, 1992, JB Lippincott, p 113. By permission of the publisher.)* **B,** Triangular fibrocartilage tear at the radial attachment with a resultant flap that catches in the joint. **C,** Suction basket trimming of triangular fibrocartilage tear. **D,** Suction shaver débridement of triangular fibrocartilage tear. *(B, C, and D, From Poehling GG, Chabon SJ, Siegel DB: Diagnostic arthroscopy. In Gelberman RH, editor: The wrist, New York, 1994, Raven Press. By permission of the publisher.)*

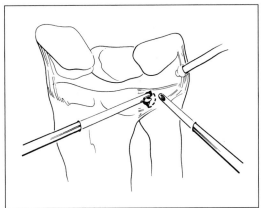

C

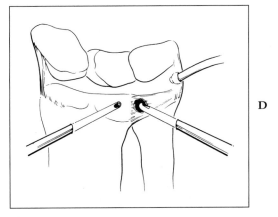

B

D

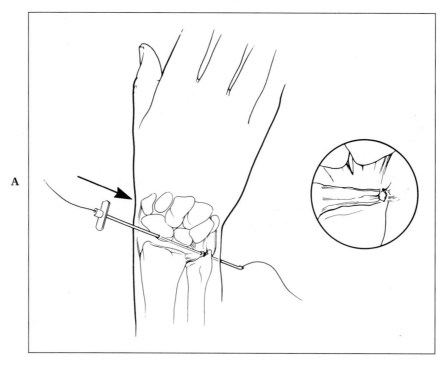

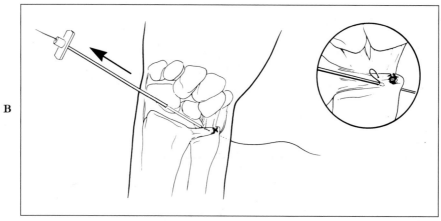

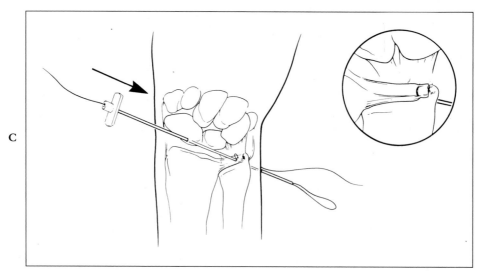

FIGURE 30-20

A, Tuohy needle inserted from the 1-2 portal through the triangular fibrocartilage tear. A 2-0 PDS is passed retrograde through the needle. **B,** While the suture is held at the ulnar side of the wrist, the needle is withdrawn and passed again through the triangular fibrocartilage 2 to 3 mm from the previous insertion. **C,** The needle is passed through the skin, and the suture end is retrieved. A small longitudinal incision is made and the suture ends are brought through and tied over the capsule. (*A, B,* and *C, From Poehling GG, Chabon SJ, Siegel DB:* Diagnostic arthroscopy. *In Gelberman RH, editor:* The wrist, *New York, 1994, Raven Press. By permission of the publisher.*)

2-0 Dacron suture is inserted through the needle. A second pass of the Tuohy needle is performed radial to ulnar again through the free edge of the TFC. The Tuohy needle is passed through the skin adjacent to the other suture end. Several sutures can be placed in the TFC with this technique. A small ulnar incision is performed at the base of the ulnar styloid to tie down the repair sutures. The tightness of the repair can be examined arthroscopically within the joint and the resilience of the TFC can be checked to determine the tightness of the repair. Whipple and Geissler[85] have developed a different approach to the peripheral TFC repair with specialized instruments. The repair technique is otherwise similar to that described above.

ARTHROSCOPIC TREATMENT OF DEGENERATIVE TEARS

For most cases of degenerative tears of the TFC, joint arthroscopic débridement is necessary before beginning the definitive procedure. With the scope in the dorsal 3-4 portal and the radial side shaver in the 4-5 portal, the radiocarpal joint is first débrided. This usually involves the radial styloid area, palmar aspect of the radiocarpal joint, and the ulnar aspect of the wrist near the meniscal homologue. With the chronic degenerative tears, the edges of the TFC are cleaned up with the suction punch and, when necessary, the central 3 to 4 mm of the TFC is excised. The unstable edges of the TFC are excised.

Ulna carpal impingement[25,32] should be assessed by unloading traction across the wrist and, as possible, radially and ulnarly deviating the wrist. Rotation of the ulna should also be performed to determine if there are changes of chondromalacia on the head of the ulna.[28] If there is ulnocarpal abutment, the surgeon can choose to perform excision of the head of the ulna arthroscopically or by open technique (Feldon procedure).[30] Ulna recession is an alternative procedure. Resection of 2 mm of the ulna by any of these techniques changes the loadbearing characteristics of the wrist.

Resection of the ulna arthroscopically must be performed carefully and with excellent visualization. The TFC must be resected enough to see the entire head of the ulna. Dorsal 3-4 and 4-5 portals are used for scope placement and for power instruments and each should be alternated between the two portals. First the scope is placed in the 3-4 portal and the ulna head is rotated. The power abrader (bur) is used to remove the articular cartilage and subchondral bone. The radial side cutting shaver is used intermittently to help clean the joint and to fine tune the work of the bur when necessary. The power resector should also be inserted through the radial portal to complete the resection. Fluoroscopy is needed to judge the depth of the abrasion-excision and the completeness of the

peripheral excision. Final inspection with the scope in the 4-5 portal also assists in reviewing the extent of resection.

When there is an associated lunotriquetral tear with ulna-carpal impaction, the choices of ulna recession or distal ulna excision are now balanced with the need to débride, repair, or fuse the lunotriquetral joint. It is not clear if débridement alone is sufficient, but if there is a lunotriquetral tear without a palmar intercalated segment instability deformity, resection of loose cartilage and ligament tissues may suffice. We prefer ulna recession in most of the types III, IV, and V degenerative lesions (see boxes on pp. 720 [Palmer] and 721) because it unloads the entire ulnar side of the wrist, treating the lunotriquetral lesion, ulnocarpal abutment, and TFC tear simultaneously. Arthroscopic treatment of these conditions, however, may improve with time and prove to be the treatment of choice.

AUTHOR'S PREFERRED TREATMENT

The TFC functions as a buffer between the distal end of the ulna and the radioulnar carpal joint and as a ligamentous tether connecting the distal ulna to the distal radius and ulnar carpus. Compressive force across the carpal ulnar articulation is partially transmitted through the center of the TFC to the ulnar dome, but this same force tends to separate the radius and ulna. Bowers[12] noted that the TFC resists this tendency by converting some of the compressive loading to tensile loading within the lamellar collagen of the periphery of the TFC. Schuind et al.[76] have demonstrated further the importance of the TFC to resist not only dorsal to palmar forces but lateral to medial and distal to proximal forces, agreeing with Adams and Holley[2] that the TFC has multidirectional control of stability at the DRUJ alone as well as in combination with the interosseous membrane, ECU subsheath, and pronator quadratus. Although gross loss of ligament support at the DRUJ leads to subluxation or dislocation, the significance of isolated TFC tears is less clear—in particular, traumatic tears that are clinically symptomatic with painful rotation of the forearm, loss of strength, and a click or catch referable to the DRUJ. My colleagues and I think that the complex of the TFC is an important support structure of the wrist and repair of peripheral tears is the treatment of choice whenever feasible. We agree with the observations by Imbriglia and Boland[42] and others[51,75] that partial excision of central tears of the TFC is reasonable, but we question the indiscriminate resection of large portions or total removal of this structure.[21,58,82]

Based on current understanding of the function of the TFC and the anatomy and vascular supply of the various substructures of the TFC, we recommend the following approach to TFC injuries.

1) TFC avulsion with distal radius fractures: Primary treatment is of the distal radius fracture along with closed reduction of the DRUJ. Immobilize the DRUJ in neutral rotation to supination. If wide displacement of the ulnar styloid is present after closed reduction, then open reduction and tension band wire fixation of the ulnar styloid should be performed.

2) TFC avulsion with Galeazzi's fracture: Treatment involves open reduction of the Galeazzi fracture and closed reduction with percutaneous pinning of the DRUJ with the forearm in supination. If the DRUJ cannot be reduced or if wide displacement of the ulnar styloid is present, open reduction of the DRUJ is recommended with internal fixation of the ulnar styloid.

3) TFC tear with distal radius fracture: Primary treatment is of the distal radius fracture and closed reduction in midrotation to supination of the DRUJ. Open repair of the TFC is done if incongruity of the DRUJ is observed or if there is gross instability of the DRUJ (most commonly dorsal subluxation).

4) TFC tears, isolated without fracture.

Type IA (Palmer) or Type II tear (Mayo): In the symptomatic patient, the central tears of the TFC are treated with arthroscopic resection of the central tear with débridement of the free edge. If there is a positive ulna variance of greater than 2 mm, ulna recession should be considered. If the TFC tear is near the ulnar border of the distal radius (a Mayo type I radial rim tear), we recommend open repair of the TFC back to the radius with freshening of

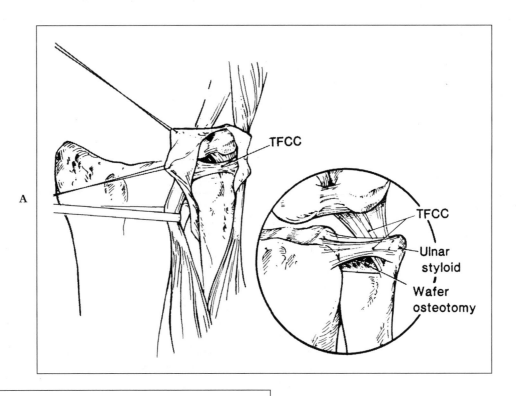

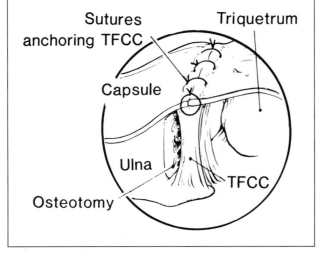

FIGURE 30-21

Feldon procedure. **A,** The flap of capsule is reflected radially to expose the distal ulna, the distal radioulnar joint, the triangular fibrocartilage complex (*TFCC*), and the lunate and triquetrum. *Inset,* A 2- to 4-mm wafer of cartilage and subchondral bone is resected from the distal ulna. **B,** The TFCC is sutured to the dorsal capsule with a row of sutures, suspending the TFC and restoring its normal tension. *(From Feldon et al.[30] Copyright, American Society for Surgery of the Hand, by permission of Churchill Livingstone.)*

the border of the distal radius and edge of the TFC.[24] An arthroscopic technique of repair of the Mayo Type I radial border tear has been described. We have had limited successful experience. After this type of repair, immobilization for 6 weeks is required with the forearm in supination, followed by gradual return of forearm rotation over 3 to 4 weeks.

Type IB tear (Palmer) or Type III tear (Mayo): In the patient with tenderness at the base of the ulnar styloid with symptoms of pain with rotational stress, direct repair of the TFC to the distal ulna is recommended by open or arthroscopic repair; the choice depends on the surgeon's experience and the ability to replace the ulnar border of the TFC back to its origin near the base of the ulnar styloid.[39] We have preferred the open repair technique[39] in late presentations because excision of granulation tissue is more reliable and the location of reattachment of the TFC can be varied by the resilience or tension present. Arthroscopic repair is less precise but certainly an alternative for experienced surgeons.

Type IC tear (Palmer) or Type IV tear (Mayo): A dorsal approach to the TFC combined with ulnar osteotomy is preferred in the repair of tears of the palmar edge of the TFC. The operative technique often involves repairing the ulnotriquetral and ulnolunate ligaments and adjacent collateral ligament complex at the ulnar edge of the distal ulna out to the pisiform with mattress plicating sutures. The tear is best visualized by arthroscopy of the wrist which can help delineate other intracarpal pathologic conditions. However, simple arthroscopic excision or débridement of such a lesion of the palmar edge of the TFC or adjacent ulnocarpal ligaments alone does not seem sufficient to address the pathology involved.[57]

During the dorsal approach, other areas of injury such as the ECU subsheath, DRUJ surface, and lunotriquetral ligament should be examined. The palmar approach is reserved for cases of clinically evident palmar instability of the distal ulna on the radius. We have not used it for isolated palmar TFC tears.

Type ID tear (Palmer): Open reduction of the distal radius to reduce and pin radius fracture fragments that enter the DRUJ is the treatment of choice.[15] Both the lunate fossa of the distal radius and the sigmoid fossa and articulation of the head of the ulna with the sigmoid fossa are critically examined for anatomic alignment. Kirschner-wire fixation of fracture fragments appears best, but if there are associated intra-articular fractures of the radius that are amenable to plate fixation, then a combination of plate and Kirschner wires may be an excellent choice for fracture fixation. Ligamentotaxis reduction alone is probably insufficient. However, arthroscopic-assisted reduction with traction across the wrist may prove to be a valuable technique worth pursuing. We have had limited experience with arthroscopy in Type ID injuries, using closed reduction and percutaneous pinning when feasible.

5) Degenerative tears of the TFC: For stage I and II presentations of ulnocarpal impaction syndrome,[63] it is necessary to show dynamic contact of the ulna with the triquetrum and lunate on grip view posteroanterior radiographs of the wrist and related abnormalities on wrist arthroscopy. If the patient is clinically symptomatic and there is neutral to positive ulna variance, then ulna recession is the treatment of choice: 2 to 3 mm of the ulna. For stage III and IV in which there is a perforation within the central portion of the TFC with chondromalacia of the lunate or ulna, our preference is ulna recession. Arthroscopic excision of the TFC free edge and arthroscopic resection of 1 to 2 mm of the head of the ulna are an acceptable alternative provided that there is no damage to the articular surface of the head of the ulna within the sigmoid notch of the distal radius. The third alternative is open resection of the distal articular surface of the head of the ulna (Feldon procedure) (Fig. 30-21), but we have noted continued symptoms in several patients after this operation as the rough edge of bone of the distal ulna rubs against the undersurface of the TFC.

REFERENCES

1. Adams BD: Partial excision of the triangular fibrocartilage complex articular disk: a biomechanical study, *J Hand Surg [Am]* 18:334-340, 1993.
2. Adams BD, Holley KA: Strains in the articular disk of the triangular fibrocartilage complex: a biomechanical study, *J Hand Surg [Am]* 18:919-925, 1993.
3. af Ekenstam F: The distal radioulnar joint: an anatomical, experimental, and clinical study. *Acta Univ Abstr Uppsala,* Dissertation from the Faculty of Medicine, 505:1-55, Uppsala ISBN 91-554-161H-7, 1984.
4. af Ekenstam F, Hagert CG: Anatomical studies on the geometry and stability of the distal radio ulnar joint, *Scand J Plast Reconstr Surg* 19:17-25, 1985.
5. Aulicino PL, Siegel JL: Acute injuries of the distal radio-ulnar joint, *Hand Clin* 7:283-293, 1991.
6. Bednar MS, Arnoczky SP, Weiland AJ: The microvasculature of the triangular fibrocartilage complex: its clinical significance, *J Hand Surg [Am]* 16:1101-1105, 1991.
7. Bell MJ, Hill RJ, McMurtry RY: Ulnar impingement syndrome, *J Bone Joint Surg Br* 67:126-129, 1985.
8. Berger RA, Blair WF, el-Khoury GY: Arthrotomography of the wrist. The triangular fibrocartilage complex, *Clin Orthop* 172:257-264, 1983.
9. Botte MJ, Cooney WP, Linscheid RL: Arthroscopy of the wrist: anatomy and technique, *J Hand Surg [Am]* 14:313-316, 1989.
10. Boulas HJ, Milek MA: Ulnar shortening for tears of the triangular fibrocartilaginous complex, *J Hand Surg [Am]* 15:415-420, 1990.
11. Bowers WH: Problems of the distal radioulnar joint, *Adv Orthop Surg* 7:289-303, 1984.
12. Bowers WH: *The distal radioulnar joint.* In Green DP, editor: *Operative hand surgery,* ed 2, vol 2, New York, 1988, Churchill Livingstone, pp 939-989.
13. Bowers WH, Whipple TL: *Arthroscopic anatomy of the wrist.* In McGinty JB, Caspari RB, Jackson RW, et al., editors: *Operative arthroscopy,* New York, 1991, Raven Press, pp 613-623.
14. Boyd HB, Stone MM: Resection of the distal end of the ulna, *J Bone Joint Surg* 26:313-321, 1944.
15. Bradway JK, Amadio PC, Cooney WP: Open reduction and internal fixation of displaced, comminuted intra-articular fractures of the distal end of the radius, *J Bone Joint Surg Am* 71:839-847, 1989.
16. Burkhart SS, Wood MB, Linscheid RL: Posttraumatic recurrent subluxation of the extensor carpi ulnaris tendon, *J Hand Surg [Am]* 7:1-3, 1982.
17. Cerofolini E, Luchetti R, Pederzini L, et al.: MR evaluation of triangular fibrocartilage complex tears in the wrist: comparison with arthrography and arthroscopy, *J Comput Assist Tomogr* 14:963-967, 1990.
18. Chidgey LK: Histologic anatomy of the triangular fibrocartilage, *Hand Clin* 7:249-262, 1991.
19. Chidgey LK, Dell PC, Bittar E, et al.: Tear patterns and collagen arrangement in the triangular fibrocartilage (abstract), *J Hand Surg [Am]* 15:826, 1990.
20. Chidgey LK, Dell PC, Bittar ES, et al.: Histologic anatomy of the triangular fibrocartilage, *J Hand Surg [Am]* 16:1084-1100, 1991.
21. Coleman HM: Injuries of the articular disk at the wrist, *J Bone Joint Surg Br* 42:522-529, 1960.
22. Cooney WP: Evaluation of chronic wrist pain by arthrography, arthroscopy, and arthrotomy, *J Hand Surg [Am]* 18:815-822, 1993.
23. Cooney WP, Bussey R, Dobyns JH, et al.: Difficult wrist fractures. Perilunate fracture-dislocations of the wrist, *Clin Orthop* 214:136-147, 1987.
24. Cooney WP, Linscheid RL, Dobyns JH: Triangular fibrocartilage tears, *J Hand Surg [Am]* 19:143-154, 1994.
25. Darrow JC Jr, Linscheid RL, Dobyns JH, et al.: Distal ulnar recession for disorders of the distal radioulnar joint, *J Hand Surg [Am]* 10:482-491, 1985.
26. Dingman PVC: Resection of the distal end of the ulna (Darrach operation): an end-result study of twenty-four cases, *J Bone Joint Surg Am* 34:893-900, 1952.
27. Edwards GS Jr, Jupiter JB: Radial head fractures with acute distal radioulnar dislocation. Essex-Lopresti revisited, *Clin Orthop* 234:61-69, 1988.
28. Epner RA, Bowers WH, Guilford WB: Ulnar variance—the effect of wrist positioning and roentgen filming technique, *J Hand Surg [Am]* 7:298-305, 1982.
29. Essex-Lopresti P: Fractures of the radial head with distal radioulnar dislocation: report of two cases, *J Bone Joint Surg Br* 33:244-247, 1951.
30. Feldon P, Terrono AL, Belsky MR: Wafer distal ulna resection for triangular fibrocartilage tears and/or ulna impaction syndrome, *J Hand Surg [Am]* 17:731-737, 1992.
31. Fernandez DL: Radial osteotomy and Bowers arthroplasty for malunited fractures of the distal end of the radius, *J Bone Joint Surg Am* 70:1538-1551, 1988.
32. Friedman SL, Palmer AK: The ulnar impaction syndrome, *Hand Clin* 7:295-310, 1991.
33. Fulkerson JP, Watson HK: Congenital anterior subluxation of the distal ulna. A case report, *Clin Orthop* 131:179-182, 1978.
34. Gilula LA, Hardy DC, Totty WG: Distal radioulnar joint arthrography, *AJR* 150:864-866, 1988.
35. Golimbu CN, Firooznia H, Melone CP Jr, et al.: Tears of the triangular fibrocartilage of the wrist: MR imaging, *Radiology* 173:731-733, 1989.
36. Hagert C-G: Functional aspects on the distal radioulnar joint (abstract), *J Hand Surg* 4:585, 1979.
37. Hanker GJ: Diagnostic and operative arthroscopy of the wrist, *Clin Orthop* 263:165-174, 1991.
38. Hardy DC, Totty WG, Carnes KM, et al.: Arthrographic surface anatomy of the carpal triangular fibrocartilage complex, *J Hand Surg [Am]* 13:823-829, 1988.
39. Hermansdorfer JD, Kleinman WB: Management of chronic peripheral tears of the triangular fibrocartilage complex, *J Hand Surg [Am]* 16:340-346, 1991.
40. Hughston JC: Fracture of the distal radial shaft: mistakes in management, *J Bone Joint Surg Am* 39:249-264, 1957.

41. Hui FC, Linscheid RL: Ulnotriquetral augmentation tenodesis: a reconstructive procedure for dorsal subluxation of the distal radioulnar joint, *J Hand Surg [Am]* 7:230-236, 1982.

42. Imbriglia JE, Boland DS: Tears of the articular disk of the triangular fibrocartilage complex: results of the excision of the articular disk (abstract), *J Hand Surg* 8:620, 1983.

43. Kapandji IA: *The inferior radioulnar joint and pronosupination.* In Tubiana R, editor: *The hand,* vol 1, Philadelphia, 1981, WB Saunders.

44. Kapandji IA: The Kapandji-Sauve operation. Its techniques and indications in non-rheumatoid diseases, *Ann Chir Main* 5:181-193, 1986.

45. Kauer JMG: The articular disk of the hand, *Acta Anat* 93:590-605, 1975.

46. King GJ, McMurtry RY, Rubenstein JD, et al.: Computerized tomography of the distal radioulnar joint: correlation with ligamentous pathology in a cadaveric model, *J Hand Surg [Am]* 11:711-717, 1986.

47. King GJ, McMurtry RY, Rubenstein JD, et al.: Kinematics of the distal radioulnar joint, *J Hand Surg [Am]* 11:798-804, 1986.

48. Lewis OJ, Hamshere RJ, Bucknill TM: The anatomy of the wrist joint, *J Anat* 106:539-552, 1970.

49. Linscheid RL: Symposium on the distal radioulnar joint, *Contemp Orthop* 7:81, 1983.

50. Linscheid RL: Ulnar lengthening and shortening, *Hand Clin* 3:69-79, 1987.

51. Menon J, Schoene HR: Isolated tear of the triangular fibrocartilage of the wrist joint: result of excision (abstract), *J Hand Surg* 7:421, 1982.

52. Menon J, Wood VE, Schoene HR, et al.: Isolated tears of the triangular fibrocartilage of the wrist: results of partial excision, *J Hand Surg [Am]* 9:527-530, 1984.

53. Mikic Z: The blood supply of the human distal radioulnar joint and the microvasculature of its articular disk, *Clin Orthop* 275:19-28, 1992.

54. Mikic ZD: Age changes in the triangular fibrocartilage of the wrist joint, *J Anat* 126:367-384, 1978.

55. Mikic ZD: Arthrography of the wrist joint. An experimental study, *J Bone Joint Surg Am* 66:371-378, 1984.

56. Mino DE, Palmer AK, Levinsohn EM: The role of radiography and computerized tomography in the diagnosis of subluxation and dislocation of the distal radioulnar joint, *J Hand Surg [Am]* 8:23-31, 1983.

57. Mooney JF, Poehling GG: Disruption of the ulnolunate ligament as a cause of chronic ulnar wrist pain, *J Hand Surg [Am]* 16:347-349, 1991.

58. Mossing N: Isolated lesions of the radio-ulnar disk treated with excision, *Scand J Plast Reconstr Surg* 9:231-233, 1975.

59. Neviaser RJ, Palmer AK: Traumatic perforation of the articular disk of the triangular fibrocartilage complex of the wrist, *Bull Hosp Jt Dis Orthop Inst* 44:376-380, 1984.

60. Osterman AL: Arthroscopic debridement of triangular fibrocartilage complex tears, *Arthroscopy* 6:120-124, 1990.

61. Osterman AL, Terrill RG: Arthroscopic treatment of TFCC lesions, *Hand Clin* 7:277-281, 1991.

62. Palmer AK: Symposium on distal ulnar injuries, *Contemp Orthop* 7:81, 1983.

63. Palmer AK: Triangular fibrocartilage complex lesions: a classification, *J Hand Surg [Am]* 14:594-606, 1989.

64. Palmer AK: Triangular fibrocartilage disorders: injury patterns and treatment, *Arthroscopy* 6:125-132, 1990.

65. Palmer AK, Levinsohn EM, Kuzma GR: Arthrography of the wrist, *J Hand Surg [Am]* 8:15-23, 1983.

66. Palmer AK, Neviaser R: Triangular fibrocartilage complex abnormalities: results of surgical treatment. Second International Congress—International Federation of Societies for Surgery of the Hand, Abstract 129, p 62, Boston, MA, 1983.

67. Palmer AK, Werner FW: The triangular fibrocartilage complex of the wrist—anatomy and function, *J Hand Surg* 6:153-162, 1981.

68. Palmer AK, Werner FW, Glisson RR, et al.: Partial excision of the triangular fibrocartilage complex, *J Hand Surg [Am]* 13:391-394, 1988.

69. Pederzini L, Luchetti R, Soragni O, et al.: Evaluation of the triangular fibrocartilage complex tears by arthroscopy, arthrography, and magnetic resonance imaging, *Arthroscopy* 8:191-197, 1992.

70. Poehling GG: *Arthroscopy of the wrist and elbow,* New York, 1994, Raven Press.

71. Poehling GG, Siegel DB, Komen LA, et al.: *Arthroscopy of the wrist and elbow.* In Green DP, editor: *Operative hand surgery,* ed 3, vol 1, New York, 1993, Churchill Livingstone, pp 189-214.

72. Reinus WR, Hardy DC, Totty WG, et al.: Arthrographic evaluation of the carpal triangular fibrocartilage complex, *J Hand Surg [Am]* 12:495-503, 1987.

73. Resnick D, Andre M, Kerr R, et al.: Digital arthrography of the wrist: a radiographic-pathologic investigation, *AJR* 142:1187-1190, 1984.

74. Roth JH: *Wrist arthroscopy: radiocarpal arthroscopy: technique and selected cases.* In Lichtman DM, editor: *The wrist and its disorders,* Philadelphia, 1988, WB Saunders, pp 108-128.

75. Sanders RA, Hawkins B: Reconstruction of the distal radioulnar joint for chronic volar dislocation. A case report, *Orthopedics* 12:1473-1476, 1989.

76. Schuind F, An KN, Berglund L, et al.: The distal radioulnar ligaments: a biomechanical study, *J Hand Surg [Am]* 16:1106-1114, 1991.

77. Shaw JA, Bruno A, Paul EM: Ulnar styloid fixation in the treatment of posttraumatic instability of the radioulnar joint: a biomechanical study with clinical correlation, *J Hand Surg [Am]* 15:712-720, 1990.

78. Snook GA, Chrisman OD, Wilson TC, et al: Subluxation of the distal radio-ulnar joint by hyperpronation, *J Bone Joint Surg Am* 51:1315-1323, 1969.

79. Taleisnik J: The ligaments of the wrist, *J Hand Surg [Am]* 1:110-118, 1976.

80. Taleisnik J: Symposium on distal ulnar injuries, *Contemp Orthop* 7:81-116, 1983.

81. Thiru RG, Ferlic DC, Clayton ML, et al.: Arterial anatomy of the triangular fibrocartilage of the wrist and its surgical significance, *J Hand Surg [Am]* 11:258-263, 1986.

82. van der Linden AJ: Disk lesion of the wrist joint, *J Hand Surg [Am]* 11:490-497, 1986.

83. Weigl K, Spira E: The triangular fibrocartilage of the wrist joint, *Reconstr Surg Traumatol* 11:139-153, 1969.

84. Whipple TL, Cooney WP, Poehling GG: *Intra-articular fractures.* In McGinty JB, Caspari RB, Jackson RW, et al., editors: *Operative arthroscopy,* New York, 1991, Raven Press, pp 651-654.

85. Whipple TL, Geissler WB: Arthroscopic management of wrist triangular fibrocartilage complex injuries in the athlete, *Orthopedics* 16:1061-1067, 1993.

86. Wnorowski DC, Palmer AK, Werner FW, et al.: Anatomic and biomechanical analysis of the arthroscopic wafer procedure, *Arthroscopy* 8:204-212, 1992.

87. Zachee B, De Smet L, Fabry G: Arthroscopic suturing of TFCC lesions, *Arthroscopy* 9:242-243, 1993.

88. Zlatkin MB, Chao PC, Osterman AL, et al.: Chronic wrist pain: evaluation with high-resolution MR imaging, *Radiology* 173:723-729, 1989.

ADDITIONAL READING

De Smet L, De Ferm A, Steenwerckx A, et al.: Arthroscopic treatment of triangular fibrocartilage complex lesions of the wrist, *Acta Orthopaedica Belgica* 62:8-13, 1996.

Hauck RM, Skahen J III, Palmer AK: Classification and treatment of ulnar styloid nonunion, *J Hand Surg [Am]* 21:418-422, 1996.

Jantea CL, Baltzer A, Ruther W: Arthroscopic repair of radial-sided lesions of the triangular fibrocartilage complex, *Hand Clin* 11:31-36, 1995.

Melone CP Jr, Nathan R: Traumatic disruption of the triangular fibrocartilage complex. Pathoanatomy, *Clin Orthop Rel Res* 275:65-73, 1992.

Mikic ZD: Treatment of acute injuries of the triangular fibrocartilage complex associated with distal radioulnar joint instability, *J Hand Surg [Am]* 20:319-323, 1995.

Minami A, Ishikawa J, Suenaga N, et al.: Clinical results of treatment of triangular fibrocartilage complex tears by arthroscopic debridement, *J Hand Surg [Am]* 21:406-411, 1996.

Sennwald GR, Lauterburg M, Zdravkovic V: A new technique of reattachment after traumatic avulsion of the TFCC at its ulnar insertion, *J Hand Surg [Br]* 20:178-184, 1995.

Zachee B, De Smet L, Fabry G: Arthroscopic suturing of TFCC lesions, *Arthroscopy* 9:242-243, 1993.

FRACTURES OF THE DISTAL RADIOULNAR JOINT

John M. Rayhack, M.D.
William P. Cooney, M.D.

EMBRYOLOGY
ANATOMY
   MUSCLE ATTACHMENTS
   STRUCTURAL SUPPORT OF THE DISTAL ULNA
PEDIATRIC ULNAR FRACTURES
   TORUS FRACTURE
   GREENSTICK FRACTURE
   TREATMENT

PHYSEAL INJURY
COMPLICATIONS OF PHYSEAL INJURIES TO THE ULNA
PLASTIC DEFORMATION OF THE ULNA
ULNAR FRACTURES IN THE ADULT
   STRESS FRACTURES OF THE ULNA
   COMPLICATIONS OF ADULT ULNAR FRACTURES
   SYNOSTOSIS OF THE DISTAL ULNA TO RADIUS

Although fractures of the distal ulna often occur in tandem with fractures of the distal radius, it is the latter that attracts most of our attention. Despite this bias, it is well known that distal ulnar fractures often lead to significant dysfunction of the forearm and of the distal radioulnar joint in particular. If disorders of this joint secondary to ulnar fractures are to be avoided, our attention to this pivotal joint must not be minimized.

EMBRYOLOGY

The ulna, like the other bones of the axial skeleton, develops by endochondral ossification of the central mesenchymal anlage of cells. The primary ossification center develops into the diaphysis and metaphysis. The distal ulnar epiphysis develops from a secondary ossification center which ossifies at age 5 years. The significance of this delay in ossification resides in the fact that a fracture through the ulnar epiphyseal cartilage in a child may become evident only in retrospect as an osteochondral fracture after ossification of this center. A separate ossification center for the ulnar styloid is rare but it does occur.[21] This leads to the radiographic appearance of accessory ossicles.[2] The most well known

is the os triangulare, which may be difficult to distinguish from ulnar styloid chip fractures.[3]

Physiologic epiphysiodesis occurs at age 16 years in boys and 14 years in girls. The physiologic difference and the difference in fracture characteristics necessitate a distinction between childhood and adult ulnar fractures.

ANATOMY

MUSCLE ATTACHMENTS

No muscles take origin or have their insertion on the distal palmar aspect of the distal ulna, with the sole exception of the origin of the pronator quadratus muscle (Fig. 31-1). The distal ulnar diaphysis is the site of origin of the extensor indicis proprius dorsally (Fig. 31-2) and the flexor digitorum profundus more proximally. However, these muscles play little role in the deformation of distal ulnar fractures. In discussions concerning the role played by the overlying muscles in determining the direction of angulation of distal forearm fractures, attention centers primarily on the radius. Because the distal ulna is intimately attached to and works in concert with the distal radius, it seems prudent to briefly mention these forces.

In general, muscles with a proximal ulnar origin and radial insertion, such as the flexor carpi radialis, tend to pronate the distal radius. Dorsal muscles, such as the brachioradialis, abductor pollicis longus, extensor pollicis brevis, and extensor pollicis longus, tend to supinate the distal radius. The extensor carpi ulnaris is the only muscle connected to the distal ulna, and it resides alone in the sixth dorsal compartment (Fig. 31-2). This tendon imparts stability to the distal radioulnar joint through a strong fibro-osseous tunnel overlying 1.5 to

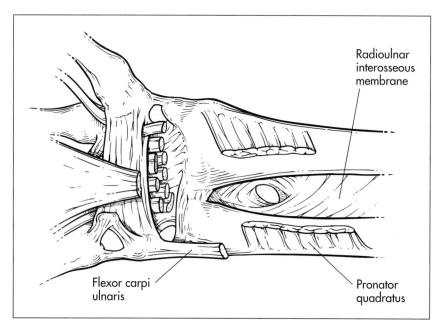

FIGURE 31-1

Palmar dissection of the distal forearm. Note that the pronator quadratus is the only muscle with origin or insertion on the palmar distal ulna.

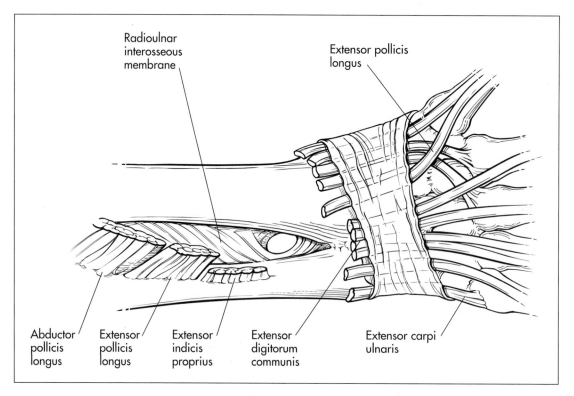

FIGURE 31-2

Dorsal dissection of the distal forearm demonstrates the origin of finger extensors (extensor indicis proprius, extensor pollicis longus, extensor digiti quinti) and the broad attachments of the interosseous membrane.

2.0 mm of the distal ulna in the extensor carpi ulnaris sulcus.[31] Two layers of the infratendinous portion of the extensor retinaculum envelop this tendon (see Chapter 3).[33]

STRUCTURAL SUPPORT OF THE DISTAL ULNA

As previously stated, the distal ulna is intimately held in the sigmoid fossa of the distal radius. The primary stabilizers of the ulnar head to the distal radioulnar joint are the triangular fibrocartilage and the radioulnar ligaments.[11,24,27] The triangular fibrocartilage originates from the distal rim of the sigmoid fossa and extends to insert on the base of the ulnar styloid.[23] Dorsally, the triangular fibrocartilage is attached to the dorsal radioulnar ligament and palmarly, to the ulnocarpal ligaments. Distally, the triangular fibrocartilage is also attached to the articular meniscus and the ulnar collateral ligament complex. The dorsal portion of the triangular fibrocartilage and dorsal radioulnar ligament are taut in pronation. The significance of this point is evident in the frequency of ulnar styloid fractures seen in association with distal radial fractures. These fractures commonly occur during falls on outstretched and pronated forearms. This is true for children as well as adults, although it may not be readily apparent in children, as already discussed[21] (Ogden JA, personal communication). The depth of the sigmoid fossa of the distal radius imparts significant geometric stability by virtue of its dorsal and palmar lips, which partially envelop the distal ulnar articular surface.

The interosseous ligament (or membrane) (Fig. 31-2) is also an important stabilizer of the forearm. Fiber direction suggests a distal ulnar insertion and a proximal radial origin. Although the arrangement of these oblique fibers imparts significant proximodistal stability, it is often insufficient to prevent radial migration in cases of radial head resection. With this exception, it is the triangular fibrocartilage that usually garners the majority of attention in discussions of stability of the distal radioulnar joint.[24]

PEDIATRIC ULNAR FRACTURES

Fractures to the distal ulna (and radius) are among the most common injuries to the developing skeleton (Fig. 31-3).[19]

TORUS FRACTURE

Pediatric fracture types generally include the torus, greenstick, and completely displaced fractures. The *torus fracture* has buckling of one cortex of the ulna, with

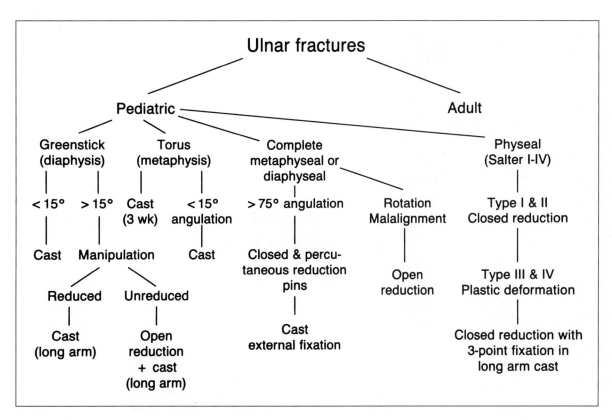

FIGURE 31-3

Treatment algorithm for pediatric patients.

minimal evidence of trabecular disruption. This traditionally occurs through the metaphysis about 2 to 3 mm proximal to the physis. The mechanism of injury is usually axial loading with cortical buckling on the compression side. The opposite cortex and periosteal sleeve remain intact in the true torus fracture. No angulation of the ulna occurs, and redeformation should not occur during the healing process. Treatment usually consists of immobilization for 3 weeks in a short arm cast.

GREENSTICK FRACTURE

In contradistinction to the true torus fracture, the *greenstick fracture* of the ulna involves both cortices with a noticeable deformity of the bone. This type of fracture is fascinating in concept and vexing to the clinician. Progressive deformity and recurrence of angulation during the healing process have been observed. In many respects this fracture is analogous to the displaced adult radial fracture that, when reduced, has the propensity to redisplace. In the case of the radius, at least the clinician is forewarned with the knowledge that recurrence of deformity to the original displaced position of the distal radius may occur. In the greenstick fracture, however, the physician may not know the degree of original displacement of the fracture segments. One must be fully aware that the static picture at the time of the radiograph does not represent the more severely displaced dynamic fracture at the time of the original injury.[22] It is the fracture's return to its original displaced position that must be prevented during the healing process.

The mechanism of injury of the greenstick fracture is longitudinal compression and torsional forces that usually result from a fall on an outstretched hand. The bone fractures through the tensile cortex, with bowing by plastic deformation of the opposite (compressive) cortex. Both greenstick and torus fractures thus have the capacity to dissipate the energy of the ulnar fracture before the second cortex is fractured.

TREATMENT

Treatment of greenstick fractures of the ulna is controversial. If such a fracture is seen in association with a distal radial fracture, the amount of angulation of the bones is critical. Greater than 10° to 15° of residual angulation usually requires gentle manipulation of the fracture under general anesthesia to complete the fracture of the intact cortex. Completion of the fracture helps prevent recurrence of deformity by eliminating the tensile force stored up in the fractured bone. With completion of the fracture (through both cortices) care must be taken to avoid tearing of the periosteum so as to prevent a completely displaced fracture. Some authors[6] believe that a three-point casting technique

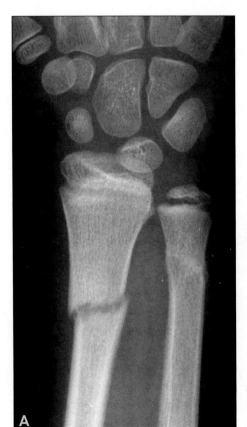
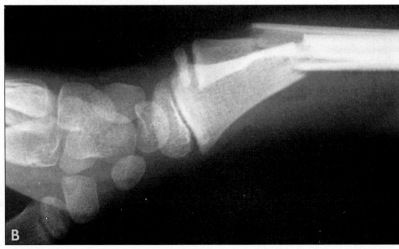

FIGURE 31-4

Displaced distal radius and distal ulna (diaphyseal fractures demonstrate complete displacement). **A,** Posteroanterior radiograph; satisfactory alignment. **B,** Lateral radiograph; palmar angulation apex dorsal to both radius and ulna.

can prevent redisplacement during the healing process. Although this may be true in some cases, the clinician must be alert to the propensity of these fractures to redisplace.

Complete fractures of the ulna (Fig. 31-4) are frequently seen in association with complete fractures of the radius. These fractures fail in both tension and compression. These are often seen as overriding fractures, which are difficult to reduce as well as difficult to maintain. A displaced fracture of the radius with a greenstick fracture of the ulna may be difficult to reduce. It is frequently necessary to complete the greenstick fracture of the ulna in order to reduce the overriding fracture of the radius. It is not uncommon to see the association of a distal radial epiphyseal injury with an overriding fracture of the ulna.[22]

Displaced and overriding radial and ulnar fractures that are unstable may be treated with a single percutaneous pin in each bone in order to secure fixation. Although this is obviously more aggressive treatment than cast treatment alone, the surgeon must consider whether the risk of infection from a single smooth pin outweighs the risk of a second anesthetic and attendant family consternation if the fractures redisplace. It has become increasingly accepted to add percutaneous pins at the time of reduction of unstable distal radial and ulnar fractures. Good fracture immobilization and removal of the percutaneous pin(s) at the earliest moment limit the chances of pin-tract infection. Overriding or bayonet position of a fracture of 1/4 to 1/2 in. is sometimes accepted because of the common occurrence of bone overgrowth in the fractured bone, with restoration of bone length in 9 to 12 months.[8] Irreducible fractures of the radius and ulna occasionally occur and necessitate open reduction and internal fixation. Occasionally, soft tissues (muscle tissue and periosteal flaps) become interposed between the fractured bone surfaces, necessitating open reduction.

Fracture reduction of the distal forearm can accept a degree of loss of length and malangulation (dorsal-palmar). Malrotation of distal forearm fractures, however, cannot be accepted. The most common late cause of problems from forearm fractures in children is the failure to identify and to correct malrotation of the radius, the ulna, or, occasionally, both bones of the forearm.

PHYSEAL INJURY

Physeal injuries to the distal ulna may occur[29] in association with distal radial physeal fractures, but the occurrence is considered rare (Fig. 31-5) (see Chapter 42).[22] Similarly, an isolated fracture-separation of the ulnar physis not associated with a radial fracture is considered an unusual injury. In general, physeal fractures result from hyperextension forces applied at the radiocarpal joint. These fractures may be irreducible by closed means and may require open reduction because of interposed periosteum. Although the majority of ulnar epiphyseal fractures are type I or II

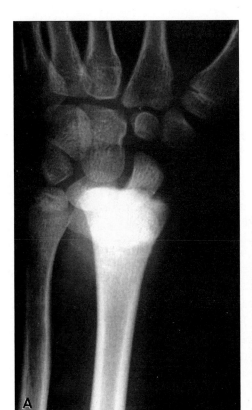

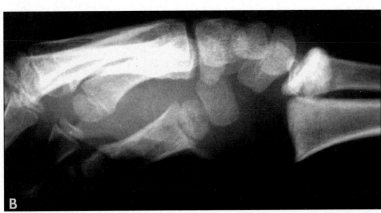

FIGURE 31-5

Complete displacement of radial epiphysis with an ulnar epiphysis fracture-separation. **A,** Posteroanterior radiograph demonstrates shortening of the wrist-forearm. **B,** Lateral view confirms a physeal injury (Salter II) with dorsal displacement of the wrist, radial epiphysis, and distal ulna.

shear fractures,[29] occasionally type III and IV injuries are seen in more violent injuries associated with extreme ulnar deviation or displaced epiphyseal radial fractures.[39] Type V injuries are diagnosed in retrospect. It often takes 6 to 12 months of follow-up to determine if a physis has been obliterated.[20,32] Salter type I fractures are often diagnosed on clinical grounds alone. Tenderness at the site of the physis should be treated as a fracture, with short arm casting for 3 weeks and reevaluation for tenderness at that time to determine if continued protection is indicated. Displaced physeal fractures should be reduced promptly. After 10 to 14 days, however, forceful attempts to reduce the physis may lead to further damage and arrest of growth.

COMPLICATIONS OF PHYSEAL INJURIES TO THE ULNA

Arrest of growth of the distal ulna has been well documented by Nelson et al.[20] In four patients ages 7 to 13 years with ulnar epiphyseal arrest, bowing of the radial diaphysis, ulnar translation of the radial epiphysis, and increased angulation of the distal radiocarpal joint were noted. Interestingly, not only were growth discrepancies noted in the ulna but also secondarily in the radius. Despite the absence of pain in these children, the displeasing cosmetic appearance and functional limitations were indications for surgical intervention. Options for surgical management include a closing wedge osteotomy of the radius, ulnar lengthening, distal radial epiphysiodesis, and stapling of the lateral side of the distal radial physis.[39] It is clear that soft-tissue tethering of the radius as a result of the short ulna should not be underestimated. From the work of Stahl and Karpman,[32] growth prediction charts for the radius and ulna have been developed and may aid in treatment if differential bone growth occurs secondary to arrest of ulnar growth.

PLASTIC DEFORMATION OF THE ULNA

Just as arrest of distal ulnar epiphyseal growth may result in compensatory radial bowing, as seen above, plastic deformation of the ulna secondary to injury may also result in bowing and altered rotation of the forearm. Although first recognized by Barton in 1821, it was not until 1975 that Borden's paper[3] emphasized the difficulty in diagnosis and treatment of plastic deformation. Interestingly, the ulna is the bone that most frequently undergoes plastic deformation.[7] The radius may be fractured in addition to the ulna and similarly have plastic deformation. A child's bone is more flexible because of the larger Haversian canals, thus rendering the bone more porous.[15] Therefore,

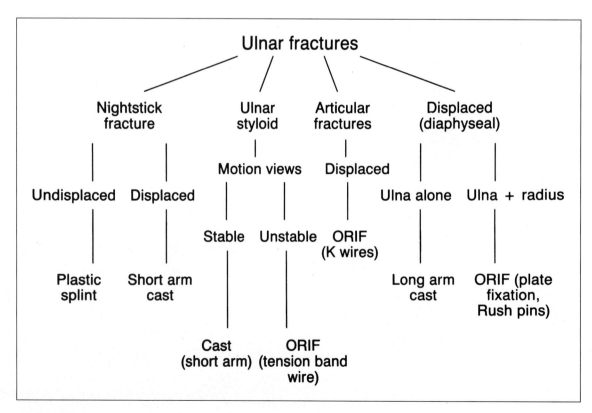

FIGURE 31-6

Treatment algorithm for adult patients. *ORIF*, open reduction and internal fixation.

the plastic response to stress allows the bone to bend. Microfractures occur along the concave border of the bone, which is longitudinally compressed.

The diagnosis of plastic deformation is made clinically by noting tenderness over the involved bone and loss of forearm rotation if both bones are involved. A bone scan can help to determine if a fresh fracture has occurred, but it will not help in the case of an old fracture, nor will plain films demonstrate periosteal new bone.

Treatment of plastic deformation consists of remodeling the bone under general anesthesia with a significant force placed along the convex border of the bone(s). If seen in association with a displaced fracture, the bone with a plastic deformation must first be reduced, and then the displaced fracture may be reduced. Lack of full forearm rotation after reduction may indicate lack of full reduction of the bone with a plastic deformation. In addition, late dislocation of the distal radioulnar joint has also been reported[1] to result from an ulna with a plastic deformation. A long arm cast should be applied for 6 weeks to allow full bone healing. Molding must be carefully performed to maintain pressure on the convex surface while avoiding the complication of skin irritation or necrosis. Some authors (Ogden JA, personal communication) believe that a forearm bone with plastic deformation in a child requires no reduction because of the bone's capacity to remodel.

ULNAR FRACTURES IN THE ADULT

The *nightstick fracture* (Fig. 31-6) is well known to the practicing clinician. This fracture results from a direct blow on the exposed subcutaneous border of the ulna. Frequently, the cause of injury is a direct blow to the forearm in an attempt to ward off a strike to the head. An indirect cause of injury in nightstick fracture is a fall on an outstretched hand. Treatment of these nondisplaced or minimally displaced fractures has become quite cavalier. Short arm casts have generally been replaced by the use of functional braces popularized by Sarmiento et al. in 1976.[30] Circumferential thermoplastic sleeves held with Velcro straps are easily made by occupational therapists and permit significant comfort. Nonunions are seen infrequently with this type of treatment.

Ulnar styloid fractures represent another fracture that has been treated with benign neglect. Frequently seen in association with fractures of the distal radius, ulnar styloid fractures are provoked by rotatory stresses and also by forced radial deviation. They are generally considered avulsion injuries. Despite the innocuous appearance of the majority of ulnar styloid fractures, it is clear that many of these fractures indicate tears of the peripheral attachment of the triangular fibrocartilage. Tears of the triangular fibrocartilage should be considered when the ulnar styloid is displaced in a radial direction (Fig. 31-7). Up to 25% of ulnar styloid fractures fail to unite or heal by fibrous union. It is sometimes helpful to view radial and ulnar deviation on radiographs to determine if motion is present as a source of the patient's pain. Magnetic resonance imaging, diagnostic fluoroscopy, and arthroscopy have been recommended[1,15,16] for evaluation of ulnar styloid fractures in the high-performance athlete but are otherwise usually not warranted. Significantly displaced ulnar styloid fractures and nonunion of the ulnar styloid (Fig. 31-7) are occasionally symptomatic, and these may require tension band wiring[9] or perhaps subperiosteal excision of the styloid.[42]

Displaced distal ulnar fractures are often the result of high-velocity automobile injuries or high-energy industrial injuries. These fractures may be associated with distal radial fractures and many are open injuries. *Open displaced ulnar fractures* must be treated with the same degree of care as any other fracture of a long bone. Débridement of the contaminated skin margins, excision of devitalized tissue, irrigation of the wound, and delayed closure are the main principles. Immediate fixation of open fractures is often indicated, although this may be delayed for 1 to 3 weeks to allow soft-tissue healing.

Plate fixation of displaced ulnar fractures has been advocated since the early work by Lane[18] in England and by Lambotte[17] in Belgium. Once early difficulties with metallurgy were overcome by the electrolysis work of Venable et al.[35] in 1937, plate fixation gained popularity.

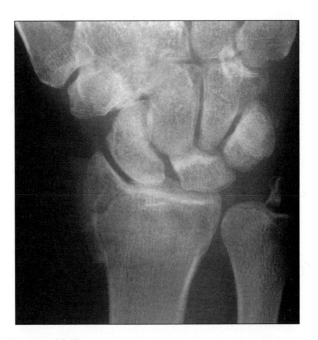

FIGURE 31-7

Radial displacement of an ulnar styloid avulsion fracture.

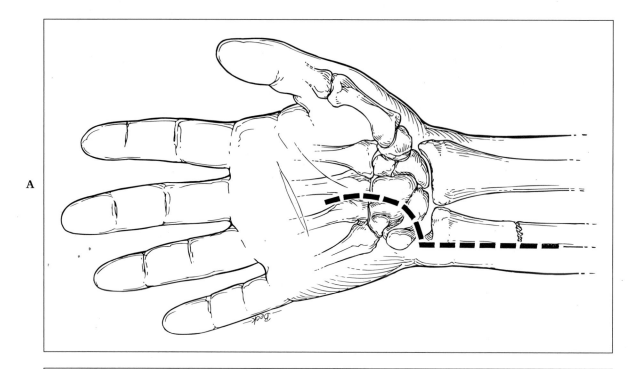

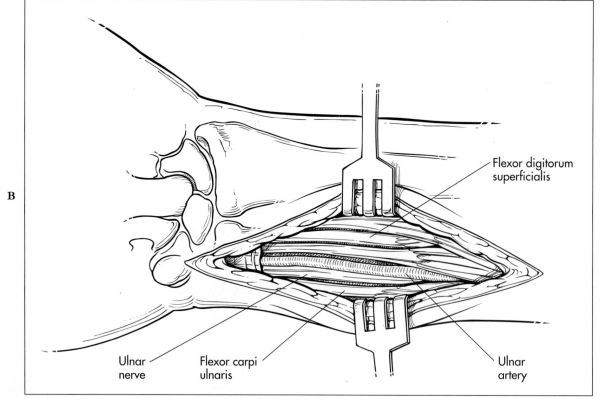

FIGURE 31-8

A, Palmar approach to the ulna. Skin incision follows the ulnar nerve and artery, curving distally to the ulnar border of the carpal tunnel and radial border of Guyon's canal. **B,** Deeper dissection of palmar approach demonstrates the plane of dissection down to the ulnar nerve and artery.

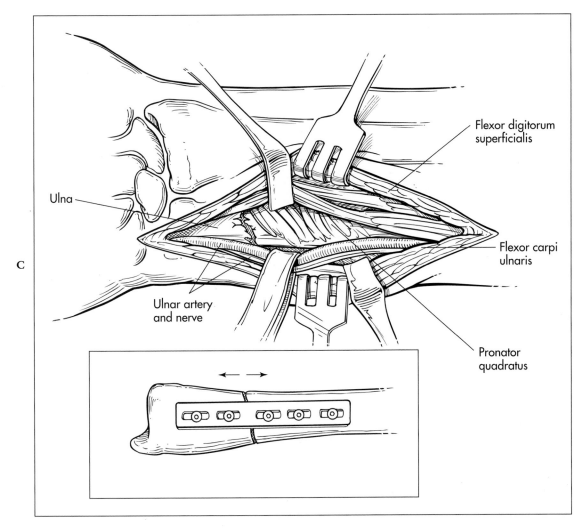

FIGURE 31-8, CONT'D.

C, After retraction of the ulnar neurovascular bundle medially, the pronator quadratus is exposed and reflected between the flexor digitorum superficialis and flexor carpi ulnaris from its ulnar origin. *Inset,* A five- to six-hole dynamic compression plate is applied for internal fixation of the distal ulna; the pronator quadratus is reapproximated to its origin, covering the plate.

It is generally accepted that the dynamic compression plate system developed by Muller in 1958 that uses a modified Danis plate remains the most efficacious technique of plate fixation of distal ulnar fractures.[39] Although Teipner and Mast[34] evaluated double-plating techniques, it is clear that distal ulnar fractures may be adequately treated by a single plate, which may be palmarly, dorsally, or medially placed. The palmar approach to the ulna, radial to the ulnar nerve and artery and flexor carpi ulnaris and ulnar to the flexor digitorum superficialis, can be selected for plate fixation of distal ulnar metaphyseal or diaphyseal fractures (Fig. 31-8). Dorsal plating of the ulna (dorsal-medial) is most commonly chosen and can be done through a medial (ulnar) approach (Fig. 31-9). If exploration of the articular surface is necessary, the second portion of the incision (Fig. 31-9) may be

used. If further dissection is needed to explore the triangular fibrocartilage complex and ulnar carpus, the third portion of the incision may be used. This zigzag skin approach avoids crossing the dorsal skin creases at a right angle, as has been stressed.[41] The dorsal branch of the ulnar sensory nerve passes around the distal ulna dorsally and distally in this interval. It is not generally stressed, however, that a rather well-developed transverse branch often crosses the triquetrum toward the lunate, and this branch should be carefully preserved during this exposure. In communication of the ulna involving more than 30% of the cortex, it is recommended that additional cancellous bone graft be placed at the fracture site to hasten bone healing.

Rush pinning of displaced ulnar fractures enjoyed early popularity and is still done today. A 16.6% nonunion rate has been reported with Rush rods. If a

A

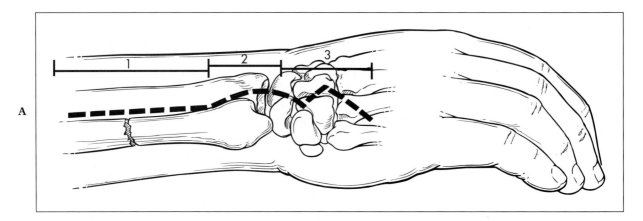

B

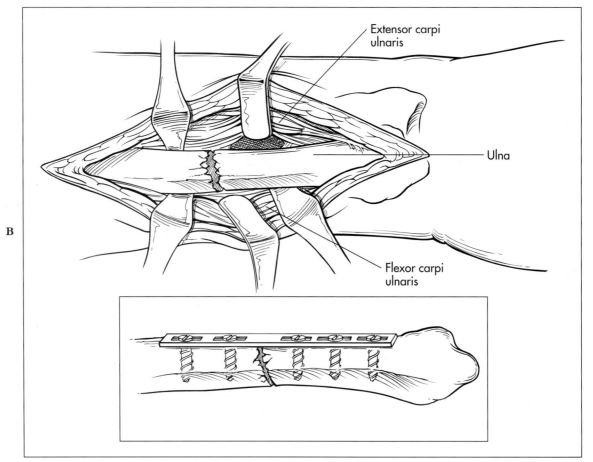

FIGURE 31-9

A, Dorsal-medial approach to the ulna. The skin incision has three components: distal third (Z incision over the wrist); middle third (curvilinear incision over the distal ulnar head); and proximal third (straight incision over the dorsal ulna). **B,** Deep surgical exposure is between the extensor carpi ulnaris and flexor carpi ulnaris, exposing the medial and dorsal shaft of the ulna. Subperiosteal Bennett-type retractors assist in exposure. *Inset,* Dorsal compression plate applied to the distal third of the ulna.

Rush pin is to be used, it is imperative that the anatomic congruency of the distal ulnar articular surface is maintained in the ulnar notch of the radius. Failure to reduce ulnar fractures (Fig. 31-10) into an anatomic position may ultimately require a Sauvé-Kapandji fusion or excision of the distal ulna (Darrach resection) to treat pain at the distal radioulnar joint. Sage nails have been touted by some[28] as a more successful method to treat displaced ulnar fractures because of their triangular shape, but the use of this nail is rare today.

Articular fractures of the ulna at the distal radioulnar joint are also known to occur alone sometimes.[14] As in any articular fracture, restoration of congruency by early internal fixation of significant fracture fragments, if possible, is indicated. The late result of an unrecognized osteochondral articular fracture in association with an ulnar styloid fracture (Fig. 31-11) illustrates the problem of misdiagnosis. At this stage the joint is destroyed and only a hemiresection interposition arthroplasty (see Chapters 34 and 35) or distal radioulnar arthrodesis (see Chapter 34) has any chance of overcoming the pain resulting from this destroyed joint.[4,10] Although a complete resection of the distal

ulna (Darrach resection) appears to be fairly successful in rheumatoid and elderly patients, the results are not as encouraging for younger patients with traumatic destruction of the distal radioulnar joint.[38] Articular fractures of the distal ulna have also been seen in association with traumatic dislocations of the distal radioulnar joint.[36] These dislocations may be missed and significant joint instability, including palmar dislocations (Figs. 31-12 and 31-13) and joint destruction with irreversible arthritis (Fig. 31-14), may result. Early computed tomograms are quite beneficial in determining the absence or presence of a dislocation and possibly associated intra-articular abnormality (Fig. 31-15).[40]

STRESS FRACTURES OF THE ULNA

Although stress fractures of the upper extremity are extremely rare compared to those in the lower extremity, they do occur. To date, eight stress fractures of the ulna have been documented[25] in athletes who exert substantial force on their upper extremities. Signs of stress fractures of the ulna on plain radiographs include periosteal reactions, sclerosis, cortical lysis, and overt fractures. If in doubt, a bone scan may

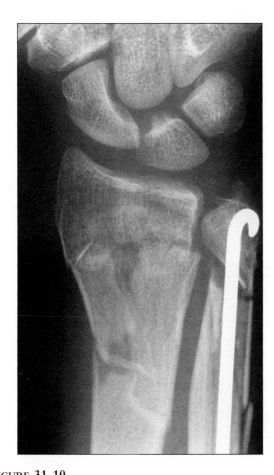

FIGURE 31-10

Improper pinning of a displaced ulnar fracture with a Rush rod.

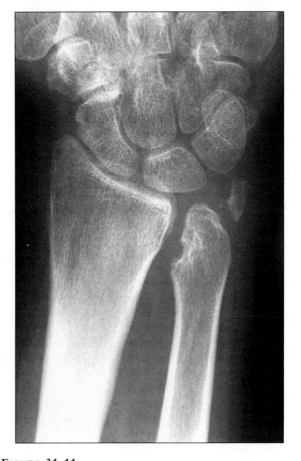

FIGURE 31-11

Late result of an osteochondral ulnar articular fracture.

be necessary to demonstrate increased bone activity. A period of rest is all that is necessary for complete healing of the stress fracture when only a periosteal reaction, cortical sclerosis, or cortical lysis is present.[25] A complete fracture can be treated with cast bracing, as described above.

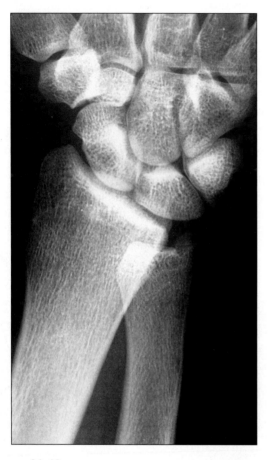

FIGURE 31-12

Palmar dislocation of the ulna related to avulsion of the triangular fibrocartilage from the ulnar styloid.

COMPLICATIONS OF ADULT ULNAR FRACTURES

As in any open fracture, osteomyelitis may result from the original open fracture or be secondary to open reduction and internal fixation. Standard treatment consists of surgical débridement of necrotic bone, irrigation and débridement of infected soft tissue, and judicious use of intravenously administered antibiotics. Although small bone defects can be bridged with firm fixation and iliac crest graft, larger defects may require a vascularized fibular graft.[13]

Pathologic fractures or impending fractures of the ulna are not common, but they have been reported.[12] These should be treated as in any other long bone with cast immobilization or possibly by internal fixation with plates or nails. Methyl methacrylate augmentation may be necessary in instances in which excessive bone substance has been lost.[13] Alternative complete excision of the distal ulna for tumor has been reported.[5]

SYNOSTOSIS OF THE DISTAL ULNA TO RADIUS

Synostosis of the articular portion of the distal ulna to the radius has been described in 4 patients of the 28 documented in 1987 by Vince and Miller.[37] Although usually associated with multiple trauma, open fractures, and surgical intervention, three of these four "type I" synostoses (after Vince and Miller) occurred after closed treatment of a closed fracture. When the synostosis occurs just proximal to the articular surface, these distal ulnar fractures are categorized as type II; however, this can include synostoses of any portion of the diaphysis, which is clearly outside the scope of this chapter. However, Razemon[26] postulated that the combination of a distal radial fracture with a slightly more proximal ulnar fracture predisposes to a synostosis because of increased tearing of the interosseous membrane. Yet in the article by Vince and Miller,[37] all type II synostoses followed fractures that occurred at the same level.

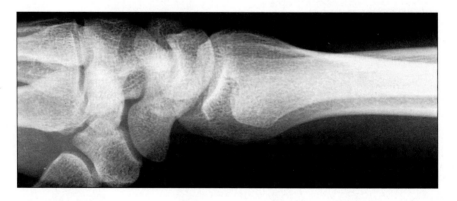

FIGURE 31-13

Palmar dislocation. Lateral view demonstrates the head of the ulna inferior to the midline of the radius.

Treatment of type I (articular) synostoses has been unsuccessful by resection of the synostoses. In three of the four cases cited, synostosis recurred. A resection of the ulna just proximal to this articular site seems to be the most logical approach. Slightly more good results occurred proximally with excision alone in 10 cases cited by Vince and Miller.[37] Free-fat interposition has also been advocated as an effective treatment modality.

Synostoses complicating forearm fractures in children are rare complications. No reports to date document type I synostoses in children. Type II synostoses are rare as well, and only two cases were reported after open reduction and internal fixation. Results after excision of the synostosis are inconclusive because of the paucity of cases.

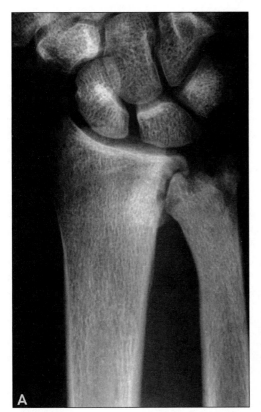

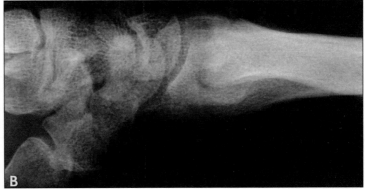

FIGURE 31-14

A, Posteroanterior radiograph of late palmar instability with degenerative changes at the distal radioulnar joint. **B,** Lateral view shows palmar dislocation reduced.

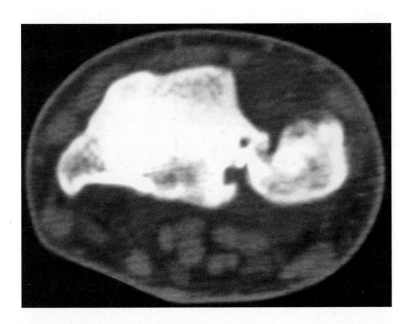

FIGURE 31-15

Instability of the distal radioulnar joint shown on computed tomographic scan: palmar dislocation of the ulna with an osteochondral fracture.

REFERENCES

1. Albert MJ, Engber WD: Dorsal dislocation of the distal radioulnar joint secondary to plastic deformation of the ulna, *J Orthop Trauma* 4:466-469, 1990.
2. Bogart FB: Variations of the bones of the wrist, *Am J Roentgenol Rad Ther* 28:638-646, 1932.
3. Borden S: Roentgen recognition of acute plastic bowing of the forearm in children, *Am J Roentgenol* 125:524-530, 1975.
4. Bowers WH: Distal radioulnar joint arthroplasty: the hemiresection-interposition technique, *J Hand Surg [Am]* 10:169-178, 1985.
5. Cooney WP, Damron TA, Sim FH, et al.: *En bloc* resection of tumors of the distal end of the ulna, *J Bone Joint Surg Am* 79:406-412, 1997.
6. Davis DR, Green DP: Forearm fractures in children: pitfalls and complications, *Clin Orthop* 120:172-184, 1976.
7. Demos TC: Radiologic case study: traumatic (plastic) bowing of the ulna, *Orthopedics* 3:1108, 1112-1114, 1121, 1980.
8. Derian PS: Extremity fractures in children. 2. Upper extremity, *Postgrad Med* 48:132-138, Oct 1970.
9. Fernandez DL: Irreducible radiocarpal fracture-dislocation and radioulnar dissociation with entrapment of the ulnar nerve, artery and flexor profundus II-V—case report, *J Hand Surg [Am]* 6:456-461, 1981.
10. Fernandez DL: Radial osteotomy and Bowers arthroplasty for malunited fractures of the distal end of the radius, *J Bone Joint Surg Am* 70:1538-1551, 1988.
11. Heiple KG, Freehafer AA, Van't Hof A: Isolated traumatic dislocation of the distal end of the ulna or distal radioulnar joint, *J Bone Joint Surg Am* 44:1387-1394, 1962.
12. Huber DF, Weis LD: Metastatic carcinoma of the distal ulna from an occult pancreatic carcinoma, *J Hand Surg [Am]* 10:725-727, 1985.
13. Hurst LC, Mirza MA, Spellman W: Vascularized fibular graft for infected loss of the ulna: case report, *J Hand Surg* 7:498-501, 1982.
14. Ishibe M, Ogino T, Sato Y, Nojima T: Osteochondritis dissecans of the distal radioulnar joint, *J Hand Surg [Am]* 14:818-821, 1989.
15. King RE: *Fractures of the shafts of the radius and ulna.* In Rockwood CA Jr, Wilkins KE, King RE, editors: *Fractures in children,* vol 3, Philadelphia, 1984, JB Lippincott, pp 301-356.
16. Koman LA, Mooney JF III, Poehling GC: Fractures and ligamentous injuries of the wrist, *Hand Clin* 6:477-491, Aug 1990.
17. Lambotte A: *Chirurgie operatoire dans les fractures,* Paris, 1913, Masson and Cie.
18. Lane WA: On the operative treatment of simple fractures, *Lancet* 1:1489-1493, 1900.
19. Levinthal DH: Fractures in the lower one-third of both bones of the forearm in children: manipulative reduction, *Surg Gynecol Obstet* 57:790-799, 1933.
20. Nelson OA, Buchanan JR, Harrison CS: Distal ulnar growth arrest, *J Hand Surg [Am]* 9:164-170, 1984.
21. Ogden JA: *Skeletal injury in the child,* Philadelphia, 1982, Lea & Febiger.
22. O'Brien ET: *Fractures of the hand and wrist.* In Rockwood CA Jr, Wilkins KE, King RE, editors: *Fractures in children,* vol 3, Philadelphia, 1984, JB Lippincott, pp 229-296.
23. Palmer AK: The distal radioulnar joint, *Orthop Clin North Am* 15:321-335, Apr 1984.
24. Palmer AK, Werner FW: The triangular fibrocartilage complex of the wrist—anatomy and function, *J Hand Surg* 6:153-162, 1981.
25. Patel MR, Irizarry J, Stricevic M: Stress fracture of the ulnar diaphysis: review of the literature and report of a case, *J Hand Surg [Am]* 11:443-445, 1986.
26. Razemon JP: *Kienböck's disease: radiographic and therapeutic study: a review of 22 cases of shortening of the radius.* In Razemon JP, Fisk GE, editors: *The wrist,* Edinburgh, 1988, Churchill Livingstone, pp 188-193.
27. Rose-Innes AP: Anterior dislocation of the ulna at the inferior radio-ulnar joint: case reports, with a discussion of the anatomy of rotation of the forearm, *J Bone Joint Surg Br* 42:515-521, 1960.
28. Sage FP: *Fractures of the shaft of the radius and ulna in the adult.* In Adams JP, editor: *Current practice in orthopaedic surgery,* St. Louis, 1963, Mosby.
29. Salter RB, Harris WR: Injuries involving the epiphyseal plate, *J Bone Joint Surg Am* 45:587-622, 1963.
30. Sarmiento A, Kinman PB, Murphy RB, et al.: Treatment of ulnar fractures by functional bracing, *J Bone Joint Surg Am* 58:1104-1107, 1976.
31. Spinner M, Kaplan EB: Extensor carpi ulnaris: its relationship to the stability of the distal radio-ulnar joint, *Clin Orthop* 68:124-129, 1970.
32. Stahl EJ, Karpman R: Normal growth and growth predictions in the upper extremity, *J Hand Surg [Am]* 11:593-596, 1986.
33. Taleisnik J, Gelberman RH, Miller BW, et al.: The extensor retinaculum of the wrist, *J Hand Surg [Am]* 9:495-501, 1984.
34. Teipner WA, Mast JW: Internal fixation of forearm diaphyseal fractures: double plating versus single compression (tension band) plating—a comparative study, *Orthop Clin North Am* 11:381-391, July 1980.
35. Venable CS, Stuck WG, Beach A: The effects on bone of the presence of metals; based upon electrolysis: an experimental study, *Ann Surg* 105:917-938, 1937.
36. Veseley DG: The distal radio-ulnar joint, *Clin Orthop* 51:75-91, 1967.
37. Vince KG, Miller JE: Cross-union complicating fracture of the forearm, *J Bone Joint Surg Am* 69:640-653, 1987.

38. Watson HK, Ryu J, Burgess RC: Matched distal ulnar resection, *J Hand Surg [Am]* 11:812-817, 1986.

39. Weber BG, Brunner C, Frueler F: *Treatment of fractures in children and adolescents,* Berlin, 1980, Springer-Verlag.

40. Wechsler RJ, Wehbe MA, Rifkin MD, et al.: Computed tomography diagnosis of distal radioulnar subluxation, *Skel Radiol* 16:1-5, 1987.

41. Wehbé MA: Surgical approach to the ulnar wrist, *J Hand Surg [Am]* 11:509-512, 1986.

42. Zemel NP: The prevention and treatment of complications from fractures of the distal radius and ulna, *Hand Clin* 3:1-11, 1987.

32

DORSAL AND PALMAR DISLOCATIONS OF THE DISTAL RADIOULNAR JOINT

Marc Garcia-Elias, M.D.
James H. Dobyns, M.D.

LITERATURE REVIEW
TERMINOLOGY
STABILIZING MECHANISMS OF THE DRUJ
    ORIENTATION AND CONGRUITY OF THE
      ARTICULAR SURFACES
    SOFT-TISSUE CONSTRAINTS
      THE TRIANGULAR FIBROCARTILAGE
      THE ULNOCARPAL LIGAMENTOUS COMPLEX
      THE INFRATENDINOUS EXTENSOR
        RETINACULUM
      THE PRONATOR QUADRATUS MUSCLE
      THE INTEROSSEOUS MEMBRANE
CLASSIFICATION

TYPE I
TYPE II
TYPE III
PATHOMECHANICS
DIAGNOSIS
TREATMENT AND COMPLICATIONS
    TYPE I: PURE DRUJ DISLOCATIONS
    TYPE II: INTRA-ARTICULAR DRUJ FRACTURE
      DISLOCATIONS
    TYPE III: EXTRA-ARTICULAR DRUJ FRACTURE
      DISLOCATIONS
SUMMARY

Traumatic dislocations or subluxations of the distal radioulnar joint (DRUJ), with or without associated fractures of the radius, are common.[4,16,30,51,66] The majority of these injuries consist of a spectrum of bony and ligamentous damage resulting in DRUJ instability, that is, in a loss of a normal anatomic or kinematic relationship between the two forearm bones and the carpus during physiologic loads.[9,34]

An early and accurate diagnosis of the acute injury and a precise reduction and continuous stabilization of the reduced position until ligamentous and osseous healing is complete have the best chance of achieving a satisfactory restoration of function.[2,8,51,58] Unfortunately, such injuries, particularly in the absence of a fracture of the distal radius, are often overlooked or misdiagnosed as "sprained wrists," resulting in chronic instabilities. In such situations, late treatment is difficult and not always satisfactory.[8,16,51,66]

In this chapter, the pertinent anatomy and the pathomechanics of DRUJ dislocations are discussed. Emphasis is placed on making the proper diagnosis in the acutely injured DRUJ and on the techniques to ensure and to maintain an adequate reduction. Treatment options for chronic DRUJ instabilities from unreduced dislocations,[20,34,46] excessive distal ulnar recessions,[5,7] or systemic disease such as rheumatoid arthritis[66] are dealt with in other chapters of this book.

LITERATURE REVIEW

Numerous studies have addressed fractures of the distal radius producing instability of the DRUJ. In his paper on fractures of the radius published in 1814,[13] Abraham Colles already noted "...the facility with

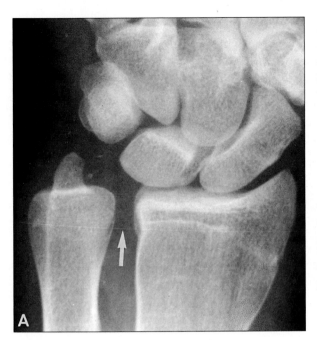 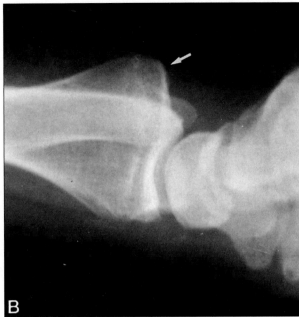

FIGURE 32-1

Dislocation of the distal radioulnar joint (ulna dorsal). **A,** The posteroanterior view shows marked widening of the joint space (*arrow*). **B,** The true lateral view (with superimposition of the lunate, proximal pole of the scaphoid, and triquetrum) shows a dorsally displaced ulna (*arrow*) relative to the radius.

which… the ulna can be moved backward and forward [after this type of fracture]." In 1880, Moore[50] reported three cases of a DRUJ derangement in connection with a Colles fracture and stated that derangement occurs if, once the fracture is completed, "…the hand, with its broken fragment of the radius, is [further] forced backward, the strain is often sufficient to rupture the connection between the two bones…." Since then, there have been numerous publications[1,9,54] documenting the different aspects of such common associated injuries. In 1959, Lidström[42] reviewed the long-term results of 515 Colles' fractures treated conservatively and found that about 15% had persistent laxity of the DRUJ. Frykman,[24] in 1967, found a disturbance of the DRUJ in 80 of 430 patients (18.6%) after a Colles fracture. Cooney and associates,[14] in an end-result study of 565 Colles' fractures seen at the Mayo Clinic, reported 27 patients with serious malalignment of the DRUJ, leading to a painful wrist.

Instabilities of the DRUJ have also been found in association with other fractures of the distal radius: palmar fractures of the distal radius (Smith's fractures),[9,54,66] fractures of the radial shaft (Galeazzi's fracture dislocation),[33,35] and proximal radial head fracture resulting in a radioulnar length discrepancy (Essex-Lopresti's injury).[10,22]

DRUJ dislocations in the absence of an accompanying fracture of the radius were first described in 1791 by Desault.[19] His case consisted in postmortem

findings and no history of the injury was given. Cotton and Brickley[15] mention Dupuytren as having reported a series of these cases in his book in 1834. Darrach,[17,18] Milch,[47] Eliason,[20] and many others agreed with Cotton and Brickley[15] who, in 1912, stated that "the lesion is rare; it occurs only as the result of much force, applied suddenly or slowly." Despite the rarity of the lesion, however, the literature is full of case reports.* An extensive review of the world literature performed by Birch-Jensen[8] in 1951 identified no more than 100 cases of an acute isolated DRUJ dislocation; the dorsal variety (Fig. 32-1) was more frequent than the palmar variety.[17,34,43,59] Since that report, a series of such injuries has been reported by Dameron[16] (10 cases), Hui and Linscheid[34] (8 cases), and Mino et al.[49] (9 cases).

Various forms of treatment of the disability created by the chronically subluxed DRUJ have been proposed: ligamentous reconstruction,[20,34,46,47] resection arthroplasties,[11,38] ulna resections,[17,18] corrective osteotomy of the distal radius,[1,29] and hemiresection arthroplasties.[9,54] A consensus agreement, however, is not present as to what is the best treatment for the different types of DRUJ instabilities. In review of the pertinent literature, the treatment proposed in 1913 by Darrach,[18] which consists in the resection of the distal end of the ulna, probably still is the most widely used, but not without secondary complications.[5,7]

---

* References 3,15,28,30,31,44,51.

TERMINOLOGY

Traditionally, descriptions of DRUJ dislocations refer to the ulna as the mobile bone dislocating from the radius. Phrases such as "dorsal or palmar dislocation of the distal ulna" have been used quite extensively.[17,31,44,46,59] However, as already pointed out by Desault,[19] and later by Darrach,[18] Milch,[47] and many others,[7,11,16,58] this is not anatomically correct because it is not the ulna that dislocates, but rather it is the distal radius (usually together with the carpal bones) that undergoes an abnormal displacement. It would be more appropriate to refer to these injuries as "dorsal or palmar dislocations of the radiocarpal unit relative to the ulna." However, in order not to create confusion in the description of DRUJ instability and yet use an anatomically accurate terminology, the terms "DRUJ dislocation-ulna dorsal, or ulna palmar," as suggested by Dameron,[16] will be used in this chapter.

STABILIZING MECHANISMS OF THE DRUJ

During pronation and supination of the forearm, rotation of the radius about the ulna is accompanied by a variable degree of dorsopalmar sliding movement. In supination the radius rotates and translates dorsally, and in pronation the radius translates toward the palmar edge of the sigmoid notch.[1,9,41,48,53] During load-bearing, such a complex kinematic behavior could easily destabilize the DRUJ unless a precise interaction of osseous architecture and soft-tissue constraints was present.[41,56,62]

Two factors need to be considered when discussing DRUJ instabilities: the orientation and congruity of the articular surfaces and the integrity of the soft-tissue (ligaments, muscles, and retinacula) constraints (Fig. 32-2).

ORIENTATION AND CONGRUITY OF THE ARTICULAR SURFACES

The DRUJ has been defined as a diarthrodial trochoid articulation formed by the head of the ulna and the shallow sigmoid cavity of the lower end of the radius.[1,39,56] The two articular surfaces are inclined toward the long axis of the ulna an average of 18°, ranging from 11° to 27°.[1] The ulnar head has cartilage over an average of 111° (range, 90°-135°) of its lateral surface, whereas the sigmoid notch has only an average articular sector of 71° (47°-80°).[1] The curvatures of the two articulating surfaces are not equal. The radius of curvature of the distal ulna appears to be about one-third shorter than that of the sigmoid notch concavity.[29] For this reason, a full congruity of the two articular surfaces is not possible (Fig. 32-3, A). In neutral forearm rotation, approximately 60% of the overall articular surface of the sigmoid notch is in contact with the ulnar head. This percentage is significantly reduced in both extremes of forearm rotation to about a 10% contact. Consequently, the deeper the sigmoid notch, the greater the osseous stability.[9,66] If the sigmoid notch cavity is shallow, with hypoplastic palmar or dorsal margins, or if these margins had been displaced by a fracture of the distal radius (Fig. 32-4, C), the chances of the DRUJ becoming unstable in full pronation or supination are high.

SOFT-TISSUE CONSTRAINTS

Five different structures are important in ensuring stability at the DRUJ: 1) the triangular fibrocartilage (TFC), 2) the ulnocarpal ligamentous (UCL) complex, 3) the infratendinous extensor retinaculum, 4) the pronator quadratus muscle, and 5) the interosseous membrane (IOM).* Their relative contributions, however, remain controversial. What follows is a brief review of the pertinent anatomy of these structures and the mechanisms by which DRUJ stability is achieved.

The Triangular Fibrocartilage. The TFC is part of the so-called TFC complex[56] and one of the most important DRUJ stabilizers.[9,16,61] The TFC has two components: the discus articularis and the distal radioulnar ligaments.

1) The discus articularis is a semicircular fibrocartilaginous biconcave structure, variable in thickness, interposed between the ulnar dome and the ulnar part of the carpal condyle[12,23,56] (Fig. 32-2). It arises from the distal margin of the sigmoid notch of the radius and consists of two zones: 1) an avascular central zone, formed by loosely organized collagen fibers, and 2) a peripheral sector, formed by dense semicircular-oriented collagen fibers[6,12,25] (see Chapter 30). Most authors[1,41,56] agree that the discus articularis basically has a shock-absorbing function and little effect on DRUJ stability.

2) The distal radioulnar ligaments (DRUL) are the primary support for the DRUJ. From the dorsal edge of the distal radius, often indistinguishable from the peripheral fibers of the discus articularis, emerges a bundle of densely organized, longitudinally oriented fibers, called the dorsal DRUL. Most of its fibers insert ulnarly into a rough and depressed oval notch, referred to as the "basistyloid fovea,"[45] located close to the center of the distal aspect of the ulna[12,25] (Fig. 32-3, B). The rest of the ligament continues toward the base of the ulnar styloid process where it inserts and wraps into the ulnocollateral ligament complex.[25]

Poorly identifiable as a separate structure from the peripheral fibers of the discus articularis is the palmar DRUL, although several authors[9,29] reported the

---

* References 1,27,37,41,48,58,61-63,65,66.

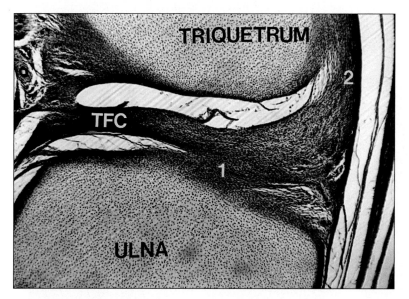

FIGURE 32-2

Parasagittal section through the ulnotriquetral joint of a 90-mm crown-rump length human fetus. Separating the triquetrum from the head of the ulna is the triangular fibrocartilage (*TFC*). The palmar ulnotriquetral fascicle (*2*) emerges from the TFC, which in turn is attached to the basistyloid fovea (*1*). In pronation, this ligament tightens, preventing the ulna from dislocating dorsally relative to the radius.

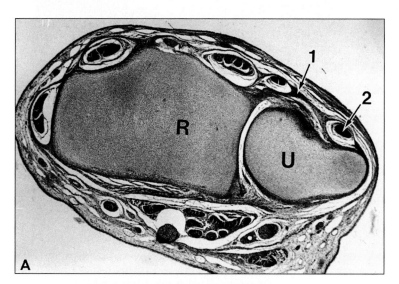

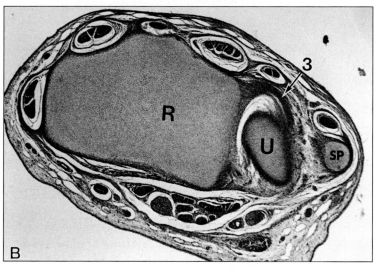

FIGURE 32-3

Transverse sections through the head of the ulna (*U*) **(A)** and the basistyloid fovea **(B)** of a 110-mm crown-rump length human fetus. *R*, radius; *SP*, ulnar styloid process; *1*, intratendinous extensor retinaculum; *2*, extensor carpi ulnaris tendon and sheath; *3*, dorsal radioulnar ligament.

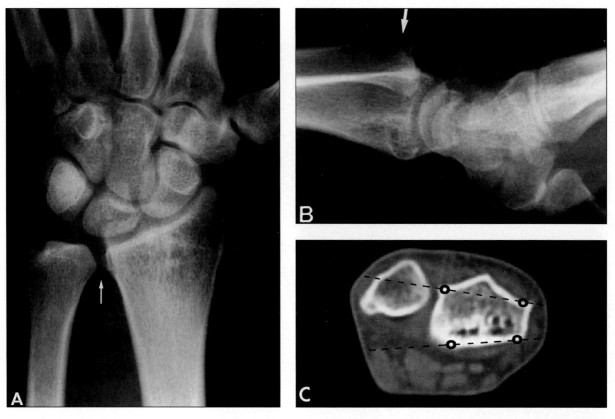

FIGURE 32-4

Chronic distal radioulnar joint (DRUJ) subluxation (ulna dorsal) demonstrated by an increasing joint diastasis (*arrow*) on a posteroan-terior view (**A**), by a dorsal prominence (*arrow*) of the ulna on a true lateral radiograph (**B**), and by a transverse computed tomographic scan (**C**) where the ulnar head appears subluxed relative to the radius according to the method of tracing radioulnar lines from Mino et al.[48] Note the abnormal (convex) shape of the sigmoid notch, secondary to an old malunited articular fracture of the radius (type II DRUJ dislocation).

ligament as a discrete anatomic structure. It emerges from the palmar corner of the distal radius and inserts into the basistyloid fovea, blending with fibers of its dorsal counterpart.[12,25,56] It serves as the origin of the palmar ulnocarpal ligaments (ulnolunate and ulnotri-quetral ligaments).

Much has been discussed about the constraining effects of the two DRULs. There is experimental evi-dence suggesting that both palmar and dorsal DRULs need to be intact for maintenance of complete stabil-ity of the joint throughout the whole range of fore-arm rotation.[1,29,62] Shaw et al.,[62] in a series of cadaver experiments, clearly demonstrated that the stabilizing influence of the two DRULs is more important than the combined effects of the palmar capsule, pronator quadratus, and IOM with the forearm in neutral rota-tion and pronation but not in supination where the palmar capsule and the pronator quadratus muscle would be more important stabilizers. Most authors consider that the TFC plays an important role to pre-vent dorsal or palmar translation of the radius leading to radioulnar dislocations, and research in our labora-tory demonstrates that the palmar ligament is taut in

supination and the dorsal ligament, in pronation. There is evidence of that instability of the DRUJ toward palmar translation of the ulna with respect to the radius in supination, and dorsal translation of the ulna occurs in pronation. Complete dislocation is pre-vented by progressive tension of the DRUL in supination and the progressive tension in the palmar ligament in pronation. These ligaments must rupture for dislocation to occur.

As already noted by Gemmill in 1900,[27] there is a change in relative length of the radius relative to the ulna during forearm rotation. Pronation gives a rela-tive lengthening of the ulna and supination, a relative shortening.[21,56] Because of this "piston movement,"[58] tension in both the palmar and the dorsal DRUL increases at both extremes of forearm rotation for dif-ferent mechanical reasons: in pronation, because they would be tented over the underlying ulnar head; in supination, because they would be pulled distally by the radius (Fig. 32-5). Such an increasing tension of the ligaments is likely to enhance DRUJ coaptation, compensating for the dramatic reduction in joint contact present in the two extreme positions.

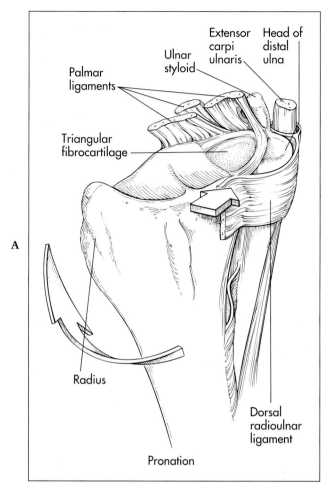 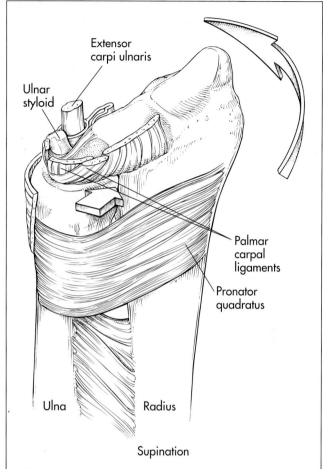

A

B

FIGURE 32-5

Schematic representation of the stabilizing mechanisms of the distal radioulnar joint. **A,** In full pronation, the tightening (*curved arrow*) of the palmar radioulnar and ulnocarpal ligaments, together with the constraining effect of the dorsal extensor retinaculum and supination, results in articular coaptation (*straight arrow*) of the ulnar head against the dorsal margin of the sigmoid notch. **B,** In full supination, the combined action of the dorsal radioulnar ligament and that of the pronator quadratus and interosseous membrane ensures articular coaptation (*straight arrow*).

The Ulnocarpal Ligamentous Complex. The UCL complex originates from the palmar edge of the TFC (discus articularis). There are two groups of longitudinally oriented collagen fibers that form: 1) the ulnotriquetral ligament that courses distally until inserting into the palmar aspect of the triquetrum and 2) the ulnolunate ligament that takes an oblique course until its distal insertion into the lunate. Neither one of these two ligaments emerges directly from the ulna but from the periphery of the TFC[26] (Fig. 32-2). A third group of ligament fibers, more superficial than the ulnotriquetral and ulnolunate ligaments, forms the ulnocapitate ligament. It arises not from the TFC but directly from the basistyloid fovea of the ulna, and it courses distally until attaching to the capitate bone[26] (Fig. 32-5).

In addition to ensuring a proper axial alignment between the ulna and the medial carpus, the UCL complex also has a major role in the stabilization of the DRUJ.[9] During maximal pronation, the UCL becomes extremely taut, thus resisting the tendency of the radiocarpal unit toward dislocating palmarly relative to the ulna. In full supination tension also increases on the UCL complex.[9,60] If the dorsal DRUL is intact, tension on the UCL has a positive effect on DRUJ stability by promoting a greater articular coaptation of the ulnar head against the anterior margin of the sigmoid notch (Fig. 32-5, *B*).[9] Conversely, if the dorsal DRUL is injured, tightening of the UCL complex has a destabilizing effect by forcing the ulna to displace palmarly, thus promoting a DRUJ dislocation (ulna palmar).

The Infratendinous Extensor Retinaculum. The infratendinous extensor retinaculum is also an important stabilizer of the DRUJ. During pronation and supination, the extensor carpi ulnaris tendon is maintained in a close relationship with the head of the ulna by a fibrous tunnel (sixth extensor compartment). The latter is formed by fibers of the infratendinous extensor retinaculum[34,40,63,64] (Fig. 32-3), which inserts on the ulnar margin of a vertical groove located just dorsal to the ulnar styloid process. Radially, the infratendinous extensor retinaculum crosses transversely the dorsal aspect of the DRUJ, deep to the fifth dorsal extensor compartment, and attaches to the dorsal margin of the sigmoid notch of the radius with the fifth and sixth extensor compartment retinacular septa.[64]

Using cadaver specimens, Spinner and Kaplan,[63] and later King et al.[41] showed that for a complete dislocation of the DRUJ (ulna dorsal) to occur the infratendinous extensor retinaculum needs to be severed and the extensor carpi ulnaris freed from its fibro-osseous tunnel. Our investigations tend to confirm their findings. At full pronation, the infratendinous retinaculum is effectively on stretch, giving passive viscoelastic resistance to the tendency of the ulna toward dorsal dislocation.[34,61] This, combined with the action of an intact palmar DRUL, promotes coaptation of the ulna against the dorsal rim of the sigmoid cavity, thus securing DRUJ stability.[1,9,29] In full supination, the dorsally located extensor carpi ulnaris tendon may also add dynamic stability to the DRUJ by resisting any abnormal palmar displacement of the ulnar head.

The Pronator Quadratus Muscle. The pronator quadratus has proved to be an additional important stabilizing component of the DRUJ.[37,62] It arises from the palmar crest (pronator ridge) of the ulna, immediately proximal to the palmar aspect of the DRUJ capsule. From its proximal ulnar origin, this quadrilateral muscle courses obliquely to its distal broad insertion into the flat palmar aspect of the metaphysis of the radius.[37] In pronation, the pronator quadratus tightens, actively supporting DRUJ stabilization, whereas in supination, the muscle is at maximum length, providing dynamic DRUJ stabilization by holding the distal ulna in the geometric constraints of the sigmoid notch. This dynamic force increases DRUJ articular coaptation and prevents lateral displacement (Fig. 35-5).[37,56,62]

The Interosseous Membrane. The IOM is the final stabilizer of the DRUJ. It has long been recognized as playing an important role in transmitting axial forces from the radius to the ulna while preventing lateral separation of the lower ends of the two forearm bones.[22,27,32] As shown by Hotchkiss et al.,[32] the IOM contains a central band of ligamentous tissue responsible for 71% of the longitudinal stiffness of the IOM after radial head excision. This band arises from a crest on the ulnar aspect of the mid-shaft of the radius, and it courses obliquely until its distal attachment to the lateral aspect of distal ulna (approximately 3.2 cm from the ulnar styloid process[32]).

As already noted by Gemmill[27] in 1900, most fibers of the IOM tighten in supination because the radial origin of the IOM is displaced dorsally, while its distal insertion wraps over the underlying ulnar metaphysis. Therefore, in this position the IOM shares a role with the pronator quadratus muscle in preventing abnormal dorsal translation of the distal radius relative to the ulna, a stabilizing effect of equal or greater importance than the action of the TFC and the two radioulnar ligaments, according to investigations by Shaw et al.[62]

Injury of the IOM, when associated with a defect of the proximal radial head secondary to fracture or surgical excision, may create radioulnar length discrepancy,[10,22] resulting in ulnocarpal impaction,[23,54] a syndrome known as the Essex-Lopresti lesion.[22]

CLASSIFICATION

Many different types of DRUJ dislocation have been described.[4,9,28,52,66] They may be the result of a single (acute) or multiple (repetitive) trauma. They can affect different anatomic structures (bone, ligaments, or muscles) or be the consequence of a local or systemic joint disease (congenital, developmental, metabolic, infectious, degenerative). Different patterns of radio-ulno-carpal malalignment may appear and cause occasional DRUJ dysfunction (during certain loading conditions) or permanent dysfunction, if unreduced, regardless of the forearm position or the amount of load being applied.

Vesely,[66] in 1967, listed more than 50 pathologic conditions that can affect this joint. Bowers[9] found 19 different categories of DRUJ instability. Because of such a multiplicity of conditions, a simple, clinically usable comprehensive classification for all types of DRUJ instability problems would be useful.[52] If only acute traumatic cases are considered, DRUJ dislocations may be conveniently classified into three major groups.

TYPE I

Pure dislocations of the DRUJ, secondary to a major disruption of the primary soft-tissue retaining structures. A) Soft-tissue injury (e.g., TFC tear). B) Bone injury (e.g., displaced ulnar styloid fracture).

TYPE II

Intra-articular DRUJ fracture dislocations, with alteration of the congruency of the articular surfaces.

TYPE III

Extra-articular DRUJ fracture dislocations, resulting in an abnormal joint surface orientation (type IIIa) or a radioulnar length discrepancy (type IIIb).

Each group may be further subclassified according to the direction of the created instability: ulna dorsal, ulna palmar, ulna distal, and multidirectional.

PATHOMECHANICS

The most frequent mechanism of acute DRUJ dislocations combines a rotational injury to the forearm (forced pronation or supination) and a hyperextension injury to the wrist.[16,30,44,51] Typical causes are a fall of a rotating body on the outstretched hand[4,28] or the forearm being twisted by rotating machinery (or a crank handle).[51,59]

Pronation not only implies rotation but also a palmar translation of the radius relative to the ulna.[1,53] Consequently, forced hyperpronation may result in a rupture or an avulsion of the palmar DRUL as well as in an abnormal stretching of the infratendinous extensor retinaculum (extensor carpi ulnaris subsheath). An associated hyperextension would increase tension on the palmar ulnocarpal ligaments, thus promoting avulsion of all the basistyloid fovea inserted structures (Fig. 32-5, *A*). As found in different laboratory studies,[51,55,62] without the constraining effects of these three stabilizing structures (palmar DRUL, UCL complex, and dorsal infratendinous extensor retinaculum), the DRUJ becomes unstable and easily dislocates, the ulna displacing dorsally with respect to the radius (Fig. 32-1 and 32-4).

Conversely, forced hypersupination implies an abnormal dorsal translation of the distal radius (ulna palmar dislocation), eventually causing a disruption or an avulsion of the dorsal DRUL while promoting an abnormal stretching of the pronator quadratus muscle and the distal part of the IOM (Fig. 32-5, *B*). This association of injuries increases the likelihood of a DRUJ dislocation (ulna palmar).[37,41,62]

If the wrist is involved in a high-energy hyperextension and axial rotation injury, a fracture of one of the two forearm bones may appear in combination with a variable-degree radioulnar ligamentous disruption. Fractures may directly affect the articular joint surfaces, impairing DRUJ congruity (type II dislocations) (Fig. 32-4)[13,14,24,43,54] or alter the axial alignment of the two forearm bones, resulting in a type III DRUJ dislocation (Fig. 32-6).[9,22,33,35] In the latter cases, disruption of the DRUJ constraining ligaments usually is complete, and therefore the created instability is multidirectional.

Sometimes, an axial loading mechanism on a hypersupinated and extended forearm may eventually end with a combination of injuries (fracture of the

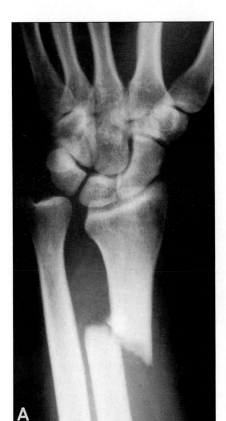

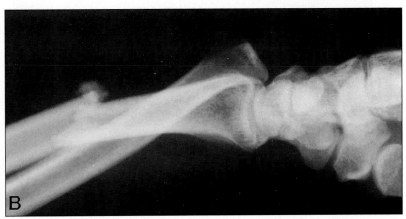

FIGURE 32-6

A and **B**, Posteroanterior and lateral views of type IIIa (Galeazzi) fracture dislocation. All distal radioulnar joint (DRUJ) stabilizing capsuloligamentous structures, except for the interosseous membrane, need to be disrupted for such an injury to occur. Treatment priorities are: 1) DRUJ reduction and reattachment of the triangular fibrocartilage complex, 2) reconstruction of the fibro-osseous tunnel for the extensor carpi ulnaris with an extensor retinaculum fascial flap,[63] and 3) anatomic reduction and stabilization of the radial fracture.

radial head, disruption of the IOM, and avulsion or perforation of the TFC), resulting in an acute type IIIb DRUJ dislocation, ulna distal,[10,22] causing an ulnocarpal impaction syndrome.[23]

DIAGNOSIS

The patient with an acute DRUJ subluxation or dislocation (with no associated fracture) usually complains of pain over the ulnar aspect of the wrist that is accentuated by any attempt at pronosupination of the forearm. Moderate swelling and tenderness may be present over the DRUJ. Loss of wrist motion and weakness of grip are associated findings. In dorsal dislocations, the prominence of the distal ulna (piano key sign[58]) is evident clinically, particularly if the wrist is flexed. In palmar dislocations, swelling may obscure the ulnar head prominence. In those cases, however,

ulnar nerve dysesthesias may appear from compression of the displaced ulnar head.

The diagnosis of chronic DRUJ dislocations with or without associated malunion of fractures of the distal radius continues to be missed frequently.[43,46] Clinically, in addition to checking for abnormal dorsal-palmar instability of the distal ulna relative to the radius, one should look for painful subluxations in the extremes of rotation, often with an audible snap, and weakness of grip (Fig. 32-7).

DRUJ subluxations may be extremely difficult to diagnose on routine radiographs.[16,30,48,51] A dorsal or palmar displacement of the distal ulna relative to the radius is only of value when observed on a *true lateral radiograph* of the wrist (complete superimposition of the lunate, proximal pole of the scaphoid, and triquetrum) and in the absence of any deformity of the distal radius (Figs. 32-1, *B*, 32-7, *A*, and 32-8, *B*).[48] As shown by Mino et al.,[49] minor degrees

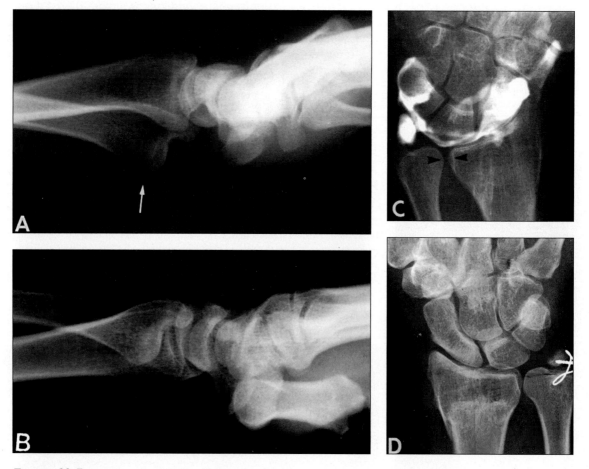

FIGURE 32-7

Habitual unilateral distal radioulnar joint (DRUJ) dislocation (ulna palmar) in a 46-year-old woman with no history of trauma. Probably the dislocation was secondary to a flattened sigmoid notch cavity and subluxation of the extensor carpi ulnaris (ECU) tendon. True lateral views show the dislocated joint (*arrow*) in forced supination (**A**) and the joint self-reduced once pronation is started (**B**). DRUJ dysfunction in this case has always been well tolerated and does not require surgical treatment. **C,** Interposition of ECU tendon produces an irreducible DRUJ (*arrowheads*). **D,** Ulnar styloid reattachment for acute instability after distal radius fracture.

of forearm rotation may frequently lead to an inaccurate diagnosis.

A posteroanterior radiograph may show a greater than normal distance (gap) between the head of the ulna and the radius if the ulna is dorsally subluxed (Figs. 32-1, *A* and 32-4, *A*), while a superimposition of the two bones may be present in DRUJ dislocations-ulna palmar (Fig. 32-8, *A*).[16,51] Comparison views with both forearms in the same degree of forearm rotation may help in the diagnosis, particularly if there is ulna positive variance secondary to an unstable distal radius fracture[23] or fracture malunion. Standard

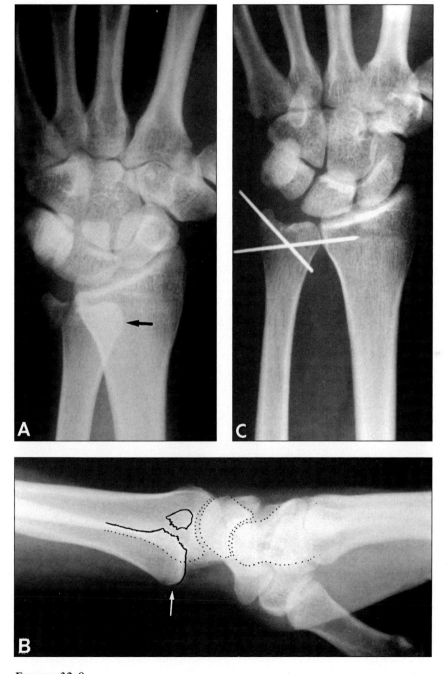

FIGURE 32-8

Acute distal radioulnar joint dislocation (ulna palmar). **A,** Posteroanterior (PA) view shows overlap (*arrow*) of the distal radius and ulna. **B,** True lateral view shows palmar displacement (*arrow*) of the ulnar head (*solid line*) and a palmar intercalated segment instability pattern of carpal malalignment (*dotted lines*) probably from increasing tension on the ulnocarpal ligaments. **C,** PA view shows the joint after reduction and stabilization with Kirschner wires of the dislocation and the styloid fracture.

posteroanterior radiographs, however, are not consistently diagnostic (false-negative rate of 60% according to Mino et al.[49]), except for the diagnosis of associated fractures (Fig. 32-6, *A*). Stress views in different positions of forearm rotation searching for abnormal translational motion of the radius relative to the ulna may help to identify subtle dynamic DRUJ subluxations.[57]

If concern exists in spite of normal-appearing radiographs, further evaluation by means of transverse computed tomography or magnetic resonance imaging scans may be warranted. According to criteria from Mino et al.,[49] the ulnar head of a normal DRUJ lies between two lines defining the dorsal and palmar borders of the radius (Fig. 32-4, *C*). The arcs made by the ulnar head and sigmoid notch must be congruous throughout the whole range of pronosupination. Another way to assess DRUJ congruity using transverse computed tomographic scans is the so-called epicenter method described by Wechsler et al.[67] In normal wrists, the perpendicular line from the center of the ulnar head to the chord of the sigmoid notch lies in the middle half of the joint. In the subluxed DRUJ, it lies outside the central part of the sigmoid notch.[67]

TREATMENT AND COMPLICATIONS

TYPE I: PURE DRUJ DISLOCATIONS

Pure dislocations of the DRUJ are frequently easy to reduce if the patient is seen early. With an appropriate anesthesia, the dorsally dislocated joint (ulna dorsal) is reduced by digital pressure on the distal ulna and forceful supination. Conversely, palmar dislocations are reduced by forcing pronation of the forearm and manipulation of the ulna in an ulnar and dorsal direction to neutralize the pull of the pronator quadratus muscle. Immobilization in a long arm cast with the forearm in neutral rotation and the wrist slightly ulnar deviated for 6 weeks usually leads to a satisfactory result. Occasionally, closed reduction is not successful, particularly if treatment is delayed or if interposition of soft tissue (TFC rupture, extensor carpi ulnaris entrapment, or osteochondral fragment) locks the joint.[58] Open reduction through a dorsal incision, repair of the damaged ligaments, and temporary Kirschner-wire fixation is then recommended (Fig. 32-7, *C*).

Isolated fractures of the base of the ulnar styloid associated with an abnormal translational motion of the distal ulna relative to the radius should alert one to the possible existence of a complete avulsion of the ulnar styloid with the TFC intact.[55] To avoid late instability problems, an open reattachment of the ulnar styloid process should be done[4,62] (Fig. 32-7, *C*).

Complications after ligament injuries of the DRUJ are not uncommon. Recurrent DRUJ instability, limited range of forearm rotation, and painful degenerative

arthritis have been noted. Different operative methods of stabilization of the chronically unstable DRUJ have been described.[20,34,38,46] They will be discussed in subsequent chapters of this book (see Chapter 35).

TYPE II: INTRA-ARTICULAR DRUJ FRACTURE DISLOCATIONS

Treatment of displaced intra-articular fractures of the distal radius associated with a variable amount of DRUJ ligamentous damage may result in instability of the DRUJ. The amount of instability varies with the location of the fracture, the degree of displacement, and the severity of associated soft-tissue injury.[9,35,42]

Reduction of the DRUJ (and distal radius fracture) is usually achieved by longitudinal traction followed by gentle manipulation of the fracture site, forearm supination, and application of a support splint (sugar tongs) or a long arm cast.[54] If postreduction radiographs show an anatomic alignment of the radio-ulno-carpal joint, normal joint congruity, and a normal radial length, immobilization continues until consolidation of the distal radius fracture is complete. Alternatively, percutaneous Kirschner-wire fixation or external fixation of the fracture with transfixion of the previously reduced DRUJ may be appropriate. At 3 weeks after treatment, assessment of DRUJ stability is performed to determine if a longer period of forearm immobilization is needed.

If malalignment remains, or if an articular step-off greater than 2 mm persists, the fracture may lead to improper healing and persistent subluxed deformity of the DRUJ.[14,24] In cases in which anatomic reduction is not present, the injury may benefit from open repair of the injured ligaments, reduction of the articular osseous architecture, and stabilization by means of an internal, external, or combination of fixation methods.[54]

Malunion of the distal radius with distal or dorsal subluxation (or both) of the distal ulna is perhaps the most common complication of this type of injury (Fig. 32-4). In those cases, we recommend a corrective osteotomy at the site of the malunited radius fracture and repair of the damaged ligaments of the TFC. Alternatively, we would perform a hemiresection arthroplasty of the DRUJ.[9,29,54]

TYPE III: EXTRA-ARTICULAR DRUJ FRACTURE DISLOCATIONS

Metaphyseal or diaphyseal fractures of the radius are the result of high-energy forces involving hypertension of the wrist and forearm rotation. The combination of forces leads to a complete disruption of most DRUJ stabilizers (type IIIa injuries). This injury results in fracture dislocations commonly referred to as the Galeazzi fractures[33] (Fig. 32-6). Proximal one-third fractures of the radius may also cause a DRUJ instability problem. In those, however, not only the distal DRUJ stabilizer ligaments may have failed but also the central band of the IOM may be disrupted. In such cases, a severe radioulnar length discrepancy with or without dorso-palmar DRUJ dislocation may appear (type IIIb injuries, often referred to as the Essex-Lopresti fractures[22]).

The creation of a severe alteration of the DRUJ congruity suggests that these fractures should be considered as true articular injuries.[29] Therefore, in both IIIa and IIIb injuries not only the radial fracture but also the DRUJ needs to be carefully reduced and internally fixed for optimal results.

In type IIIa injuries (fracture with abnormal joint alignment), incongruity or instability of the DRUJ should be addressed first through a dorsoulnar approach. The TFC complex and the extensor carpi ulnaris subsheath (fibro-osseous tunnel) are repaired. The joint is next pinned with Kirschner wires in neutral rotation, after openly reducing and plating the radial fracture.[36,62] In type IIIb injuries (fracture with increased ulnar length), treatment should also include reducing the proximal migration of the radial diaphysis by longitudinal traction, repairing the TFC complex,

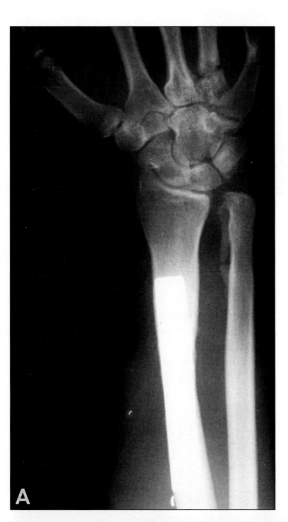

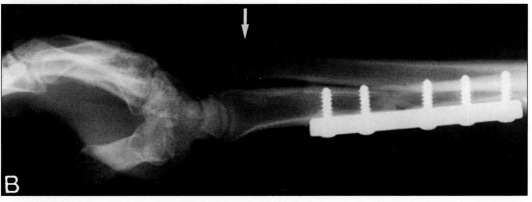

FIGURE 32-9

A and **B,** Posteroanterior and lateral views of an improperly treated Galeazzi's fracture dislocation. Distal radioulnar joint (DRUJ) disruption was not addressed at operation. The radius healed malrotated, thus explaining the persistence of a chronic DRUJ dislocation, ulna dorsal (*arrow*). Treatment options at this moment should include corrective osteotomy of the radius and stabilizing ligamentoplasty of the DRUJ.

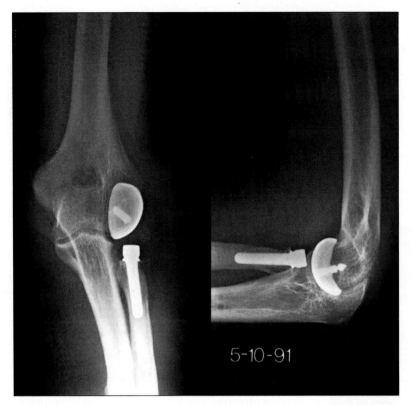

5-10-91

FIGURE 32-10

Prosthetic replacement of the radial head and capitellum for treatment of a patient with chronic proximal-distal radioulnar dissociation[65]—the Essex-Lopresti lesion.[22] Ulnar recession and stabilization of the distal radioulnar joint procedures were unsuccessful.

fixation of radial head fracture (if present), and stabilizing the forearm with two Steinmann pins, transfixing both forearm bones.[22]

In the Galeazzi fracture dislocation, the radial fracture must always be treated by open reduction and plate fixation followed by reduction and pinning of the DRUJ. If the DRUJ does not easily reduce or if the reduction is not anatomic (posteroanterior-lateral radiographs), open reduction of the DRUJ is required. For injuries with fracture at the base of the ulnar styloid, we recommend open fixation of the ulnar styloid (Fig. 32-7, *D*).

The most frequent complication of a Galeazzi fracture dislocation is malunion of the radius and residual DRUJ subluxation (Fig. 32-9).[33] This usually results from: 1) failure to recognize the severity of the DRUJ problem and 2) unsatisfactory reduction of the radius, particularly in the transverse plane, leading to a malrotated and angulated radial shaft. In those cases, a DRUJ-stabilizing tenodesis cannot restore a normal functioning joint unless a corrective osteotomy of the malunited radius is performed.[9,33]

If unsuccessfully treated, type IIIb injuries often result in disabling wrist pain from a severe ulnocarpal impingement problem. This cannot be solved unless the full length of the radius is reestablished and the integrity of the proximal DRUJ achieved. We recommend radial head replacement (if it is excised), ulnar recession (if positive ulna variance is the problem), and repair or reconstruction of DRUJ instability. The important role of the IOM as the major stabilizer of the proximal-distal relationship of the two bones[32] is difficult to restore short of radioulnar fusion (one-bone forearm). Efforts to date to reconstruct or right the IOM have been fruitless.[65] Radial head prosthetic replacement and hemiarthroplasty of the elbow can prevent proximal radius migration, thereby decreasing instability of the DRUJ (Fig. 32-10). Long-term success of such procedures is uncertain. At this time there are no well-established methods to treat axial instability of the forearm. Prevention is the best means of avoiding these significant complications.

SUMMARY

Acute dislocations of the DRUJ can be identified early by careful history and physical examination as well as radiographic examination in difficult planes of forearm rotation. Axial computed tomography, comparing the injured and uninjured extremities, provides the most sensitive method of determining dorsal and palmar instability. Three major types of DRUJ dislocations have been identified: I) pure dislocation, a) soft-tissue injury, b) ulnar styloid fracture; II) intra-articular fracture dislocation; and III) extra-articular fracture dislocation, a) radius fractures, ulna dislocation, b) axial radioulnar length discrepancy.

Specific treatment alternatives are recommended for each of these problem areas; late reconstruction is significantly more complicated and predictable than with acute injuries.

REFERENCES

1. af Ekenstam F, Hagert CG: Anatomical studies on the geometry and stability of the distal radio ulnar joint, *Scand J Plast Reconstr Surg* 19:17-25, 1985.

2. Albert SM, Wohl MA, Rechtman AM: Treatment of the disrupted radio-ulnar joint, *J Bone Joint Surg Am* 45:1373-1381, 1963.

3. Alexander AH: Bilateral traumatic dislocation of the distal radioulnar joint, ulna dorsal: case report and review of the literature, *Clin Orthop* 129:238-244, 1977.

4. Aulicino PL, Siegel JL: Acute injuries of the distal radioulnar joint, *Hand Clin* 7:283-293, 1991.

5. Bell MJ, Hill RJ, McMurtry RY: Ulnar impingement syndrome, *J Bone Joint Surg Br* 67:126-129, 1985.

6. Benjamin M, Evans EJ, Pemberton DJ: Histological studies on the triangular fibrocartilage complex of the wrist, *J Anat* 172:59-67, 1990.

7. Bieber EJ, Linscheid RL, Dobyns JH, et al.: Failed distal ulna resections, *J Hand Surg [Am]* 13:193-200, 1988.

8. Birch-Jensen A: Luxation of the distal radio-ulnar joint, *Acta Chir Scand* 101:312-317, 1951.

9. Bowers WH: Instability of the distal radioulnar articulation, *Hand Clin* 7:311-327, 1991.

10. Brockman EP: Two cases of instability of the wrist joint following excision of the head of the radius, *Proc R Soc Med* 24:904, 1930.

11. Buck-Gramcko D: On the priorities of publication of some operative procedures on the distal end of the ulna, *J Hand Surg [Br]* 15:416-420, 1990.

12. Chidgey LK: Histologic anatomy of the triangular fibrocartilage, *Hand Clin* 7:249-262, 1991.

13. Colles A: On the fracture of the carpal extremity of the radius, *Edinburgh Med Surg J* 10:182-186, 1814.

14. Cooney WP III, Dobyns JH, Linscheid RL: Complications of Colles' fractures, *J Bone Joint Surg Am* 62:613-619, 1980.

15. Cotton FJ, Brickley WJ: Luxation of the ulna forward at the wrist (without fracture), *Ann Surg* 55:368-374, 1912.

16. Dameron TB Jr: Traumatic dislocation of the distal radioulnar joint, *Clin Orthop* 83:55-63, 1972.

17. Darrach W: Anterior dislocation of the head of the ulna, *Ann Surg* 56:802-803, 1912.

18. Darrach W: Partial excision of lower shaft of ulna for deformity following Colles's fracture, *Ann Surg* 57:764-765, 1913.

19. Desault P: Sur la luxation de l'extrémité inférieure du radius, *J Chir* 1:78-87, 1791.

20. Eliason EL: An operation for recurrent inferior radioulnar dislocation, *Ann Surg* 96:27-35, 1932.

21. Epner RA, Bowers WH, Guilford WB: Ulnar variance—the effect of wrist positioning and roentgen filming technique, *J Hand Surg [Am]* 7:298-305, 1982.

22. Essex-Lopresti P: Fractures of the radial head with distal radio-ulnar dislocation: report of two cases, *J Bone Joint Surg Br* 33:244-247, 1951.

23. Friedman SL, Palmer AK: The ulnar impaction syndrome, *Hand Clin* 7:295-310, 1991.

24. Frykman G: Fracture of the distal radius including sequelae—shoulder-hand-finger syndrome, disturbance in the distal radio-ulnar joint and impairment of nerve function, *Acta Orthop Scand Suppl* 108:1-153, 1967.

25. Garcia-Elias M, Domènech-Mateu JM: The articular disc of the wrist. Limits and relations, *Acta Anat (Basel)* 128:51-54, 1987.

26. Garcia-Elias M, Domènech-Mateu JM: Anatomy of the ulno-carpal ligaments. Presented at the 46th Annual Meeting of the American Society for Surgery of the Hand, Orlando, Florida, October, 1991.

27. Gemmill F: On the movement of the lower end of the radius in pronation and supination and on the interosseous membrane, *J Anat Physiol* 35:101-109, 1900.

28. Graham HK, McCoy GF, Mollan RA: A new injury of the distal radio-ulnar joint, *J Bone Joint Surg Br* 67:302-304, 1985.

29. Hagert CG: The distal radioulnar joint, *Hand Clin* 3:41-50, 1987.

30. Hamlin C: Traumatic disruption of the distal radioulnar joint, *Am J Sports Med* 5:93-97, 1977.

31. Heiple KG, Freehafer AA, Van't Hof A: Isolated traumatic dislocation of the distal end of the ulna or distal radioulnar joint, *J Bone Joint Surg Am* 44:1387-1394, 1962.

32. Hotchkiss RN, An KN, Sowa DT, et al.: An anatomic and mechanical study of the interosseous membrane of the forearm: pathomechanics of proximal migration of the radius, *J Hand Surg [Am]* 14:256-261, 1989.

33. Hughston JC: Fractures of the distal radial shaft: mistakes in management, *J Bone Joint Surg Am* 39:249-264, 1957.

34. Hui FC, Linscheid RL: Ulnotriquetral augmentation tenodesis: a reconstructive procedure for dorsal subluxation of the distal radioulnar joint, *J Hand Surg [Am]* 7:230-236, 1982.

35. Hyman G, Martin FRR: Dislocation of the inferior radio-ulnar joint as a complication of fracture of the radius, *Br J Surg* 27:481-491, 1940.

36. Jenkins NH, Mintowt-Czyz WJ, Fairclough JA: Irreducible dislocation of the distal radioulnar joint, *Injury* 18:40-43, 1987.

37. Johnson RK, Shrewsbury MM: The pronator quadratus in motions and in stabilization of the radius and ulna at the distal radioulnar joint, *J Hand Surg [Am]* 1:205-209, 1976.

38. Kapandji IA: The Kapandji-Sauvé operation. Its techniques and indications in non rheumatoid diseases, *Ann Chir Main* 5:181-193, 1986.

39. Kaplan EB: *Functional and surgical anatomy of the hand*, ed 2, Philadelphia, 1965, JB Lippincott.

40. Kauer JM: The articular disc of the hand, *Acta Anat (Basel)* 93:590-605, 1975.

41. King GJ, McMurtry RY, Rubenstein JD, et al.: Computerized tomography of the distal radioulnar joint: correlation with ligamentous pathology in a cadaveric model, *J Hand Surg [Am]* 11:711-717, 1986.

42. Lidström A: Fractures of the distal end of the radius. A clinical and statistical study of end results, *Acta Orthop Scand Suppl* 41:1-95, 1959.

43. Lippmann RK: Laxity of the radio-ulnar joint following Colles' fracture, *Arch Surg* 35:772-786, 1937.

44. Mestdagh H: Luxation habituelle de la tête cubitale en avant. A propos d'un cas, *Ann Chir Main* 3:253-257, 1984.

45. Mikic ZD: Detailed anatomy of the articular disc of the distal radioulnar joint, *Clin Orthop* 245:123-132, 1989.

46. Milch H: Dislocation of the inferior end of the ulna; suggestion for a new operative procedure, *Am J Surg* 1:141-146, 1926.

47. Milch H: So-called dislocation of the lower end of the ulna, *Ann Surg* 116:282-292, 1942.

48. Mino DE, Palmer AK, Levinsohn EM: The role of radiography and computerized tomography in the diagnosis of subluxation and dislocation of the distal radioulnar joint, *J Hand Surg [Am]* 8:23-31, 1983.

49. Mino DE, Palmer AK, Levinsohn EM: Radiography and computerized tomography in the diagnosis of incongruity of the distal radio-ulnar joint. A prospective study, *J Bone Joint Surg Am* 67:247-252, 1985.

50. Moore EM: Three cases illustrating luxation of the ulna in connection with Colles' fractures, *Medical Record* 17:305-308, 1880.

51. Morrissy RT, Nalebuff EA: Dislocation of the distal radioulnar joint: anatomy and clues to prompt diagnosis, *Clin Orthop* 144:154-158, 1979.

52. Nathan R, Schneider LH: Classification of distal radioulnar joint disorders, *Hand Clin* 7:239-247, 1991.

53. Olerud C, Kongsholm J, Thuomas KA: The congruence of the distal radioulnar joint. A magnetic resonance imaging study, *Acta Orthop Scand* 59:183-185, 1988.

54. Palmer AK: *Fractures of the distal radius.* In Green DP, editor: *Operative hand surgery,* ed 2, vol 2, New York, 1988, Churchill Livingstone.

55. Palmer AK: Triangular fibrocartilage complex lesions: a classification, *J Hand Surg [Am]* 14:594-606, 1989.

56. Palmer AK, Werner FW: The triangular fibrocartilage complex of the wrist—anatomy and function, *J Hand Surg [Am]* 6:153-162, 1981.

57. Pirela-Cruz MA, Goll SR, Klug M, et al.: Stress computed tomography analysis of the distal radioulnar joint: a diagnostic tool for determining translational motion, *J Hand Surg [Am]* 16:75-82, 1991.

58. Regan JM: Derangement of the inferior radio-ulnar joint, Thesis, Mayo Graduate School of Medicine (University of Minnesota), Rochester, 1945.

59. Rose-Innes AP: Anterior dislocation of the ulna at the inferior radio-ulnar joint: case reports, with a discussion of the anatomy of rotation of the forearm, *J Bone Joint Surg Br* 42:515-521, 1960.

60. Savelberg HH, Kooloos JG, De Lange A, et al.: Human carpal ligament recruitment and three-dimensional carpal motion, *J Orthop Res* 9:693-704, 1991.

61. Schuind F, An KN, Berglund L, et al.: The distal radioulnar ligaments: a biomechanical study, *J Hand Surg [Am]* 16:1106-1114, 1991.

62. Shaw JA, Bruno A, Paul EM: Ulnar styloid fixation in the treatment of posttraumatic instability of the radioulnar joint: a biomechanical study with clinical correlation, *J Hand Surg [Am]* 15:712-720, 1990.

63. Spinner M, Kaplan EB: Extensor carpi ulnaris. Its relationship to the stability of the distal radio-ulnar joint, *Clin Orthop* 68:124-129, 1970.

64. Taleisnik J, Gelberman RH, Miller BW, et al.: The extensor retinaculum of the wrist, *J Hand Surg [Am]* 9:495-501, 1984.

65. Trousdale RT, Amadio PC, Cooney WP, et al.: Radioulnar dissociation. A review of twenty cases, *J Bone Joint Surg Am* 74:1486-1497, 1992.

66. Vesely DG: The distal radio-ulnar joint, *Clin Orthop* 51:75-91, 1967.

67. Wechsler RJ, Wehbe MA, Rifkin MD, et al.: Computed tomography diagnosis of distal radioulnar subluxation, *Skeletal Radiol* 16:1-5, 1987.

33

ULNOCARPAL ABUTMENT

Owen J. Moy, M.D.
Andrew K. Palmer, M.D.

ETIOLOGY
BIOMECHANICS
CLASSIFICATION
DIAGNOSIS
TREATMENT
ULNA RECESSION-SURGICAL PROCEDURE
SUMMARY

Ulnocarpal abutment is a degenerative condition associated with a discrepancy in the relative length of the distal articular surfaces of radius and ulna. The discrepancy is one of increased ulnar length in relation to the radius. This discrepancy increases the transmission of force across the ulnocarpal articulation. A sequence of events follows, including wearing of the triangular fibrocartilage complex (TFCC), chondromalacia of the ulnar head and proximal ulnar aspect of the lunate, and disruption of the lunotriquetral ligament.[8,18,26] This condition is referred to by several interchangeable names—ulnar impaction, ulnar impingement, ulnocarpal impingement, and ulnocarpal loading. Other conditions are known by the same names but are different entities and require different treatments.[1,53]

ETIOLOGY

Ulnocarpal abutment may be acquired or congenital. Acquired deformities, which are usually the result of trauma, include fractures of the distal radius with residual shortening and angulation, fractures with associated ligamentous injuries at the distal radioulnar joint (DRUJ) such as Galeazzi and Essex-Lopresti fractures, excision of the radial head with subsequent proximal migration of the radius, and epiphyseal injuries affecting the palmar-ulnar portion of the distal radial epiphysis.[13,15,27,30,31] Recently, ulnocarpal abutment has been described as a consequence of wrist arthrodesis.[50] Congenital etiologies include local dyschondroplasia such as Madelung's deformity[13,41] as well as naturally occurring ulna plus variance in association with overuse.[5,11]

As part of an examination of the evolution of the primate wrist joint and DRUJ, Lewis et al.[23,24] described the changes associated with an increasingly mobile wrist joint. There has been a progressive regression of the distal ulna from its pisotriquetral articulation, with formation of the ulnar styloid process and the homogeneous TFCC.[35,39] The evolutionary regression of the distal ulna is replicated in the development of the human fetus.[54] An apparent result of this regression is the variation of ulnar length in relation to the distal radial articular surface. Described by Hültén[22] as ulna variance, this variation has been implicated in Kienböck's disease and disruption of the intercarpal ligaments as well as ulnocarpal abutment.[9,11,20,22]

BIOMECHANICS

Biomechanical and anatomic studies of the DRUJ have shown that the radius encompasses three-quarters

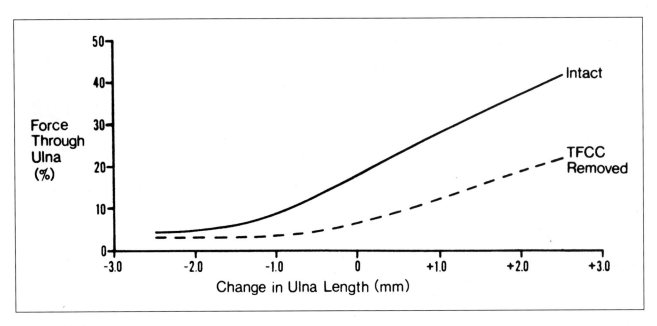

FIGURE 33-1

Axial load transmission through the ulnar column as a consequence of change in ulnar length. *TFCC*, triangular fibrocartilage complex.

of the distal joint surface of the forearm. The remaining one-quarter is composed of the TFCC and underlying ulnar head.[46] Studies of the transmission of force have shown that during axial loading of the forearm, approximately 80% of the load is transmitted through the radius and 20% through the distal ulna.[36,49] Slight variations in ulnar length produce significant alteration in the ratio of transmitted load. Palmer and Werner[40] demonstrated that shortening the ulna by 2.5 mm redistributes the ratio of load between radius and ulna to 95.7% and 4.8%, respectively. If the ulna is lengthened by 2.5 mm, the ratio of transmission is 58.1% through the radius and 41.9% through the ulna (Fig. 33-1). Additional studies[38] revealed that an inverse relationship exists between positive ulna variance and the thickness of the articular component of the TFC. This inverse relationship suggests that the central portion of the articular disk, which functions as a compressive cushion,[7,28,39] is thinner in people with ulna plus variant wrists and, therefore, more prone to perforation. Additional anatomic studies by Mikic[29] and Viegas and Ballantyne[52] have identified an age-related degeneration of this relatively avascular central disk. In his anatomic studies of 180 wrist joints and 19 fetuses, Mikic[29] did not detect perforations until the 3rd decade of life, after which perforations steadily increased to 40% in the 5th decade. Viegas and Ballantyne[52] noted similar findings in their evaluation of 100 wrist joints. No perforations were noted in those age 45 years or younger whereas older specimens showed a 27.6% incidence of perforations.

Darrow et al.[11] and Uchiyama and Terayama[51] have documented the radiographic changes in wrists with ulna plus variance (Fig. 33-2). Both groups noted that when degenerative changes were confined to the ulnar aspect of the wrist, the vast majority occurred at the distal ulna and proximal ulnar aspect of the lunate. These findings correlate with previous studies by Palmer and Werner,[39] who noted that 73% of wrists with perforated TFCC and erosions of the ulna-lunate interface had ulna neutral or ulna plus variance. Further, Palmer and Werner[39] observed that 70% of wrists with TFCC perforations had disruptions of the lunotriquetral interosseous ligament.

Ulnar abutment may also be caused by alteration of the transmission of the radial-ulnar load with changes in the distal radial inclination, as seen in displaced fractures of the distal radius. Short et al.[47] demonstrated that ulnocarpal loading increased from 21% to 67% when palmar inclination of the distal radius decreased to 45° of dorsal angulation.

CLASSIFICATION

From the evaluation of different abnormalities affecting the ulnar side of the wrist, ulnocarpal abutment has been considered a degenerative process involving the TFC, ulnar head, and lunotriquetral aspect of the proximal carpal row. In Palmer's classification of TFC lesions (see box on p. 775), ulnocarpal abutment is considered a degenerative lesion. The treatment alternatives to be mentioned correlate with the degree of advancing degenerative change that this classification presents. Ulnocarpal abutment usually stands alone as a cause of ulnar wrist pain but, as explained

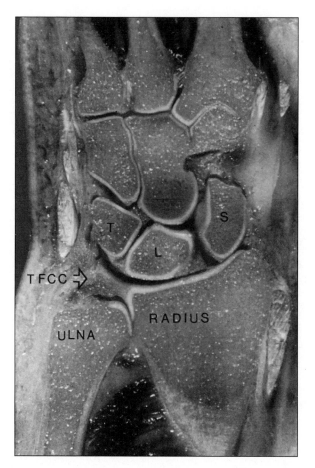

FIGURE 33-2

Anatomy of the distal radioulnar joint. The head of the ulna covers 80% of the surface and articulates with the sigmoid notch of the distal radius (radially) and with the inferior surface of the triangular fibrocartilage complex (*TFCC*). *L*, lunate; *S*, scaphoid; *T*, triquetrum.

TRIANGULAR FIBROCARTILAGE COMPLEX ABNORMALITIES

Class I—Traumatic
A.   Central perforation
B.   Ulnar avulsion
      With distal ulnar fracture
      Without distal ulnar fracture
C.   Distal avulsion
D.   Radial avulsion
      With sigmoid notch fracture
      Without sigmoid notch fracture

Class II—Degenerative (ulnocarpal abutment syndrome)
Stage
   1   TFCC wear
   2   TFCC wear + lunate or ulnar chondromalacia
   3   TFCC perforation + lunate or ulnar chondromalacia
   4   TFCC perforation + lunate or ulnar chondromalacia + L-T ligament perforation
   5   TFCC perforation + lunate or ulnar chondromalacia + L-T ligament perforation + ulnocarpal arthritis

L-T, lunotriquetral; *TFCC*, triangular fibrocartilage complex.
From Bowers WH: *The distal radioulnar joint.* In Green DP, editor: *Operative hand surgery,* ed 3, vol 2, New York, 1988, Churchill Livingstone, p 942. By permission of the publisher.

---

below, may be associated with dorsal-palmar instability, derangement of the DRUJ, TFC tears with instability, and lunotriquetral dissociation. See Chapter 35 for a broader view of disorders of the DRUJ.

DIAGNOSIS

Diagnosing the cause of ulnar wrist discomfort is challenging. Linscheid and Dobyns noted that even after a most careful examination by a discerning observer, it is not always possible to elicit all the characteristics of ulnar column pain or to give proper weight to the various findings.[12,26] The differential diagnosis of the patient with ulnar wrist discomfort should include, but not be limited to, subluxation of the extensor carpi ulnaris, calcific tendinitis, dysfunction of the DRUJ, intercarpal pathology and instability, and pisotriquetral dysfunction. Despite anticipated overlap in presentation and physical findings, ulnocarpal abutment can be identified through a careful history, physical examination, and adjuvant diagnostic studies.

Patients typically present with chronic or subacute pain localized to the dorsal aspect of the wrist over the DRUJ of the forearm (see Chapter 12). Extremes of rotation and ulnar deviation aggravate discomfort. Patients may complain of an intermittent clicking sensation as well as activity-related swelling and decreased strength and motion. In patients with findings of ulnocarpal abutment secondary to an inherent ulna plus variance, there may not be a history of trauma. The traumatic injury usually results in residual deformity in the form of radial shortening, premature epiphyseal closure, or DRUJ instability. Increased ulnocarpal loading is the basic pathologic feature in all of these conditions.

Positive physical findings are observed with direct palpation and stress loading of the ulnar side of the wrist. Pain and tenderness between the ulnar head and triquetrum or lunate are generally present on physical examination. The discomfort can be exacerbated with ulnar deviation while the forearm is pronated and the ulnar head is displaced palmarward. Ballottement (dorsal and palmar displacement) of the distal ulna with the wrist in ulnar deviation accentuates symptoms (Fig. 33-3). Concomitant lunotriquetral disruption, which can be present in the later

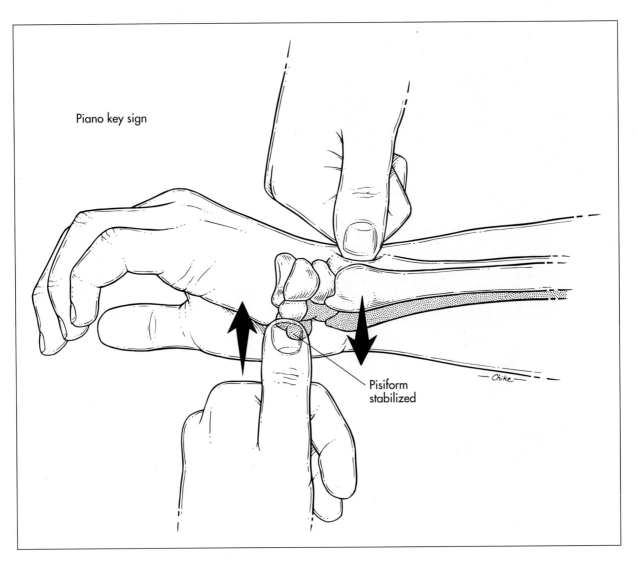

Piano key sign

Pisiform stabilized

— Ohike —

Figure 33-3

Ballottement test reducing dorsal displacement of ulna, which accentuates symptoms at the distal radioulnar joint.

stages, results in discomfort with stress loading of the lunotriquetral joint (direct pressure over the joint). It is important to distinguish ulnocarpal abutment from pathology intrinsic to the DRUJ, in which there is pain throughout the range of motion of pronation-supination. In addition, primary DRUJ pathology has increased discomfort consistently reproduced with DRUJ translation and compression.

Radiographic evaluation is essential to the correct diagnosis of ulnocarpal abutment. Routine posteroanterior and lateral radiographs show an ulna neutral or ulna plus variant wrist. In more advanced cases, there is perforation of the TFC, with sclerosis and cystic changes at the ulnar head and the proximal ulnar border of the lunate (Fig. 33-4).

In judging the degree of ulnocarpal abutment, arm position must be standardized for radiographs. Studies by Palmer et al.[37] and Epner et al.[14] have shown that forearm rotation alters the magnitude of ulna variance. During forearm supination, the radius moves distally, decreasing ulna variance, whereas with forearm pronation there is the opposite effect of increased ulna variance.[14,37] Other investigators have also observed a dynamic ulna plus variance where ulna variance increases with power grip, a factor that may explain ulnar abutment in the patient with an ulnar neutral or minus wrist.[19] Radial deviation in the supinated forearm (which produces proximal radius migration against a fixed ulna) increases ulna variance; when the wrist is brought into ulnar deviation, variance decreases. Radial and ulnar deviation with the pronated forearm, however, do not have a significant effect on variance. Based on their findings, Epner et al.[14] and Palmer et al.[37] recommended standardized

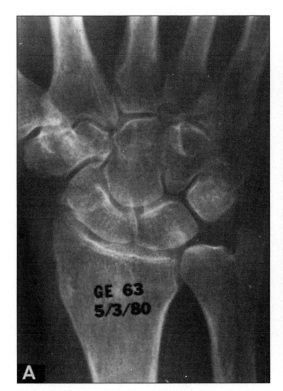
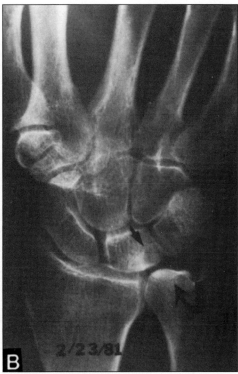

FIGURE 33-4

A, Presentation of ulnocarpal abutment in a 63-year-old worker (*GE*) with mid-ulnar wrist pain. **B,** About 1 year later with continued work. The degenerative changes progressed to demonstrate a cyst in the ulnar aspect of the lunate with associated sclerosis of the distal articular surface of the ulna. *(From Darrow et al.[11] By permission of the American Society for Surgery of the Hand.)*

positions for wrist radiographs, consisting of an x-ray beam (Fig. 33-5, *A*) perpendicular to the wrist, with the shoulder placed in 90° abduction, elbow flexed to 90°, and forearm pronated. Although Epner et al. recommended that the wrist be placed in ulnar deviation, Palmer et al. suggested neutral deviation. Both of these studies are significant in that they demonstrate the need for a standard, reproducible, radiographic technique so that radiographs can be reliably compared.

Ulna variance is measured by one of two methods. The first extends a line from the distal articular surface of the radius toward the ulna. This line should be perpendicular to the long axis of the radius. The distance between this projected line and the distal articular surface of the ulna is then measured[11] (Fig. 33-5, *B*). An alternative method, devised by Palmer et al.,[37] uses a template of concentric semicircles at 1-mm intervals (Fig. 33-5, *C* [Parts *A* and *B*]). The semicircle that most closely approximates the concavity of the distal radius is aligned to contour the radial articular surface. The number of semicircles separating the aligned semicircle from the caput ulna represents the amount of ulna variance in millimeters (Fig. 33-5, *C*).[37]

Arthrography is helpful in determining the presence of ligamentous pathology such as lunotriquetral interosseous ligament disruption as well as perforations of the TFC (Fig. 33-6). Arthrography can also be helpful in determining the degree of ulna variance and results of ulna recession in relieving stress on the distal ulna lunotriquetral space. Linscheid recommended triple-injection arthrography commencing at the midcarpal joint and moving proximally.[36]

With advances in technique and expertise, arthroscopy is now an accepted component of evaluation and treatment. It is most helpful in difficult cases in which less invasive studies are inconclusive. Arthroscopy allows clear identification of chondromalacia of the lunate and the presence of TFCC or lunotriquetral ligamentous disruption (see Chapter 14).[4,34,43]

TREATMENT

Initial treatment of the patient with ulnocarpal abutment consists of modification of activity, rest, and nonsteroidal anti-inflammatory drugs. Surgical alternatives aim to correct the primary source of pathology and to

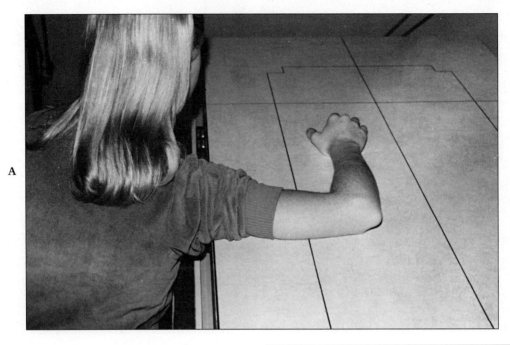

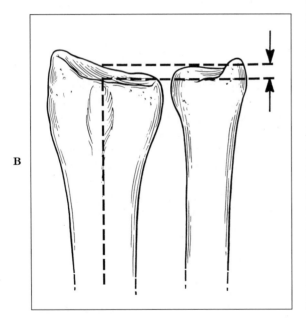

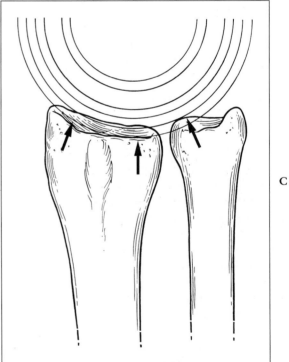

FIGURE 33–5

A, Standard positioning for wrist radiographs to measure ulna variance. The shoulder is abducted, the elbow is flexed 90°, and the wrist is placed in neutral forearm pronation-supination. **B,** Articular surface method. A line from the articular surface of the lunate fossa of the distal radius is drawn toward the ulna. This line should be perpendicular to the longitudinal axis of radius. **C,** Concentric semicircle method. A semicircular template is aligned closely to the contour of the articular surface of the distal radius. The ulnar head is outlined (*right arrow*) and compared to the distal radius articular surface lines (*arrows on the left*). In this case, 2.6 mm of positive ulna variance is measured.

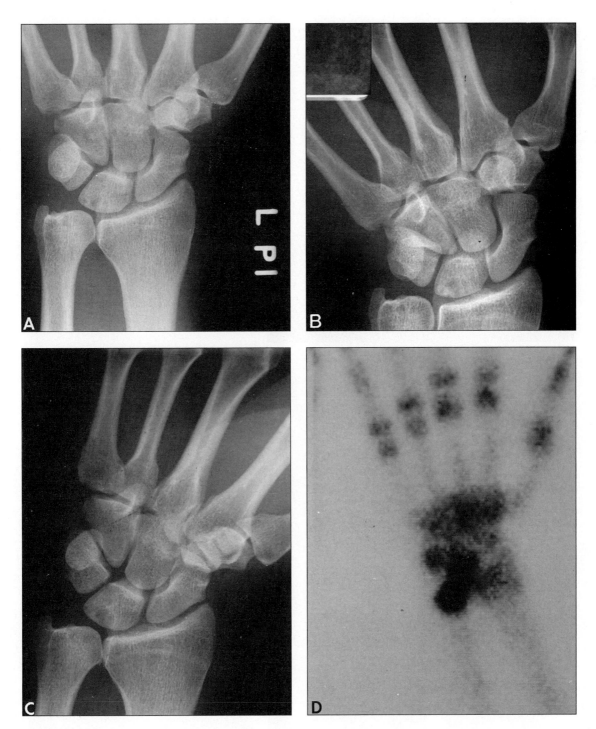

FIGURE 33-6

Ulna positive variance with associated interosseous ligament tear. **A,** Anteroposterior view of wrist. Positive ulna variance in a 47-year-old industrial worker with progressive ulnar-sided wrist pain. **B** and **C,** Radial-ulnar deviation views. Note cystic changes in the proximal lunate with greater potential for ulnocarpal abutment in radial deviation than ulnar deviation. Note 2 to 3 mm positive ulna variance. **D,** Technetium-99m bone scan. Increased uptake at the ulnolunate area (ulnolunate abutment).   *Continued.*

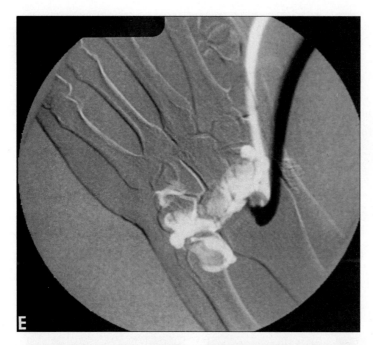

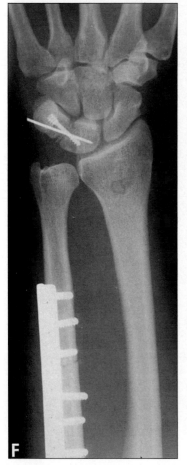

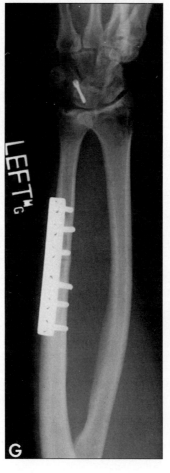

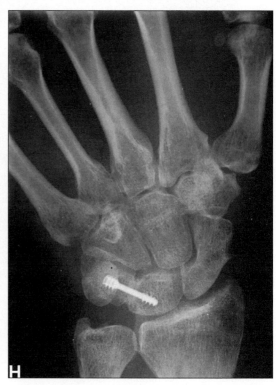

FIGURE 33-6, CONT'D.

E, Digital subtraction arthrogram shows lunotriquetral interosseous ligament tear and a tear of the triangular fibrocartilage. **F,** Ulna recession combined with lunotriquetral fusion (Herbert screw, Kirschner wire with interposition cancellous bone graft). **G** and **H,** Healed ulna osteotomy and lunotriquetral fusion site. Excellent relief of symptoms.

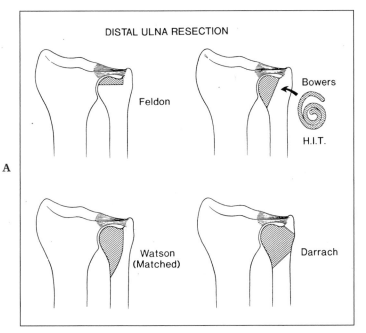

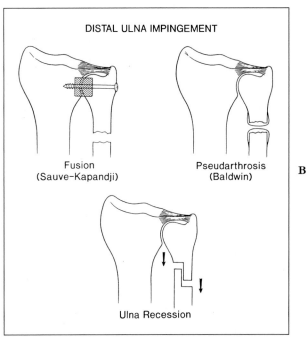

FIGURE 33-7

Methods of distal ulna recession, resection, or fusion. **A,** *Top left:* Feldon procedure of open resection of the articular surface of the ulna. *Top right:* Hemi-interposition transposition (*H.I.T.*) (after Bowers[6]). Resection of articular surface of the ulna and soft tissue (tendon or capsule). *Bottom left:* Resection of articular surface (after Watson[53]) with preservation of the ulna border. *Bottom right:* Darrach[10] resection of the distal ulna; preserve attachment of triangular fibrocartilage to ulnar styloid. **B,** *Top left:* Fusion of the distal radioulnar joint, proximal pseudarthrosis (after Sauvé-Kapandji[32,48]). *Top right:* Pseudarthrosis of distal ulna. *Bottom:* Recession of distal ulna (step-cut shortening of the ulna shaft).

unload the ulnocarpal joint. There are several effective procedures that can accomplish this goal (Fig. 33-7): resection of the distal ulna (Darrach,[10] Bowers,[6] Feldon,[17] and Watson[53] techniques); fusion of the DRUJ (the Sauvé-Kapandji[32,48] procedure); pseudarthrosis technique (Baldwin); ulnar recession shortening procedures; or arthroscopic resection of the distal ulnar surface beneath the TFC, also known as the wafer procedure.[17,18]

Each of these procedures has the potential benefit of relieving stress from the ulnar side of the wrist by effectively shortening the ulna, but each also may result in residual symptoms that bother the patient and may be difficult to treat. Residual weakness and instability of the remaining ulnar shaft have been described after the Darrach procedure.[2,33] Hemiresections of the DRUJ may also result in impingement of the resected ulna at the level of the sigmoid notch and at the ulnar styloid-carpal interface if there was a significant ulna plus variance before resection.[4] Similarly, the Sauve-Kapandji procedure can produce problems associated with instability at the site of pseudarthrosis.[21,42,44]

We believe that ulna recession (shortening) is the procedure of choice for most cases of ulnar carpal abutment (Fig. 33-8). Ulnar recession has the advantage of maintaining the articular surfaces of the ulnocarpal joint and the DRUJ. In addition, shortening the ulna tightens the ulnocarpal ligaments (and TFC), providing

a stabilizing effect for those with ligamentous laxity or injury. Ulnar recession was first described by Milch[30,31] for the treatment of patients with deformity secondary to distal radius malunion. Since then, several modifications have been described using transverse, step-cut, or oblique osteotomies with various fixation devices (Fig. 33-9). Darrow et al.,[11] Linscheid,[25] and Boulas and Milek[5] have used a transverse osteotomy and fixation with a 3.5-mm dynamic compression plate. Chun and Palmer[8] advocated an oblique osteotomy with the addition of a compression screw to minimize delayed unions and nonunions.

The preferred technique of ulnar recession is based on experiences of the surgeon, but recent advances in plate design and alignment jigs suggest that the oblique osteotomy may be preferred (Fig. 33-10). If there are small, defined areas of concomitant pathology at the DRUJ, ulnar recession is still applicable. As the ulnar head recedes in relation to the radius, it also displaces laterally as it follows the obliquity of the sigmoid notch.[26] This shortening and lateral displacement decompress the distal radioulnar articulation and change the weightbearing surface (Fig. 33-11). In the presence of dorsal subluxation of the DRUJ, as in Madelung's deformity and some cases of malunited distal radius fractures, the osteotomy should be angulated palmarly to correct alignment at the DRUJ in the lateral projection.

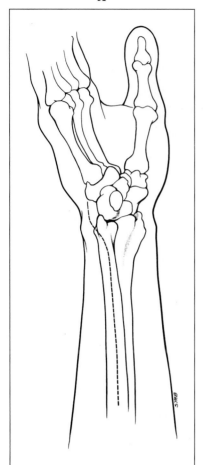

A

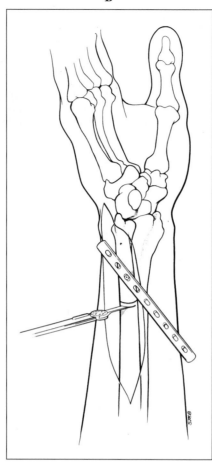

B

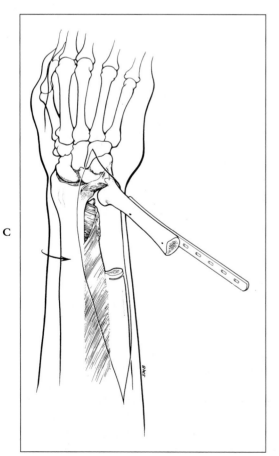

C

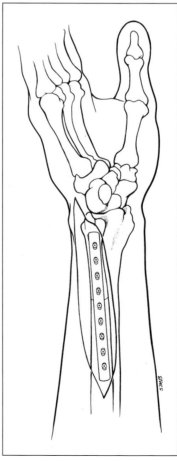

D

FIGURE 33-8

Surgical technique for shortening of the ulna. **A,** Incision is made over the subcutaneous border of the ulna and curved dorsally for exploration of the distal radioulnar (DRUJ) and ulnocarpal joints. **B,** After subperiosteal exposure of the ulna, a dynamic compression plate is applied with two screws distally marking alignment; the plate is then loosened by removing one screw and rotated for performing the osteotomy at the desired level. **C,** For exposure of the DRUJ (to determine arthritis at the DRUJ, for triangular fibrocartilage repair, or to assess the amount of ulna shortening), the plate is reapplied distally, and the distal ulna is swung outward after releasing attachments of the interosseous membrane. **D,** Completion of procedure involves application proximally of the compression plate (minimal screw holes 6 to 8) with dynamic compression applied through consecutive screw holes. *(From Darrow et al.[11] By permission of Mayo Foundation.)*

A

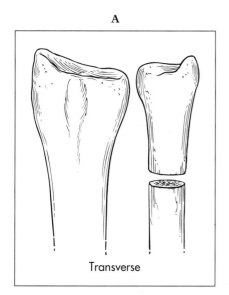

B

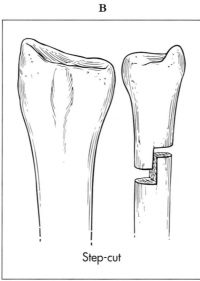

C

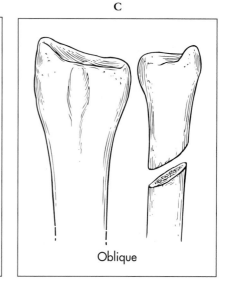

Transverse

Step-cut

Oblique

FIGURE 33-9

Ulnar recession osteotomy. **A,** Transverse osteotomy[5,11] provides for exact measurement of ulna shortening. **B,** Step-cut osteotomy[31] maximizes contact. **C,** Oblique osteotomy[8] (Rayhack J, unpublished data) adds a compression screw to the longitudinal plate.

ULNA RECESSION-SURGICAL PROCEDURE

The surgical procedure (Fig. 33-8) consists of a straight line incision over the distal one-third of the ulnar aspect of the ulnar shaft. If arthrotomy of the ulnocarpal joint is anticipated, the incision curves dorsally and distally just proximal to the ulnar head. Care is taken to avoid injury to the dorsal branch of the ulnar sensory nerve. A subperiosteal dissection exposes the ulnar aspect of the ulnar shaft. The shaft can be stripped of its interosseous membrane and pronator quadratus insertion to allow the ulna to swing outwardly to permit inspection of the TFC. In most cases this is unnecessary and such soft-tissue stripping should be unnecessary.

A prebent six- to eight-hole dynamic compression plate is applied first to the distal ulna by using two of the distal holes. One of the screws is then removed, and the plate is rotated away from the cortical surface. The osteotomy site is identified, and a longitudinal marker is placed in the bone with the use of a bone scribe to provide a guide for rotational alignment after the osteotomy is completed. An intraoperative arthrogram can determine the results of ulna recession with respect to the distal radius, sigmoid notch, lunate, and triquetrum.

A predetermined amount of bone is then removed, and the dynamic compression plate is placed in its original position. The osteotomy site is manually closed down, and the plate is fixed to the bone in compressive fashion. If it is necessary to expose the TFC, the forearm is placed in the pronated position, and the interval between the extensor carpi ulnaris and extensor digiti minimi is used to gain access to the ulnocarpal joint.

The extensor retinaculum is reflected as a radially based flap with its ulnar margin at the fourth and fifth dorsal compartment interface. The capsule is then entered by using an inverted "L" incision that is ulnarly based. Repair of the TFC to the distal radius, palmar carpal ligaments, or ulnar styloid is possible through this approach. Excision of a central TFC tear can also be considered. For closure, a small cuff of tissue is left at the level of the sigmoid notch; extensor carpi ulnaris extensor compartment and common wrist extensor retinaculum are closed in layers after capsule repair of DRUJ and radiocarpal joint.

Rayhack (Rayhack J, unpublished data) reported an alternative technique for an exact oblique osteotomy with controlled bone resection and potentially greater bone contact with internal fixation (Fig. 33-10). Others suggest a step-cut osteotomy just proximal to the ulna head. Screws are used for fixation.

Postoperatively, the extremity is immobilized in a Munster type of cast for 6 weeks to control forearm rotation, followed by a removable Orthoplast splint until complete union is obtained.

If ulna plus variance is mild, the wafer procedure (excision of distal ulna articular surface) may provide another alternative.[3,17] The procedure involves resection of the distal 2 to 3 mm of the ulnar head. The ulnar styloid and TFC are preserved. The procedure should be avoided if there is marked ulna plus variance because the residual ulnar styloid can be a source of impingement. The greatest advantage of the wafer procedure is that an osteotomy is unnecessary and, therefore, delayed unions or nonunions are avoided. The exposure is slightly different from that used for ulnar recession because only the distal third of the incision is needed to

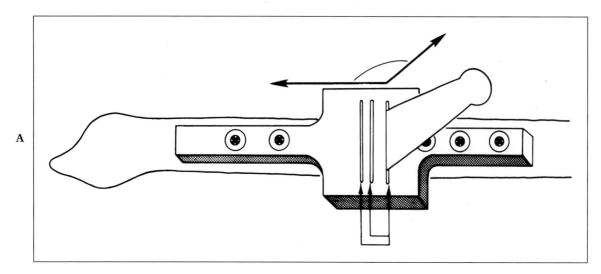

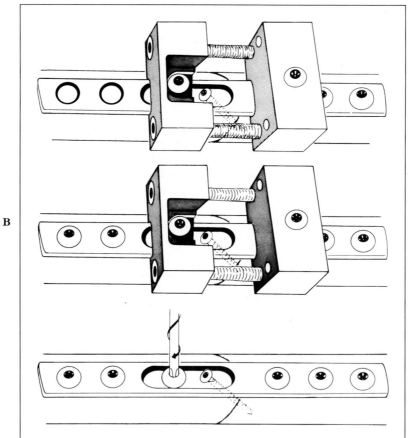

FIGURE 33-10

Rayhack technique of ulna recession. **A,** Oblique osteotomy of the ulna using a precision cutting guide. This allows removal of bone segments at 2.5, 3.5, and 5.5 cm. **B,** Application of plate and compression device. The technique provides for compression through the overlying compression device; plate application with cortical bone screws and a cortical intrafragmentary lag screw. *Top,* Lag screw placement; *middle,* distal cortical bone screws; *bottom,* removal of compression device and insertion of final cortical bone screw.

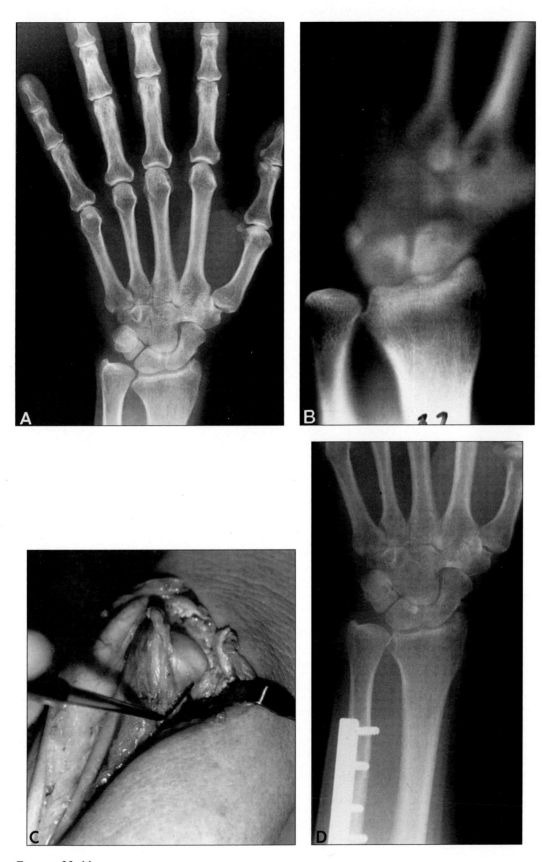

FIGURE 33-11

A, Ulna-carpal abutment with incongruity of the distal radioulnar joint. Note 4 mm of ulna positive variance. **B,** Polytomography of the wrist demonstrates a prominent proximal osteophyte within the distal radioulnar joint impinging on the ulnar head. **C,** Intraoperative appearance of ulnar head shows wear on the ulnar head. The osteophyte was resected and the joint cartilage of the sigmoid notch was undercut and flattened to provide a smooth articular surface after ulna recession. **D,** Ulna recession after contouring the distal radioulnar joint provided satisfactory relief of symptoms.

approach the DRUJ. The joint capsule can be opened without dividing capsule or ligaments of the radiocarpal joint. With retraction of the TFC and dorsal DRUJ joint capsule, a "wafer" of ulnar head, usually 2 to 4 mm thick, is excised. Bilos and Chamberland[3] recommended use of a cut-back osteotomy perpendicular to the main osteotomy site and adjacent to the ulnar styloid to prevent iatrogenic fracture of the styloid, whereas Feldon et al.[17] performed a straight osteotomy of the distal ulnar head. Postoperatively, the limb is immobilized by a short arm cast for 3 weeks, after which protective range of motion exercise begins. In an attempt to avoid a formal arthrotomy, Friedman and Palmer[18] have described an arthroscopic wafer procedure involving resection of the distal ulnar head via the defect in the TFC.

In the presence of injury to the TFC, Schuind et al.[45] showed that the central portion of the TFC is not essential to the preservation of the DRUJ stability and, therefore, can be excised. Treatment of associated injury of the lunotriquetral interval disruption is addressed elsewhere (see Chapter 22). Alternatives to consider include interosseous ligament repair, ligament reconstruction by tendon graft, or lunotriquetral fusion.[16,42] If fusion is to be performed, the addition of a compressive device such as the Herbert screw may be helpful in enhancing bony fusion and decreasing the incidence of nonunion (Figs. 33-6, A through D). Others have suggested that tightening of the ulnocarpal ligaments via ulnar recession alone is sufficient treatment for lunotriquetral instability.[36]

SUMMARY

Ulnar abutment syndrome, as a well-defined source of pain on the ulnar side of the wrist, occurs as a result of increased loading at the ulnocarpal articulation. The cause may be positive ulna variance, which is acquired, congenital, or dynamic. With repetitive loading, the TFC deteriorates and produces ulnolunate abutment and subsequent degenerative changes. The final stage is lunotriquetral interosseous ligament disruption.

There are several treatment options that depend, in part, on the etiology of the increased ulnar load and the extent of pathology. If there is significant DRUJ involvement, distal ulnar hemiresection and the Darrach procedure may be of use. In the absence of such involvement, ulnar recession is the preferred treatment, although newer techniques such as the wafer procedure are also useful in milder cases of ulna plus variance.

REFERENCES

1. Bell MJ, Hill RJ, McMurtry RY: Ulnar impingement syndrome, *J Bone Joint Surg Br* 67:126-129, 1985.
2. Bieber EJ, Linscheid RL, Dobyns JH, et al.: Failed distal ulna resections, *J Hand Surg [Am]* 13:193-200, 1988.
3. Bilos ZJ, Chamberland D: Distal ulnar head shortening for treatment of triangular fibrocartilage complex tears with ulna positive variance, *J Hand Surg [Am]* 16:1115-1119, 1991.
4. Bora FW Jr, Osterman AL, Maitin E: The role of arthroscopy in the treatment of disorders of the wrist, *Contemp Orthop* 12:28-30, 1986.
5. Boulas HJ, Milek MA: Ulnar shortening for tears of the triangular fibrocartilaginous complex, *J Hand Surg [Am]* 15:415-420, 1990.
6. Bowers WH: Distal radioulnar joint arthroplasty: the hemiresection-interposition technique, *J Hand Surg [Am]* 10:169-178, 1985.
7. Chidgey LK, Dell PC, Bittar ES, et al.: Histologic anatomy of the triangular fibrocartilage, *J Hand Surg [Am]* 16:1084-1100, 1991.
8. Chun S, Palmer AK: The ulnar impaction syndrome: follow-up of ulnar shortening osteotomy, *J Hand Surg [Am]* 18:46-53, 1993.
9. Czitrom AA, Dobyns JH, Linscheid RL: Ulnar variance in carpal instability, *J Hand Surg [Am]* 12:205-208, 1987.
10. Darrach W: Partial excision of the lower shaft of the ulna for deformity following Colles' fracture, *Ann Surg* 57:764-765, 1913.
11. Darrow JC Jr, Linscheid RL, Dobyns JH, et al.: Distal ulnar recession for disorders of the distal radioulnar joint, *J Hand Surg [Am]* 10:482-491, 1985.
12. Dobyns JH, Linscheid RL: *Fractures and dislocations of the wrist,* In Rockwood CA Jr, Green DP, editors: *Fractures,* vol 1, Philadelphia, 1975, JB Lippincott.
13. Dwyer FC: Treatment of traumatic Madelung's deformity by shortening ulna, *Proc R Soc Med* 48:100-103, 1955.
14. Epner RA, Bowers WH, Guilford WB: Ulnar variance—the effect of wrist positioning and roentgen filming technique, *J Hand Surg [Am]* 7:298-305, 1982.
15. Essex-Lopresti P: Fractures of radial head with distal radio-ulnar dislocation; report of 2 cases, *J Bone Joint Surg Br* 33:244-247, 1951.

16. Favero KJ, Bishop AT, Linscheid RL: Lunotriquetral ligament disruption: a comparative study of treatment methods. Proceedings of the Annual Meeting of the American Society for Surgery of the Hand, Orlando, Florida, 1991.

17. Feldon P, Terrono AL, Belsky MR: Wafer distal ulna resection for triangular fibrocartilage tears and/or ulna impaction syndrome, *J Hand Surg [Am]* 17:731-737, 1992.

18. Friedman SL, Palmer AK: The ulnar impaction syndrome, *Hand Clin* 7:295-310, 1991.

19. Friedman SL, Palmer AK, Short WH, et al.: The change in ulnar variance with grip, *J Hand Surg [Am]* 18:713-716, 1993.

20. Gelberman RH, Salamon PB, Jurist JM, et al.: Ulnar variance in Kienbock's disease, *J Bone Joint Surg Am* 57:674-676, 1975.

21. Gordon L, Levinsohn DG, Moore SV, et al.: The Sauve-Kapandji procedure for the treatment of posttraumatic distal radioulnar joint problems, *Hand Clin* 7:397-403, 1991.

22. Hültén O: Über anatomische Variationen der Handgelenkknochen ein. Ein Beitrag zur Kenntnis der Genese zwei verschiedener mondbeinveränderungen, *Acta Radiol* 9:155-168, 1928.

23. Lewis OJ: Evolutionary change in the primate wrist and inferior radio-ulnar joints, *Anat Rec* 151:275-285, 1965.

24. Lewis OJ, Hamshere RJ, Bucknill TM: The anatomy of the wrist joint, *J Anat* 106:539-552, 1970.

25. Linscheid RL: Ulnar recession for disorders of the distal radioulnar joint (abstract), *Orthop Trans* 6:475, 1982.

26. Linscheid RL: Ulnar lengthening and shortening, *Hand Clin* 3:69-79, 1987.

27. McDougall A, White J: Subluxation of the inferior radioulnar joint complicating fracture of the radial head, *J Bone Joint Surg Br* 39:278-287, 1957.

28. Menon J, Wood VE, Schoene HR, et al.: Isolated tears of the triangular fibrocartilage of the wrist: results of partial excision, *J Hand Surg [Am]* 9:527-530, 1984.

29. Mikic ZD: Age changes in the triangular fibrocartilage of the wrist joint, *J Anat* 126:367-384, 1978.

30. Milch H: So-called dislocation of lower end of ulna, *Ann Surg* 116:282-292, 1942.

31. Milch H: Treatment of disabilities following fracture of the lower end of the radius, *Clin Orthop* 29:157-163, 1963.

32. Millroy P, Coleman S, Ivers R: The Sauve-Kapandji operation. Technique and results, *J Hand Surg [Br]* 17:411-414, 1992.

33. Minami A, Ogino T, Minami M: Treatment of distal radioulnar disorders, *J Hand Surg [Am]* 12:189-196, 1987.

34. North ER, Meyer S: Diagnosis of instability on the ulnar side of the wrist: a comparative study of clinical and arthroscopic findings (abstract), *Orthop Trans* 14:165, 1990.

35. Palmer AK: Triangular fibrocartilage disorders: injury patterns and treatment, *Arthroscopy* 6:125-132, 1990.

36. Palmer AK, Taleisnik J, Fisk G: Symposium: Distal ulnar injuries, *Contemp Orthop* 7:81-94, 1983.

37. Palmer AK, Glisson RR, Werner FW: Ulnar variance determination, *J Hand Surg [Am]* 7:376-379, 1982.

38. Palmer AK, Glisson RR, Werner FW: Relationship between ulnar variance and triangular fibrocartilage complex thickness, *J Hand Surg [Am]* 9:681-682, 1984.

39. Palmer AK, Werner FW: The triangular fibrocartilage complex of the wrist—anatomy and function, *J Hand Surg [Am]* 6:153-162, 1981.

40. Palmer AK, Werner FW: Biomechanics of the distal radioulnar joint, *Clin Orthop* 187:26-35, 1984.

41. Ranawat CS, DeFiore J, Straub LR: Madelung's deformity: an end-result study of surgical treatment, *J Bone Joint Surg Am* 57:772-775, 1975.

42. Reagan DS, Linscheid RL, Dobyns JH: Lunotriquetral sprains, *J Hand Surg [Am]* 9:502-514, 1984.

43. Roth JH, Haddad RG: Radiocarpal arthroscopy and arthrography in the diagnosis of ulnar wrist pain, *Arthroscopy* 2:234-243, 1986.

44. Sanders RA, Frederick HA, Hontas RB: The Sauve-Kapandji procedure: a salvage operation for the distal radioulnar joint, *J Hand Surg [Am]* 16:1125-1129, 1991.

45. Schuind F, An KN, Berglund L, et al.: The distal radioulnar ligaments: a biomechanical study, *J Hand Surg [Am]* 16:1106-1114, 1991.

46. Schulte LA: Anomalies of the distal radio-ulnar joint, *Arch Chir Neerl* 11:311-326, 1959.

47. Short WH, Palmer AK, Werner FW, et al.: A biomechanical study of distal radial fractures, *J Hand Surg [Am]* 12:529-534, 1987.

48. Taleisnik J: The Sauve-Kapandji procedure, *Clin Orthop* 275:110-123, 1992.

49. Trumble T, Glisson RR, Seaber AV, et al.: Forearm force transmission after surgical treatment of distal radioulnar joint disorders, *J Hand Surg [Am]* 12:196-202, 1987.

50. Trumble TE, Easterling KJ, Smith RJ: Ulnocarpal abutment after wrist arthrodesis, *J Hand Surg [Am]* 13:11-15, 1988.

51. Uchiyama S, Terayama K: Radiographic changes in wrists with ulnar plus variance observed over a ten-year period, *J Hand Surg [Am]* 16:45-48, 1991.

52. Viegas SF, Ballantyne G: Attritional lesions of the wrist joint, *J Hand Surg [Am]* 12:1025-1029, 1987.

53. Watson HK, Brown RE: Ulnar impingement syndrome after Darrach procedure: treatment by advancement lengthening osteotomy of the ulna, *J Hand Surg [Am]* 14:302-306, 1989.

54. Weigl K, Spira E: The triangular fibrocartilage of the wrist joint, *Reconstr Surg Traumatol* 11:139-153, 1969.

34

ARTHRITIS DEFORMITY: RESECTION ARTHROPLASTY AND FUSION

Julio Taleisnik, M.D.
Leonard K. Ruby, M.D.

DIAGNOSIS
TREATMENT
RESECTION ARTHROPLASTY
TECHNIQUE OF EXCISION OF THE DISTAL
  ULNA (DARRACH)
PRONATOR QUADRATUS INTERPOSITION

PARTIAL RESECTION ARTHROPLASTIES
HEMIRESECTION INTERPOSITION TECHNIQUE
TECHNIQUE OF MATCHED DISTAL ULNAR
  RESECTION
RADIOULNAR FUSION AND ULNAR OSTEOTOMY
OPERATIVE TECHNIQUE

This chapter is limited to discussion of the treatment of degenerative arthritis involving the distal radioulnar joint (DRUJ). Although we believe that chondromalacia is a precursor of degenerative arthritis, it will not be discussed here, because in our opinion, the treatment of choice for chondromalacia is ulna shortening, a technique covered elsewhere in this book (see Chapter 35). The differential diagnosis of pain at the DRUJ includes arthritic deformity, instability, or ulnocarpal impaction. The last two conditions each have options for treatment that are different from those for arthritic deformity, the subject of this chapter. Other DRUJ problems, including subluxations, dislocations, DRUJ instability, and inflammatory (i.e., rheumatoid) arthritis, are discussed elsewhere in the book (see Chapters 31, 32, 33, 36, and 48).

Degenerative arthritis of the DRUJ is a troublesome cause of severe disability for which a single, reliable solution does not exist.[22,72] This explains the plethora of operations that have been proposed for this problem. A patient presenting with ulnar wrist pain requires a careful history and an accurate determination of the location of symptoms, followed by a detailed examination and by appropriate radiographs and ancillary tests. The DRUJ is but one of the many structures contained within this small area, each of which may produce similar symptoms and findings. One must decide first if the DRUJ is indeed the source of the patient's disability and second if the disability is severe enough to warrant an operation.[18,21,24,71,123] Once this decision is made, the surgeon must exercise critical judgment to decide which operation will be most likely to succeed. This operation must be performed with rigorous attention to surgical detail, because failure to do so may create an even more vexing problem than the initial one.

DIAGNOSIS

The presenting symptom of chondromalacia and degenerative arthritis of the DRUJ is pain projected to the dorsum of the DRUJ. Limitation of forearm rotation may be present. There is a consistent reproduction of pain by forced passive rotation of the forearm beyond the active range available. Swelling is rare. Crepitation or snapping commonly occurs during forearm rotation. Symptoms develop gradually over a period of years, as is typical for degenerative arthritis in other joints. Both extensor and flexor tendon ruptures have been reported.[81]

Pain and tenderness must be localized to the DRUJ. Because the distal radioulnar, ulnocarpal, lunotriquetral, triquetrohamate, and pisotriquetral joints are within such a small area, it may be difficult to pinpoint tenderness.[18] Using one's fingertip or a small soft object, such as the eraser end of a pencil, may be of assistance.[106] Each of the joints mentioned must be individually manipulated to detect abnormal roughness, crepitus, or snaps that reproduce the patient's pain. DRUJ pain may be produced by rotation applied to the proximal forearm or compression of the ulna against the radius. Location may be verified by relief of pain and improvement in grip strength after injection of a small amount of a local anesthetic into the DRUJ. It is helpful to use radiography with or without contrast material in the injection to localize the needle precisely in the joint.

In chondromalacia, routine radiographs are negative, although ulna plus variant is not infrequent. A posteroanterior view of a wrist with degenerative osteoarthritis in neutral rotation shows joint narrowing, sclerosis of articular surfaces, and spur and cyst formation; however, subtle changes require comparison views of affected and unaffected wrists (Figs. 34-1, *A*, *B*, and *D*).[25] A bone scan may show well-delineated radioactive uptake in the distal radioulnar area (Fig. 34-1, *C*). A computed tomographic scan is often diagnostic (Fig. 34-1, *D*). Other diagnostic techniques include arthrography, arthroscopy, and magnetic resonance imaging.[*] The last often discloses effusion within the joint.

TREATMENT

The procedures available for correction of painful osteoarthritis of the DRUJ are similar to those for other osteoarthritic joints: resection arthroplasty, arthrodesis, and replacement arthroplasty.

Resection arthroplasty of the head of the ulna is commonly known as the Darrach operation (Fig. 34-2). Recent modifications include procedures that may be classified as hemiresection or partial resection arthroplasties, in which only the articulating surface of the ulna is excised, leaving intact the ulnar shaft-to-styloid and the remaining support mechanisms.[20,22,122]

Arthrodesis of the DRUJ is known as the Sauvé-Kapandji operation (Fig. 34-3). This provides for restoration of the forearm rotation by an excisional arthroplasty of the ulna just proximal to the fusion.

The most frequent complication arising from the use of these techniques is instability of the distal ulnar stump. Its treatment is difficult and unreliable. This is a complication that is best avoided by careful patient selection and by strict adherence to surgical detail and to postoperative protocol.

Prosthetic arthroplasty of the DRUJ has been attempted in small numbers of patients by a few individuals. There are problems inherent in fixation and in reproducing the correct alignment of the components (Fig. 34-4).

Ulna shortening or osteotomies of the distal radius (or both)[13,44,46,89,106] are not within the scope of this chapter and are not indicated for the full blown, degenerative osteoarthritis of the DRUJ.

RESECTION ARTHROPLASTY

In 1880, Moore[85] described a resection of the distal end of the ulna in connection with a distal radioulnar fracture dislocation in which the ulna protruded through the skin. The ulnar head was sawed off to allow reduction. In 1886, von Lesser[119] performed the first elective excision of the head of the ulna. He successfully restored pronation and supination to the forearm of a 19-year-old locksmith who had developed a distal radioulnar ankylosis 9 months after a fracture of the wrist. Lauenstein,[70] spurred by von Lesser's experience, did a similar elective excision in 1887 to restore forearm rotation in a 36-year-old seaman with a distal radioulnar ankylosis. Van Lennep,[113] in 1897, and Angus,[5] in 1909, also reported this procedure, the latter for a 15-year-old with a chronic dislocation of the ulnar head. This technique was later popularized by Darrach[37-39] and now carries his name. The confusion of who described what operation on the distal ulna and when is the subject of a review by Buck-Gramcko.[28]

Darrach[38,39] stressed three major technical features of this operation: excision limited to the distal 1 in. (2.5 cm) of the ulna, subperiosteal removal of the ulnar head, and preservation of the styloid process (Figs. 34-2, *A right* and *B*). Preservation of the ulnar styloid was deemed to be important to protect the integrity of the ulnar collateral ligament. This was later supported by other authors.[36,42] Although controversy exists as to whether this structure should be called an ulnar collateral ligament, it does not invalidate this rationale.[40,64,108] Preserving the ulnar styloid assists in stabilizing the extensor carpi ulnaris (ECU) within its fibrous tunnel. Excision of the distal ulna in patients with rheumatoid arthritis was first reported by Smith-Petersen and coauthors[97] in 1943 and has since become an accepted procedure for the surgical treatment of rheumatoid wrists, although this also may lead to drastic complications.[*]

In 1972, Swanson[102] introduced the use of a silicone rubber implant, first developed in 1966, for the capping of the ulna after excision of the ulnar head (Fig. 34-5). This was an attempt to facilitate postoperative management of ulnar head resections, improve

---

* References 40,50,68,71,78,106,123.

* References 8,9,32,34,54,55,59,66,67,73,84,101.

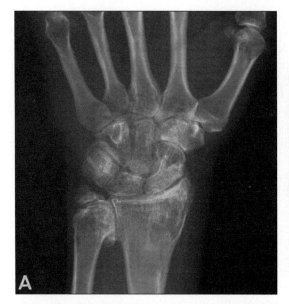

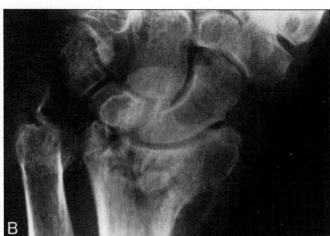

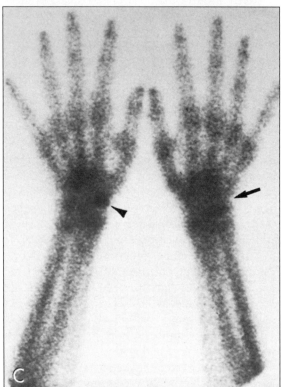

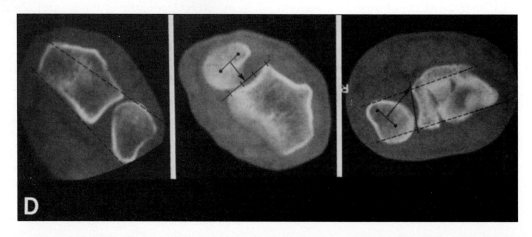

FIGURE 34-1

Degenerative arthritis of the distal radioulnar joint after distal radial fractures. **A,** Posteroanterior radiograph shows joint space narrowing and osteophyte formation. Note the fibrous nonunion of the ulnar styloid. **B,** Posteroanterior radiograph shows marked joint space malalignment associated with a late displaced distal radius fracture; displaced ulnar styloid. **C,** Bone scan of the wrist shows increased uptake on the left at the scaphotrapezial joint (*arrowhead*) and on the right from degenerative arthritis at the distal radioulnar joint (*arrow*). **D,** Computed tomographic scans of the wrist in supination (*left*) and pronation (*center*) and normal opposite wrist (*right*) show the joint space narrowing associated with degenerative arthritis.

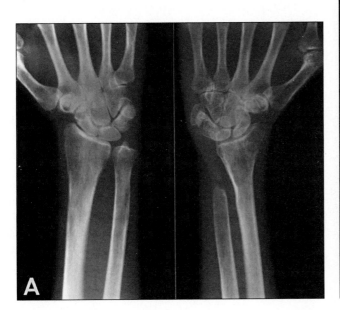

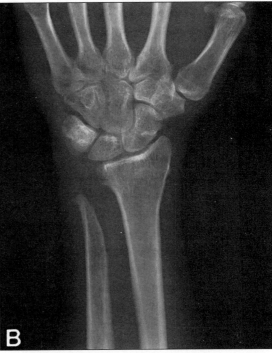

FIGURE 34-2

Darrach resection of the distal ulna associated with shortening of the radius. **A,** *Left:* Ulna positive variance with ulnocarpal impingement. *Right:* Excision of the distal ulna 2 cm proximal to the distal articular surface. Note the bone regeneration along the periosteal sleeve associated with ulna stump stability. **B,** Preferred method and length of Darrach resection of the distal ulna; the osteotomy cut is oblique radially to match the slope of the distal radius. Pronator quadratus interposition was performed to assist in stabilizing the distal ulna.

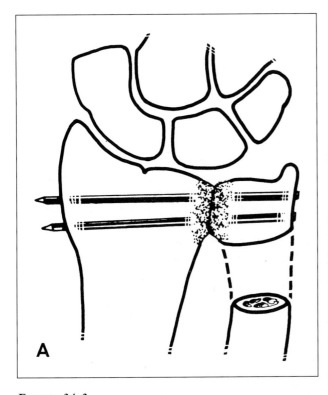

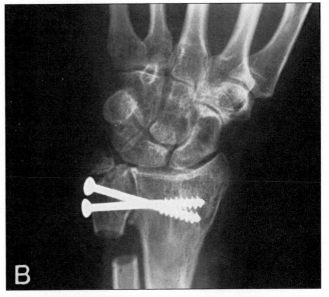

FIGURE 34-3

A, The Sauvé-Kapandji procedure involving fusion of the distal radioulnar joint combined with proximal ulna resection to produce a pseudarthrosis. **B,** Compression arthrodesis of the distal radioulnar joint with two cancellous lag screws.

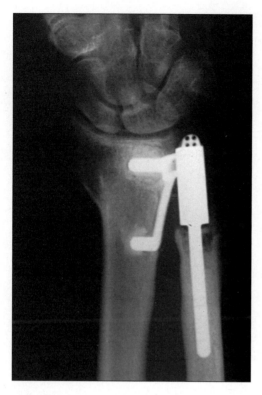

FIGURE 34-4

Prosthetic replacement of the distal radioulnar joint using a custom-designed, metallic modular component for the distal ulna that duplicates the convexity of the ulnar head, which is seated against the concave polyethylene surface of the sigmoid fossa of the distal radius. Both components are held in place with bone cement (polymethyl methacrylate). The ulnar collateral ligament complex is reattached to the distal end of the ulnar component with nonresorbable sutures.

on the reliability of the procedure, and decrease the potential for complications.[108] The success of bone capping had been demonstrated in amputation stumps in animals and in the control of overgrowth of long bones in juvenile amputees. According to Swanson,[103] benefits from ulnar capping include a more economical bone resection, maintenance of physiologic ulna length, and prevention of ulnocarpal shift. It would also provide a smooth surface for articulation with the radius and the carpus, aid gliding of overlying extensor tendons, and decrease the potential for bony overgrowth.[8,96,104,108] Recovery of function after operation would be less painful. After several years of experience, some authors concluded that this was an unnecessary addition to the simple excision of the distal ulna.* Complications of ulnar capping, which include subluxation or dislocation of the implant, excessive bone resorption under the implant, and silicone particulate synovitis, are frequent and difficult to correct (Fig. 34-6). Therefore, ulnar caps are infrequently used today (Fig. 34-7).

---

* References 14,33,35,77,86,97.

Darrach's technique has enjoyed an excellent reputation, until recently. In patients with rheumatoid arthritis and older patients with discomfort at the DRUJ after radial fracture who have relatively low demand, relief of wrist pain and improved motion are usually achieved.[75] Even in athletes there have been reports of satisfactory outcomes.[31]

In younger more vigorous patients, especially in women with lax ligamentous habitus, moderate to severe dysfunction may occur after resection of all or part of the ulnar head (Fig. 34-8). Bieber et al.[15] reported on 20 patients who had from one to seven later operations to try to improve a failed Darrach resection. af Ekenstam et al.[1] carefully evaluated a group of older patients with post-Colles' fracture ulnar head resections. They noted residual postoperative pain, decreased grip strength, and cosmetic deformities in approximately 50% and suggested that previous reports may have been unduly optimistic. Bell et al.[13] reported a small group of patients with painful snapping on pronation and supination in whom a "scallop sign" developed on the medial metaphyseal cortical surface from impingement of the ulnar stump.

Complications of the various forms of ulnar head resection include instability of the ulnar stump, ulnar stump impingement, carpal supination, ulnar translation, snapping tendons, and extensor tendon rupture. Often these problems occur together and are interrelated. It is also worth noting that even in the elderly the narrowed forearm with prominent ulnar carpus may be cosmetically disturbing.

Bell et al.,[13] McKee and Richards,[75] and Bieber et al.[15] have each pointed out the dynamic radioulnar convergence that occurs with gripping. In addition, the normal dorsal translation of the ulna with pronation and palmar translation with supination are often enhanced with the loss of the ulnar head constraints. This leads to snapping and impingement with rotation. The narrowing of the interosseous space also relaxes the interosseous membrane, further reducing axial stability. Direct impingement against the radial metaphysis leads to the erosive scallop sign.[13,15]

These problems probably account for the controversy that exists regarding the amount of ulna to be removed, preservation of the styloid, and extraperiosteal versus subperiosteal dissection. The risk of these complications may be minimized by minimal resection and careful reconstruction of the soft-tissue support. This includes the periosteal sleeve and fascial layers dorsal to the ulna. A palmar capsular restraint of ligament or muscle has also been proposed to stabilize the ulna.[18,61] In patients with rheumatoid arthritis with diminished functional demands and generalized disease, good results are anticipated, except progressive ulnar translation may be encouraged.

In younger, more vigorous patients, complications may be expected more frequently. Therefore, alternative

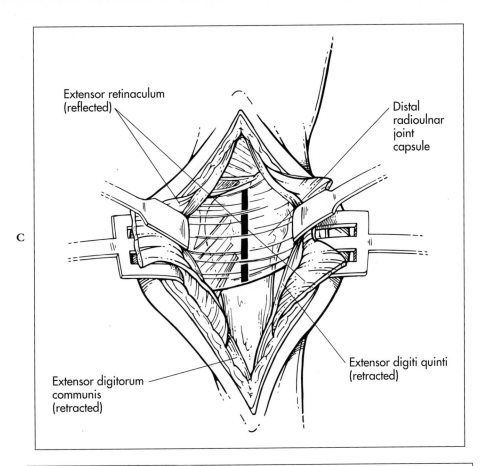

C

Extensor retinaculum
(reflected)

Distal
radioulnar
joint
capsule

Extensor digiti quinti
(retracted)

Extensor digitorum
communis
(retracted)

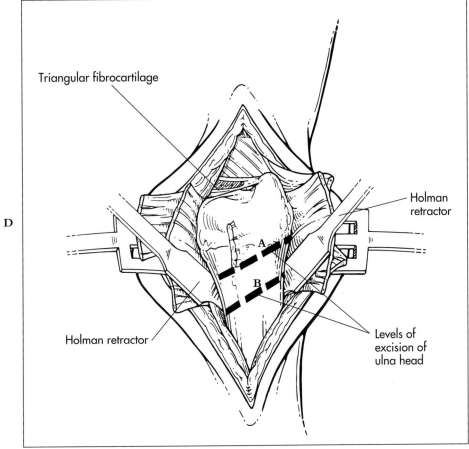

D

Triangular fibrocartilage

Holman
retractor

A

B

Holman retractor

Levels of
excision of
ulna head

FIGURE 34-9, CONT'D.

C, After the extensor retinaculum flaps are elevated and reflected, the underlying capsule and synovial sac are divided longitudinally (*dashed line*). **D,** The neck of the ulna is exposed subperiosteally and is divided along an oblique plane (*dashed line*) either (*A*) just proximal to the proximal rim of sigmoid cavity or (*B*) 2.5 cm proximal to ulnar head.

Continued.

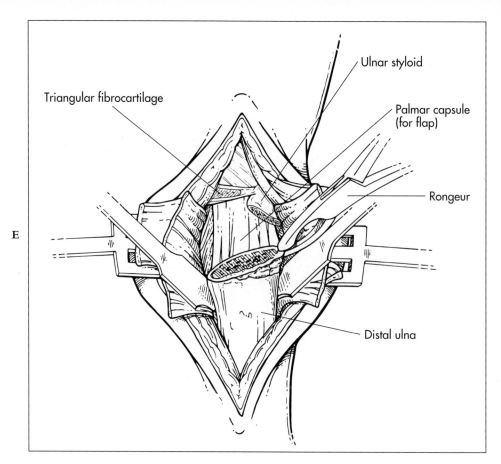

E

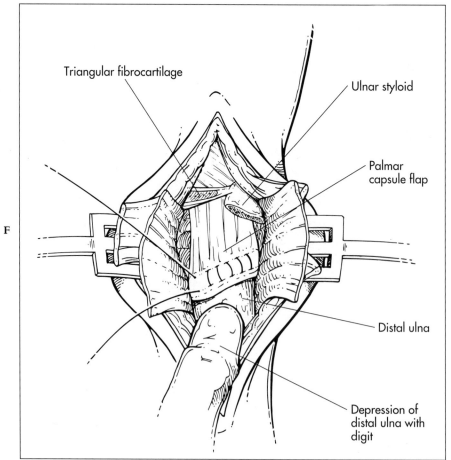

F

FIGURE 34-9, CONT'D.

E, The sharp margins of the cut end of the ulna are rounded off. A palmar capsular flap can be created to attach to the distal ulna. **F,** The palmar capsular flap is freed, divided proximally and left attached distally, and brought over the dorsum of the ulna to which it is sutured while an assistant holds the ulna depressed in a palmar direction.

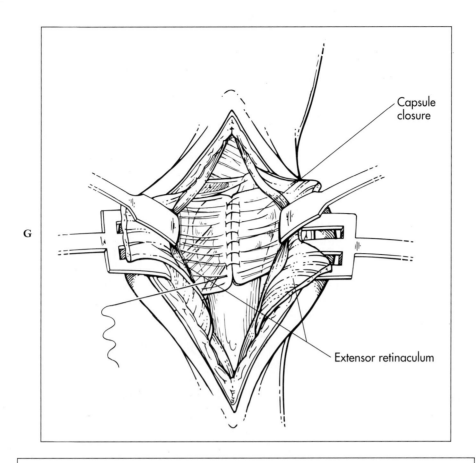

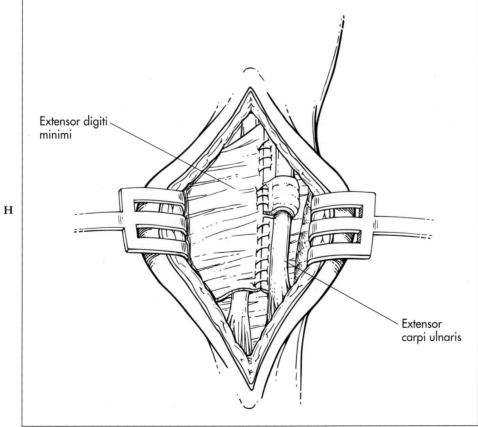

FIGURE 34-9, CONT'D.

G, Dorsal capsule and retinaculum are imbricated and closed with sutures. **H,** A loop of retinaculum is passed around the ECU tendon and is sutured to itself to stabilize the ECU tendon. *(Modified from Taleisnik J.[105] By permission of the publisher.)*

A cut along a plane directed distally and radially allows a more economical excision, decreases the likelihood of impingement against the radius, and leaves a longer medial support mechanism. Others have used a minimal resection, a fraction of the inch recommended by Darrach, giving the remaining ulna a bullet shape and, again, carefully repairing the periosteum and all dorsal support.[41] The edges of the ulnar stump are carefully rounded off until no sharp areas can be felt by palpation (Fig. 34-9, E). The periosteal sleeve, which has remained attached to the triangular fibrocartilage, should be securely plicated.[88,112] Blatt and Ashworth[18] proposed that a capsular flap based distally be raised from the palmar capsule (Fig. 34-9, F), brought over the dorsal rim of the ulna, and sutured through drill holes by using nonabsorbable material, while the ulna is depressed palmarward. If on hyperpronation, release of the pressure on the ulna shows the fixation remains firm, no additional support is used. The DRUJ capsule is then closed (Fig. 34-9, G). If there are any questions as to stability, the forearm is kept supinated throughout the remainder of the procedure and early postoperative period.

There are many variations on resection of the distal ulna, including direction of osteotomy (Fig. 34-10, A), length (Fig. 34-10, B), and preservation of periosteal sleeve (Fig. 34-10, C). Most authorities now recommend a short rather than long length of distal ulna resection, preservation of all distal ulna attachments (including periosteum and ulnar styloid), and oblique radial osteotomy to enhance ulna length and encourage periosteal sleeve regeneration. Stabilization of the ulnar stump may also be achieved by the use of one-half of the flexor carpi ulnaris, which is divided proximally and reflected back to the pisiform.[26,27,57] The free end is then placed through a drill hole in the resected surface of the distal ulna and then back onto itself at the pisiform (Fig. 34-11). An alternative procedure uses the ECU, which is freed proximally and reflected to its insertion.[111] The free end is then passed through the ulnar collateral ligament and dorsal capsule, through the end of the distal ulna, and finally into the interosseous membrane (Fig. 34-12). Both of these procedures accomplish three objectives: 1) elevate the ulnar carpus, 2) stabilize the distal ulna, and 3) support the distal ulna to the medial or ulnar side of the wrist. The second procedure also maintains the ECU in a corrected dorsal position. Tethering the mobile carpus to a detached ulnar stump is marginally sufficient for stabilization and may restrict radial deviation. In addition, such tenodesis becomes inefficient in ulnar deviation, as the tenodesis becomes slack. Clayton[33] recommended suture of the ulnopalmar capsule to the dorsum of the distal radius to elevate and derotate the ulnar carpus. This capsuloplasty more closely reproduces the direction and function of the ulnocarpal complex. A large Kirschner wire across the ulna and radius may be used to maintain supination until stability is achieved at approximately 3 weeks postoperatively.

The rest of the soft-tissue repair is completed with the forearm in supination. The capsule dorsal to the ulna can usually be securely repaired over the ulnar stump. The tunnel of the EDQ tendon is reapproximated. The wound is closed in layers, and a well-padded dressing is applied. Drains are rarely required. Immobilization in supination for the first 7 to 10 days decreases postoperative pain and discomfort. This is followed by a program of gradual exercises from the resting position of supination to full pronation. A short arm splint is used for an additional 3 weeks if there is any question as to the stability of the ulnar stump. Immobilization is discontinued after 6 weeks.

PRONATOR QUADRATUS INTERPOSITION

An alternative approach for stabilization of the distal ulna that is preferred by one of us (L.K.R.) is use of the pronator quadratus as an interposition material and dynamic depressor of the ulna on the radius (Fig. 34-13). Johnson and Shrewsbury[62] demonstrated that the pronator quadratus has two heads superficial and deep and that contracture of the pronator quadratus causes compression of the ulna against the radius. By transfer of the pronator quadratus from the palmar to the dorsal aspect of the ulna after distal ulna resection, one decreases radioulnar compression and improves stability of the distal ulna.[61]

The operative procedure is similar to that described above for distal ulna resection (Darrach resection) with sharp dissection of the pronator quadratus from the distal ulna. The ulna is further dissected subperiosteally and resected within 1.5 to 2.0 cm proximal to the ulnar head. The pronator quadratus is then redirected dorsally from the palmar aspect and sutured over the distal stump of the ulna (Fig. 34-13).

PARTIAL RESECTION ARTHROPLASTIES

In an attempt to solve the problems associated with the Darrach operation, Bowers,[20] in 1985, and Watson and co-workers,[122] in 1986, proposed very similar procedures consisting of a limited resection of the articulating surfaces of the ulnar head, leaving intact the ulna-ulnar styloid axis and its soft-tissue support.[22] Essentially identical principles, attributed to John C. Colwill, were applied to the treatment of patients with rheumatoid arthritis by Vázquez Vela in 1973.[116]

Minami and coauthors[80] observed that pain relief may not be as complete with partial resection arthroplasties as with the Darrach procedure, but stability and strength are better preserved. Partial resection arthroplasties require even more meticulous attention

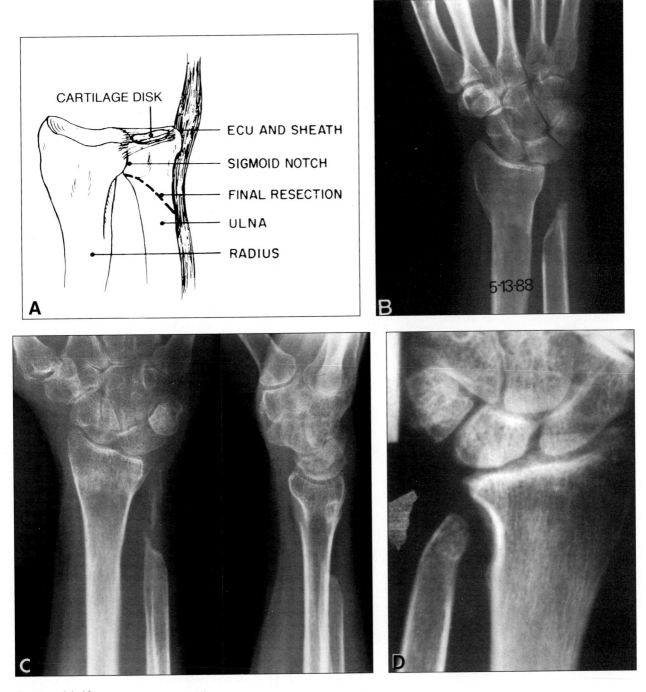

FIGURE 34-10

Darrach resection. **A,** The original technique of distal ulna resection has the osteotomy beveled proximally and ulnarly as recommended by Nolan and Eaton.[88] **B,** Preferred technique of distal ulna resection with the osteotomy angled distally away from the radius and the ulna divided 2 cm proximal to the distal end of the radius, preserving a periosteal hinge to the carpus. **C,** Darrach resection 3 cm proximal to the distal end of the radius has good stability, no impingement, and periosteal regeneration. This result questions the concept of the "limited" or short resection of the distal ulna. **D,** Impingement sign of scalloping of the distal radius. *ECU,* extensor carpi ulnaris. *(A and D, From Nolan WB III, Eaton RG.[88] By permission of JB Lippincott.)*

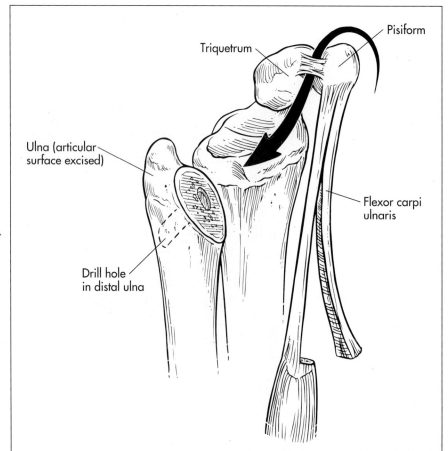

A

Triquetrum

Pisiform

Ulna (articular surface excised)

Flexor carpi ulnaris

Drill hole in distal ulna

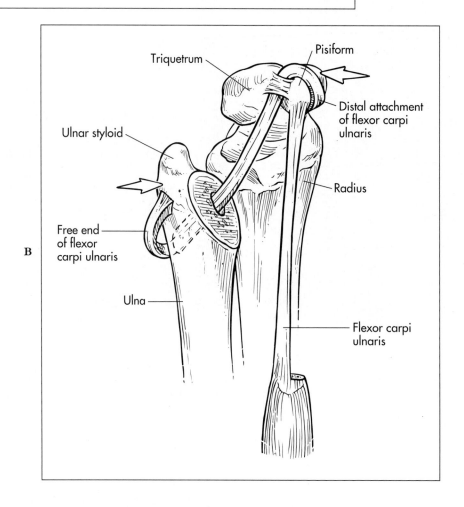

B

Triquetrum

Pisiform

Ulnar styloid

Distal attachment of flexor carpi ulnaris

Radius

Free end of flexor carpi ulnaris

Ulna

Flexor carpi ulnaris

FIGURE 34-11

Stability of the ulna stump produced by the Hui-Linscheid[57] techniques. **A,** Half of the flexor carpi ulnaris is reflected distally at the pisiform. **B,** The free tendon end is then passed through the base of the distal ulna (ulnar articular surface excised). Arrows indicate direction of tendon graft from pisiform through distal ulna and back to pisiform.

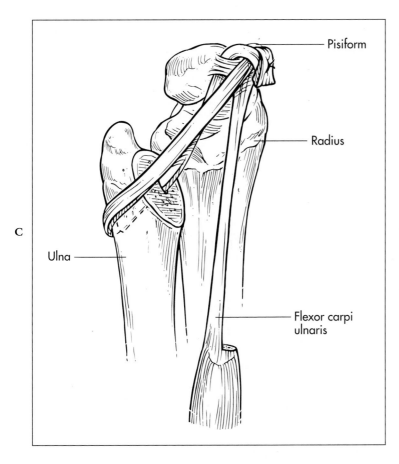

C

Pisiform

Radius

Ulna

Flexor carpi
ulnaris

Figure 34-11, cont'd.

C, The free end is then passed back onto itself to lift and correct carpal supination and stabilize the distal ulna. *(Modified from Hui FC, Linscheid RL.[57] Copyright, American Society for Surgery of the Hand, by permission of Churchill Livingstone.)*

to detail than simple excisions. Because the palmar portion of the remaining ulna is often poorly visualized at operation, insufficient bone may be removed from this area, leading to painful postoperative impingement between ulna and radius during forearm rotation.[48] This problem may be prevented if intraoperative radiographs are routinely obtained. After operation, radioulnar impingement is best visualized on axial computed tomographic images.[48]

Even when meticulously performed, these techniques may present problems. Distal radioulnar convergence necessarily occurs, particularly during forearm rotation and gripping, as a result of muscular contraction. Deletion of the ulna prevents transverse as well as axial loadbearing, a problem shared with the Darrach operation.[22,110]

Bowers[22] discussed his experience with the procedure he described: 1) the hemiresection interposition technique (Fig. 34-14) requires a functional triangular fibrocartilage to succeed, although repair of triangular fibrocartilage lesions may be adequate[79]; 2) styloid-carpal impingement must be anticipated and corrected; 3) in nonrheumatoid wrists, it is advantageous to elevate the ECU tendon within its intact sheath, to be replaced after the hemiarthroplasty is completed; 4) the procedure does not restore stability to an already unstable

DRUJ; and 5) hemiarthroplasty may fail to restore rotation to long-standing pronation contractures, because of the loss of ligamentous and interosseous membrane flexibility.

It is apparent from these stipulations that, other than for less-demanding wrists with rheumatoid arthritis, the hemiresection interposition finds its best application in the treatment of osteoarthritis of the DRUJ.[10,20,44,58,82] In this situation, there is pain during pronation or supination and limited forearm rotation, but with satisfactory DRUJ stability from well-preserved support mechanisms, particularly the interosseous membrane and triangular fibrocartilage.

HEMIRESECTION INTERPOSITION TECHNIQUE

Bowers[20] cautioned "the surgeon must understand the functional goals of reconstruction and be willing to vary the technique according to the lesion presenting in each individual case." DRUJ osteoarthritis lends itself to a simplified technique; the goal is to ablate the contiguous surfaces involved in patients without ulnar instability. The surgical approach is similar to that described for the Darrach procedure. It is best to elevate the ECU

Text continued on p. 808.

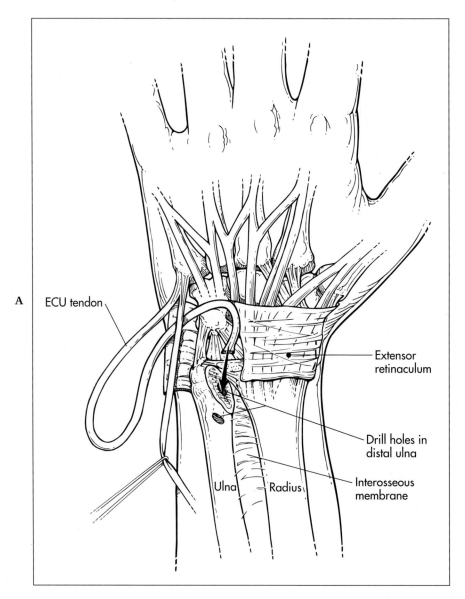

FIGURE 34–12

Stability of the ulna by using the extensor carpi ulnaris (*ECU*) (Tsai) technique. **A,** The ECU is free proximally and reflected distally to its insertion. The extensor retinaculum was previously reflected.

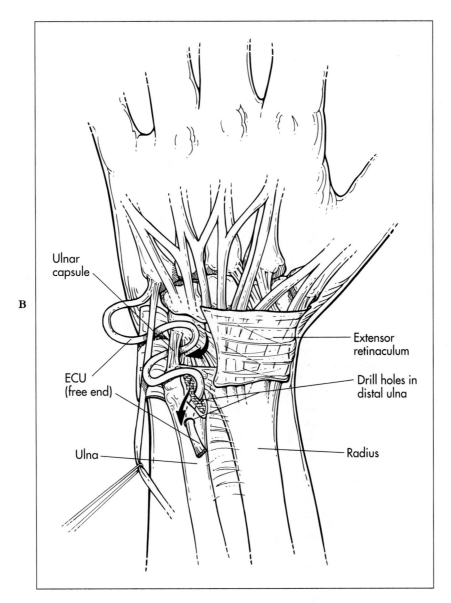

B

FIGURE 34-12, CONT'D.

B, The free tendon end is passed through the ulnar collateral ligament and dorsal capsule. It is then passed through the free end of the distal ulna, after ulna resection, and then passed through a drill hole in the dorsal cortex.   *Continued.*

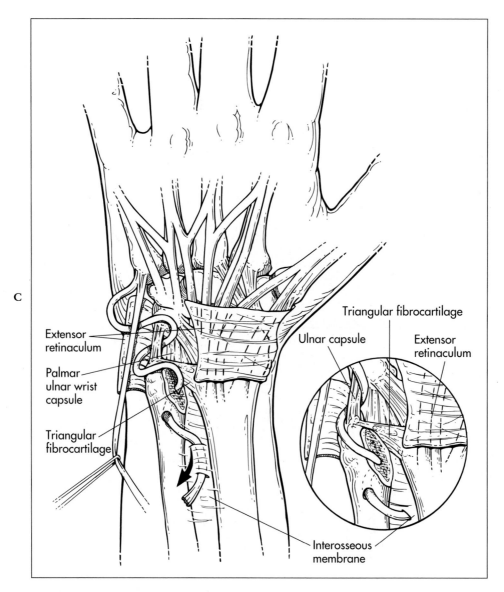

FIGURE 34-12, CONT'D.

C, It is woven through the interosseous membrane, and the free end is tightened with the ulnar head depressed and the forearm in midrotation.

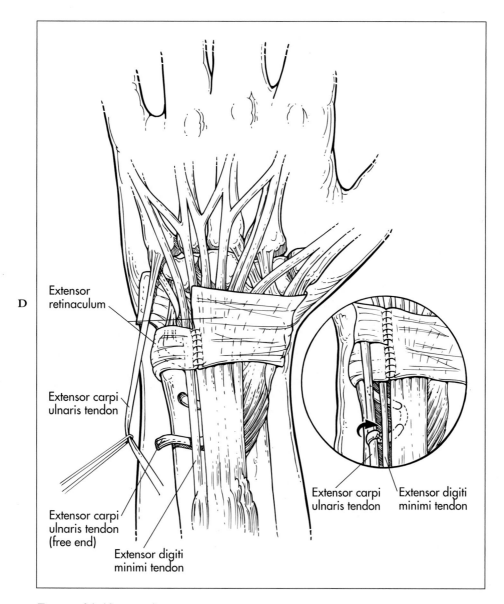

D

Extensor
retinaculum

Extensor carpi
ulnaris tendon

Extensor carpi
ulnaris tendon
(free end)

Extensor digiti
minimi tendon

Extensor carpi
ulnaris tendon

Extensor digiti
minimi tendon

FIGURE 34–12, CONT'D.

D, The remaining strip is placed dorsal to the ulna around the ECU tendon. The extensor retinaculum stabilizes the ECU tendon over the dorsal aspect of the distal ulna. *(From Tsai T-M et al.[111] Copyright, American Society for Surgery of the Hand, by permission of Churchill Livingstone.)*

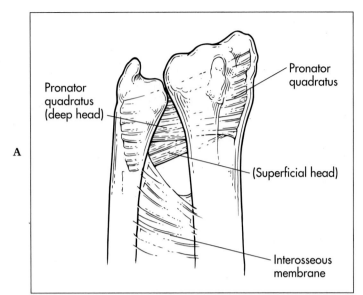

A

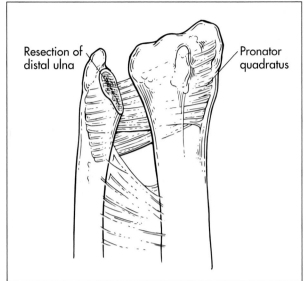

B

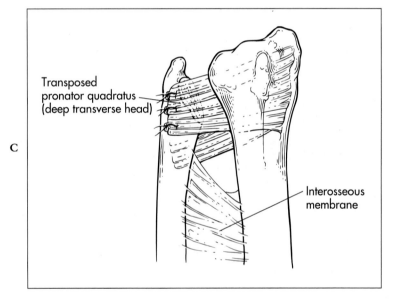

C

FIGURE 34-13

Pronator quadratus interposition. **A,** Dorsal view of the wrist shows the pronator quadratus with superficial and deep heads, originating from the pronator crest. **B,** Dorsal view shows resected distal ulna and normal position of the pronator quadratus. **C,** Dorsal view after the pronator quadratus is transposed between the distal radius and resected head of the distal ulna and resutured on the dorsal surface of the ulna with the ulnar head depressed.

tendon within its intact sheath (Fig. 34-14).[21,22] Exposure through the EDQ compartment allows division of the dorsal capsule longitudinally, close to its insertion on the radius. Soft-tissue attachments along the medial surface of the ulna and ulnar styloid are preserved to avoid ulnar instability. Next, the ulnar head is osteotomized obliquely from the base of the styloid to the radial aspect of the shaft. The pronator quadratus is stripped from the bone with a narrow fascial-periosteal band and tagged. The shaft, particularly along the palmar surface, is shaped to a rounded cross section tapering distally. Osteophytes arising from the radius are sought and excised. Restoration of free pronation and supination is now checked.

Bowers[21,22] recommended that a ball of tendon or muscle approximating the size of the resected head be placed in the void left by the bony excision to maintain the radioulnar space. This "soft-tissue" implant, obtained from the palmaris longus, ECU, or flexor carpi ulnaris, is held in place with a few sutures and closure of the overlying soft tissue. An alternative is to suture the previously tagged pronator quadratus to the dorsal margin of the ulna to serve as both interposition and palmar stabilizer for the ulna (Johnson procedure) (Fig. 34-13). Closure is completed. A short arm splint is sufficient for postoperative immobilization. This is worn continuously for 2 to 3 weeks, then decreasingly as the patient regains forearm rotation and confidence.

TECHNIQUE OF MATCHED DISTAL ULNAR RESECTION

Watson et al.[121,122] performed this procedure through a transverse incision proximal to the radioulnar joint (Fig. 34-15). A "spread technique" is used

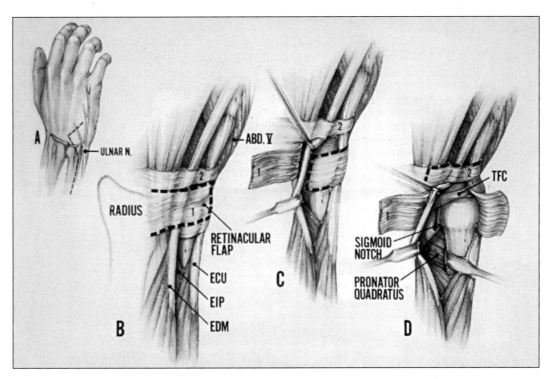

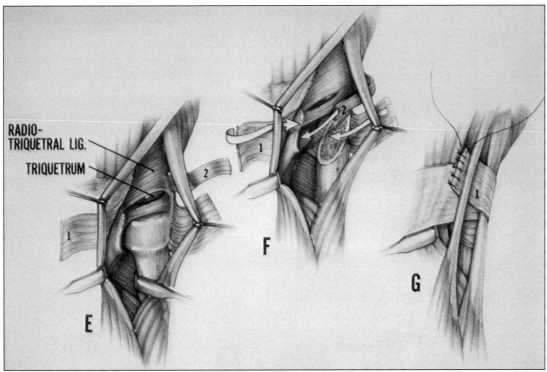

FIGURE 34-14

A, Hemiresection arthroplasty after Bowers. Operative exposure of the distal radioulnar joint. The incision, emphasizing the location of the ulnar sensory nerve (*N.*). **B,** The dorsal retinacular structures and outline of the first retinacular flap with capsule beneath. *ABD.,* abductor; *ECU,* extensor carpi ulnaris; *EDM,* extensor digiti minimi; *EIP,* extensor indicis pollicis. **C,** The proximal retinacular flap (*1*) and capsular incision (*dashed line*). **D,** The capsular flap reflected with exposure of the sigmoid notch, using retractors or a baby lamina spreader. *TFC,* triangular fibrocartilage. **E,** Retinacular flap (*2*) is developed and reflected to expose the radiotriquetral ligaments (*LIG.*) and the TFC and its carpal face. The ECU should be left in its sheath and the tendon and sheath reflected as a unit to avoid potential dorsal destabilization. **F,** The ulnar head has been resected and the capsular flap covers the cancellous resection area. The dorsal capsule is sutured to the palmar capsule as interposition material. Retinacular flap (*2*) is used to cover the radioulnar articulation by suturing it to the previous capsular attachment on the radius. **G,** The first retinacular flap (*1*) is used to stabilize the ECU tendon. This step is unnecessary if the ECU has been left undisturbed. Interposition of soft tissue is a modification of the original description of the procedure and is performed because of the tendency of the radial and ulnar shafts to approximate one another after resection of the ulnar head. The basis of this procedure is a functionally adequate or reconstructable TFC. (*From Bowers WH.*[21] *By permission of the publisher.*)

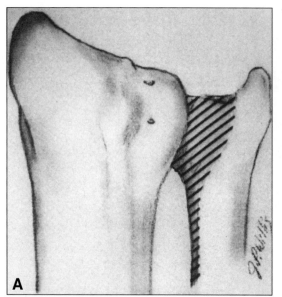

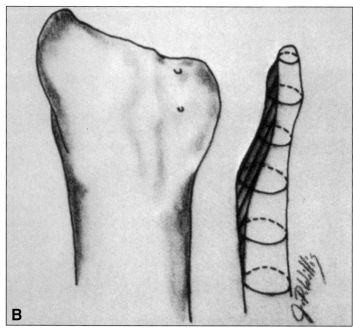

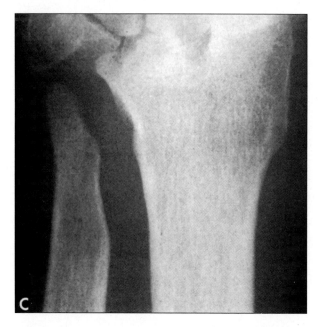

FIGURE 34-15

Matched resection of the distal ulna. The technique is performed through a transverse incision made just proximal to the distal radio-ulnar joint. The soft tissues are spread to separate the cutaneous nerves. **A,** The ulna is resected in a convex arc matching the concave metaphysis of the distal radius. One retains the full length of the ulna, including the ulnar styloid. **B,** The resection leaves a sloping cylinder of ulna with the same distance between the radius and the ulna from full pronation to full supination. If there is impingement during rotation of the forearm, only the necessary amount of distal ulna is removed to allow for clearance. The periosteum and ligament attachments to the ulna are left intact. There is no soft-tissue interposition with this procedure. **C,** An example of a successful result 6.5 years after matched ulnar resection procedure. *(From Watson HK et al.[122] Copyright, American Society for Surgery of the Hand, by permission of Churchill Livingstone.)*

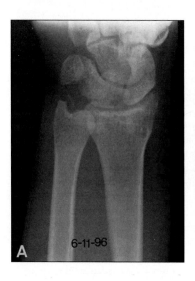

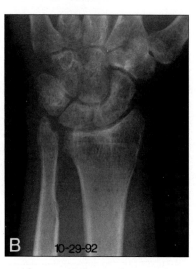

FIGURE 34-16

Painful left distal radioulnar joint in a patient with a previous distal radius fracture and ulnar styloid fracture. **A,** Preoperative radiograph shows reactive bone at the distal radioulnar joint and ulnar styloid fracture repair. **B,** Matched resection of the distal ulna was performed with the addition of soft-tissue interposition with pronator quadratus muscle flap. Improved pain and forearm rotation resulted with an increase in motion from a total 45° preoperatively to 120° postoperatively forearm rotation.

to protect superficial nerves and veins and to provide satisfactory exposure. The three-quarter arc of ulnar head, which articulates with the radius during pronation and supination, is resected along a segment of ulnar shaft approximately 4.5 cm long. The resection creates a long, sloping convex curve which "matches" the opposite concave curve of the radius in three dimensions (Figs. 34-15, *A* and *B*). This diminishes frictional disparities between radius and ulna during forearm rotation by improving congruence of the sigmoid notch. This excision leaves behind a 90° arc of the ulnar medial wall, the ulnar styloid, and its support mechanisms (Fig. 34-16). Scar formation surrounding the end of the ulna adds to its stability and coats the opposing bony surfaces. Only if the remaining ulna is too long and impacts against the carpus is a minimal resection of the distal ulna performed subperiosteally to retain ligamentous support. Range of motion exercises are allowed at 1 week postoperatively.

RADIOULNAR FUSION AND ULNAR OSTEOTOMY

In 1935, Bazy and Galtier[12] reported a technique to create an abutment for the carpus after excision of the ulnar head. The sigmoid notch of the radius and its underlying bony support were turned distally on an intact distal cortical hinge "like a drawbridge" to cover the ulnocarpal complex to which this bony flap was sutured. A year later, Sauvé and Kapandji[95] observed that this small bony shelf was rather fragile and prone to break at its hinge as it was rotated. They proposed a radioulnar fusion combined with a proximal pseudarthrosis to allow for restoration of forearm pronation and supination for isolated dislocations of the DRUJ. This technique was erroneously attributed by Steindler[98,99] and Steindler and Marxer[100] and later by Gonçalves[52] to Lauenstein. Steindler omitted a reference to Lauenstein's alleged description of this technique.[107] Lauenstein[70] described an excision of the ulnar head, the procedure we now erroneously attribute to Darrach.

In 1937, Vergoz and Choussat[117] reported their experience using "the new technique of Sauvé and Kapandji." Bunnell[29] also noted the head of the ulna may be fused to the radius, and a segment of the neck of the ulna excised to restore pronation and supination. Baldwin,[11] in 1921, proposed a similar technique to preserve the head of the ulna but without distal radioulnar arthrodesis. Baldwin's operation was mentioned by McMurray in his textbook *Practice of Orthopedic Surgery*[76] and was resurrected by Kersley[65] and by Thomas and Matthewson.[109] According to Gonçalves,[52] both operations share the advantages of the Darrach procedure but avoid its potential

complications of progressive ulnar translation of the carpus, ulnar deviation, and instability with pain and weakness of grip. Gonçalves recommended that the Baldwin operation be used for blocked forearm rotation secondary to malunion of radial fractures with an intact radioulnar joint and that what he called the Lauenstein (Darrach) procedure be reserved for the abnormal DRUJ that is subluxed, dislocated, or arthritic. Alnot and Leroux[4] used the Sauvé-Kapandji operation for treatment of the rheumatoid wrist, further recommended in subsequent reports.[3,105,118]

Although in our experience complications are less frequent with the Sauvé-Kapandji operation than with the simple excision of the ulnar head, the potential problem of the unstable ulnar stump remains.[19,83,120] There are several factors that support preservation of the ulnar head.[105,107] First, an uninterrupted surface is maintained for articulation with the carpal condyle (Figs. 34-17, *A* and *B*). Second, a more physiologic pattern of transmission of forces from the hand to the forearm is preserved (see Chapter 11).[90] The anatomic relationships among radius, ulna, and carpus are precise, and even minor modifications lead to significant changes in the load patterns.[90] Therefore, keeping the ulnar head in a normal alignment with the radius is desirable.

Third, the triangular fibrocartilage and the contiguous structures are responsible for distal radioulnar and ulnocarpal stabilization. The dorsal-ulnar corner of the radius anchors the origins of the dorsal distal radioulnar ligament and the insertion of the fifth retinacular septum for the EDQ. The ECU and its fibrous tunnel provide for ulnocarpal support regardless of forearm rotation.[40,60,64,108] This distinct tunnel is further strengthened proximally by a discrete band of transverse fibers that fuse with the epimysium of the ECU muscle and longitudinal fibers to form the "linea jugata."[40] The linea jugata originates distally from the base of the ulnar styloid, and it spreads obliquely proximal in a dorsal and medial direction to coalesce with the supratendinous retinaculum and the pars profunda of the antebrachial fascia (Fig. 34-18).[108]

With the forearm in full pronation, the ECU tendon lies in a groove within the ulnar head. In supination and ulnar deviation, this tendon tends to bend like a bowstring from its groove over the ulnar styloid. In this position, the medial wall and the linea jugata establish a block to abnormal displacement during forced supination. Maintenance of the carpal support provided by the triangular fibrocartilage and of the fibrous system that surrounds the ECU tendon is helpful in maintaining a normal ulnocarpal relationship. Retaining the ulnar head assists in minimizing the potential for the development of two complications of simple excision of the ulnar head: the palmar subluxation of the carpus and painful subluxation of the ECU over the ulna stump during pronation and

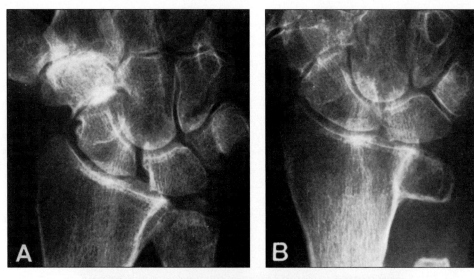

FIGURE 34-17

A wrist in a patient with rheumatoid arthritis who presented with synovitis and painful radioulnar joint motion. Treatment included radioulnar fusion and proximal pseudarthrosis (Sauvé-Kapandji procedure). **A,** Preoperative radiograph shows ulnar carpal translation combined with cystic resorption at the distal radioulnar joint. **B,** Postoperative radiograph shows solid fusion of the distal radioulnar joint and support of the ulnar translocated lunate. **C,** Preferred fusion technique includes joint resection, cancellous bone grafting, and internal fixation with two or more Kirschner wires. *(From Taleisnik J.[105] By permission of the publisher.)*

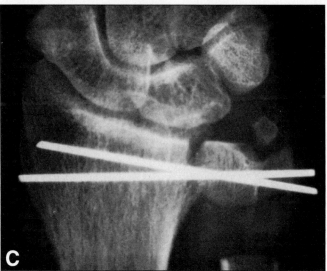

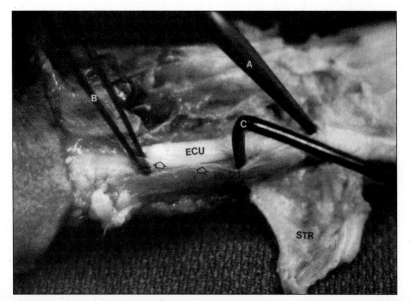

FIGURE 34-18

Anatomic specimen. The examining probe (*A*) is introduced within fibrous tunnel of extensor carpi ulnaris (*ECU*) tendon sheath. Supratendinous retinaculum (*STR*) reflected ulnarward. Linea jugata (*arrows*) elevated between forceps (*B*) and probe (*C*). *(From Taleisnik J.[107] By permission of Lippincott-Raven.)*

supination of the forearm. Finally, preservation of the ulnar head results in a more normal wrist contour, which is cosmetically more acceptable.

The Sauvé-Kapandji procedure retains an undesirable feature of the Darrach operation, the potential for an unstable proximal ulnar stump (Fig. 34-19) and regeneration of bone (ossification).[19,83,120] A review[107] of 40 Sauvé-Kapandji operations showed such instability in 7. Three responded to prolonged splinting and three more to surgical stabilization. Only 1 of the 40 wrists showed a persistent instability. In theory, preservation of a fixed distal anchor point (the ulnar head) for the dorsal support mechanism of the ulna should minimize the seriousness and frequency of this complication. Therefore, a meticulous surgical technique and a longer period of postoperative immobilization when ulnar instability is present intraoperatively may minimize this problem. This review indicated that when this operation is used for clearly unstable distal radioulnar articulations, the likelihood of postoperative instability is the greatest. This problem is shared to a large extent by all excisional arthroplasties of the distal ulna. The Sauvé-Kapandji operation provides a reasonably satisfactory answer to the problem of the osteoarthritic DRUJ.[7,63,69,105]

OPERATIVE TECHNIQUE

The surgical approach is similar to that described for the Darrach operation (Fig. 34-20, *A*). After the neck of the ulna is exposed, the periosteum along the intended site for the pseudarthrosis is excised. The ulnar head is grasped with a large towel clip to manipulate the head of the ulna after the osteotomy and to preserve its orientation in relation to the radius and the ECU tunnel. An osteotomy is performed transversely proximal to the margin of the flare of the ulnar head, 1 to 2 mm from the border of its articular cartilage (Fig. 34-20, *B*). When an ulna plus variant needs correction, the ulnar head is recessed proximally in the sigmoid cavity of the radius.[63,105] After this radioulnar relationship is reestablished, a 12-mm segment of ulna is excised. The head of the ulna is then hinged away from

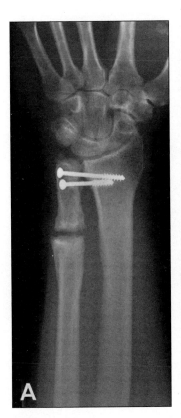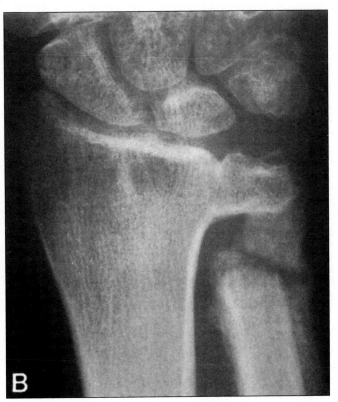

FIGURE 34-19

Sauvé-Kapandji procedure must be performed properly. It consists of at least 1 cm of bone resection at the proximal pseudarthrosis site and internal fixation of the distal radioulnar joint with two cortical cancellous lag screws. Bone graft from the distal radius or the iliac crest is placed into the denuded distal radioulnar joint, which is then compressed with the lag screws. Failure to bone graft may lead to incomplete fusion of radioulnar joint. **A,** Short length of pseudarthrosis and failed fusion at the distal radioulnar joint produced a painful result with restricted motion. **B,** Postoperative ossification at the site of the pseudarthrosis. *(From Taleisnik J.[107] By permission of Lippincott-Raven.)*

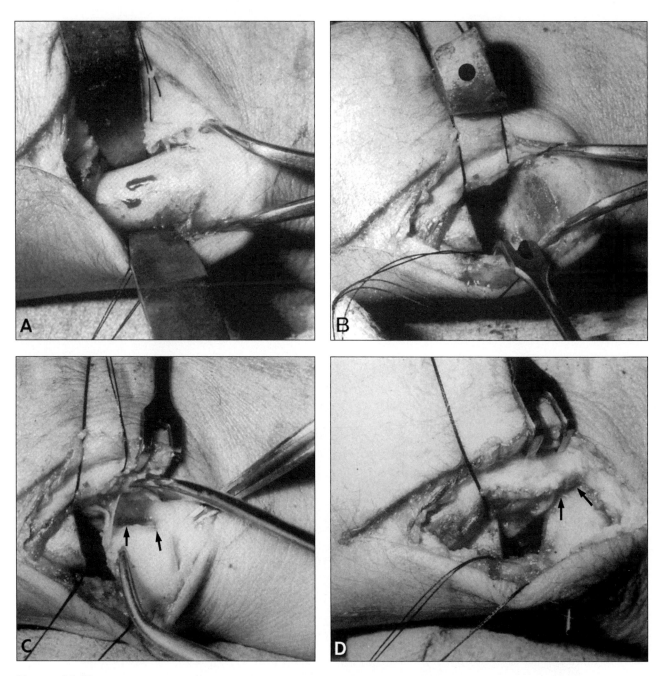

FIGURE 34-20

Surgical technique. **A,** The head and neck of the distal ulna are exposed through a longitudinal incision centered over the ulnar head between the extensor carpi ulnaris and the extensor digiti quinti. The dorsal branch of the ulnar nerve remains distal to the incision. The pretendinous retinaculum is exposed and incised along the compartment of the extensor digiti quinti, leaving the entire tunnel of the extensor carpi ulnaris undisturbed. **B,** A segment of ulna 12 to 15 mm (*black dot*) is excised, with the distal line of incision just proximal to the distal radioulnar joint. **C,** Distal radioulnar articulation (*arrows*) is exposed by rotating the distal ulna with a towel clip or bone-holding forceps. The excision of sub-chondral bone includes both ulnar head and sigmoid notch of the distal radius down to subchondral cancellous bone. A bone graft may be indicated. **D,** The ulnar head (*arrows*) is brought against the distal radius and pinned in position with two 0.54-in. or 0.45-in. Kirschner wires driven from the ulna through both cortices of the radius. The pronator quadratus attached to sutures is next brought into the pseudarthrosis gap and sutured through drill holes placed in the distal margin of the ulnar stump. This serves to preserve the pseudarthrosis and stabilize the ulnar stump. (*From Taleisnik J.[107] By permission of Lippincott-Raven.*)

the radius to expose both opposing radioulnar articular surfaces. These are denuded until cancellous bone is exposed (Fig. 34-20, *C*). The ulnar head is then brought against the radius and pinned by using two Kirschner wires driven from the ulna and through the radius until their tips are palpable under the skin on the radial aspect of the wrist (Figs. 34-17, *C* and 34-20, *D*). On the medial side, they are cut flush with the cortex of the head of the ulna. One or two lag screws may be used instead to provide compression (Figs. 34-3, *B* and 34-19, *A*).[63,94] The Kirschner wires may be removed easily after the fusion becomes solid, which occurs usually by 6 weeks. Bone grafts obtained from the portion of the ulna that was excised may be inserted into the fusion site or bone graft may be harvested from the

distal radius proximal to the fusion site. The pronator quadratus is next brought into the pseudarthrosis gap, from its palmar position, and is sutured to holes drilled through the dorsal margin of the ulnar stump. This serves two purposes: preserving the pseudarthrosis and stabilizing the ulna.

Below-elbow immobilization postoperatively is usually sufficient. If the ulnar stump appears unstable, however, the elbow may also be included for the first 3 weeks with the forearm in supination. A more proximal pseudarthrosis with minimal bone resection may preserve more stability through the interosseous membrane support. Comparative studies regarding different methods of performing the Sauvé-Kapandji procedure have not been performed.

REFERENCES

1. af Ekenstam F, Engkvist O, Wadin K: Results from resection of the distal end of the ulna after fractures of the lower end of the radius, *Scand J Plast Reconstr Surg* 16:177-181, 1982.

2. Albert SM, Wohl MD, Rechtman AM: Treatment of the disrupted radio-ulnar joint, *J Bone Joint Surg Am* 45:1373-1381, 1963.

3. Alnot JY, Fauroux L: La synovectomie réaxation stabilisation du poignet rhumatoïde. A propos d'une serie de 104 cas avec un recul moyen de 5 ans, *Rev Rhum Mal Ostéoartic* 59:196-206, 1992.

4. Alnot JY, Leroux D: Realignment stabilization synovectomy in the rheumatoid wrist. A study of twenty-five cases, *Ann Chir Main* 4:294-305, 1985.

5. Angus: Dislocation of head of ulna, caused by a "backfire" in starting a motorcar, *Northumberland Durham Med J* 18:23, 1908-1909.

6. Apfelbach G, Weinstein L, Moshein J: Ulnar resection for malunited Colles' and Smith's fractures, *Quart Bull Northwestern Univ Med School* 27:1, 1953.

7. Baciu C, Kapandji IA: L'opération de Kapandji-Sauvé dans le traitement des cals vicieux de l'extrémité inferieure du radius, *Ann Chir* 31:323-329, 1977.

8. Backdähl M: The caput ulnae syndrome in rheumatoid arthritis: a study of the morphology, abnormal anatomy and clinical picture, *Acta Rheum Scand Suppl* 5:1-75, 1963.

9. Backhouse KM, Harrison SH, Hutchings RT: *Color atlas of rheumatoid hand surgery,* Chicago, 1981, Year Book Medical Publishers.

10. Bain GI, Pugh DM, MacDermid JC, et al.: Matched hemiresection interposition arthroplasty of the distal radioulnar joint, *J Hand Surg [Am]* 20:944-950, 1995.

11. Baldwin WI: *Orthopaedic surgery of the hand and wrist.* In Jones R, editor: *Orthopaedic surgery of injuries,* London, 1921, Henry Frowde.

12. Bazy L, Galtier M: Traitement sanglant de la luxation isolée de l'extrémité inférieure du cubitus en avant, *J Chir* 45:868-876, 1935.

13. Bell MJ, Hill RJ, McMurtry RY: Ulnar impingement syndrome, *J Bone Joint Surg Br* 67:126-129, 1985.

14. Berg E: Indications for and results with the Swanson distal ulnar prosthesis, *South Med J* 69:858-861, 1976.

15. Bieber EJ, Linscheid RL, Dobyns JH, et al.: Failed distal ulna resections, *J Hand Surg [Am]* 13:193-200, 1988.

16. Black RM, Boswick JA Jr, Wiedel J: Dislocation of the wrist in rheumatoid arthritis. The relationship to distal ulna resection, *Clin Orthop* 124:184-188, 1977.

17. Blaimont P, Buchin R, Geens M, et al.: La résection de l'extrémité distale du cubitus dans les séquelles des fractures de l'avant-bras et du poignet, *Acta Orthop Belg* 29:641-651, 1963.

18. Blatt G, Ashworth CR: Volar capsule transfer for stabilization following resection of the distal end of the ulna (abstract), *Orthop Trans* 3:13, 1979.

19. Bowers WH: Problems of the distal radioulnar joint, *Adv Orthop Surg* 7:289, 1981.

20. Bowers WH: Distal radioulnar joint arthroplasty: the hemiresection-interposition technique, *J Hand Surg [Am]* 10:169-178, 1985.

21. Bowers WH: *The distal radioulnar joint.* In Green DP, editor: *Operative hand surgery,* ed 2, vol 2, New York, 1988, Churchill Livingstone.

22. Bowers WH: Distal radioulnar joint arthroplasty. Current concepts, *Clin Orthop* 275:104-109, 1992.

23. Boyd HB, Stone MM: Resection of the distal radioulnar joint, *Adv Orthop Surg* 7:289-303, 1984.

24. Boyes JH: *Bunnell's surgery of the hand,* ed 5, Philadelphia, 1970, JB Lippincott.

25. Braun RM: The distal joint of the radius and ulna. Diagnostic studies and treatment rationale, *Clin Orthop* 275:74-78, 1992.

26. Breen TF, Jupiter J: Extensor carpi ulnaris and flexor carpi ulnaris tenodesis of the unstable distal ulna, *J Hand Surg [Am]* 14:612-617, 1989.

27. Breen TF, Jupiter J: Tendodesis of the chronically unstable distal ulna, *Hand Clin* 7:355-363, 1991.

28. Buck-Gramcko D: On the priorities of publication of some operative procedures on the distal end of the ulna, *J Hand Surg [Br]* 15:416-420, 1990.

29. Bunnell S: *Surgery of the hand,* Philadelphia, 1944, JB Lippincott.

30. Campbell RD Jr, Straub LR: Surgical considerations for rheumatoid disease in the forearm and wrist, *Am J Surg* 109:361-367, 1965.

31. Carroll RE: Resection of the distal ulna in athletes (abstract), *Orthop Trans* 11:505, 1987.

32. Clayton ML: Surgical treatment at the wrist in rheumatoid arthritis. A review of thirty-seven patients, *J Bone Joint Surg Am* 47:741-750, 1965.

33. Clayton ML: *The caput ulnae syndrome: update.* In Strickland JW, Steichen JB, editors: *Difficult problems in hand surgery,* St. Louis, 1982, CV Mosby.

34. Cracchiolo A III, Marmor L: Resection of the distal ulna in rheumatoid arthritis, *Arthritis Rheum* 12:415-422, 1969.

35. Czarkowski R, Strickland J: Long term results of ulnar head implant resection arthroplasty for post-traumatic disabilities of the distal radio-ulnar joint (abstract), *Orthop Trans* 11:586, 1987.

36. Dameron TB Jr: Traumatic dislocation of the distal radio-ulnar joint, *Clin Orthop* 83:55-63, 1972.

37. Darrach W: Anterior dislocation of the head of the ulna, *Ann Surg* 56:802, 1912.

38. Darrach W: Fractures of the lower extremity of the radius. Diagnosis and treatment, *J Am Med Assoc* 89:1683-1685, 1927.

39. Darrach W, Dwight K: Derangements of the inferior radioulna articulation, *Med Rec* 87:708, 1915.

40. De Leeuw B: The stratigraphy of the dorsal wrist region as basis for an investigation of the position of the m. extensor carpi ulnaris in pronation and supination of the forearm. Thesis, Leiden, Luctor et Embergo, 1962.

41. DiBenedetto MR, Lubbers LM, Coleman CR: Long-term results of the minimal resection Darrach procedure, *J Hand Surg [Am]* 16:445-450, 1991.

42. Dingman PVC: Resection of the distal end of the ulna (Darrach operation). An end-result study of twenty-four cases, *J Bone Joint Surg Am* 34:893-900, 1952.

43. Douglas J: Resection of the head of the ulna for anterior displacement accompanying unreduced Colles's fracture, *Ann Surg* 60:388-389, 1914.

44. Faithfull DK, Kwa S: A review of distal ulnar hemi-resection arthroplasty, *J Hand Surg [Br]* 17:408-410, 1992.

45. Feldon P, Terrono AL, Belsky MR: Wafer distal ulna resection for triangular fibrocartilage tears and/or ulna impaction syndrome, *J Hand Surg [Am]* 17:731-737, 1992.

46. Feldon P, Terrono AL, Belsky MR: The "wafer" procedure. Partial distal ulnar resection, *Clin Orthop* 275:124-129, 1992.

47. Flatt AE: *Care of the arthritic hand,* ed 4, St. Louis, 1983, CV Mosby.

48. Fletcher D, Palmer AK: Failed Bower's procedure (hemi-resection interposition technique). Presented at the 45th Annual Meeting of the American Society for Surgery of the Hand, Toronto, Canada, September 1990.

49. Freese CF: Treatment of comminuted Colles' fracture by ulnar styloid resection, *N Y State J Med* 49:2540, 1949.

50. Geissler WB, Fernandez DL, Lamey DM: Distal radio-ulnar joint injuries associated with fractures of the distal radius, *Clin Orthop* 327:135-146, 1996.

51. Goldner JL, Hayes MG: Stabilization of the remaining ulna using one-half of the extensor carpi ulnaris tendon after resection of the distal ulna (abstract), *Orthop Trans* 3:330, 1979.

52. Gonçalves D: Correction of disorders of the distal radio-ulnar joint by artificial pseudarthrosis of the ulna, *J Bone Joint Surg Br* 56:462-464, 1974.

53. Hartz CR, Beckenbaugh RD: Long-term results of resection of the distal ulna for post-traumatic conditions, *J Trauma* 19:219-226, 1979.

54. Henderson ED, Lipscomb PR: Rehabilitation of the rheumatoid hand by surgical means, *Arch Phys Med Rehabil* 42:58-62, 1961.

55. Henderson ED, Lipscomb PR: Surgical treatment of rheumatoid hand, *JAMA* 175:431-436, 1961.

56. Hucherson DC: The Darrach operation for lower radio-ulnar derangement, *Am J Surg* 53:237-241, 1941.

57. Hui FC, Linscheid RL: Ulnotriquetral augmentation tenodesis: a reconstructive procedure for dorsal subluxation of the distal radioulnar joint, *J Hand Surg [Am]* 7:230-236, 1982.

58. Imbriglia JE, Matthews D: Treatment of chronic post-traumatic dorsal subluxation of the distal ulna by hemiresection-interposition arthroplasty, *J Hand Surg [Am]* 18:899-907, 1993.

59. Jackson IT, Milward TM, Lee P, et al.: Ulnar head resection in rheumatoid arthritis, *Hand* 6:172-180, 1974.

60. Jensen CM: Synovectomy with resection of the distal ulna in rheumatoid arthritis of the wrist, *Acta Orthop Scand* 54:754-759, 1983.

61. Johnson RK: Stabilization of the distal ulna by transfer of the pronator quadratus origin, *Clin Orthop* 275:130-132, 1992.

62. Johnson RK, Shrewsbury MM: The pronator quadratus in motions and in stabilization of the radius and ulna at the distal radioulnar joint, *J Hand Surg* 1:205-209, 1976.

63. Kapandji IA: The Kapandji-Sauve operation. Its techniques and indications in non rheumatoid diseases, *Ann Chir Main* 5:181-193, 1986.

64. Kauer JMG: The collateral ligament function in the wrist joint, *Acta Morphol Neerl Scand* 17:252-253, 1979.

65. Kersley JB: Baldwin's operation for malunited Colles' fracture (abstract), *J Bone Joint Surg Br* 60:136, 1978.

66. Kessler I, Hecht O: Present application of the Darrach procedure, *Clin Orthop* 72:254-260, 1970.

67. Kessler I, Vainio K: Posterior (dorsal) synovectomy for rheumatoid involvement of the hand and wrist, *J Bone Joint Surg Am* 48:1085-1094, 1966.

68. Kihara H, Short WH, Werner FW, et al.: The stabilizing mechanism of the distal radioulnar joint during pronation and supination, *J Hand Surg [Am]* 20:930-936, 1995.

69. Konkel PD, Muniz RE, Dell PC: The Sauvé-Kapandji procedure: clinical evaluation. Presented at the 45th Annual Meeting of the American Society for Surgery of the Hand, Seattle, Washington, October 1989.

70. Lauenstein C: Zur Behandlung der nach karpaler Vorderarmfraktur zurückbleibenden Störung der Pro- und Supinations-Bewegung, *Zentralbl Chir* 14:433-435, 1887.

71. Leibovic SJ, Bowers WH: Arthroscopy of the distal radioulnar joint, *Orthop Clin North Am* 26:755-757, 1995.

72. Linscheid RL: Biomechanics of the distal radioulnar joint, *Clin Orthop* 275:46-55, 1992.

73. Lipscomb PR: Surgery of the arthritic hand: Sterling Bunnell Memorial Lecture, *Mayo Clin Proc* 40:132-164, 1965.

74. Lugnegård H: Resection of the head of the ulna in posttraumatic dysfunction of the distal radio-ulnar joint, *Scand J Plast Reconstr Surg* 3:65-69, 1969.

75. McKee MD, Richards RR: Dynamic radio-ulnar impingement following the Darrach procedure: a long-term follow-up study (abstract), *Orthop Trans* 15:67-68, 1991.

76. McMurray TP: *Practice of orthopedic surgery,* ed 3, Baltimore, 1949, Williams & Wilkins.

77. McMurtry RY, Paley D, Marks P, et al.: A critical analysis of Swanson ulnar head replacement arthroplasty: rheumatoid versus nonrheumatoid, *J Hand Surg [Am]* 15:224-231, 1990.

78. Mikic ZD: Treatment of acute injuries of the triangular fibrocartilage complex associated with distal radioulnar joint instability, *J Hand Surg [Am]* 20:319-323, 1995.

79. Minami A, Kaneda K, Itoga H: Hemiresection-interposition arthroplasty of the distal radioulnar joint associated with repair of triangular fibrocartilage complex lesions, *J Hand Surg [Am]* 16:1120-1125, 1991.

80. Minami A, Ogino T, Minami M: Treatment of distal radioulnar disorders, *J Hand Surg [Am]* 12:189-196, 1987.

81. Minami A, Ogino T, Tohyama H. Multiple ruptures of flexor tendons due to hypertrophic change at the distal radio-ulnar joint. A case report, *J Bone Joint Surg Am* 71:300-302, 1989.

82. Minami A, Suzuki K, Suenaga N, et al.: Hemiresection-interposition arthroplasty for osteoarthritis of the distal radioulnar joint, *Int Orthop* 19:35-39, 1995.

83. Minami A, Suzuki K, Suenaga N, et al.: The Sauvé-Kapandji procedure for osteoarthritis of the distal radioulnar joint, *J Hand Surg [Am]* 20:602-608, 1995.

84. Møller M: Forty-eight cases of caput ulnae syndrome treated by synovectomy and resection of the distal end of the ulna, *Acta Orthop Scand* 44:278-282, 1973.

85. Moore EM: Three cases illustrating luxation of the ulna in connection with Colles' fracture, *Med Rec* 17:305-308, 1880.

86. Nicolle FV, Dickson RA: *Surgery of the rheumatoid hand. A practical manual,* London, 1979, Heinemann Medical Books.

87. Noble J, Arafa M: Stabilisation of distal ulna after excessive Darrach's procedure, *Hand* 15:70-72, 1983.

88. Nolan WB III, Eaton RG: A Darrach procedure for distal ulnar pathology derangements, *Clin Orthop* 275:85-89, 1992.

89. Oskam J, Kingma J, Klasen HJ: Ulnar-shortening osteotomy after fracture of the distal radius, *Arch Orthop Trauma Surg* 112:198-200, 1993.

90. Palmer AK, Werner FW: The triangular fibrocartilage complex of the wrist—anatomy and function, *J Hand Surg [Am]* 6:153-162, 1981.

91. Rana NA, Taylor AR: Excision of the distal end of the ulna in rheumatoid arthritis, *J Bone Joint Surg Br* 55:96-105, 1973.

92. Rasker JJ, Veldhuis EF, Huffstadt AJ, et al.: Excision of the ulnar head in patients with rheumatoid arthritis, *Ann Rheum Dis* 39:270-274, 1980.

93. Rowland SA: Stabilization of the ulnar side of the rheumatoid wrist, following radiocarpal Swanson's implant arthroplasty and resection of the distal ulna, *Bull Hosp Jt Dis Orthop Inst* 44:442-448, 1984.

94. Sanders RA, Frederick HA, Hontas RB: The Sauve-Kapandji procedure: a salvage operation for the distal radioulnar joint, *J Hand Surg [Am]* 16:1125-1129, 1991.

95. Sauvé L, Kapandji M: Nouvelle technique de traitement chirurgical des luxations récidivantes isolées de l'extrémité inferieure du cubitus, *J Chirurgie* 47:589-594, 1936.

96. Schernberg F, Gerard Y, Collin JP, et al.: Arthroplasty of the rheumatoid wrist by silicone implants. Experience with forty cases, *Ann Chir Main* 2:18-26, 1983.

97. Smith-Petersen MN, Aufranc OE, Larson CB: Useful surgical procedures for rheumatoid arthritis involving joints of the upper extremity, *Arch Surg* 46:764-770, 1943.

98. Steindler A: *Orthopedic operations: indications, technique and end results,* first printing, Springfield, Illinois, 1940, Charles C Thomas.

99. Steindler A: *Orthopedic operations: indications, technique and end results,* fourth printing, Springfield, Illinois, 1947, Charles C Thomas.

100. Steindler A, Marxer JL: *The traumatic deformities and disabilities of the upper extremity,* Springfield, Illinois, 1946, Charles C Thomas.

101. Straub LR, Wilson EH Jr: Spontaneous rupture of the extensor tendons in the hand associated with rheumatoid arthritis, *J Bone Joint Surg Am* 38:1208-1217, 1956.

102. Swanson AB: The ulnar head syndrome and its treatment by implant resection arthroplasty (abstract), *J Bone Joint Surg Am* 54:906, 1972.

103. Swanson AB: Flexible implant resection arthroplasty in the hand and extremities, St. Louis, 1973, Mosby.

104. Swanson AB: Implant arthroplasty for disabilities of the distal radioulnar joint. Use of a silicone rubber capping implant following resection of the ulnar head, *Orthop Clin North Am* 4:373-382, 1973.

105. Taleisnik J: *The wrist,* New York, 1985, Churchill Livingstone.

106. Taleisnik J: Pain on the ulnar side of the wrist, *Hand Clin* 3:51-68, 1987.

107. Taleisnik J: The Sauvé-Kapandji procedure, *Clin Orthop* 275:110-123, 1992.

108. Taleisnik J, Gelberman RH, Miller BW, et al.: The extensor retinaculum of the wrist, *J Hand Surg [Am]* 9:495-501, 1984.

109. Thomas TL, Matthewson MH: Habitual anterior subluxation of the head of the ulna treated by Baldwin's operation. A case report, *Hand* 14:67-70, 1982.

110. Trumble T, Glisson RR, Seaber AV, et al.: Forearm force transmission after surgical treatment of distal radioulnar joint disorders, *J Hand Surg [Am]* 12:196-202, 1987.

111. Tsai T-M, Shimizu H, Adkins P: A modified extensor carpi ulnaris tenodesis with the Darrach procedure, *J Hand Surg [Am]* 18:697-702, 1993.

112. Tulipan DJ, Eaton RG, Eberhart RE: The Darrach procedure defended: technique redefined and long-term follow-up, *J Hand Surg [Am]* 16:438-444, 1991.

113. Van Lennep GA: Dislocation forward of the head of the ulna at the wrist-joint. Fracture of the styloid process of the ulna, *Hahneman Month* 32:350-354, 1897.

114. Vaughan-Jackson OJ: Rupture of the extensor tendons by attrition at the inferior radio-ulnar joint. Report of two cases, *J Bone Joint Surg Br* 30:528-530, 1948.

115. Vaughan-Jackson OJ: Rheumatoid hand deformities considered in the light of tendon imbalance, *J Bone Joint Surg Br* 44:764-775, 1962.

116. Vázquez Vela SE: Nuevo Método de artroplastia radiocubital distal en el paciente reumático, *An Ortop Traum (México)* 9:217-220, 1973.

117. Vergoz, Choussat: Luxation palmaire isolée de l'extrémité inférieure du cubitus, traitée par la nouvelle technique de Sauvé et Kapandji, *Mem Acad Chir* 63:992-1000, 1937.

118. Vincent KA, Szabo RM, Agee JM: The Sauve-Kapandji procedure for the reconstruction of the rheumatoid distal radioulnar joint (abstract), *J Hand Surg [Am]* 15:811-812, 1990.

119. von Lesser L: Zur Behandlung fehlerhaft geheilter Brüche der karpalen Radius epiphyse, *Zentralbl Chir* 14:265-270, 1887.

120. Waizenegger M, Schranz P, Barton NJ: The Kapandji procedure for post-traumatic problems, *Injury* 24:662-666, 1993.

121. Watson HK, Gabuzda GM: Matched distal ulna resection for posttraumatic disorders of the distal radioulnar joint, *J Hand Surg [Am]* 17:724-730, 1992.

122. Watson HK, Ryu JY, Burgess RC: Matched distal ulnar resection, *J Hand Surg [Am]* 11:812-817, 1986.

123. Whipple TL: Arthroscopy of the distal radioulnar joint. Indications, portals, and anatomy, *Hand Clinics* 10:589-592, 1994.

ADDITIONAL READING

Kleinman WB, Greenberg JA: Salvage of the failed Darrach procedure, *J Hand Surg [Am]* 20:951-958, 1995.

Rothwell AG, O'Neill L, Cragg K: Sauve-Kapandji procedure for disorders of the distal radioulnar joint: a simplified technique, *J Hand Surg [Br]* 21:771-777, 1996.

Ruby LK, Ferenz CC, Dell PC: The pronator quadratus interposition transfer: an adjunct to resection arthroplasty of the distal radioulnar joint, *J Hand Surg [Am]* 21:60-65, 1996.

35

DISORDERS OF THE DISTAL RADIOULNAR JOINT

Ronald L. Linscheid, M.D.

ANATOMY AND PHYSIOLOGY
  TRIANGULAR FIBROCARTILAGE
  FOREARM KINEMATICS
  DORSAL RADIOULNAR JOINT
  RADIOCARPAL ROTATION AND STABILITY
CHRONIC INSTABILITIES OF THE DISTAL
  RADIOULNAR JOINT
  DORSAL SUBLUXATION OR DISLOCATION OF THE
    ULNA
      PATHOGENESIS
      TREATMENT
  PALMAR SUBLUXATION AND DISLOCATION
    PATHOGENESIS
    TREATMENT
TRIANGULAR FIBROCARTILAGE INJURIES AND
  STYLOID FRACTURES
CHONDROMALACIA AND DEGENERATIVE ARTHRITIS

JOINT CONTRACTURE
ULNA VARIANCE CONDITIONS
  ULNAR IMPACTION (ABUTMENT) SYNDROME
  TREATMENT
PROXIMAL MIGRATION OF THE RADIUS
ULNAR STYLOID IMPINGEMENT AND LOOSE BODIES
GYMNAST'S WRIST
ULNA MINUS CONDITIONS
CONGENITAL MALFORMATION AFFECTING THE
  DISTAL RADIOULNAR JOINT
SALVAGE PROCEDURES FOR THE DISTAL
  RADIOULNAR JOINT
  ULNAR HEAD EXCISION (DARRACH PROCEDURE)
  RADIOULNAR SYNOSTOSIS WITH PROXIMAL
    SEGMENT EXCISION (KAPANDJI PROCEDURE)
TENDONITIS AND TENDON SUBLUXATION
MISCELLANEOUS

That a strong highly mobile wrist and hand capable of manipulating the objects presented by nature would prove to have a price in susceptibility to injury and disease is hardly surprising. The distal radioulnar joint (DRUJ) is after all a markedly complex mechanical arrangement modified over aeons from a basic primitive amphibian precursor. The human DRUJ developed in a long series of modifications from the supportive role of the quadrupedal stance of early primates through the suspensory function of the brachiating apes of the late Miocene epoch. Simultaneously, lengthening of the forearm, increasing mobility of the shoulder and elbow, and especially increasing forearm rotation occurred. This resulted in recession of the ulnar head, reduction in size of the styloid, a more mobile radioulnar joint, and a thicker triangular fibrocartilage (TFC) interposed between the ulna and the carpus. These adaptations, when presented with the boon of bipediality, allowed the development of the essential functional upper extremity of humankind.[12,127,132]

The transfer of torque from the strong forearm muscles to the hand empowered with the ability to grasp tool objects is a primary functional adaptation in the evolutionary process.[138] The DRUJ is the pivotal joint connecting the functions of these two units, and by its position, it is readily vulnerable (Fig. 35-1). It is somewhat surprising therefore that this joint remained in relative obscurity for many years. It has come under increased scrutiny in the last two decades as its importance to good performance for both the forearm and wrist has become increasingly apparent. As we have become more exacting in our diagnostic assessment of

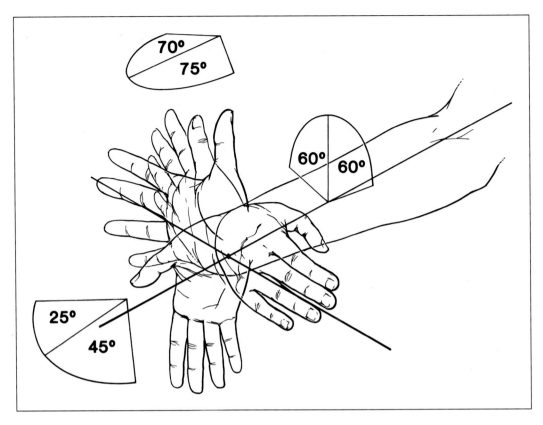

FIGURE 35-1

The wrist owes its remarkable adaptive positioning response to the radiocarpal and the dorsal radioulnar joints. The latter allows the transmission of torque from the powerful forearm motors to various grasp configurations of the hand.

it, we have learned more about the subtle complexities of the anatomy and function of this joint that is the essential linkage between hand and forearm. This has led to new procedures for diagnosis and preservation of the joint, but problems remain to be identified and solved.[15,25,202]

ANATOMY AND PHYSIOLOGY

The DRUJ is the distal articulation in the biarticular rotational arrangement of the forearm; it is distinctly different from the proximal radioulnar joint (PRUJ).[84] In the latter, the radial head transmits direct compressional loading to the capitellum as it rotates about the axes of rotation of the forearm that pass through its center.[13] At the DRUJ, the radius rotates eccentrically about the parallel articular surface component (seat) of the ulnar head (Fig. 35-2). Compressional loading at the wrist passes in large measure through the expanded articular surface of the distal radius, where in the forearm it is variably diverted to the ulna through the interosseous membrane (IOM). This force transmission through the IOM depends on the rotational attitude of the forearm and the amount of force applied. The

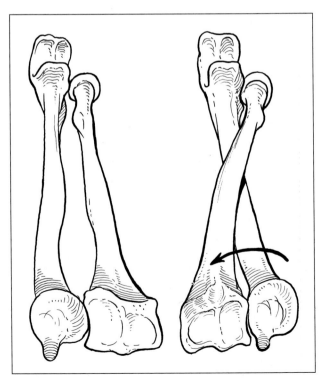

FIGURE 35-2

Left, Supination alignment of forearm. *Right*, Pronation crossover.

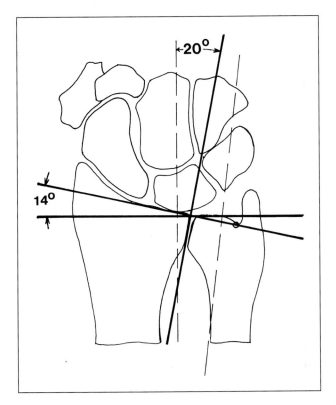

FIGURE 35-3

Relationship of radius and ulna to carpus with an ulna neutral variance. The ulnar slope of the radius tangential to the lunate fossa approximates 14°, and from radial styloid to ulnar margin it approximates 20°. If the ulnar dome is level with or perpendicular to the longitudinal axis of the radius at the ulnar margin, the condition is said to be a neutral variance when the shoulder and elbow are in 90° abduction and 90° flexion, respectively. The radioulnar joint slope of this position averages 20°. It becomes less with ulna positive and more with ulna negative conditions.

compressive load transmitted directly to the ulnar head through its distal articular surface (pole) also varies depending on the relative length of the ulna with respect to the articular surface of the distal radius, a condition originally noted by Hultën as ulna variance (Fig. 35-3).[98] This force transmission is also modified by the status of the TFC and the rotational position of the forearm.*

TRIANGULAR FIBROCARTILAGE

The TFC is central to understanding the interrelation between wrist and forearm function (see Chapter 30). The triangular component of the name is descriptive of its coronal appearance. The TFC originates from the distal edge of the sigmoid notch as a thin fibrocartilaginous sheet confluent with the articular cartilage of the lunate fossa. At the dorsal and palmar margins where the origins turn proximally it becomes increasingly collagenous, assuming the histologic appearance of ligament. This provides a shallow socket for the ulnar head before the dorsal and palmar elements converge to insert at the basistyloid fovea and the adjacent base of the styloid process. These two structures are called, respectively, the dorsal and palmar radioulnar ligaments (DRUL and PRUL) (Fig. 35-4). Those fibers providing the lamina inserting into the fovea are separated radially for a short interval from those inserting into the styloid by an areolar vascular tissue called the *ligamentum subcruentum* by Henle.[92] Because the lengths of the two laminae are slightly different as a result of their insertions, they may serve somewhat different constraint functions. The DRUL has the stoutest attachment to the

---

* References 8,22,40,95,120,130,164,185,207,211.

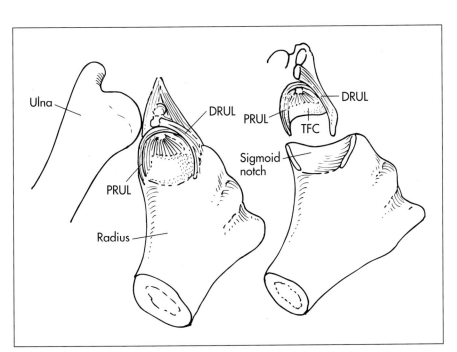

FIGURE 35-4

The dorsal (*DRUL*) and palmar (*PRUL*) distal radioulnar ligaments arise from the respective rims of the sigmoid notch of the radius. As they converge medially, a proximal lamina inserts into the basistyloid fovea adjacent to the styloid and the distal lamina inserts into the styloid base. The interval between consists of a vascular areolar connective tissue, "the ligamentum subcruentum of Henle." *TFC,* triangular fibrocartilage.

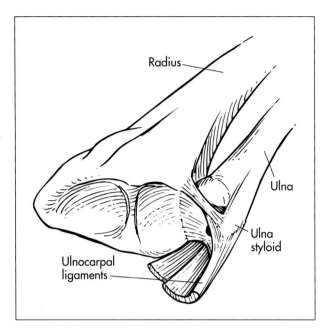

FIGURE 35-5

Schematic illustration of the triangular fibrocartilage and ulno-carpal ligaments in normal alignment in neutral forearm position. This axial or "end-on" view demonstrates the close relationship of the ulnocarpal ligaments with the palmar aspect of the triangular fibrocartilage.

styloid, whereas the PRUL gives rise to the ulnocarpal ligaments extending to the lunate and triquetrum (Fig. 35-5), which will be examined under dorsal instability below.* A separate more superficial fascicle originating on the styloid base and inserting on the capitate as the ulnocapitate ligament (UCL) has been identified in some specimens.

The central portion of the TFC is composed of wavy collagenous fibers oriented perpendicularly and embedded in a cartilage matrix sparsely populated by cartilage cells. This appears well designed to accommodate carpal compressive stresses. It becomes progressively thicker as it approaches the styloid where the prestyloid recess, a perforation lined with synovial tissue, leads to the hyaline cartilaginous cap of the styloid process.[41,111,145] This too is an atavistic remnant of the earlier functional ulnotriquetral joint. The structure is then joined by fibers originating from the periosteum of the styloid process and the infratendinous floor of the extensor carpi ulnaris (ECU) tendon sheath to continue on to attach to the ulnopalmar aspect of the triquetrum. Lewis et al.[127] envisioned the evolutionary recession of the ulnar styloid occurring in primates as leading to a tissue interposition between the interosseous fibrocartilage and the carpus designated as the "meniscus homologue." Palmer and Werner[163] introduced the

term "triangular fibrocartilaginous complex" (TFCC) to acknowledge the disparate portions of the structure. These components are the central disk and the DRUL and PRUL constituting the discus articularis, the meniscus homologue, and the ECU floor and periosteal extension from the styloid process. The last two make up, although incorrectly, strictly speaking, an ulnar collateral ligament. Studies of embryologic material, however, show differentiation occurs from a single mesenchymal nidus between the ulnar head and carpus; therefore, the term should not be interpreted as indicating differentiation rather than an amalgamation of structures.[74,111]

The TFC undergoes multiaxial stresses as it is alternately compressed and stretched between the proximal intrusions of the carpus and the translational and rotational contortions of the asymmetric ulnar head. These matrix stresses are distributed throughout the structure, with absorption and dampening being effected by the particular architectural disposition of the collagen fibers. The proximity of the carpus to the ulnar pole increases with firm grasp and ulnar deviation of the wrist. Attritional age-related changes in the disk are undoubtedly a result of cumulative wear as a result of these processes. There is a direct but nonlinear relationship between thickness of the TFC and ulna variance that has etiologic significance for several conditions and also has been exploited for some treatment options.*

FOREARM KINEMATICS

Active pronation occurs through the action of the pronator teres and pronator quadratus, each of whose point of action is distal to the midforearm. Active supination is primarily the result of tension in the supinator and biceps brachi, both acting on the proximal third of the radius. The moments supplied by the flat muscles are primarily rotational in the coronal plane, whereas the biceps and pronator teres exert moments in the transverse and sagittal planes.[13,105-107,121] This explains in part why palmar instability at the DRUJ is more apparent in supination and dorsal instability, in pronation (Fig. 35-6).

The radius and ulna have difficult to describe complex curvatures. These, combined with the mild physiologic cubitus valgus, allow the radius to pronate about the ulnar head distally without producing a marked trigonometric length disparity. This motion produces only a 1 mm apparent lengthening of the ulna in pronation. The instantaneous axis of rotation of the radius is not fixed but describes an irregular narrow cone that has its apex in the radial head and base within the ulnar head.† The loci of these axes of

---

* References 6,17,41,87,109,111,112,120,122,142,143,145,163,184,196, 210.

* References 3,4,17,50,53,69,120,129,144,154,198,206.
† References 55,117,118,120,165,172,177,215.

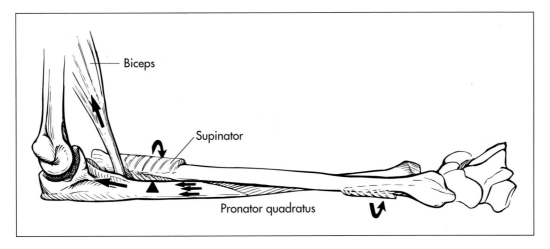

FIGURE 35-6

The stability of the forearm depends on the integrity of the proximal as well as the distal capsuloligamentous structures, the alignment of the forearm bones, the interosseous membrane, and the balance of the muscles effecting pronosupination movements. Arrows demonstrate, on the left, pull of biceps and supinator muscles for supination and, to the right, effect of pronator quadratus on pronation.

rotation lie just radial to the ulnar fovea. As Duchenne[60] pointed out in his classic studies, the ulnar head describes a small arc of counterrotation to the larger rotational arc of the radius.[106] This relationship is important to understand because it also requires a translation of the ulnar head during pronosupination, thus imparting a rolling sliding motion within the sigmoid notch (Fig. 35-7).*

Malalignment or disproportionate lengthening of the forearm bones after fracture, physeal arrest, plastic deformation, or congenital deformity has a marked effect on the kinematics of forearm rotation.[116] This most commonly results in accentuation of the eccentric movement at the DRUJ. The long-standing tenet of pediatric orthopedics that most fracture alignments undergo satisfactory remodeling in children is belied by some late results in adulthood in which limited pronosupination, cosmetic deformity, and degenerative changes in the DRUJ are apparent.[34,167,197] This is also true of adult fractures in which malunions of the distal radius may lead to displaced or eccentric incongruity at the radioulnar joint.† Every effort should be made to ensure reduction as close to anatomic restoration as possible.

DORSAL RADIOULNAR JOINT

The mean stressed dorsopalmar translation with the forearm in neutral position is 3.1 mm in men and 3.4 mm in women.[169] The ulnar head rests against a small area of the dorsal rim of the sigmoid notch in pronation where it also is dorsally displaced in reference to the

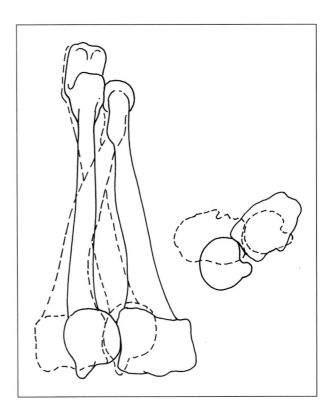

FIGURE 35-7

The radius swings about the ulnar head from pronation to supination, but the ulna describes a small rotation of its own. The loci for the instantaneous rotation axes describe a narrow cone.

ulnar carpus. Therefore, the relative lengthening of the ulna to the radius has little effect on the articulation with the carpus. The ulnar head rests against a similar small area on the palmar rim of the sigmoid notch in supination, but the inclination of the articular surface is

* References 6,13,29,76,110,118,130,157.
† References 2,7,25,38,45,56,58,59,68,72,81,89,102,113,200,208.

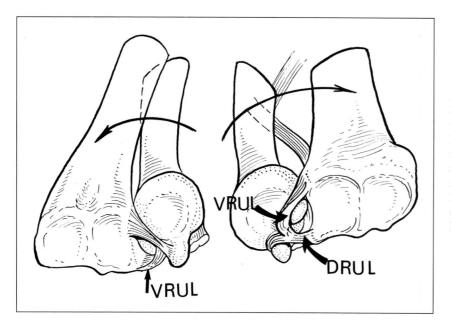

FIGURE 35-8

On the left, dorsal translation of the ulnar head occurs with forearm pronation and the concomitant tightening of the dorsal radioulnar ligament (*DRUL*). On the right, during forearm supination, the ulnar head rests against the palmar rim of the sigmoid notch and the palmar radioulnar ligament (*VRUL*) becomes taut.

slightly greater, thus affording more restraint to palmar subluxation (Fig. 35-8).[*]

The ulnar head has a modest frontal conical configuration that viewed end-on appears elliptical, with the major axis running from the base of the styloid through the center. This axis is centered in the sigmoid notch when the forearm is in neutral rotation. The radius of curvature of the ulnar head is approximately two-thirds of the radius of curvature of the sigmoid notch; thus there is limited congruence within the joint. This is least with pronation when the ulnar head is covered by only a small arc of the sigmoid notch articular surface.[157] The insertion points of the DRUL and PRUL in the fovea and on the styloid result in these ligaments being longer than the radius of curvature of the ulnar head. Therefore, the ligaments tend to remain relaxed until near the end point of either pronation or supination. This allows the dorsopalmar translation of the ulnar head over a distance of several millimeters (Fig. 35-9).[2,3,5,106,169]

The kinematic constraints of the DRUJ are the shallow concavity of the sigmoid notch, the peripheral components of the TFC (i.e., the DRUL and PRUL) and the IOM, primarily the distal portion. The ECU and its infratendinous sheath extending from its ulnar groove to the ulnopalmar aspect of the triquetrum and the ulnocarpal ligaments provide some additional support that depends on the anchorage to a stable carpus. The capsule of the DRUJ is loose and provides little additional support but is capable of fibrous contracture after injury and immobilization.[†] It is worth noting that previously there was some confusion in the literature

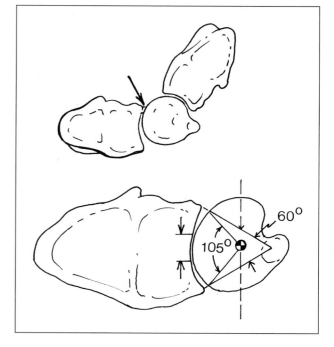

FIGURE 35-9

Different radius of curvature of the sigmoid notch (105°) and of the ulnar head (60°) results in limited congruity. The lengths of the dorsal and palmar radioulnar ligaments allow dorsopalmar translation.

when the dorsal and palmar capsules were defined as the DRUL and PRUL.[11,91,178]

The primary constraints are the DRUL and PRUL. These have strengths similar to the palmar radiocarpal ligaments.[176] Their role has at times been confused by observations in experimental situations. Several authors[31,91,120,194] have noted that the DRUL appears

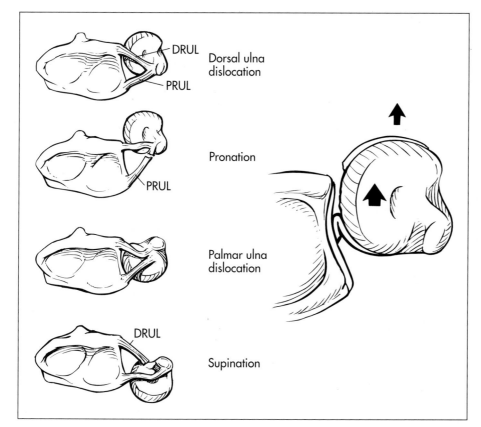

FIGURE 35-10

This drawing shows the ulna rotating within the sigmoid notch rather than the radius rotating about the ulnar head to show the translatory changes of the ulnar head with these motions. One can observe the relative tensions in the dorsal (*DRUL*) and palmar (*PRUL*) radioulnar ligaments with pronation and supination, but not the reverse tensioning of the ligament that actually restrains subluxation or dislocation. On the right, the mechanism of chondromalacia with dorsal subluxation against the dorsal radial rim is shown.

to become more taut in pronation and the PRUL, in supination, an observation recently confirmed and documented by Schuind et al.,[184] Kihara et al.,[116] and Acosta et al.[1,183] from cadaver studies. On the other hand, several authors[84,178] have suggested that it is the PRUL that prevents dorsal subluxation or dislocation of the ulnar head in pronation and the DRUL palmar dislocation in supination. This was most ably demonstrated by af Ekenstam.[5] Although these results would appear to be diametrically opposed, they are in fact readily compatible. Stuart et al.[189] have shown that the PRUL contribution to passive restraint of dorsal ulnar subluxation is greater than the remainder of the structures put together regardless of forearm position. Restraint of palmar subluxation of the ulnar head in a position of supination is more evenly divided in order by the DRUL, PRUL, and distal IOM (IOMd), ECU subsheath, and proximal IOM (IOMp).

During normal pronation, the rotation of the radius on the ulna places the fovea and styloid at a maximum distance from the dorsal rim origin of the DRUL. Were it not for the simultaneous dorsal translation of the ulnar head, the DRUL would restrain that movement. However, during an event imposing a dorsal dislocating force, the dorsal ligament is relaxed by the head translating dorsally. However, at some point the PRUL reaches its elastic limit, and when this is exceeded, dislocation may occur. The reverse is true

for palmar dislocation (Fig. 35-10).[5] There is now speculation that the foveal and styloidal components of the dorsal and palmar ligaments may act in a slightly different fashion.[84] Because the deeper portions of the ligaments are not readily seen, their tension status during pronosupination is not as readily assessed.

RADIOCARPAL ROTATION AND STABILITY

The carpus is supported primarily from the radius and is affected little by this relative motion of the ulnar head. Kuhlman[124] has described the radiocarpal stability as consisting of a deep and superficial ligamentous bridle. The superficial band is supplied by the dorsal retinaculum, which is attached dorsally between the extensor compartments before sliding over the ulnar head to insert in the triquetrum, pisiform, and abductor digiti minimi fascia before continuing on as the palmar retinaculum.[192] The deep band consists of the dorsal and palmar radiocarpal ligaments and the interposed carpal bones and radius.[124] The slack in this arrangement allows some rotation of the carpus on the radius.

The contribution of axial radiocarpal rotation to the apparent radioulnar pronosupination is rarely appreciated (Figs. 35-11 and 35-12). This laxity at the radiocarpal joint has been shown to approximate 45° in the relaxed state.[179] Kapandji,[108] experimenting on his own wrist, showed that with firm grasp the axial laxity

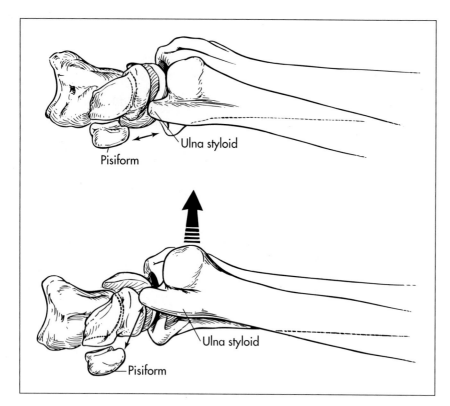

FIGURE 35-11

Top, Ulnar aspect of the distal forearm and wrist. Note alignment of radius and ulna to pisiform. *Bottom,* Dorsal subluxation of the ulnar head associated with carpal supination. The ulnar head displaces dorsally (*arrow*) while the carpus rotates (supinates) palmarly. Increased distance between pisiform and ulnar styloid.

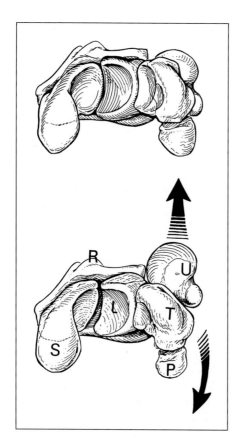

FIGURE 35-12

Top, Distal transverse aspect of the proximal carpal row superimposed on the radius and ulna. *Bottom,* Carpal supination superimposed on dorsal ulnar subluxation. *L,* lunate; *P,* pisiform; *R,* radius; *S,* scaphoid; *T,* triquetrum; *U,* ulna.

was reduced to 10°. Ritt et al.[176] showed that the dorsal radiotriquetral ligament, the palmar ulnolunate, and ECU subsheath were the primary restraint to passive carpal supination, with the dorsal retinaculum and ulnotriquetral ligament also contributing (Figs. 35-13 and 35-14). Injury to the insertion of the PRUL from which the ulnolunate and ulnotriquetral ligaments originate or to the ligaments themselves may precipitate the concomitant carpal supination seen with dorsal ulnar subluxation. This also corresponds to Palmer's 1C classification of TFC injuries.[160] The palmar radioscaphocapitate ligament is the primary restraint to passive carpal pronation; however, carpal pronation is not a known factor in DRUJ instability. These findings help to explain why it is possible to transfer marked torque from the forearm to the hand when grasping firmly and yet be able to dampen passive axial torques at the wrist during more leisurely activities.

CHRONIC INSTABILITIES OF THE DISTAL RADIOULNAR JOINT

DORSAL SUBLUXATION OR DISLOCATION OF THE ULNA

Pathogenesis. Chronic dorsal subluxation is more common than the palmar variety.[153] The misnomer of dorsal ulnar subluxation or dislocation is so firmly entrenched that reverting to the more accurate description of palmar dislocation of the radiocarpal unit would only cause confusion. Dislocation is obviously a more

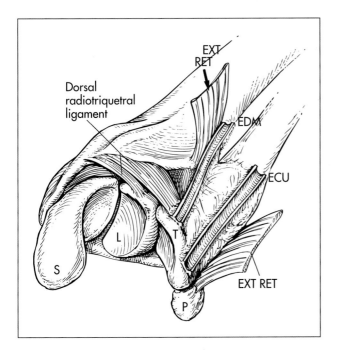

FIGURE 35-13

Schematic view with reflected dorsal retinaculum. Extensor carpi ulnaris (*ECU*) subsheath and dorsal radiotriquetral ligament are major restraints to carpal supination. *EDM*, extensor digiti minimi (subsheath); *EXT RET*, extensor retinaculum; *L*, lunate; *P*, pisiform; *S*, scaphoid; *T*, triquetrum.

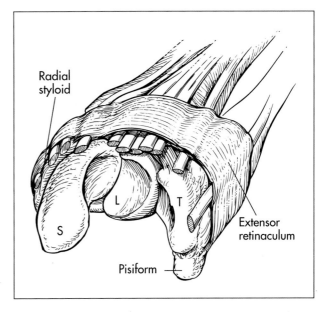

FIGURE 35-14

Schematic axial view of the proximal carpal row (scaphoid [*S*], lunate [*L*], triquetrum [*T*]) to the six extensor compartments and extensor retinaculum, which is bound to the radial styloid (laterally) and to the pisiform (medially).

severe condition than subluxation. Clinically, in the former, the ulnar head may be locked dorsally and severely compromise supination, whereas in the latter, the ulnar head is prominent and rides onto the dorsal lip of the sigmoid notch, especially in pronation. Supination is variably restricted because the radius cannot readily slip dorsally over the prominent ulnar head as one attempts to initiate this motion. There may be a distinct snap during forearm rotation. The wrist is weak and painful. The prominence of the ulnar head may be markedly enhanced when there is concomitant carpal supination, as is frequently the case in rheumatoid arthritis and is also apparent in most chronic post-traumatic cases.

Dorsal subluxation or dislocation usually occurs after an injury when the wrist is pronated and extended (Fig. 35-15).[83] In this position the ulnar styloid is in the maximum ulnopalmar position. This twists and tightens the infratendinous ECU sheath, the ulnocarpal ligaments, and the ulnar collateral component of the TFC, which act as a taut sling to lift the ulnar head against the weak dorsal capsule and dorsal rim of the sigmoid notch.[97,186] Weakening of the attachments of the TFC by styloid fracture, avulsion, or attenuation of the PRUL then allows subluxation or dislocation, depending on the severity of the injuring force. The shear stress imposed on the articular cartilage of the ulnar head as it slides past the dorsal rim of the sigmoid notch may produce a chondromalacic area that produces

painful motion even if the ulnar head spontaneously reduces (see chondromalacia) (Figs. 35-16, *A* through *C*). Although dislocation has been reported to occur without loss of the TFC insertions,[178,186] it is more likely to be associated with more extensive injury, including attenuation of the distal IOM and radial fractures.[*]

The diagnosis is usually established by the clinical appearance.[131] The forearm may be locked in pronation or have limited supination. The ulnar head is tender. Direct pressure on the ulnar head will usually produce reduction, but the ulnar head will spring back when pressure is released, a phenomenon known as the "piano key sign."[92,151,168,174] This sign may occasionally be seen in a normal wrist, particularly in lithe young women (Fig. 35-17). Occasionally, the acute dislocation is irreducible because of locking of the radius in the ECU notch from hyperpronation[186] or interposition of the displaced ECU or TFC.[77,86,103,159]

The carpus may be supinated relative to the radius, making the prominence of the ulnar head even more apparent.[97] This appearance is often heightened if the carpus has a palmar intercalated segment instability stance at the midcarpal joint (Fig. 35-17, *Bottom*).[213] The explanation for this deformity probably lies with the fact that the dorsal radiotriquetral ligament and the infratendinous sheath of the ECU, which are primary stabilizers of radiocarpal supination, have been injured or undergo attritional attenuation with time after the

---

* References 10,11,14,27,32,38,45,47,49,51,62,65,72, 75,77,90,91,109, 110,135,139,140,151,194.

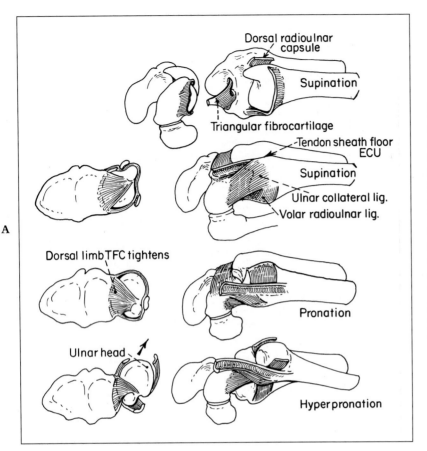

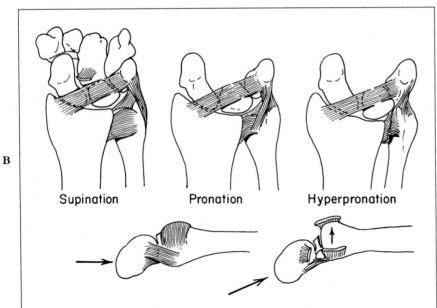

FIGURE 35-15

A, Pathomechanics of dorsal dislocation of the ulnar head. The extensor carpi ulnaris (*ECU*) subsheath and ulnar collateral ligament (*lig.*) components of the triangular fibrocartilage (*TFC*) become progressively coiled and tightened by pronation as they move ulnopalmarly. Wrist extension exerts a dorsally acting force against the shallow constraining rim of the sigmoid notch and the thin dorsal capsule of the dorsal radioulnar joint, causing dorsal ulna dislocation (*arrow*). Axial view (*left*) and medial view of wrist (*right*). Forearm supination (*top*) and pronation (*bottom*). **B,** Different ligament tensions during supination (*left*), pronation (*center*), hyperpronation (*right*). Dislocation occurs in hyperpronation.

initial insult to the TFC. Any residual tension in the ulnocarpal ligaments arising from the PRUL tends to flex the proximal carpal row as the carpus sags into supination. Compensatory extension at the midcarpal joint accounts for the palmar intercalated segment instability stance.[27,134,176,213] Viegas and colleagues[195,204] have shown that the radiocarpal contact also changes when the instability is severe.

Routine radiographic examination may be non-diagnostic unless the ulnar head is seen to be superimposed on the ulnar aspect of the distal radius on the anteroposterior view, an often subtle finding. Sagittal views are notoriously difficult to interpret because the ulna may appear either above or below the radius when the wrist is positioned but a few degrees away from true lateral.[27,29] Definite confirmation is best

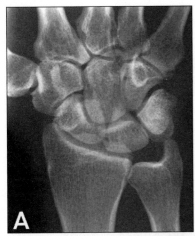

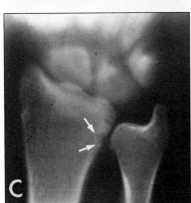

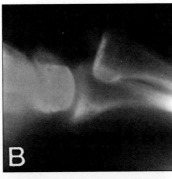

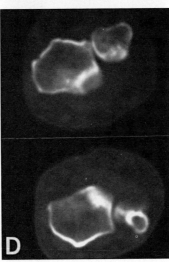

FIGURE 35-16

A, Anteroposterior appearance of wrist after patient felt a snap while pushing a boat. Slight overlap of distal ulna on the distal radius noted. **B,** Lateral polyaxial tomogram taken as true lateral. Dorsal subluxation of ulnar head. **C,** Anteroposterior trispiral tomogram shows cystic changes on dorsal rim of sigmoid notch (*arrows*). **D,** Computed tomographic scan, transverse views. *Bottom,* Normal left wrist. *Top,* Dorsal subluxation of ulnar head in pronation and narrowed joint space.

obtained with cross-sectional computed tomographic scans. Both wrists should be included so that comparison views eliminate the possibility of a normal patient with unusual dorsally positioned ulnae (Fig. 35-16, *D*). These views may also help to show carpal supination if successive views through radius and carpus are compared. Ideally, neutral and supination views are obtained at the same time to eliminate the possibility of more complex problems.* Magnetic resonance imaging studies to elucidate the status of the involved ligamentous structures may be helpful, but at this time the resolution is often insufficient for definitive application.[39]

Treatment. When dorsal subluxation or dislocation of the ulna is seen acutely, it is important to assess the length of the forearm and the situation at the radiocapitellar joint as well as the wrist.[108] Reduction is usually obtained with gentle depression and supination. Regional or general anesthesia may be necessary, especially if there is soft-tissue interposition necessitating open reduction. The stability of the reduction should be checked with gentle manipulation followed by radiographic assessment of the position of the ulnar head and the styloid if it is fractured. For the uncomplicated reduction, immobilizing the forearm in full supination and neutral flexion of the wrist for a period of 6 weeks often restores forearm rotational stability. The cast should include the flexed elbow to maintain position.[46] There is increasing interest in early open reduction and repair of injuries of the TFC to ensure satisfactory maintenance of long-term stability.* An irreducible dislocation that requires open exposure to remove or release the obstructing structure provides an opportunity for repair of the torn or fractured elements.[86]

Chronic subluxations provide a more difficult problem for which several solutions have been proposed (Fig. 35-18).[100,104,108,109] The use of a conformal distal forearm splint that exerts some relocation force on the ulnar head may be of occasional or temporary help, but it is not a satisfactory long-term solution.[26] Surgical solutions have been proposed in four broad categories: a repair or reinsertion of the TFC to the ulnar head or radial rim, a restraining tendinous loop at the level of the ulnar neck, a tendinous tether from carpus to ulna, and a dynamic muscle transfer.[85,104,109] Distal ulnar resection and distal radioulnar synostosis are described elsewhere under salvage procedures.

---

* References 25,30,36,88,117,148,149,157.

* References 11,27,30,51,91,154.

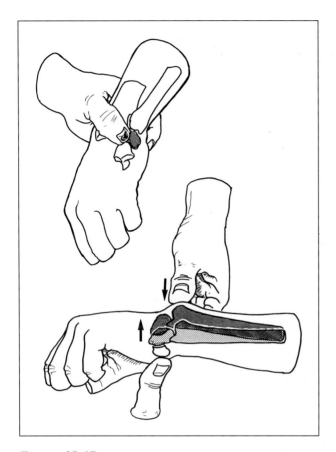

FIGURE 35-17

Top, Carpal supination is corrected by pressing up from beneath the triquetrum and pisiform and down on the distal ulna. *Bottom,* When depressed, the ulnar head relocates, but on release it springs back like a piano key.

Repair or reconstruction of the TFC is discussed in detail in Chapter 30. Repair of this structure for late instability is also appropriate as long as there are sufficient portions of the ligaments remaining to be anatomically repositioned. This may require some lysis of contracted scar tissue to free the TFC adequately. Often the TFC has been avulsed from the ulnar head with the styloid, in which case reattachment may be accomplished by osteosynthesis of a styloid nonunion (Figs. 35-18, 35-19, and 35-20). If not, reattachment of the TFC to the fovea or the styloid base or repair of the avulsion from the rim of the sigmoid notch is possible (Fig. 35-12).* Ligamentous augmentation of or replacement of a DRUL has recently been suggested. Scheker et al.[183] have described an intra-articular tendinous replacement for the DRUL based on previous experimental work showing that ligament at its greatest tension in pronation (Fig. 35-21). More recent evidence[189] suggests that the PRUL is the most important passive structure in stabilization of a chronic dorsal subluxation, and the

---
* References 14,26,38,140,141,181.

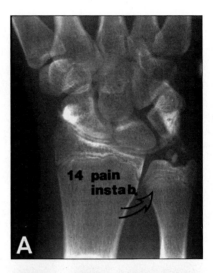

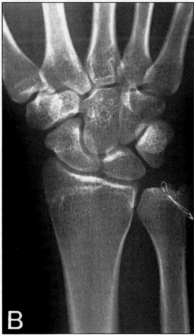

FIGURE 35-18

A, A 14-year-old girl with a tennis injury, unstable with forehand. Avulsion foveal attachment. **B,** After excision of loose body and transosseous wiring of foveal attachment, recovery was satisfactory. *instab.,* instability.

technique is readily revisable to re-create the PRUL or both components of the TFC. Melone and Nathan[140] noted the additional frequent avulsion of the infratendinous ECU sheath and suggested simultaneous repair.

Several ingenious methods have been used to create a restraining loop around the ulnar neck. Ideally, this loop should exert its tension increasingly during pronation as ulnar head displacement increases. Various strips of tendon or fascia lata have been used for this purpose, usually being anchored in drill holes in the radial metaphysis (Fig. 35-22). Long-term follow-up

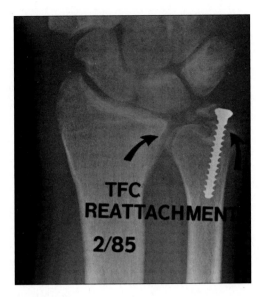

FIGURE 35-19

Triangular fibrocartilage (*TFC*) detachment dorsally and radially from sigmoid notch rim and ulnar styloid. Note unreduced fragments from foveal area as well as styloid. Styloid reattached with screw and transosseous suture on dorsoulnar aspect radial rim. Osteochondral fragments should have been excised. A smaller screw with compression lag effect is recommended.

of an adequate series is unfortunately not available. Some of these reconstructions were originally designed for anterior subluxation reconstructions but are used to illustrate surgical techniques for dorsal subluxations as well. These reconstructions do not address the carpal supination problem.* During the healing period of 6 to 10 weeks, supination immobilization needs to be imposed to prevent stretching of the devascularized tendon strips. Even then, increasing laxity of the construct is not infrequent. This is likely the result of the forces acting on the radius during pronation. The crossover of the radius on the ulna occurs between the proximal third of the two bones. The line of action of the pronator teres as well as the wrist and finger flexors lies palmar to this crossover, thus imparting a palmar displacement of the radius in relation to the ulnar head. This force acting on constraints weaker than the normal ones can induce attenuation with repetition. An instability may also develop at the PRUJ in these chronic situations that favors the "teeter-totter" effect at the point of crossover (Fig. 35-6). This may explain

---

* References 26,32,54,91,99,128,151,166,174,186.

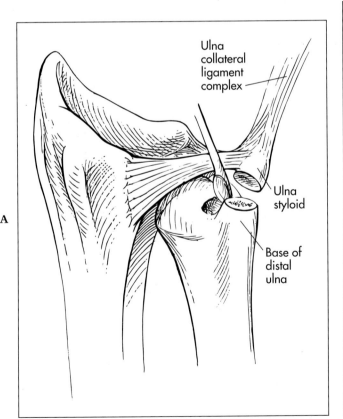

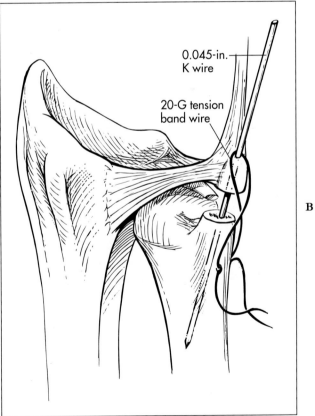

FIGURE 35-20

A, Repair of the triangular fibrocartilage can be accomplished by freshening the foveal area and suturing the remnant of triangular fibrocartilage securely through drill holes in the metaphyseal cortex or **(B)** by reattaching the avulsed ulnar styloid using a tension band wiring technique or small cancellous screw.

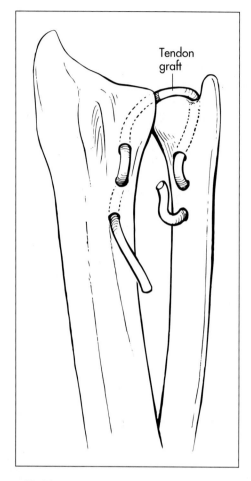

FIGURE 35-21

Reconstruction of the dorsal radioulnar ligament for dorsal sub-luxation as proposed by Scheker et al.[183] uses an ingenious technique to thread a tendon through multiple drill holes to ensure a taut reconstruction with firm bony anchorage.

why some patients with DRUJ instability also complain of elbow discomfort from PRUJ instability.

Ulnocarpal tendinous tethers have been created using portions of the ECU or flexor carpi ulnaris (FCU). These are usually left attached distally and then inserted under tension into the ulnar diaphysis or ulnar head. This approach has the advantage of addressing the frequent concomitant carpal supination, but it has a poorer mechanical advantage at the radioulnar joint.[94,97,199] There is also decreased tension in the tether with ulnar deviation. In one method we have used in a series of 12 patients, a strip of FCU is brought intra-articularly through the pisotriquetral capsule and passed through a drill hole in the fovea of the ulnar head (Figs. 35-23, *Left* and 35-24). The tendon can be passed through the thick ulnar portion of the TFC at the same time to reanchor the detached radioulnar ligaments (Fig. 35-23, *Right*). The long-term results have been generally satisfactory although restricted pronation has

been noted as a result of the prolonged immobilization in supination. A revision of this technique to reconstruct the PRUL simultaneously is being studied experimentally (Fig. 35-24). A revision of the original Bunnell technique in the fifth edition of *Surgery of the Hand*[33] edited by J.H. Boyes illustrates a tendon loop addition to the ulnocarpal tether procedure. An ulnocarpal tether using a strip of distally attached FCU passed through a drill hole at the base of the styloid and then attached to the radial rim is also illustrated by Bowers.[28] This has the advantage of augmenting the DRUL in the same procedure.

Dynamic constraint options include advancement of the pronator quadratus (Fig. 35-25), transfer of the FCU to the triquetral area dorsally (Fig. 35-26), and sling tenodeses using the FCU or ECU (see Darrach procedure).

Advancement of the pronator quadratus to the dorsum of the ulna ideally results in transferring the line of action of that muscle to produce palmar displacement of the ulnar head with pronation activity. To stretch the muscle origin to the dorsum of the ulna with minimal tension, the forearm needs to be pronated.[104] A careful subperiosteal dissection of the fibrous origin is required for adequate tissue to ensure reattachment dorsally. Multiple small drill holes are desirable to aid fixation. The pronator quadratus is composed of a short-fibered deep head lying between the two bones that primarily aids coaption and a longer-fibered superficial head that provides most of the rotational moment.[105] Changes in length, direction, and origin may result in loss of at least one grade of muscle function. A reduced position of the forearm bones should be transfixed by large transosseous Kirschner wires during the early healing period.

Hamlin[85] described a transfer of the insertion of the FCU to the dorsoulnar carpus with the rationale that the tension in the muscle crossing the ulnar neck would depress the ulnar head while elevating the ulnar carpus (Fig. 35-26). This is an intriguing concept, particularly with marked carpal supination. Unfortunately, long-term results are unknown.

Maintenance of the ECU in a dorsal position relative to the distal ulna to act as a depressor to the ulnar head has been attempted with several techniques. Spinner and Kaplan[187] created a retinacular pulley by splitting an ulnar portion of the dorsal retinaculum, looping it under the ECU, and suturing it back on itself. A tendon loop around the ECU and FCU tendons is less predictable,[125] but a strip of FCU left attached distally may be tethered through a hole in the ulna and then wrapped around the ECU to create both an ulnocarpal and an ECU tether.[80] At times, two or more of these surgical approaches may be combined in an effort to ensure stability. They may also be

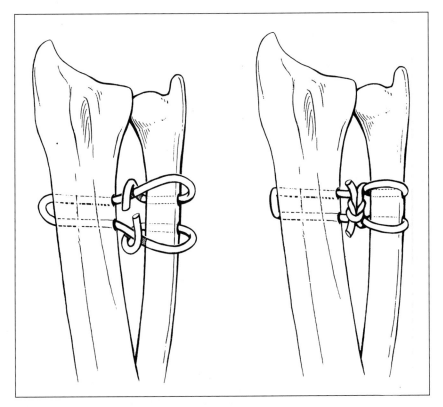

FIGURE 35-22

Hunter and Kirkpatrick[99] designed a Dacron silicone ligamentous tether that tightens during pronation to depress the ulnar head.

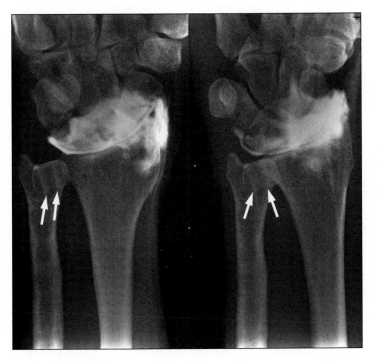

FIGURE 35-23

Left, Arthrogram of a 37-year-old woman after ligament augmentation. Arrows show bone tunnel. *Right*, Arthrogram shows competent distal radioulnar joint.

used with an unstable ulnar stump in the radioulnar impingement syndrome (see Chapter 34).

Petersen and Adams[166] compared several of the techniques listed above on cadaver forearms in a biomechanical setting. Although they found the Fulkerson-Watson technique the most stable in that passive situation, it is readily apparent that this class of radioulnar ligamentous slings is nonphysiologic in design and subject to dynamic stresses in vivo, as are all techniques using tendon strips.[73] Several of the techniques originally designed for palmar subluxation are used inappropriately for dorsal reconstructions. At this

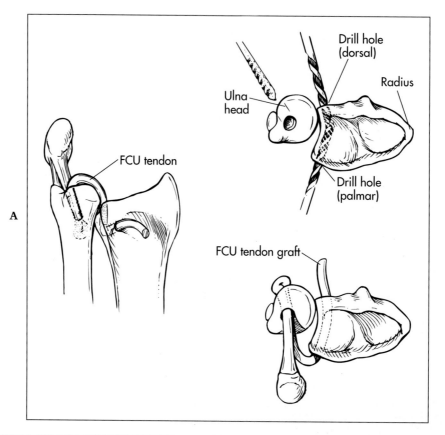

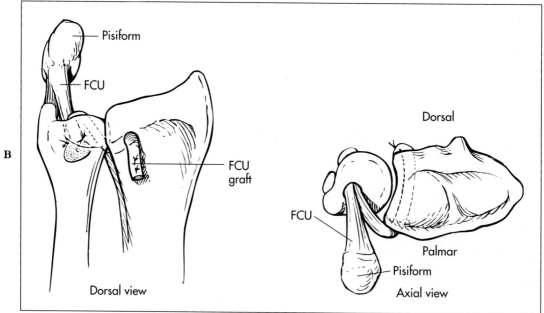

FIGURE 35-24

A, A ligamentous augmentation meant to simultaneously correct dorsal subluxation of the ulnar head and carpal supination uses a doubled strip of flexor carpi ulnaris (*FCU*) pulled into a hole drilled from the ulnopalmar corner of the radius to the dorsum, and the free end of the tendon strip is pulled through the hole. **B,** The forearm is turned into supination, reducing dorsal subluxation and carpal supination. The tendinous ligament is then tightened at both ends and fixed firmly to bone. Immobilization is continued for 6 weeks.

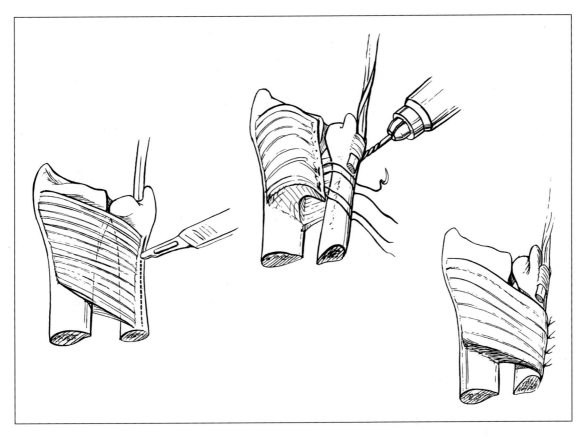

FIGURE 35-25

Advancement of the pronator quadratus as a dynamic stabilizer was proposed by Johnson.[104] *Left*, The superficial layer of the muscle should be elevated with a strip of periosteum. *Middle*, Drill holes for secure fixation are made dorsally on the ulna and the surface is roughened. *Right*, The forearm is pronated to relax the muscle while it is advanced and sutured. It should be held in that position for 6 weeks.

time, I recommend, as the foremost consideration, correction of any anatomic malalignment of the bones of the forearm. A second consideration is reattachment of the TFC to re-create the normal constraint pattern. If these options are limited, then one or a combination of the reconstructive procedures is appropriate. For dorsal subluxation, an attempt at reconstructing the PRUL is recommended. If there is obvious carpal supination as well, an ulnocarpal tether or augmentation of the radiotriquetral ligament is reasonable. The dynamic techniques of pronator quadratus advancement and FCU transfer work best when the muscle is contracting, but the resting tension may be insufficient to maintain reduction against persisting subluxation forces.

Salvage operations—ulnar head resection and its variants, including distal radioulnar arthrodesis—are described in Chapter 34. Chondromalacia of the seat of the ulnar head is not necessarily an indication for these procedures. If it is possible to restore and stabilize the ulnar head in the sigmoid notch, the joint usually tolerates the condition well (Fig. 35-16).

PALMAR SUBLUXATION AND DISLOCATION

Pathogenesis. This condition is generally considered to occur less commonly than dorsal instability and is easy to overlook, with perhaps 50% of cases being missed initially. The mechanism of injury is usually a fall on the outstretched supinated hand, but injury may occur from marked exertional lifting with the forearm supinated or when forced into hypersupination.[*] In this position the ulnar styloid with the ECU intervening lies next to the dorsal border of the radius where they offer little support to the palmar aspect of the joint. The thin palmar capsule is stretched out, affording little resistance when impact on the heel of the hand drives the radius dorsally. Although the PRUL is the more taut of the two structures in supination, DRUL failure is the likely critical event that allows the dislocation to occur according to af Ekenstam and Hagert.[6] Kihara et al.[116] found marginal differences in the support of the PRUL and DRUL. Stuart et al.[189]

---

* References 20,48,49,57,78,146,150,171,181,212.

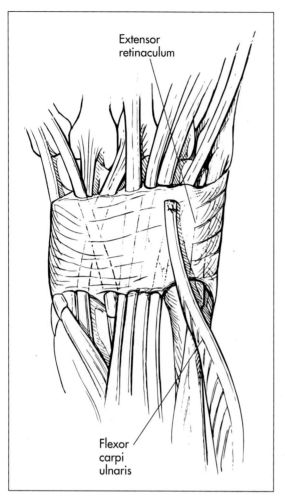

FIGURE 35-26

Advancement of the flexor carpi ulnaris from the pisiform to the dorsum of the triquetrum was proposed by Hamlin.[85] This places a bowstringing tension from the muscles to depress the ulnar head and relieves some tension from the pisiform which might induce carpal supination.

showed on sequential sectioning of the various structures during load displacement stress testing that the PRUL and IOMd exerted almost as much restraint as the DRUL. The infratendinous ECU sheath and IOMp exerted somewhat less.

Clinically, in palmar dislocation the forearm is narrowed when viewed from above and widened at the wrist when seen laterally. The forearm is held in a supinated position, and pronation is quite limited (Fig. 35-27). Forced pronation is painful and a block to motion is noted. Ulnar dysesthesias may occur. Subluxation of the ulnar head usually develops after a similar injury, but the sensation of the ulnar head slipping out of place occurs with supination. It usually spontaneously relocates with pronation. The ulnar head can be readily palpated on the ulnopalmar aspect of the wrist in both instances.[46]

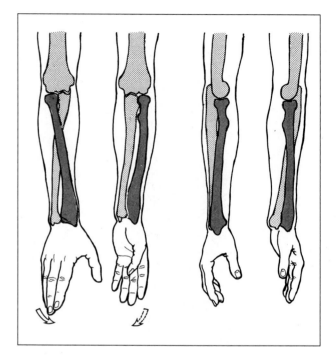

FIGURE 35-27

Left, Anteroposterior view. Pronation, left forearm restricted by palmar dislocation of ulnar head. *Right*, Lateral view, ulnar head locked under palmar rim of the sigmoid notch.

Radiographic examination using standard films is usually diagnostic if the condition is suspected. On the anteroposterior view, the dislocated ulnar head overlaps the ulnar margin of the radius. An ulnar styloid fracture is apparent in more than half the cases (Figs. 35-28, *A* through *C*). The lateral view is often dramatic, with the ulnar head located under the palmar rim of the radius. A subluxated ulnar head may require both anteroposterior and lateral views in supination to show the ulnar head displaced. A computed tomographic scan is sometimes helpful as well because there may be an indented fracture in the ulnar head where it is locked under the ulna (similar to a Hill-Sachs lesion).[115] A fracture or an erosion of the palmar lip of the sigmoid notch, especially in a long-standing subluxation, may help explain persistent instability.

Treatment. Closed reduction of a dislocation when seen acutely is not always possible. Sometimes these are seen days to months after injury. If initial supination and manual displacement followed by pronation are insufficient to initiate the distinct sound and feel of relocation, open reduction should be considered to avoid further osteochondral damage to the ulnar head. Ulnar nerve function should also be assessed before and after reduction. Entrapment of the ulnar neurovascular complex is rare but possible. If reduction is achieved,

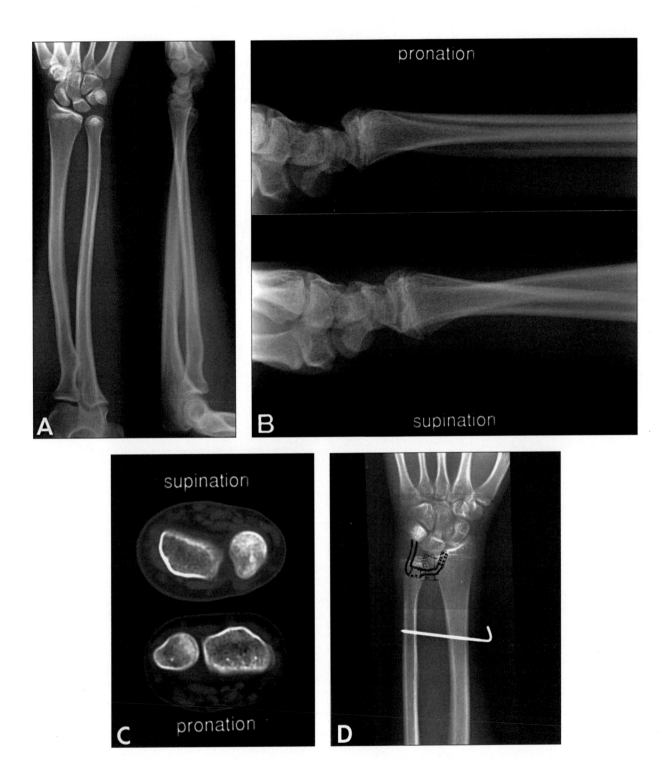

FIGURE 35–28

Palmar subluxation of ulnar head. **A,** A 14-year-old girl fell playing basketball. *Left,* Anteroposterior view in supination was nondiagnostic. *Right,* Palmar prominence of ulnar head. **B,** Lateral radiographs. *Top,* Pronation is normal. *Bottom,* Supination shows palmar subluxation. **C,** Computed tomographic scan. Palmar subluxation in supination and reduced pronation. **D,** Postoperative radiograph shows palmar capsular imbrication and tendinous augmentation.

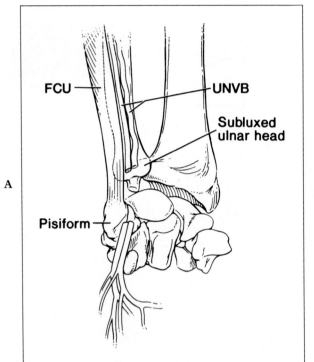

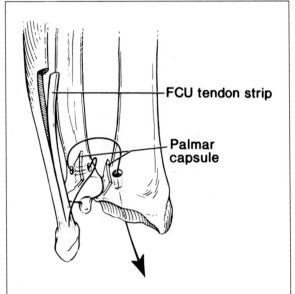

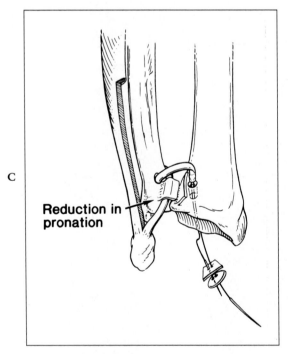

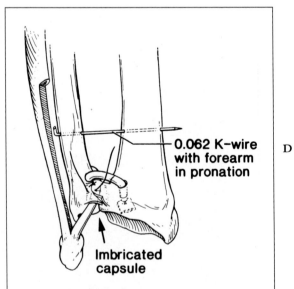

FIGURE 35-29

Reduction and ligamentous augmentation for palmar subluxation of the dorsal radioulnar joint (DRUJ). **A,** Schematic diagram of structures at palmar aspect of DRUJ. **B,** Raise strip of flexor carpi ulnaris (*FCU*) attached distally. Expose palmar capsule of DRUJ. **C,** Transverse drill hole in the distal ulnar neck and a palmodorsal drill hole in the ulnopalmar corner. **D,** Pass tendon strip through ulnar hole using double-armed nonabsorbable suture. Then pass needles through radius and retrieve them percutaneously. Tie suture over felt bolster. Pronate forearm to neutral. Pull tendon strip taut and suture at ulnar neck. Imbricate palmar capsule. Supination progressively tightens construct and prevents palmar subluxation. *UNVB,* ulnar neurovascular bundle.

the postreduction film should be closely inspected for transarticular shear fractures.

Open reduction is done through an incision paralleling the radial border of the FCU. The ulnar neurovascular bundle is held ulnarly, and the ulnar head is exposed by sweeping the finger flexor fascia radially. Ecchymosis in the surrounding areolar tissue is displaced, exposing the rent in the palmar capsule and the ulnar head. If finger pressure is insufficient to effect reduction, a small cervical laminectomy spreader inserted between radius and ulna will produce sufficient distraction to unlock the ulnar head from its perch on the palmar rim of the radius. It is difficult to inspect the dorsal aspect of the articular surface adequately through this approach. Reflection of the capsule affords a partial view of the TFC for evaluation. It should lie in its anatomic position so healing can occur. Repair may be considered if the joint seems unstable on manipulation. This may require styloid fixation or transosseous suturing of the TFC insertion. Arthroscopic assistance or a secondary dorsal incision may be needed. A tight closure of the palmar capsule and 2 to 3 weeks of neutral or partially pronated immobilization are sufficient to avoid redislocation.

Recurrent chronic subluxation requires some form of reconstruction. Radiographs help eliminate the possibility of malalignment of the radius and ulna. Corrective osteotomies are necessary before soft-tissue repair. The status of the TFC is checked by arthrography or arthroscopy. A large styloid fragment suggests the possibility of styloid reattachment. This can be accomplished through a longitudinal incision over the styloid, freshening of the fracture facets, and fixation using a compression screw or tension band wiring. Reattachment of the DRUL to the radius is also possible with an open or arthroscopic technique.

When TFC repair is not feasible there are several reconstructive procedures described. Several of the radioulnar tendinous loops described above were initially used for habitual palmar subluxation.[63,73,136,174] Because the subluxation usually occurs as the forearm is supinated, the loop should tighten on supination and relax on pronation. This can be controlled by adjusting the anchor point on the radius somewhat dorsally. Sanders and Hawkins[181] described a combination procedure using a palmaris longus tendon radioulnar loop and then added an ulnocarpal tether by using the distal ECU tendon passed through a hole in the ulnar head and then reanastomosed to its proximal stump.

The following procedure, plication of the palmar capsule augmented with a strip of FCU, has been effective in a series of six patients in whom there did not appear to be a reconstructible TFC (Fig. 35-29). The ulnopalmar approach with the forearm supinated is used to expose the redundant capsule (Fig. 35-28, D). The capsule is incised longitudinally and reflected. The

ulnar head and palmar aspect of the TFC are inspected. A transverse drill hole is made at the base of the ulnar neck and another is directed dorsally from the ulnopalmar corner of the radius immediately adjacent to the articular rim. A strip of FCU is detached proximally and left attached at the pisiform. The end is passed through the drill hole in the ulnar neck. A double-armed suture is then woven through the end of the tendon and the needles are fed through the hole in the radius and exit through the dorsal skin. Finger motion is checked to be sure an extensor tendon has not been pierced. The suture is tied over a felt bolster. The slack is removed from the tendon while the forearm is returned to a neutral position. It is then sutured to the ulnar half of the capsule and the capsule is plicated in a pants-over-vest fashion. Immobilization is protected for 6 weeks, during which time the transcutaneous dorsal suture is removed. Progressive supination exercises are then begun and done until full rotation is achieved in an anticipated 8 to 12 weeks (Fig. 35-28).

The rationale of the procedure relies on the capsular reconstruction becoming increasingly taut with progressive supination. The FCU slip also acts to augment the buttressing effect of the palmar rim of the sigmoid notch because the latter is often eroded from chronic subluxation.

A depressed lesion in the ulnar head is not a contraindication to a stabilization procedure. If the ulnar head can be maintained in its normal relationship with the sigmoid notch, the lesion is well tolerated. A salvage procedure is rarely needed.

TRIANGULAR FIBROCARTILAGE INJURIES AND STYLOID FRACTURES

The TFC is a complex structure that subserves several functions: apposition of the radius to the ulna, dorsopalmar restraint, joint compressive load transference, and separation of the radiocarpal joint from the DRUJ.[29,185] It is frequently injured with sprains of the wrist and fractures of the distal forearm. The components of the TFC, although subserving different functions, to some extent, are held closely organized so that distinction in symptoms or diagnosis related to a specific area is seldom possible.

When disruption of the TFC occurs medially, there is often a fracture of the ulnar styloid as well. The degree of disruption that takes place is a function of the energy dissipation occurring at the joint and the net displacement that occurs between ulna and radius. Palmer[160] classified TFC injuries as noted in Table 35-1. The site of styloid fracture provides some indication of the extent or severity of the injury as this relates to the insertional areas of the components of the TFC. A fracture distal to the midpoint of the styloid is unlikely to indicate disruption of the attachments to the base. A fractured tip may indicate styloidal carpal impaction or avulsion associated with the periosteal sleeve. A fracture at the base destabilizes the styloidal attachment of the TFC and can also be associated with soft-tissue avulsion of the foveal element. A fracture through the base that

Table 35-1. Abnormalities of the Triangular Fibrocartilage Complex

Class 1: Traumatic
Stage
A: Central perforation
B: Ulnar avulsion
      With distal ulnar fracture
      Without distal ulnar fracture
C: Distal avulsion
D: Radial avulsion
      With sigmoid notch fracture
      Without sigmoid notch fracture

Class 2: Degenerative (Ulnocarpal Abutment Syndrome)
Stage
A: TFCC wear
B: TFCC wear
      + Lunate or ulnar chondromalacia or both
C: TFCC perforation
      + Lunate or ulnar chondromalacia or both
D: TFCC perforation
      + Lunate or ulnar chondromalacia or both
      + Lunotriquetral ligament perforation
E: TFCC perforation
      + Lunate or ulnar chondromalacia or both
      + Lunotriquetral ligament perforation
      + Ulnocarpal arthritis

TFCC, triangular fibrocartilage complex.

includes the fovea obviously destabilizes the entire ulnar attachment of the TFC. Fractures through the ulnar neck are even more severe injuries on average and are not discussed here.[47,160]

When the styloid is fractured the periosteal sleeve that envelops the medial three-quarters of the circumference is variably disrupted. In the more severe injury, the adjacent ECU subsheath may be avulsed or stripped from its groove adjacent to the styloid.[137] Indeed the styloid on some occasions may be stripped completely of its soft-tissue attachments where its intact profile misleads the radiograph interpreter into underestimating the seriousness of the injury.

Injuries of the radial attachment of the TFC obviously also occur. The thin central attachment has only a cartilaginous continuity with poor healing potential. It may be of little clinical significance unless an intrusive flap develops or there is an element of ulnocarpal impaction. These tears may be difficult to distinguish from the central defects seen with the attrition of aging or as impaction defects. Peripheral avulsions may include a portion of the radial rim and represent more destabilizing injuries. Tears in the substance of the TFC may be stellate or intralaminar in character. There is often an element of ulnocarpal compression as well as displacement and torque in the mechanism of injury.*

Symptoms include pain aggravated by twisting or ulnar deviation. A click or snap is often heard and felt at the same time. On examination there is tenderness at the ulnotriquetral interval which may be aggravated by ballottement of the ulnar head. Direct pressure in the medial "snuffbox" just palmar to the styloid sometimes induces the click on ulnar deviation. This test also has a positive result in patients who have lunotriquetral tears.

Standard radiographic studies are often normal unless a styloid or radial rim avulsion is noted. A wrist

---

* References 4,42,47,93,144,154.

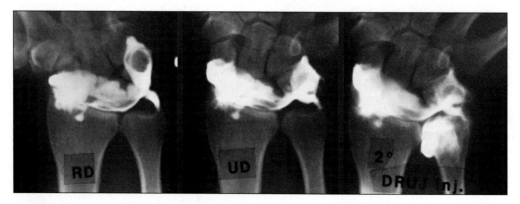

FIGURE 35–30

Radiocarpal arthrogram. *Left*, Radial deviation. *Middle*, Ulnar deviation. *Right*, Radioulnar arthrogram. Note the palmar radial bursal extension at the scapholunate fossa junction, the filling of the pisotriquetral joint, and the change in contour of the distal margin of the triangular fibrocartilage. Arthrogram read as normal. *DRUJ*, dorsal radioulnar joint; *inj.*, injection; *RD*, radial deviation; *UD*, ulnar deviation.

arthrogram is usually the most productive next exami-nation.[79,126,213] Observation of the dye flow under the image intensifier may give some extra insight into the problem (Fig. 35-30). Peripheral tears at the styloid or fovea are not likely to be apparent unless the DRUJ is injected separately. Dye filling the fovea or surrounding the styloid and infiltrating the ECU tendon sheath indicates a tear (Figs. 35-31, 35-32, and 35-33).[216] In late instances of TFC foveal disruption there is often evidence of enchondral new bone formation on the pole that has a distinct cutoff immediately adjacent to the fovea.

Arthroscopy has been cited increasingly as the diag-nostic test of choice in evaluating TFC injuries because it provides direct information on the size, extent, and severity of the injury and allows inspection of the carpus and radiocarpal ligaments at the same time. It also allows débridement of frayed tissue, and some arthroscopic-aided repairs of TFC attachments have been successful.[23,47,158,170] Examination of the radio-ulnar portion of the joint is more difficult because of the tight confines. The potential for overusing this tool should also be kept in mind.

The indications for treatment vary as a function of the duration and severity of symptoms as well as asso-ciated injuries. Ulnar styloid and TFC injuries are fre-quently associated with other injuries of the wrist. In Colles' fractures, for instance, or even in an Essex-Lopresti injury where the displacement is sufficient to ensure disruption of the TFC, if satisfactory reduction of the primary injury is adequate, late problems asso-ciated with the detachment are infrequent. Nevertheless, if operation is required for open reduc-tion and internal fixation of the radius, simultaneous fixation of the TFC injury is worth consideration,

especially if the radioulnar joint is unstable to manip-ulation when tested after radial fixation. Optimum conditions for repair are never better than at the time of the acute injury.

In the late injury, the treatment of TFC disruptions from the ulna can be repaired by exposure alongside the styloid. Freshening of the fovea or styloid fracture facets with a curette followed by tension band wiring or mini-screw fixation is usually successful (Fig. 35-20), although screw, wire, or Kirschner wire breakage readily occurs

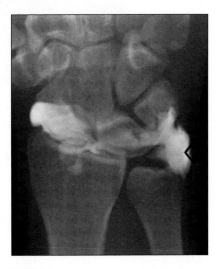

FIGURE 35-32

A 39-year-old man with a wrist sprain. Arthrogram shows trian-gular fibrocartilage styloidal detachment and dye outline within ligamentum subcruentum.

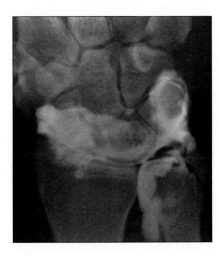

FIGURE 35-31

A 37-year-old man sustained an injury using a punching bag. Arthrogram shows central communication, partial disruption at ulnar styloid and fovea (arrow), and a lunotriquetral joint commu-nication, with possible luntotriquetral ligament tear.

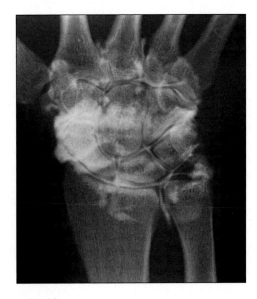

FIGURE 35-33

A 23-year-old man. Radiocarpal appearance consistent with arthro-gram showing lunotriquetral tear. Triangular fibrocartilage commu-nication and ulna positive variance. Treatment should be directed at the ulna length variance.

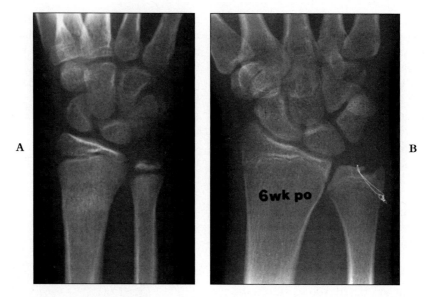

FIGURE 35-34

A, A 14-year-old girl with a tennis injury presented with unstable forehand stroke. Avulsion foveal attachment was suspected. **B,** After excision of loose body and transosseous wiring of the ulnar aspect of the triangular fibrocartilage with foveal reattachment, recovery was satisfactory.

with motion if adequate immobilization is not maintained for at least 6 weeks. Excision of the styloid and coaptation of the ligament to the raw area is also a reasonable option that obviates styloid nonunion. A nonabsorbable 2.0 suture should be passed through the thickened attachment area of the TFC and brought through drill holes in the ulnar cortex for knotting under mild tension (Fig. 35-34).[47,93]

Avulsions from the radial attachment require similar freshening of the site of attachment. Exposure from the palmar aspect is outlined in treatment for palmar subluxation. Dorsal exposure between the fourth and fifth extensor tendon compartments provides access to the dorsal rim of the radius. Small drill holes made with a 1-mm twist drill or a 0.28-in. Kirschner wire are angled to the site of detachment. Nonabsorbable sutures (3.0 or 4.0) are woven through the edge of the avulsed margin of the TFC and brought back through the holes for knotting. A bony fragment may be fixed in a similar manner. Adequate postoperative immobilization for 6 weeks is imperative. Standard physical therapy regimens are then undertaken.[47,93]

CHONDROMALACIA AND DEGENERATIVE ARTHRITIS

Chondromalacia of the ulnar head may occur on either the distal pole or the radioulnar joint laterally. The former is discussed below with ulnar impaction, and the latter has already been mentioned with dorsal

subluxation. A shearing injury of the seat of the ulnar head against the dorsal rim of the sigmoid notch during subluxation is the presumed mechanism (Figs. 35-10 and 35-16). When seen acutely, the DRUJ is tender and rotation is often limited. If the subluxation has been completely reduced, pronation is likely to be limited as the injured area on the ulnar head again approaches the dorsal rim of the radius. Conversely, if subluxation persists, pain is aggravated as the injured area attempts to slip under the radial rim. This feature can also be used in physical diagnosis by ballottement of the ulnar head as the forearm is sequentially turned through short arcs of motion.[134]

Repetitive injury eventually leads to degenerative arthritis associated with a central area of eburnation and fibrillated cartilage with underlying enchondral new bone formation to either side. The cumulative effect is to produce an irregular eccentric shape to the head that mechanically inhibits rotation (Figs. 35-35, *A* and *B*). The osteophyte produced has in some instances mirrored the problem seen in rheumatoid involvement of the DRUJ in which the osteophytes perforate the overlying capsule and rupture the extensor digiti minimi or the ECU through attrition (Figs. 35-36 and 35-37).[147]

Standard radiographs are often normal at initial examination. Computed tomographic scans may suggest dorsal subluxation or a superficial cortical injury on the ulna head (Fig. 35-38). Magnetic resonance imaging has shown joint effusions that are not readily appreciated on radiographs (Fig. 35-39). A technetium-99 scan may be negative if only cartilage damage was involved,

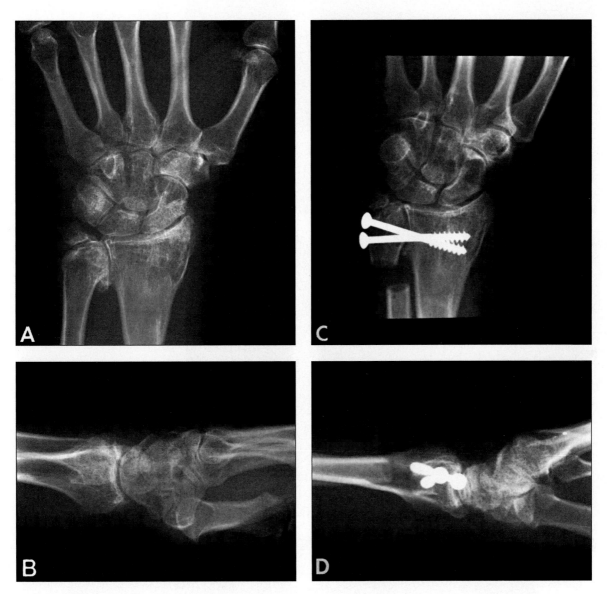

FIGURE 35-35

A, Anteroposterior view of wrist shows hypertrophic degenerative joint disease at the dorsal radioulnar joint ulnar styloid avulsion fracture. **B,** Lateral residual dorsal angulation of a distal radial fracture. **C** and **D,** After a Kapandji procedure.

but it tends to show strong localization if the bone is injured. When the chronic stage has been reached, osteophytes, subcortical cysts, and joint space narrowing are seen.

The initial episode should be treated conservatively. The area of injury should be localized by the method described above, and the forearm should be immobilized in a position in which the defect is not in contact with the opposing surface. Usually this is determined by the position of optimum comfort between neutral and supination.

In chronic conditions, the radiographs may suggest that the distal portion of the joint is more involved than the proximal. An ulnar recession of 2 to 4 mm may be

sufficient to eliminate the painful contact. With more extensive involvement, open assessment allows several options. These include proceeding to joint débridement, partial ulnar head excision, and a Darrach or Kapandji procedure (Figs. 35-35, *C* and *D*).[44,52] Tendon repair or interposition grafting may be indicated as well.

JOINT CONTRACTURE

Limitation of pronosupination after trauma is common and may result from several factors, including intra-articular damage, fracture malunion, muscular damage, and soft-tissue fibrosis. The last may affect the

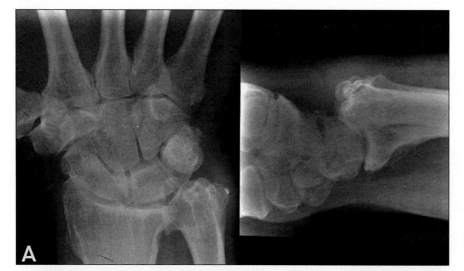

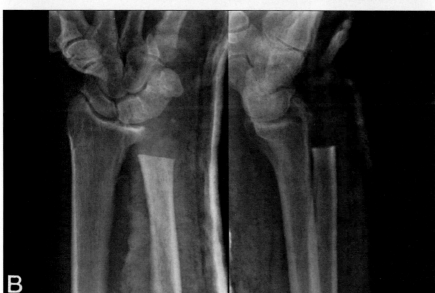

FIGURE 35-36

A, A 61-year-old man. Distal radius fracture sustained fusion of the dorsal radioulnar joint in childhood. Note arthritic changes in the distal ulna. Positive ulna variance. Recent extensor digiti quinti, extensor digitorum communis 4,5 tendon ruptures; painful limited supination. **B,** Darrach resection and tenorrhaphy of extensor tendons.

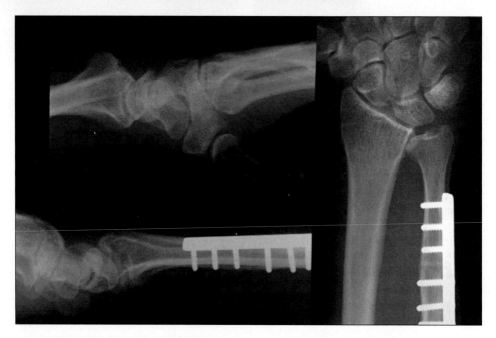

FIGURE 35-37

A 62-year-old woman with a weak wrist and loss of extension of the fifth finger. *Top left,* Dorsal prominence of ulnar head; positive piano key sign. Ruptured extensor digiti quinti. *Bottom left* and *right,* Ulnar recession realignment relieved discomfort; tendon transfer of the extensor digiti quinti to extensor digiti communis.

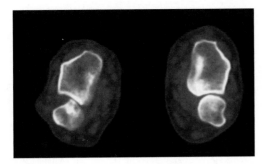

FIGURE 35-38

A 40-year-old man with pain and limited forearm supination. Computed tomographic scan, coronal view through dorsal radioulnar joint bilaterally, shows advanced degenerative joint disease on the left and hypertrophic ulnar styloid.

ordinarily loose dorsal or palmar capsules of the DRUJ. This is most likely after stretching or tearing of the capsule followed by a period of immobilization in a shortened position. The capsule may thicken and develop cross adherence between its laminar components. The IOM may also undergo some contracture from lengthy inactivity.[7]

Physical examination discloses a distinct block to further rotation not explainable on the basis of known deformity. The ulnar head is not readily ballotable.

Progressive, active-assisted rotational exercises under the supervision of a hand therapist may be adequate to overcome the contracture. Addition of a dynamic splint, particularly for leisure intervals and for sleep, may help stretch out the fibrosis. If the joint shows signs of inflammation reaction with swelling or erythema, the dynamic splinting will need to be moderated.

If contracture persists, surgical release of the tight capsule is justifiable.[7] For a pronation contracture the palmar approach detailed above allows exposure of the palmar capsule. This can be cut obliquely from the margin of the pronator quadratus to the PRUL. A periosteal elevator is then inserted to sweep open the space between the TFC and the pole of the ulnar head (recessus sacciformis). The forearm is slowly and firmly supinated while the ulnar head is observed to prevent its palmar subluxation. The wound is irrigated with bupivacaine to allow early postoperative motion after skin closure. A similar dorsal approach through the extensor retinaculum over the fifth compartment permits incision of the dorsal capsule and the distal IOM if needed. Manipulation into pronation is accomplished with thumb pressure over the ulnar head to prevent dorsal subluxation. Closure of the dorsal retinaculum may be difficult without using a Z-plastic modification. Postoperatively, a pronation splint may be necessary for several weeks between exercise periods. A useful aid in regaining motion is

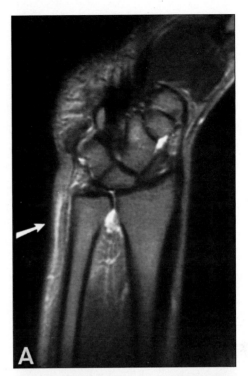

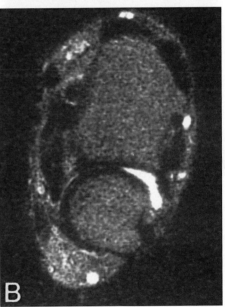

FIGURE 35-39

A, T1-weighted magnetic resonance coronal view. Effusion in dorsal radioulnar joint (DRUJ) and along extensor carpi ulnaris tendon sheaths (*arrow*). **B,** T2-weighted axial view shows effusion in DRUJ after dorsal subluxation injury. Possible chondromalacic change.

the use of a broom or long-handled hammer which, when tightly grasped with the forearm parallel to the floor while allowing the broom head to fall, imparts a torque on the joint that is easily altered by adjusting the length of the handle.[133]

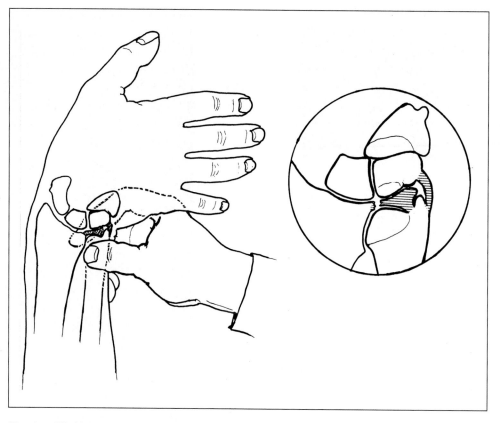

FIGURE 35–40

If the ulnar head is depressed while the forearm is pronated, ulnar deviation will compress the triangular fibrocartilage (TFC) and elicit pain if the TFC is injured.

ULNA VARIANCE CONDITIONS

ULNAR IMPACTION (ABUTMENT) SYNDROME

This condition occurs primarily in wrists exhibiting a positive ulna variance and is a result of the carpus impacting against the pole of the ulnar head when the radiocarpal joint is compressed (see Chapter 33). Schuind et al.[185] and Neviaser and Palmer[154] have shown that the radius migrates proximally about 1 mm during firm grasp. During external load, proximal radial migration as well as a bowing deflection of the radius may accentuate the ulnar projection.[207] The TFC is thinnest in the interval between the ulnar head and the ulnar aspect of the lunate, providing little dampening of impaction forces. Palmer and Werner[163] have classified the attritional changes that occur in the TFC as Class 2 lesions. These may begin on either the proximal or distal surface of the TFC—2A. Chondromalacia next occurs on the ulnar pole or ulnar aspect of the proximal lunate—2B. With continuing usage, chondromalacia is associated with perforation of the central portion of the TFC—2C. This develops more ragged edges as its size increases, and a tear may also develop in the central portion of the lunotriquetral ligament with time—2D.[160,175] This is likely the result of the shearing stress occurring with piston action

between the two bones. Koebke[120] and Mikic[144] have shown that the subcortical trabeculae initially increase in thickness below the site of impaction. Subcortical cystic degenerative changes follow. This condition is seen more commonly in the elderly and there is some evidence that positive ulna variance increases with time, possibly from settling at the radiocapitellar joint.

Symptoms are primarily pain and tenderness at the ulnocarpal area aggravated by strenuous activity, ulnar deviation, and pronosupination. The last two activities promote a shearing motion across the site of involvement. Ballottement or depression of the ulnar head, especially with ulnar deviation, usually accentuates the pain by compressing and shearing the injured structures (Fig. 35-40).[53]

Although the condition is often appreciated on standard radiographs, the 90/90 shoulder, elbow films in which the x-ray tube is precisely above the wrist provide the greatest accuracy for evaluation.[64,69,88,123,193] Measurement of ulna variance may be done using a project-a-line technique described by Hultén,[98] the concentric circle method of Palmer et al.,[161] or the perpendicular to the radial axis technique. Steyers and Blair[188] showed that the differences in technique or between observers were probably of little consequence (Fig. 35-41). A close inspection in addition to

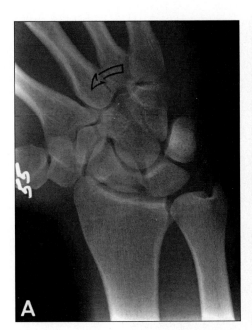

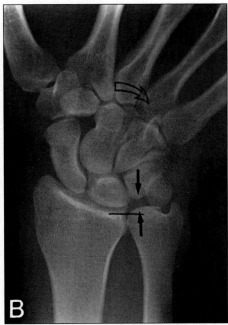

FIGURE 35-41

A, Note radiodensity of ulnar dome in radial deviation. **B,** Ulnar deviation. Ulna plus variance 2 mm (*solid arrows*).

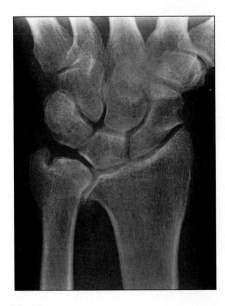

FIGURE 35-42

A 58-year-old man with probable childhood injury with premature closure of radial physis, resulting in ulna plus variance, secondary reversal of radioulnar angle, and ulnolunotriquetral impaction.

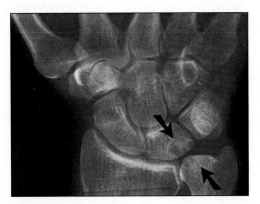

FIGURE 35-43

A 57-year-old man with ulnocarpal impaction. Anteroposterior radiograph shows previous excision of the radial head for a radial head comminuted fracture. Ulna positive variance, sclerosis of ulnar head (*bottom arrow*) and lunate, subcortical cysts at lunate (*top arrow*), and reversal slope at the radioulnar joint.

the ulna plus variance often discloses cortical sclerosis at the point of closest ulnolunate apposition (Fig. 35-42). There may be trabecular sclerosis surrounding a small cystic or osteopenic area immediately below (Fig. 35-43). This condition is more readily appreciated with polyaxial tomography or computed tomographic scans.* At times, the changes have been dramatic enough to suggest Kienböck's disease (Fig. 35-44). However, the changes in Kienböck's disease are usually over the radius rather than the ulna. Radiographs of the elbow may be indicated if there is a history of previous forearm or elbow injury (see radial head excision and gymnast's wrist). Technetium-99 scans usually show a rather intense isotopic take-up at the site (Fig. 35-45).[53]

_____

* References 36,39,43,71,87,148.

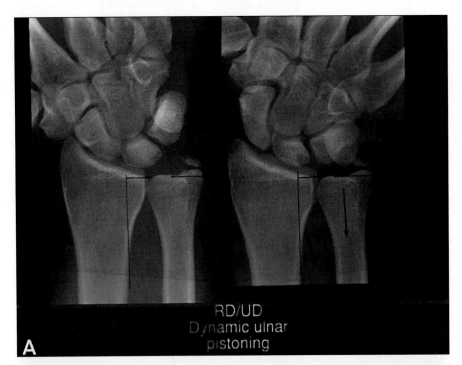

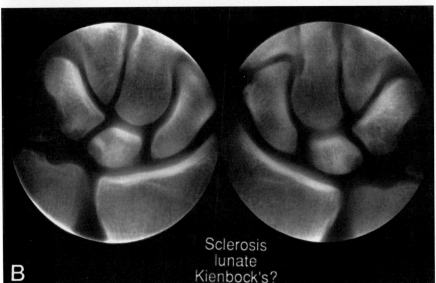

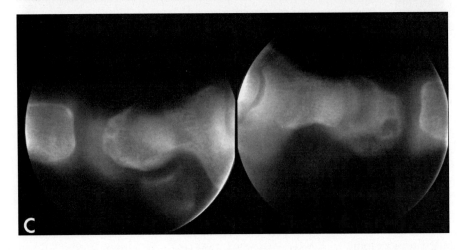

FIGURE 35-44

A, Patient referred as having bilateral Kienböck's disease. *Left* and *right*, Old fractures of the ulnar styloid and sclerotic, irregular proximal lunate with radioulnar deviation without obvious impaction. **B** and **C,** Trispiral tomograms show erosions on lunate and opposite pole of the ulnar head. Bilateral intraosseous changes in lunate and triquetrum. An ulnar recession of 2 mm resolved the clinical symptoms. *RD,* radial deviation; *UD,* ulnar deviation.

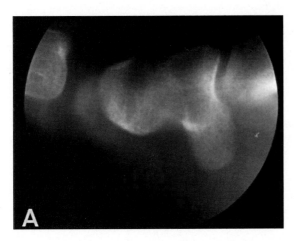 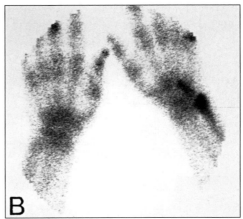

FIGURE 35-45

In a motor vehicle accident, the hand on the steering wheel twisted, extended, and ulnarly deviated. **A,** Trispiral tomogram shows impaction defect in ulnopalmar aspect of the triquetrum (sclerosis). **B,** Technetium-99 uptake is intense in left distal ulna and triquetrum.

TREATMENT

Not all patients with this condition have sufficient symptoms to justify active treatment. Open arthrotomy for partial or complete TFC excision has largely been superseded by arthroscopic débridement of the ragged central TFC defects.[201] This of course may be insufficient to decompress the ulnocarpal contact.[158,170] There are various surgical options that all follow the rationale of reducing the contact between ulna and lunate.

Ulnar recession can be accomplished by transverse, step-cut, or oblique osteotomies designed to produce an ulnar shortening to an ulna neutral or ulna minus position (Fig. 35-46). The osteotomy is best done at or distal to the junction of the distal and mid-thirds of the ulna to avoid interruption with the function of the IOM.[24,53,66,173] Another option is excision of the distal articular surface of the ulnar head ("wafer procedure"). Secondary adhesions between the roughened surface lying beneath the proximal aspect of the TFC are seldom a problem.[67] There has also been a considerable interest in arthroscopic removal of the ulnar pole, which can be accomplished through the defect in the TFC. In both instances, the articular surface between the ulnar dome and sigmoid notch of the radioulnar joint is protected.

Ulnar recession has been a successful procedure at my institution. The primary key to success is accurate measurement of the amount of bone to be removed, including that removed by the saw blade itself (the kerf). As little as 2 mm may be sufficient, and as much as 8 mm may be accomplished. Difficulty may be seen when there is a reverse radioulnar angle. This angle tends to increase with increasing ulna plus variance.[70] This may not only impede the proximal slide of the

ulnar head but also impinge against a cortical lip that projects from the inferior margin of the sigmoid notch. This projection may be undermined and forced out of the way or merely osteotomized (Figs. 35-47 and 35-48).

On several occasions at the time of ulnar osteotomy the distal portion of the IOM and pronator quadratus have been stripped from the distal ulnar fragment, allowing it to be swung aside to expose the DRUJ from the proximal aspect. With the capsule incised, the entire ulnar head, sigmoid notch, and undersurface of the TFC are readily inspected. This facilitates TFC repair, débridement, and modification of the projecting lip mentioned above (Fig. 35-46, *C*). It also relaxes the space available to inspect the ulnocarpal joint through a capsulotomy in the fifth dorsal compartment. A lunotriquetral tear may then also be repaired at the same time (Fig. 35-49). This technique has not been responsible for delayed healing of the ulna or other complications. The procedure is accomplished by applying the compression plate distally before the osteotomy is marked. Proximal alignment markings are made to ensure proper alignment as the distal fragment is later advanced and compression applied. It is possible to include a slight correction to the alignment if there is an exaggerated dorsal arc to the distal ulna that has produced excessive dorsopalmar translation in the notch.[53] Ulnar recession can be a versatile procedure for various problems at the DRUJ.

PROXIMAL MIGRATION OF THE RADIUS

Proximal migration of the radius occurs after radial head excision. This is usually done for comminuted radial head fractures.[114] The longitudinal instability of

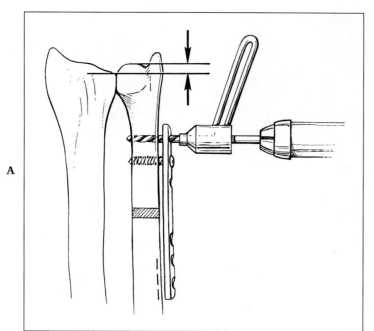

A

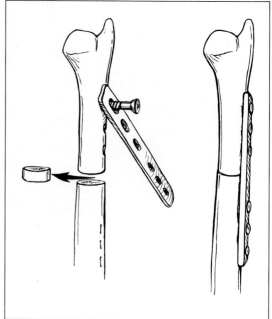

B

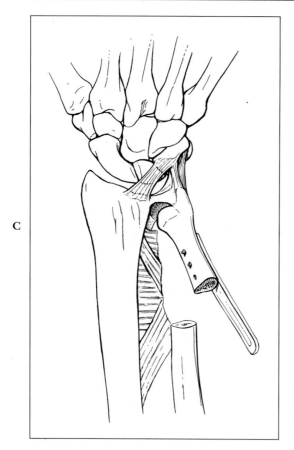

C

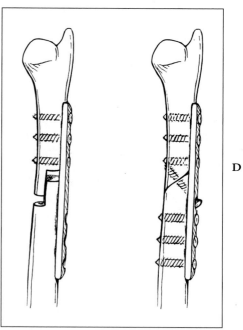

D

FIGURE 35-46

A, Ulnar recession is generally planned to render the wrist ulna neutral or slightly negative. A simple method relies on a 6-hole dynamic compression plate sized for 2.7-mm screws in smaller boned individuals or 3.5-mm screws in larger patients. The plate is contoured to shape to fit well distally. The distal two holes are drilled, tapped, and filled. Alignment marks are made along the bone proximally. **B,** One screw is removed and the other is loosened to allow rotation of the plate, and an osteotomy of predetermined size is made in the distal ulna. The plate is realigned and securely fixed in compression. **C,** Alternatively, the distal segment may be freed to swing outward on the distal soft-tissue elements. This allows an excellent view of not only the dorsal radioulnar joint but also the ulnocarpal joint through a more distal capsular incision for more extensive repairs. **D,** Alternative methods of ulnar recession include step-cut or precision oblique osteotomies using a jig (Rayhack).

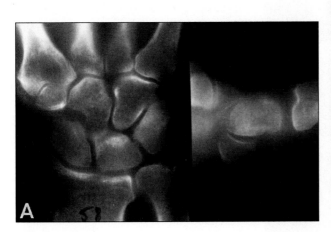
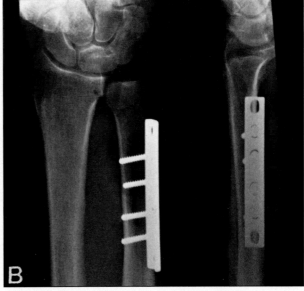

FIGURE 35-47

A 47-year-old male brewer with ulnar wrist pain after a twisting injury. **A,** *Left,* Anteroposterior tomogram with ulna plus variance. *Right,* Lateral tomogram shows pisotriquetral degenerative joint disease. At operation, we discovered a tear in the triangular fibrocartilage, intact lunotriquetral ligament, and a proximal flange in the sigmoid notch. **B,** Postoperative ulnar recession and recession of proximal lip of the sigmoid notch with pisiformectomy. Improvement in pain.

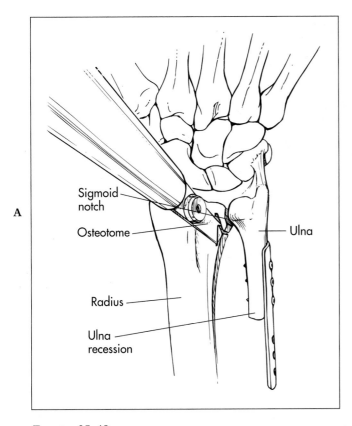
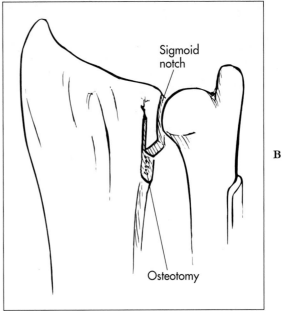

FIGURE 35-48

A, If there is a reverse slope to the sigmoid notch that impedes proximal retraction of the ulnar head, the sigmoid notch may be undercut with a saw or osteotome and **(B)** the articular fragment rotated to avoid further impingement. Procedure performed with ulnar recession.

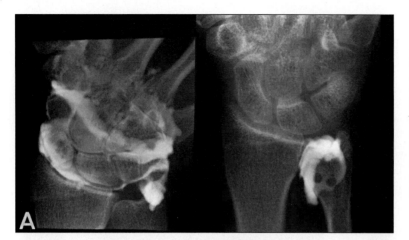

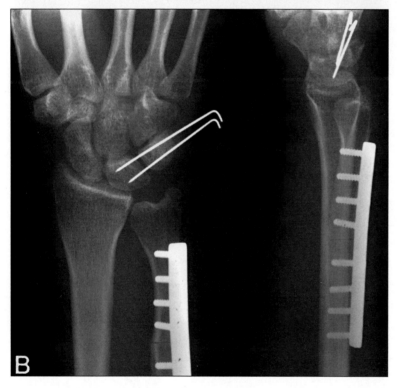

FIGURE 35-49

A, A 19-year-old female competitive tennis player with a positive arthrogram and symptoms of lunotriquetral (LT) dissociation and triangular fibrocartilage instability. **B,** Treatment by ulna recession and LT ligament repair. Exposure aided by swinging distal ulna out to increase space for repair of LT ligament (see Figure 35-46). Ulna recession with 8-hole compression plate fixation. Kirschner wires are used across the LT joint.

the forearm is probably greater after an extensive injury such as radial head fracture combined with DRUJ dislocation (Essex-Lopresti fracture dislocation) (Fig. 35-43). An ulna plus variance of 2 to 3 mm develops in most patients, but this becomes symptomatic enough to warrant treatment in a minority. The ulnar head should be resected as a last resort because this further narrows and weakens the forearm. An ulnar recession is a better choice, but persistent radial migration sometimes results in proximal radial neck capitellum impingement as well as ulnocarpal reimpaction. Efforts to create a strengthened IOM have been only marginally successful. Radial head replacements with silicone prostheses may be of temporary help in stabilizing the radius, but angulation, fragmentation, capitellar erosion, and particulate synovitis are seen as adverse reactions. The radiocapitellar joint should be preserved when feasible.

ULNAR STYLOID IMPINGEMENT AND LOOSE BODIES

In some individuals the ulnar styloid is unusually large or projects close to the triquetral surface as seen on an anteroposterior radiograph. Mechanisms of wrist injury can cause the tip of the styloid to impinge against the triquetrum (Figs. 35-45 and 35-50). This can result in a localized painful area that slowly improves with time without any apparent radiographic findings. At other times, a small impacted area is seen in the triquetrum, and in some circumstances it has been suggested as an element in fractures to the dorsal triquetral rim. The tip of the styloid is covered with an articular cartilaginous cap. If a portion of this is sheared off, it can grow and develop partial ossification, as is seen in many other joints. This usually stays in the

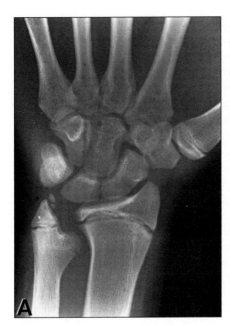 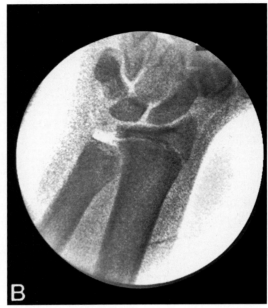

FIGURE 35-50

A 15-year-old boy 12 months postinjury. **A,** Anteroposterior radiograph shows premature physeal closure under pole of the ulnar head with continued growth of the ulnar styloid; residual of fracture distally. Ulnar styloid-triquetral impingement. **B,** Postoperative styloid excision and repair of ulnar attachment of the triangular fibrocartilage.

prestyloid recess where it is labeled an "os secondarium" or an "os Daubentonni." It may also impinge between styloid and triquetrum in some situations, acting as a loose body. Occasionally, two or more symptomatic loose bodies develop. The distal fragment of a styloid nonunion may hypertrophy with time and also induce an impingement. Excision is usually curative.[35] A few instances of synovial osteochondritis have been reported. Excision of these is not as easy as it might seem. An intraoperative image intensifier may be helpful even if an arthroscope is used. Excision of the distal portion of the styloid is without substantial risk.

GYMNAST'S WRIST

With the marked increased interest in gymnastics worldwide, there has been an alarming increase in wrist problems in young students (see Chapter 45).[9,180,214] The increased compressional stress imposed on the wrist by handstands, floor exercises, and pommel horse routines appears to be responsible for physeal changes that are most marked at the distal radius. Pain, weakness, and swelling at the distal radius are symptoms that resolve with rest but often return with resumption of exercise. Radiographs show a widening zone of osteopenia proximal to the physis with some adjacent small areas of sclerosis and irregularity of the physeal line. This seems to promote a premature epiphysiodesis of the radius that, with continued growth of the ulna, produces

the ulnolunate impaction syndrome described above, except the patient presents in adolescence or young adulthood (Fig. 35-42). The physis proximal to the lunate fossa may be at greater risk because a pseudo-Madelung's deformity has been noted to occur.

A variant of this condition may be seen in individuals who specialize in events that produce distraction forces such as the uneven bars of girls' gymnastics. Petersen and Adams[166] have noted that a special glove worn to transmit some of the force from the fingers directly to the wrist may be a factor. Radiographs show a widened physis with some irregularity and metaphyseal osteopenia.

Treatment of these conditions is primarily modification of the training routines after a suitable period of rest and recovery. If symptoms persist after growth termination, surgical intervention is warranted.

ULNA MINUS CONDITIONS

An ulna minus is the normal status for the majority of wrists and is probably of little significance to most individuals. As the degree of minus variant increases, there is a correlation with an increased radioulnar angle so that the ulnar head is somewhat more conical.[18,64] The TFC is usually somewhat thicker, but the amount of joint compressive force transmitted through the ulnar head is decreased.[162] Hultén[98] was the first to note a correlation of Kienböck's disease with ulna minus variance. This has been disputed, but most series, including those from my institution, validate this observation. There also appears to be a disproportionate representation of ulna minus variance in patients demonstrating scapholunate dissociation, and there is a suggestion that patients with carpal instability nondissociative also show this tendency.[50,206,213]

Ulnar lengthening or radial recession has been used as a joint-leveling procedure in Kienböck's disease and in a few patients with the "catch-up clunk" seen in carpal instability nondissociative.[213] If the radioulnar angle is marked, there may be an increased shear stress placed in the radioulnar joint if the ulnar head is displaced distally without a compensatory translation of the radius.

CONGENITAL MALFORMATION AFFECTING THE DISTAL RADIOULNAR JOINT

Madelung's disease and multiple hereditary exostoses are the two primary conditions affecting the joint. The former appears to be a condition in which premature closure occurs of the portion of the distal radial physis underlying the lunate fossa. The severity of involvement varies with the age at onset and is generally worse in the

approximately 50% of patients with hereditary dyschondrosteosis. The deformity is characterized by progressive ulnopalmar angulation of the distal radius, shortening of the forearm, and dorsal and distal prominence of the ulnar head. On radiographs there is a marked increase of the ulnar and palmar slope of the distal radius; a physeal scar of the lunate fossa trailing proximally on the ulnar border of the radius; a conformal wedge shape to the carpus; a spread between radius and ulna; and a broadened, lengthened distorted ulnar head (Fig. 35-51). Vickers and Nielsen[203] described a fibrous band tethering the ulnopalmar rim of the radius as the cause of Madelung's disease. Removal of this band, if performed early, has allowed sufficient growth to resume in the physis of the lunate fossa to remodel the radius to a near-normal configuration.

A wide variety of osteotomies have been described in the more mature patient. Currently, we use an opening wedge osteotomy that parallels the physeal scar on the ulnopalmar aspect of the radial metaphysis. Exposure is gained between the ulnar neurovascular bundle and the finger flexors. The lunate fossa is wedged distally and held with a trapezoidal-shaped iliac graft. A second open wedge graft is inserted more proximally if radial bowing warrants. Temporary additional distraction with an external fixator was sometimes used to remove the load on the construct. Soft-tissue

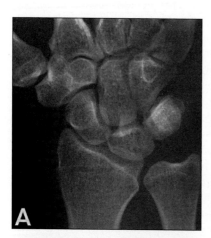

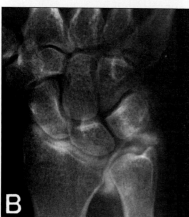

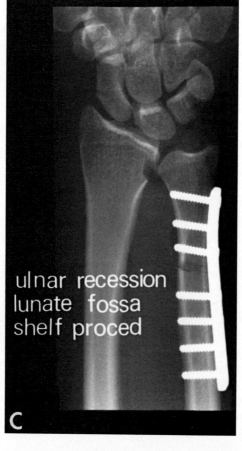

ulnar recession
lunate fossa
shelf proced

FIGURE 35-51

A 35-year-old female industrial worker had insidious progression of pain in her wrists. **A,** Forme fruste Madelung's deformity; note dorsal rim overlap, ulna plus, proximal lip sigmoid notch, and increased slant of articular surface. **B,** Arthrogram. Note increased space within the lunate fossa of the distal radius secondary to ulnocarpal abutment. **C,** Ulnar recession with undercutting of proximal sigmoid notch. *proced*, procedure.

interposition between radius and ulnar head is freed proximally and pushed distally to aid formation of support beneath the lunate and triquetrum. The ulnar head is reduced to the radius for additional support. Although a normal joint does not develop, this pseudojoint seems well tolerated.[152]

Multiple hereditary exostoses commonly affect the distal ulna.[34] The exostosis decreases the growth of the ulna. This tethers the ulnar aspect of the radius, inducing progressive ulnar bowing of the radius. The ulnar exostosis sometimes impinges against the radius and provides a further pivot point to radial bowing. Treatment of this condition was well described by Peterson.[167]

SALVAGE PROCEDURES FOR THE DISTAL RADIOULNAR JOINT

ULNAR HEAD EXCISION (DARRACH PROCEDURE)

This technique was first described by Desault in 1791[57] and was redescribed several additional times before popularization by Darrach in a series of publications beginning in 1912.[52] The results have been published in several series and indicate generally good to excellent results.[96] The indications for the procedure have included just about any problem arising at the DRUJ not readily alleviated by simple measures (see Chapter 34). Various minor modifications in technique have been proposed which would lead one to think that there were occasional unsatisfactory results (Fig. 35-52). The advised length of bone to be removed is 0.75 in., but this has been criticized as both insufficient and excessive.[44] Subperiosteal resection with closure of the periosteum to retain continuity with the ulnar styloid has been criticized for encouraging a thin spike of heterotopic new bone to form and interfere with function. Generally, the TFC and styloid are retained with the capsular remnants of the ulnar head. In vigorous defense of the procedure, Tulipan et al.[200] and DiBenedetto et al.[58] have suggested a slightly oblique osteotomy at the synovial reflection of the ulnar head combined with a Z-plasty closure that stabilizes the ulnar stump by capsulorrhaphy and dorsal positioning of the ECU with a capsuloperiosteal flap (Fig. 35-53).

Criticisms of ulnar head resection have been more specific in other studies. Patient satisfaction with the procedure is less if a detailed examination of grip strength, forearm rotation, and dexterity uses comparison with the normal arm. There are cosmetic concerns such as narrowing of the forearm as well as symptomatic complaints of continued discomfort, weakness, and occasional snapping. Some patients' radiographs

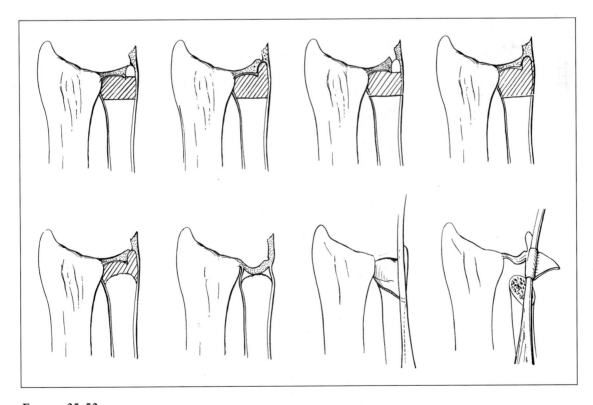

FIGURE 35-52

Several modifications of the distal ulnar resection, including the angle and length of resection of the distal ulna and treatment of the ulnar styloid, have been proposed in an effort to obviate impingement between stump and radius, stump instability, and heterotopic bone formation.

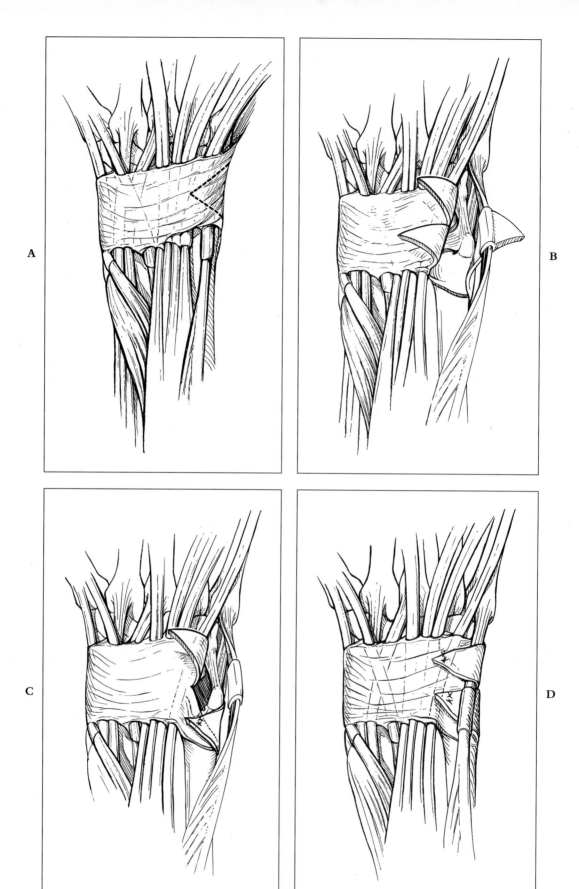

FIGURE 35-53

Modified Darrach procedure (Tulipan). **A,** A Z-plastic incision is made in the ulnar aspect of the dorsal retinaculum. **B,** The extensor carpi ulnaris (ECU) is subperiosteally reflected from its ulnar groove, and the ulnar osteotomy is made obliquely radiodistally from the ulnar aspect. The styloid process is retained with the triangular fibrocartilage. **C,** The styloid and triangular fibrocartilage are pulled proximally. The remnant of capsule and two of the retinacular flaps are oversewn. **D,** To stabilize the ulnar stump, the distal retinacular flap is looped under the ECU sheath and sewn back to the retinaculum to displace the ECU dorsally over the ulna.

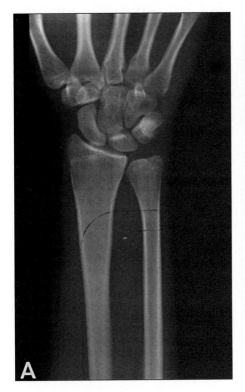
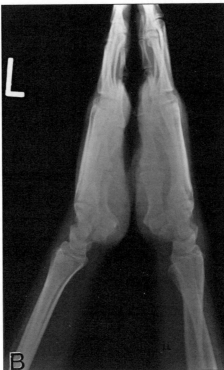
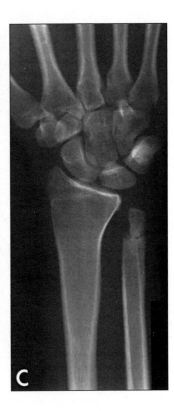

FIGURE 35-54

A 22-year-old woman with pain at the right distal radioulnar joint. **A,** Anteroposterior radiograph 2 years after operative treatment of radial fracture. **B,** Note residual angulation of radius and ulnopalmar subluxation of the right wrist. **C,** Darrach recession for progressive weakness, pain, snapping. Three subsequent operations: Silastic ulnar head capping, prosthetic removal and tenodesis procedures, and pronator quadratus transfer. Persistent symptoms. Note scalloping of ulnar border of radial metaphysis. Corrective radial osteotomy and stabilization of the triangular fibrocartilage to the distal ulna would be the initial treatment of choice.

show an erosion on the radial metaphysis secondary to ulnar impingement.[6,18,19,155] This may be quite symptomatic in a few patients, with a sensation of snapping, pain, and giving way with rotatory movements (Fig. 35-54). This problem seems more likely to occur in young lax-jointed women.

Two recent modifications of the basic procedure have retained continuity of the ulnar shaft to the styloid process to provide better stability of the ulnar stump. In the hemiresection interposition technique, the ulnar head is resected obliquely from the shaft and the resultant space is filled with adjacent soft tissue augmented with a coiled piece of tendon (Fig. 35-55).[28,29,68,100,156] In the "matched arthroplasty" procedure, the ulnar head is removed in such a way as to provide a conical remnant of shaft that allows a smooth rotation of the radius about it (Fig. 35-56).[208,209]

RADIOULNAR SYNOSTOSIS WITH PROXIMAL SEGMENT EXCISION (KAPANDJI PROCEDURE)

In 1936 Sauvé and Kapandji[182] described an operation for the DRUJ, mistakenly attributed to Lauenstein by Steindler, which preserved the support of the ulnar head while removing the underlying painful condition

by arthrodesis of the ulnar head to the radius. Rotation was restored by excising a segment of ulnar shaft just proximal to the arthrodesis. This procedure has received increased interest in recent years because the radiocarpal joint is better preserved than with ulnar head excision.[82,191,205] A similar idea was suggested by Baldwin[16] who left the radioulnar joint free while excising a segment of ulnar shaft proximally. He emphasized the importance of suturing the pronator quadratus into the defect to prevent regrowth of bone. Although these two procedures have some advantage over ulnar head excision, they both have the potential for ulnar stump instability (Fig. 35-57).

Treatment has been difficult for patients with markedly symptomatic unstable distal ulnar stumps giving rise to ulnar impingement (Fig. 35-58).[19,181] The use of silicone ulnar head caps was tried enthusiastically when they were first introduced, but displacement, fracture, and loosening of these devices have lessened their appeal.[190] Stabilization with distal to proximal tendon stabilization of the ulnar stump has provided mixed results. Strips of ECU and of FCU have been advocated.[21,156] The addition of a tendon loop around the ulnar stump and ECU tendon has the disadvantage of being effective only with

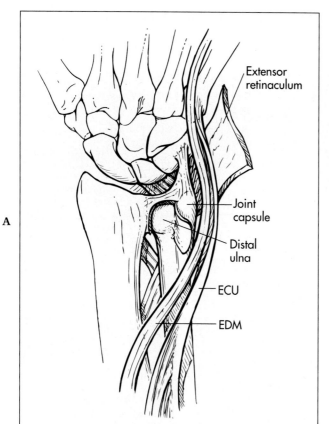

A

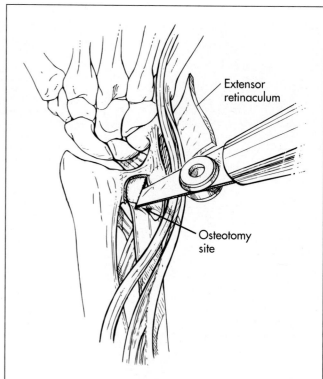

B

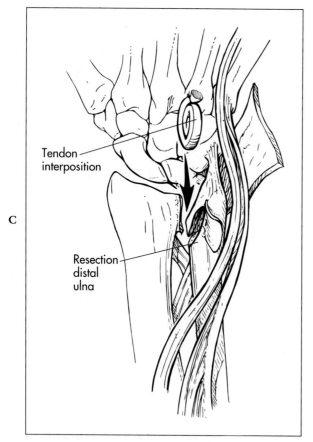

C

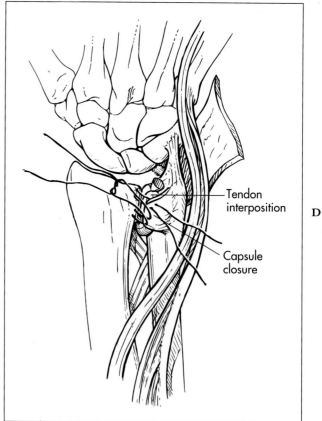

D

FIGURE 35-55

Hemiresection interposition technique (Bowers). **A,** The dorsal retinaculum is incised and the extensor carpi ulnaris (ECU) and extensor digiti minimi (EDM) are retracted ulnarly. **B,** The articular surface of the ulnar head is excised obliquely. **C,** The remnants of triangular fibrocartilage or a coil of tendon or soft tissue is interposed into the defect. **D,** The dorsal radioulnar capsule is sutured securely to the radial rim of the sigmoid notch. The retinaculum may be closed over this repair or split and partially closed over the ECU and EDM or looped under to hold the tendons in a more radial position.

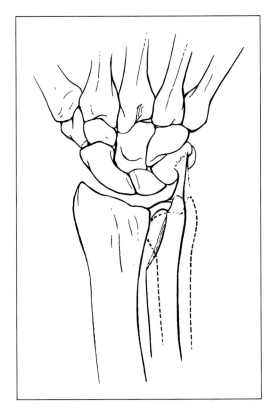

FIGURE 35-56

Matched arthroplasty (Watson). After excision of the ulnar articular surface obliquely, the osteotomized surface is rounded to allow better congruence with the sigmoid notch during forearm rotation.

active contraction. A modification of the Johnson procedure, transfer of the pronator quadratus through the interosseous space to the dorsum of the ulna, provides muscle interposition as well as a palmar stabilizing force (Fig. 35-59).[104] Kleinman and Greenberg[119] have recommended using all three techniques to effect maximum control of the ulnar stump. In some circumstances it has been necessary to resort to a radioulnar synostosis to effect relief. Prosthetic arthroplasty may offer another solution to this problem.[114]

TENDONITIS AND TENDON SUBLUXATION

Tenosynovitis in the dorsal compartments of the wrist is often seen with rheumatoid arthritis.[15] Occasionally, an isolated stenosing tenosynovitis is seen in the ECU compartment without the rheumatoid stigma. Symptoms of soreness, swelling, and catching are mentioned. Spontaneous resolution may occur with rest. Tenosynovial effusion and nodular formation within the tendon at sites of narrowing by the dorsal retinaculum can account for the snapping or, rarely, "triggering" with wrist extension or ulnar deviation. Erosion of the floor of the sixth compartment over the styloid with secondary bony roughening may produce tendon attrition or even rupture. This condition responds to cortisone injections and modification of

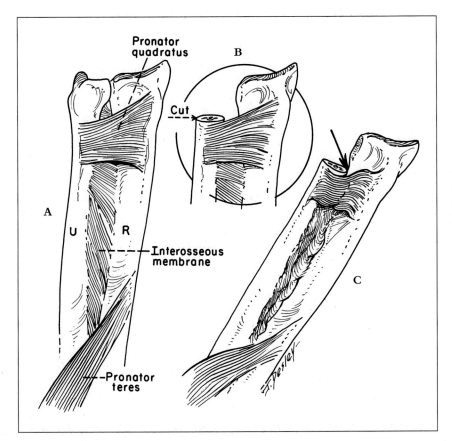

FIGURE 35-57

Effect of excision of ulnar head on the forearm. **A,** Normal interosseous width. **B,** Excision of ulnar head. **C,** Contraction of the pronator quadratus and pronator teres, in particular, close the interosseous space and cause radioulnar impingement. *R,* radius; *U,* ulna.

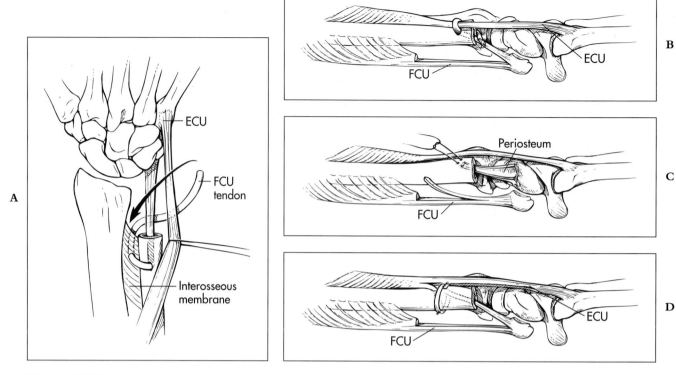

FIGURE 35-58

A, The flexor carpi ulnaris (*FCU*) tendon strip is drawn through the intramedullary shaft of the ulna and the interosseous membrane to stabilize the stump before looping over the extensor carpi ulnaris (*ECU*) for dorsal stabilization. **B,** A similar procedure stabilizes the ECU to the dorsum of ulnar stump before looping the FCU strip around the stump to be sutured to itself. **C,** The ECU sheath and periosteal remnant of the styloid region are sutured to the ulnar stump before the FCU strip is looped over the ECU (Blatt). **D,** Strips of both ECU and FCU are used to stabilize the ulnar stump and ECU (Breen and Jupiter).

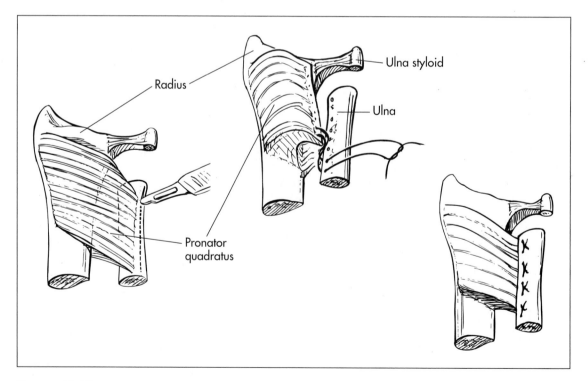

FIGURE 35-59

Transposition of the pronator quadratus through the interosseous space (modified Johnson procedure) places a soft-tissue interposition between the ulnar stump and radius and introduces a measure of dynamic stabilization to the stump.

90. Hauck RM, Skahen JR, Palmer AK: Classification and treatment of ulnar styloid non-unions. Presented at the 48th annual meeting of the American Society for Surgery of the Hand, Cincinnati, Ohio, October 1994.

91. Heiple KG, Freehafer AA, Van't Hof A: Isolated traumatic dislocation of the distal end of the ulna or distal radioulnar joint, *J Bone Joint Surg Am* 44:1387-1394, 1962.

92. Henle J: *Handbuch der Handerlehre des Menschen.* In *Handbuch der System Atischen Anatomie des Menschen,* vol 1, Braunschweig, 1856, Vieweg.

93. Hermansdorfer JD, Kleinman WB: Management of chronic peripheral tears of the triangular fibrocartilage complex, *J Hand Surg [Am]* 16:340-346, 1991.

94. Hill RB: Habitual dislocation of the distal end of the ulna: report of a case, *J Bone Joint Surg* 21:780, 1939.

95. Hotchkiss RN, An KN, Sowa DT, et al.: An anatomic and mechanical study of the interosseous membrane of the forearm: pathomechanics of proximal migration of the radius, *J Hand Surg [Am]* 14:256-261, 1989.

96. Hucherson DC: Darrach operation for lower radioulnar derangement, *Am J Surg* 53:237-241, 1941.

97. Hui FC, Linscheid RL: Ulnotriquetral augmentation tenodesis: a reconstructive procedure for dorsal subluxation of the distal radioulnar joint, *J Hand Surg [Am]* 7:230-236, 1982.

98. Hultën O: Über anatomische Variationen der handgelenkknochen. Ein Beitrag zur Kenntnis der Genese Zwei verschiedener Mondbeinveränderungen, *Acta Radiol* 9:155-168, 1928.

99. Hunter JM, Kirkpatrick WH: Dacron stabilization of the distal ulna, *Hand Clin* 7:365-371, 1991.

100. Imbriglia JE, Matthews D: Treatment of chronic posttraumatic dorsal subluxation of the distal ulna by hemiresection-interposition arthroplasty, *J Hand Surg [Am]* 18:899-907, 1993.

101. Inada Y, Fukui A, Maeda M, et al.: Reconstruction of the triangular fibrocartilage complex after surgery for treatment of synovial osteochondromatosis of the distal radioulnar joint, *J Hand Surg [Am]* 15:921-924, 1990.

102. Ishikawa JI: Kinematic studies of the distal radioulnar joint. Comparison between normal joints and joints affected by distal radial fractures, *J Jpn Soc Surg Hand* (in press).

103. Jenkins NH, Mintowt-Czyz WJ, Fairclough JA: Irreducible dislocation of the distal radioulnar joint, *Injury* 18:40-43, 1987.

104. Johnson RK: Stabilization of the distal ulna by transfer of the pronator quadratus origin, *Clin Orthop* 275:130-132, 1992.

105. Johnson RK, Shrewsbury MM: The pronator quadratus in motions and in stabilization of the radius and ulna at the distal radioulnar joint, *J Hand Surg [Am]* 1:205-209, 1976.

106. Kapandji AI: *The inferior radioulnar joint and pronosupination.* In Tubiana R, editor: *The hand,* vol 1, Philadelphia, 1981, WB Saunders, pp 121-129.

107. Kapandji AI: *The distal radio-ulnar joint, functional anatomy.* In Razemon JP, Fisk GR, editors: *The wrist,* Edinburgh, 1988, Churchill Livingstone, pp 34-44.

108. Kapandji AI: Prothese radio-cubitale inferieure, *Ann Chir Main Memb Super* 11:320-332, 1992.

109. Kapandji AI: *Dislocation and instability of the distal radioulnar joint.* In Schuind F, editor: *Advances in the biomechanics of the hand and wrist,* New York, 1994, Plenum Press, pp 401-406.

110. Kapandji AI, Martin-Bouyer Y, Verdeille S: Etude du carpe au scanner a trois dimensions sous contraintes de prono-supination, *Ann Chir Main Memb Super* 10:36-47, 1991.

111. Kauer JM: The articular disc of the hand, *Acta Anat (Basel)* 93:590-605, 1975.

112. Kauer JM: The distal radioulnar joint. Anatomic and functional considerations, *Clin Orthop* 275:37-45, 1992.

113. Kaukonen JP, Karaharju EO, Porras M, et al.: Functional recovery after fractures of the distal forearm. Analysis of radiographic and other factors affecting the outcome, *Ann Chir Gynaecol* 77:27-31, 1988.

114. Khurana JS, Kattapuram SV, Becker S, et al.: Galeazzi injury with an associated fracture of the radial head, *Clin Orthop* 234:70-71, 1988.

115. Kiene RH, Albers JA: Dislocation of the distal end of the ulna with impaction of the distal ulna into the radius: a case report, *J Trauma* 13:829-836, 1973.

116. Kihara H, Short WH, Werner FW, et al.: The stabilizing mechanism of the distal radioulnar joint during pronation and supination, *J Hand Surg [Am]* 20:930-936, 1995.

117. King GJ, McMurtry RY, Rubenstein JD, et al.: Computerized tomography of the distal radioulnar joint: correlation with ligamentous pathology in a cadaveric model, *J Hand Surg [Am]* 11:711-717, 1986.

118. King GJ, McMurtry RY, Rubenstein JD, et al.: Kinematics of the distal radioulnar joint, *J Hand Surg [Am]* 11:798-804, 1986.

119. Kleinman WB, Greenberg JA: Salvage of the failed Darrach procedure, *J Hand Surg [Am]* 20:951-958, 1995.

120. Koebke J: A biomechanical and morphological analysis of human hand joints, *Adv Anat Embryol Cell Biol* 80:1-85, 1983.

121. Koebke J, Schluter M: Zur lagebeziehung zwischen distaler Radiusepiphyse und distalem Ende der Ulna, *Z Orthop Ihre Grenzgeb* 125:82-84, 1987.

122. Koebke J, Werner J, Piening H: Der Musculus pronator quadratus—eine morphologische und funktionelle analyse, *Anat Anz* 157:311-318, 1984.

123. Kristensen SS, Thomassen E, Christensen F: Ulnar variance determination, *J Hand Surg [Br]* 11:255-257, 1986.

124. Kuhlman N: Anatomie descriptiva y functional del carpo en relation con la pathologie traumatic del mismo, *Rev Esp Chir Lo Mine* 5:103-104, 1977.

125. Lengsfeld M, Strauss JM, Koebke J: Funktionelle Bedeutung des M. extensor carpi ulnaris für das distale Radioulnargelenk, *Handchir Mikrochir Plast Chir* 20:275-278, 1988.

126. Levinsohn EM, Palmer AK, Coren AB, et al.: Wrist arthrography: the value of the three compartment injection technique, *Skeletal Radiol* 16:539-544, 1987.

127. Lewis OJ, Hamshere RJ, Bucknill TM: The anatomy of the wrist joint, *J Anat* 106:539-552, 1970.

128. Liebolt FL: A new procedure for treatment of luxation of the distal end of the ulna, *J Bone Joint Surg Am* 35:261-262, 1953.

129. Linscheid RL: Ulnar lengthening and shortening, *Hand Clin* 3:69-79, 1987.

130. Linscheid RL: Biomechanics of the distal radioulnar joint, *Clin Orthop* 275:46-55, 1992.

131. Linscheid RL: *Examination of the wrist*. In Nakamura R, Linscheid RL, Miura T, editors: *Wrist disorders: current concepts and challenges,* Tokyo, 1992, Springer-Verlag.

132. Linscheid RL: The hand and evolution, *J Hand Surg [Am]* 18:181-194, 1993.

133. Linscheid RL: *Kinematic dysfunction of the distal radioulnar joint after distal radial fractures.* In Schuind F, editor: *Advances in the biomechanics of the hand and wrist,* vol 1, New York, 1994, Plenum Press, pp 427-429.

134. Linscheid RL, Dobyns JH, Beabout JW, et al.: Traumatic instability of the wrist. Diagnosis, classification, and pathomechanics, *J Bone Joint Surg Am* 54:1612-1632, 1972.

135. Lippman RK: Laxity of radio-ulnar joint following Colles' fracture, *Arch Surg* 35:772-786, 1937.

136. Lowman CL: The use of fascia lata in the repair of disability at the wrist, *J Bone Joint Surg* 12:400-402, 1930.

137. Lyritis G: Synovial chondromatosis of the inferior radio-ulnar joint, *Acta Orthop Scand* 47:373-374, 1976.

138. Marske MW: Hominid hand use in the pliocene and pleistocene: evidence from experimental archaeology and comparative morphology, *J Hum Evolution* 15:439-460, 1986.

139. McDougall A, White J: Subluxation of the inferior radio-ulnar joint complicating fracture of the radial head, *J Bone Joint Surg Br* 39:278-287, 1957.

140. Melone CP Jr, Nathan R: Traumatic disruption of the triangular fibrocartilage complex. Pathoanatomy, *Clin Orthop* 275:65-73, 1992.

141. Menon J, Wood VE, Schoene HR, et al.: Isolated tears of the triangular fibrocartilage of the wrist: results of partial excision, *J Hand Surg [Am]* 9:527-530, 1984.

142. Mikic Z: The blood supply of the human distal radioulnar joint and the microvasculature of its articular disk, *Clin Orthop* 275:19-28, 1992.

143. Mikic Z, Somer L, Somer T: Histologic structure of the articular disk of the human distal radioulnar joint, *Clin Orthop* 275:29-36, 1992.

144. Mikic ZD: Age changes in the triangular fibrocartilage of the wrist joint, *J Anat* 126:367-384, 1978.

145. Mikic ZD: Detailed anatomy of the articular disc of the distal radioulnar joint, *Clin Orthop* 245:123-132, 1989.

146. Milch H: So-called dislocation of lower end of ulna, *Ann Surg* 116:282-292, 1942.

147. Minami A, Ogino T, Tohyama H: Multiple ruptures of flexor tendons due to hypertrophic change at the distal radio-ulnar joint. A case report, *J Bone Joint Surg Am* 71:300-302, 1989.

148. Mino DE, Palmer AK, Levinsohn EM: The role of radiography and computerized tomography in the diagnosis of subluxation and dislocation of the distal radioulnar joint, *J Hand Surg [Am]* 8:23-31, 1983.

149. Mino DE, Palmer AK, Levinsohn EM: Radiography and computerized tomography in the diagnosis of incongruity of the distal radio-ulnar joint. A prospective study, *J Bone Joint Surg Am* 67:247-252, 1985.

150. Mitchell AP: Recurrent anterior dislocation of lower end of ulna complicated by ununited fracture of styloid process of ulna, *Br J Surg* 9:555-557, 1922.

151. Morrissy RT, Nalebuff EA: Dislocation of the distal radioulnar joint: anatomy and clues to prompt diagnosis, *Clin Orthop* 144:154-158, 1979.

152. Murphy MS, Linscheid RL, Dobyns JH, et al.: Radial opening wedge osteotomy in Madelung's deformity. Presented at the 47th Annual Meeting of the American Society for Surgery of the Hand, Las Vegas, Nevada, November 1993.

153. Nathan R, Schneider LH: Classification of distal radio-ulnar joint disorders, *Hand Clin* 7:239-247, 1991.

154. Neviaser RJ, Palmer AK: Traumatic perforation of the articular disc of the triangular fibrocartilage complex of the wrist, *Bull Hosp Jt Dis Orthop Inst* 44:376-380, 1984.

155. Newmeyer WL, Green DP: Rupture of digital extensor tendons following distal ulnar resection, *J Bone Joint Surg Am* 64:178-182, 1982.

156. Noble J, Arafa M: Stabilisation of distal ulna after excessive Darrach's procedure, *Hand* 15:70-72, 1983.

157. Olerud C, Kongsholm J, Thuomas KA: The congruence of the distal radioulnar joint. A magnetic resonance imaging study, *Acta Orthop Scand* 59:183-185, 1988.

158. Osterman AL, Terrill RG: Arthroscopic treatment of TFCC lesions, *Hand Clin* 7:277-281, 1991.

159. Paley D, Rubenstein J, McMurtry RY: Irreducible dislocation of distal radial ulnar joint, *Orthop Rev* 15:228-231, 1986.

160. Palmer AK: Triangular fibrocartilage complex lesions: a classification, *J Hand Surg [Am]* 14:594-606, 1989.

161. Palmer AK, Glisson RR, Werner FW: Ulnar variance determination, *J Hand Surg [Am]* 7:376-379, 1982.

162. Palmer AK, Glisson RR, Werner FW: Relationship between ulnar variance and triangular fibrocartilage complex thickness, *J Hand Surg [Am]* 9:681-682, 1984.

163. Palmer AK, Werner FW: The triangular fibrocartilage complex of the wrist—anatomy and function, *J Hand Surg [Am]* 6:153-162, 1981.

164. Palmer AK, Werner FW: Biomechanics of the distal radioulnar joint, *Clin Orthop* 187:26-35, 1984.

165. Patrick J: A study of supination and pronation, with especial reference to the treatment of forearm fractures, *J Bone Joint Surg* 28:737-748, 1946.

166. Petersen MS, Adams BD: Biomechanical evaluation of distal radioulnar reconstruction, *J Hand Surg [Am]* 18:328-334, 1993.

167. Peterson HA: Multiple hereditary osteochondromata, *Clin Orthop* 239:222-230, 1989.

168. Peycelon R: A propos de la pathologie du fibro-cartilage de l'articulation radio-cubitale inférieure, *Rev d'orthop* 25:551-554, 1938.

169. Pirela-Cruz MA, Goll SR, Klug M, et al.: Stress computed tomography analysis of the distal radioulnar joint: a diagnostic tool for determining translational motion, *J Hand Surg [Am]* 16:75-82, 1991.

170. Poehling GG: Instrumentation for small joints: the arthroscope, *Arthroscopy* 4:45-46, 1988.

171. Rainey RK, Pfautsch ML: Traumatic volar dislocation of the distal radioulnar joint, *Orthopedics* 8:896-900, 1985.

172. Ray RD, Johnson RJ, Jameson RM: Rotation of the forearm: an experimental study of pronation and supination, *J Bone Joint Surg Am* 33:993-996, 1951.

173. Rayhack JM, Gasser SI, Latta LL, et al.: Precision oblique osteotomy for shortening of the ulna, *J Hand Surg [Am]* 18:908-918, 1993.

174. Reagan DS, Linscheid RL, Dobyns JH: Lunotriquetral sprains, *J Hand Surg [Am]* 9:502-514, 1984.

175. Regan JM, Bickel WH: Fascial sling operation for instability of lower radio-ulnar joint, *Proc Staff Meet Mayo Clin* 20:202-208, 1945.

176. Ritt MJ, Stuart PR, Berglund LJ, et al.: Rotational stability of the carpus relative to the forearm, *J Hand Surg [Am]* 20:305-311, 1995.

177. Robbin ML, An KN, Linscheid RL, et al.: Anatomic and kinematic analysis of the human forearm using high-speed computed tomography, *Med Biol Eng Comput* 24:164-168, 1986.

178. Rose-Innes AP: Anterior dislocation of the ulna at the inferior radio-ulnar joint: case reports, with a discussion of the anatomy of rotation of the forearm, *J Bone Joint Surg Br* 42:515-521, 1960.

179. Roux JL: La Rotation longitudinale radio-metacarpienne (Etude bio mechanique et application's cliniques). Theses: Presentee et publiquement soutenue devent la Faculte de Medicine de Montpellier, Juin 1992.

180. Ruggles DL, Peterson HA, Scott SG: Radial growth plate injury in a female gymnast, *Med Sci Sports Exerc* 23:393-396, 1991.

181. Sanders RA, Hawkins B: Reconstruction of the distal radioulnar joint for chronic volar dislocation. A case report, *Orthopedics* 12:1473-1476, 1989.

182. Sauve L, Kapandji M: Nouvelle technique de traitement chirurical des luxations récidivantes isolées de l'extrémité inférieure du cubitus, *J de Chir* 47:589-594, 1936.

183. Scheker LR, Belliappa PP, Acosta R, et al.: Reconstruction of the dorsal ligament of the triangular fibrocartilage complex, *J Hand Surg [Br]* 19:310-318, 1994.

184. Schuind F, An KN, Berglund L, et al.: The distal radioulnar ligaments: a biomechanical study, *J Hand Surg [Am]* 16:1106-1114, 1991.

185. Schuind FA, Linscheid RL, An KN, et al.: A normal data base of posteroanterior roentgenographic measurements of the wrist, *J Bone Joint Surg Am* 74:1418-1429, 1992.

186. Snook GA, Chrisman OD, Wilson TC, et al.: Subluxation of the distal radio-ulnar joint by hyperpronation, *J Bone Joint Surg Am* 51:1315-1323, 1969.

187. Spinner M, Kaplan EB: Extensor carpi ulnaris. Its relationship to the stability of the distal radio-ulnar joint, *Clin Orthop* 68:124-129, 1970.

188. Steyers CM, Blair WF: Measuring ulnar variance: a comparison of techniques, *J Hand Surg [Am]* 14:607-612, 1989.

189. Stuart P, Bergan R, Linscheid RL, et al.: The dorsopalmar stability of the distal radioulnar joint. Presented at the annual meeting of the American Academy of Orthopedic Surgeons, Orlando, Florida, February 1995.

190. Swanson AB: Implant arthroplasty for disabilities of the distal radioulnar joint. Use of a silicone rubber capping implant following resection of the ulnar head, *Orthop Clin North Am* 4:373-382, 1973.

191. Taleisnik J: The Sauve-Kapandji procedure, *Clin Orthop* 275:110-123, 1992.

192. Taleisnik J, Gelberman RH, Miller BW, et al.: The extensor retinaculum of the wrist, *J Hand Surg [Am]* 9:495-501, 1984.

193. Tanaka Y: Study of ulnar variance, *J Jpn Soc Surg Hand* 6:120-130, 1989.

194. Taylor GW, Parsons CL: The role of the discus articularis in Colles' fractures, *J Bone Joint Surg* 20:149-152, 1938.

195. Tencer AF, Viegas SF, Cantrell J, et al.: Pressure distribution in the wrist joint, *J Orthop Res* 6:509-517, 1988.

196. Thiru RG, Ferlic DC, Clayton ML, et al.: Arterial anatomy of the triangular fibrocartilage of the wrist and its surgical significance, *J Hand Surg [Am]* 11:258-263, 1986.

197. Trousdale RT, Linscheid RL: Operative treatment of malunited fractures of the forearm, *J Bone Joint Surg [Am]* 77:894-902, 1995.

198. Trumble T, Glisson RR, Seaber AV, et al.: Forearm force transmission after surgical treatment of distal radioulnar joint disorders, *J Hand Surg [Am]* 12:196-202, 1987.

199. Tsai TM, Stilwell JH: Repair of chronic subluxation of the distal radioulnar joint (ulnar dorsal) using flexor carpi ulnaris tendon, *J Hand Surg [Br]* 9:289-294, 1984.

200. Tulipan DJ, Eaton RG, Eberhart RE: The Darrach procedure defended: technique redefined and long-term follow-up, *J Hand Surg [Am]* 16:438-444, 1991.

201. Van der Linden AJ: Disk lesion of the wrist joint, *J Hand Surg [Am]* 11:490-497, 1986.

202. Vesely DG: The distal radio-ulnar joint, *Clin Orthop* 51:75-91, 1967.

203. Vickers D, Nielsen G: Madelung deformity: surgical prophylaxis (physiolysis) during the late growth period by resection of the dyschondrosteosis lesion, *J Hand Surg [Br]* 17:401-407, 1992.

204. Viegas SF, Pogue DJ, Patterson RM, et al.: Effects of radioulnar instability on the radiocarpal joint: a biomechanical study, *J Hand Surg [Am]* 15:728-732, 1990.

205. Vincent KA, Szabo RM, Agee JM: The Sauve-Kapandji procedure for reconstruction of the rheumatoid distal radioulnar joint, *J Hand Surg [Am]* 18:978-983, 1993.

206. Voorhees DR, Daffner RH, Nunley JA, et al.: Carpal ligamentous disruptions and negative ulnar variance, *Skeletal Radiol* 13:257-262, 1985.

207. Walker PS: *Biomechanics of the forearm.* In Walker PS, editor: *Human joints and their artificial replacement,* Springfield, Illinois, 1977, Charles C Thomas, pp 190-195.

208. Watson HK, Gabuzda GM: Matched distal ulna resection for posttraumatic disorders of the distal radioulnar joint, *J Hand Surg [Am]* 17:724-730, 1992.

209. Watson HK, Ryu JY, Burgess RC: Matched distal ulnar resection, *J Hand Surg [Am]* 11:812-817, 1986.

210. Weigl K, Spira E: The triangular fibrocartilage of the wrist joint, *Reconstr Surg Traumatol* 11:139-153, 1969.

211. Werner FW, Murphy DJ, Palmer AK: Pressures in the distal radioulnar joint: effect of surgical procedures used for Kienbock's disease, *J Orthop Res* 7:445-450, 1989.

212. Weseley MS, Barenfeld PA, Bruno J: Volar dislocation distal radioulnar joint, *J Trauma* 12:1083-1088, 1972.

213. Wright TW, Dobyns JH, Linscheid RL, et al.: Carpal instability non-dissociative, *J Hand Surg [Br]* 19:763-773, 1994.

214. Yong-Hing K, Wedge JH, Bowen CV: Chronic injury to the distal ulnar and radial growth plates in an adolescent gymnast. A case report, *J Bone Joint Surg Am* 70:1087-1089, 1988.

215. Youm Y, Dryer RF, Thambyrajah K, et al.: Biomechanical analyses of forearm pronation-supination and elbow flexion-extension, *J Biomech* 12:245-255, 1979.

216. Zinberg EM, Palmer AK, Coren AB, et al.: The triple-injection wrist arthrogram, *J Hand Surg [Am]* 13:803-809, 1988.

X
RHEUMATOID ARTHRITIS

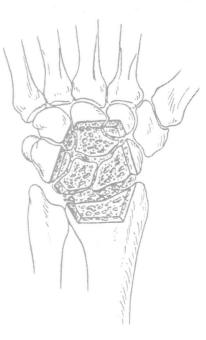

36

CLINICAL EVALUATION OF THE ARTHRITIC WRIST

James H. Dobyns, M.D.

DIFFERENTIAL DIAGNOSIS
    DISEASES AFFECTING THE LININGS OF JOINTS AND
        TENDONS
    RHEUMATOID (SEROPOSITIVE) AND
        SERONEGATIVE ARTHRITIS
        PSORIASIS
        SYSTEMIC LUPUS ERYTHEMATOSUS
        ARTHRITIS MUTILANS
        REITER'S SYNDROME
        ENTEROPATHIC ARTHRITIS
        BYPASS ARTHRITIS
        ANKYLOSING SPONDYLITIS
        ACUTE RHEUMATIC FEVER
        VIRAL ARTHRITIS
        GOUT
        PSEUDOGOUT
        LYME DISEASE
        PARTICULATE ARTHRITIS
CLINICAL EVALUATION
    SYMPTOMS, SIGNS, AND FINDINGS
        CONTACT (PALPATION AND MANUAL TESTING)
        CLUES OF RHEUMATOID INVOLVEMENT
LABORATORY FINDINGS
IMAGING FINDINGS
CLINICAL GUIDES TO TREATMENT DECISIONS
    CONFIRMING THE DIAGNOSIS
    EVALUATING THE PATHOLOGIC FEATURES
    BALANCING THE PRIORITIES OF PERSON, DISEASE,
        AND TREATMENT
SUMMARY

With luck and caution one may escape significant trauma in a lifetime, but no one escapes some degree or form of arthritis, synovitis, or rheumatism.* The American Rheumatism Association has included more than 65 disease entities in 10 major headings: polyarthritis of unknown etiology (includes rheumatoid arthritis), connective tissue disorders, rheumatic fever, degenerative joint diseases, nonarticular rheumatism, diseases with frequent arthritis association, arthritis associated with known infectious agents (includes bacterial, rickettsial, viral, fungal, parasitic), traumatic or neurogenic disorders (or both), arthritis associated with known biochemical or endocrine abnormalities, and arthritis associated with tumors.[17] Many of these conditions are to be considered in the differential diagnosis, but most can be confirmed or excluded fairly quickly. The usual diagnostic concerns are with

infectious arthritis, degenerative or post-traumatic arthritis, seropositive rheumatoid or connective tissue disorders, and seronegative arthritis (rheumatoid and rheumatoid impersonators).

A quick look at these possibilities is planned for differential diagnostic purposes, but the focus of the clinical evaluation will be on rheumatoid arthritis, which is still somewhat of a mystery disease. Taleisnik[41] summarized its gradual appearance in Western medical literature with a first mention in 1800 (Beauvais) and a fairly expansive discussion under the name of "rheumatoid gout" in 1859 (Garrod). Egyptian mummies, American Indian skeletons, and Flemish paintings have all been offered as early evidence of rheumatoid arthritis, but there is no convincing evidence that this disease was present before the 18th or 19th century. An etiologic interrelationship among infectious agents, genetics, and autoimmunity is the current presumption for this systemic disease that preferentially

---

* References 5-10,13,16,18,19,40,41.

targets synovium. Prevalence of rheumatoid arthritis is estimated at 0.3% in adults younger than age 35 years, but it is increased to 10% in persons older than age 65 years, with a 2.5:1 female-to-male ratio.[33] The initial pathologic event appears to be activation or injury to microvascular endothelial cells, possibly by an antibody-antigen reaction. This reaction results in an accumulation of leukocytes, macrophages, and other mononuclear cells in response to chemotactic factors in the rheumatoid joint fluid. A corresponding activation of other cells releases proteinases, collagenases, prostaglandins, and reactive oxidants, which inflame and damage ligaments, tendons, cartilage, and bone. Invasive fibroblastlike cells proliferate to form granulation tissue (pannus), which invades and destroys periarticular bone and cartilage. Further progression results in erosion and destruction of cartilage and rupture of ligaments, tendons, and joint capsules.[17,24,33] Although responsible for only one-quarter of the arthritis patients needing treatment, rheumatoid arthritis disables most because of its combination of severity and chronicity.[39]

DIFFERENTIAL DIAGNOSIS

DISEASES AFFECTING THE LININGS OF JOINTS AND TENDONS

Most of the 65 or more diagnoses already in the differential diagnosis of rheumatoid arthritis can target synovial tissues. Historical clues are most helpful except in childhood and the aged, when insidious or unspecified onset and other details based on a history from the patient are not forthcoming. Combined with a history of inflammatory synovitis, several common symptoms and signs assist in making the diagnosis. The most common are listed in Table 36-1.

In considering infection in the differential diagnosis, the critical finding is identification of the infecting agent, either by histopathologic identification or more commonly by positive culture results. The latter are not always easy to obtain. Multiple specimens, often surgical specimens (tissue blocks), and a laboratory skilled in handling the special requirements of infectious agents may be needed.

In considering trauma, the critical finding is from clinical examination combined with imaging of the injured wrist. Localization of pain and tenderness and provocative stress testing are important in evaluating trauma and lead to specific imaging studies. Most useful have been standard radiographs, scans, tomograms, arthrograms, motion studies (preferably on video), and magnetic resonance images. Instances in which the traumatic event is not known are common in childhood, and the subsequent symptoms can be misdiagnosed as juvenile rheumatoid arthritis.[37] Because a

fracture in young children may be through the unossified part of a carpal bone, it may not show on standard radiographs. Even if a fracture-type defect does show, it may be misinterpreted as a developmental lack of coalition between carpal segments. Not many years ago, it took surgical inspection and tissue sampling to determine some carpal area diagnoses in children. Occasionally this is still true, but the combination of arthroscopy and imaging techniques such as magnetic resonance imaging is usually sufficient for diagnosis now. It is important in children that the diagnosis of trauma be confirmed or denied, because the prognosis with properly treated trauma deformity and inflammation is still much better than that of the arthritides.

RHEUMATOID (SEROPOSITIVE) AND SERONEGATIVE ARTHRITIS

Although diagnosing the various types of arthritis is always necessary, most of them are either uncommon or rather specifically indicated by history.[8,23,40] Trauma may be either insidious or specific, and most of this book is involved with the diagnosis and management of trauma. Emphasis here will be on the more destructive and often cryptic arthritides, such as rheumatoid arthritis and the many conditions that resemble it. Although the diagnosis of seronegative rheumatoid arthritis is still made, the more severe disease is marked by the presence of the IgM autoantibody and nodules, which are never present without the presence of this rheumatoid factor. Clinical evaluation will be presented in the next section, but real confirmation of rheumatoid arthritis is by presence of the IgM autoantibody, as measured by particle agglutination (sensitized sheep cells or latex particles) or by nephelometry, a technique that uses light diffusion standards.

Rheumatoid arthritis (adult form) is a chronic autoimmune inflammatory disease whose etiology is unknown. The tissues of joints and tendon compartments, particularly the synovium, are preferred targets, but inflammatory neuropathy, vasculitis, and myositis are common; nodule formation and chronic anemia are characteristic.

Juvenile rheumatoid arthritis is similar to the adult disease except that it is modified by the potential for physis closure and the more likely response of fibrosis to the inflammatory process.[20,37] The latter results often in stiffness and limited motion of joints and tendons. Seronegative arthritis presents a clinical picture similar to rheumatoid arthritis. Symmetrical polyarthritis of greater than 6 weeks' duration is present and is associated with swollen joints, particularly in the hands and wrists. In all of these diseases, the treatment and the prognosis differ from that of rheumatoid arthritis. Some of the more common categories of seronegative arthritis are described below.

Table 36-1. Symptoms and Signs of Rheumatoid Arthritis

Cause	Pain or Weakness	Involvement			Imaging	Laboratory
		Sys	ST	B		
Infection	++	?	+	+	+	++
Trauma	+	−	+	+	+	−
CDD	?	−	+	−	+	++
Cong or dev	?	−	+	+	+	−
Seropos	+	+	+	+	+	++
Seroneg	+	+	+	+	+	?
Metabolic	+	+	+	?	+	+
Bleeding	+	?	+	+	+	+

B, bone; CDD, crystalline deposition disease; Cong, congenital; dev, developmental; Seroneg, seronegative; Seropos, seropositive; ST, soft tissue; Sys, systemic; ?, occasional; +, positive finding; ++, strongly positive finding; −, negative or not present.

Psoriasis. The clinical features of psoriasis, as opposed to rheumatoid arthritis, are the asymmetrical appearance, fewer joints involved, involvement of proximal interphalangeal rather than metacarpal joints with skin disease and with a predominance of spondylitis.[31] Joint stiffness is more common than in rheumatoid arthritis, and nail pitting is present in 80% of cases.

Systemic Lupus Erythematosus. Patients who have systemic lupus erythematosus and other similar, vascular collagen diseases can also present as if they had rheumatoid arthritis, but sometimes they have an appearance or pattern that involves several disease entities (dermatologic, nephrologic, vascular, arthritic).[6] Systemic lupus erythematosus characteristically affects the periarticular tissues of joints more than the synovium. It results in joints that can be lax, subluxed, or dislocated but with little destruction of the cartilage. Raynaud's phenomenon is common.

Arthritis Mutilans. Arthritis mutilans (erosive arthritis) is a form of advanced osteoarthritis but with intermittent and sometimes persistent inflammatory episodes that destroy joint and adjacent bone. It principally involves the hands, feet, and spine. The synovium resembles that of rheumatoid arthritis, but the type of tissue damage and the localized rather than systemic involvement distinguish the two. However, of all the forms of osteoarthritis, erosive arthritis resembles rheumatoid arthritis the most.

Reiter's Syndrome. The clinical appearance of patients with Reiter's syndrome includes the triad of arthritis, urethritis, and conjunctivitis. It is believed that the disease is a reaction to an infection, involves a high sedimentation rate (> 100 mm/h) and positive result for HLA-B27 in 80% of cases, and is most often seen in young men. There

is a limited form of Reiter's disease, still with a positive result for HLA-B27, with arthritis only.

Enteropathic Arthritis. Enteropathic arthritis associated with Crohn's disease or ulcerative colitis usually affects large joints in the lower extremities and is asymmetrical.[17]

Bypass Arthritis. Bypass arthritis is associated with the jejunoileal bypass for obesity and thought to be due to an immune reaction to the bowel bacteria.

Ankylosing Spondylitis. Ankylosing spondylitis occurs mostly in males and mostly in the spine and large joints, although involvement of peripheral joints may occur.[34]

Acute Rheumatic Fever. Acute rheumatic fever is presumed to be a reaction to an initial streptococcal disease and seldom seen now because of the common use of antibiotics. It is characterized by a migratory polyarthritis with fever and involvement of heart, skin, and neurologic systems.[34]

Viral Arthritis. Viral arthritis occurs with an acute onset of polyarthritis, is usually symmetrical, and often emphasizes the hands and feet. It is usually accompanied by a rash and is self-limited. Well-known types are rubella, parvovirus B19 (fifth disease), and hepatitis B.[17]

Gout. Gout is one of the metabolic diseases. Onset is usually acute (in 24 hours), monoarticular, and in the feet, but it may be polyarticular and involve the hands and the wrists. Diagnosis is confirmed by increased serum uric acid concentration, but this may be normal in 50% of patients during the initial phase. Crystals in the joint or tendon fluid are also diagnostic, but detection is infrequent, partly because the common search is conducted by examining a stained preparation rather than wet preparations.

Pseudogout. This is also a metabolic disease due to deposition of various types of calcium salts (calcium pyrophosphate, calcium hydroxyapatite) in or near joints and tendon sheaths. The wrist, knee, and shoulder are common sites, as are the various hand joints. It is a good, first-guess diagnosis for an acute, inflammatory flare of the wrist in a person age 60 to 70 years or older. Involvement of the triangular fibrocartilage is not uncommon.

Lyme Disease. Lyme disease is a spirochetal disease, similar to syphilis, including the three stages of skin, meningitis, and joint involvement.[14] Eosinophilia and a positive result of the enzyme-linked immunosorbent assay test (positive polymerase chain reaction for detection of *Borrelia* DNA) for immunoglobulin A are noted.[28] The causative agent is infectious (*Borrelia burgdorferi*) and the disease is transmitted by a tick vector. History of exposure to "deer" ticks can be diagnostic.

Particulate Arthritis. Small fragments of foreign materials, such as those used in joint reconstruction or replacement, are the cause of particulate arthritis. The material is a factor, but specific particle size seems to be the greatest factor in synovial reactivity.

There are, of course, other rheumatoid simulators, but the ones listed are more common.[39]

CLINICAL EVALUATION

SYMPTOMS, SIGNS, AND FINDINGS

Even with arthritis, a diagnosis may not be established when the patient is first seen by a wrist surgeon.[13] Whether or not this is the case, time should be spent in obtaining a general health history and performing a general examination of diseased joints, as may be relevant.[40] A truism about such a review is that a localized area of complaint is not nearly as likely to be associated with a systemic disease as are multiple areas of complaint. Diseased joints may occur anywhere in the upper extremity, but the hand and wrist are the usual foci. There are many tendon sheaths and many joints to be examined: first for inflammation, swelling, enlargement, or deformity; then for areas of tenderness, crepitus, or catching; finally for stiffness, limitation of motion, or ankylosis.[9,21,25,32] Disease activity in rheumatoid arthritis has early stages (deformity, but some degree of function of all joints and tendons) and late stages (destruction and fixed deformity).* The disease may progress

---

* References 19,21,22,25,35,36.

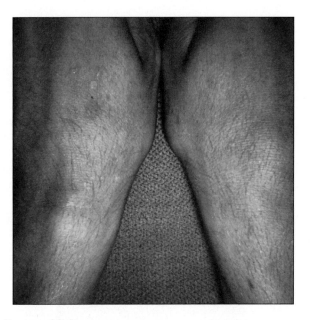

FIGURE 36-1

Bilateral, early rheumatoid arthritis of both wrists, left more involved than right, radial wrist more involved than ulnar wrist. Dorsal-radial views.

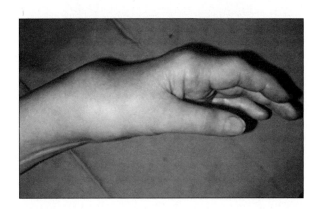

FIGURE 36-2

Radial-lateral view of rheumatoid arthritis of the left wrist and hand with a moderate amount of arthritis involving the wrist > metacarpophalangeals > interphalangeals.

through these stages gradually, persistently, and progressively; cyclically, with activity and remission alternating; or with an initial severe flare, followed by remission or a low level of activity.

Visible evidence and clues at the wrist level include: early swelling in one or more of the extensor tendon sheaths[25] (Fig. 36-1) dorsally; swelling and tenderness just proximal to the transverse carpal ligament palmarly or diffuse swelling of the entire wrist joint area, visible medially (Fig. 36-2), dorsally (Fig. 36-3), and laterally (Fig. 36-4); or a combination of these.[15] Inflammation may or may not be visible (it is often more detectable by noting the skin temperature in contact with the examiner's hand). Later, deformity may become visible, usually one of the following.

1. Dorsal, distal, and then ulnar displacement of the distal ulna (the "caput ulna syndrome")[3] (Figs. 36-4 and 36-5): this condition is secondary to laxity or attenuation, with eventual disruption of the triangular fibrocartilage and support ligaments between the distal radius and ulna and associated synovitis and fibrinous degeneration (Fig. 36-6).

2. Subluxation of the carpus, usually palmarly with supination and radial deviation leading to a zigzag collapse of the wrist and secondary increased ulnar drift[28,40] (Fig. 36-7): this condition indicates attenuation of the palmar radiocarpal and ulnocarpal support ligaments.[22,26,29,38,41]

3. Foreshortening and widening of the carpus indicate

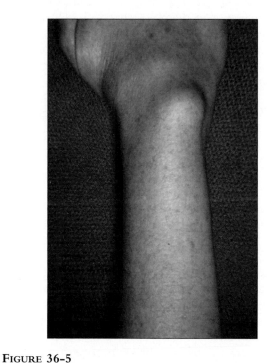

FIGURE 36-5

Dorsal view of another forearm and wrist displaying the "caput ulna" deformity in rheumatoid arthritis.

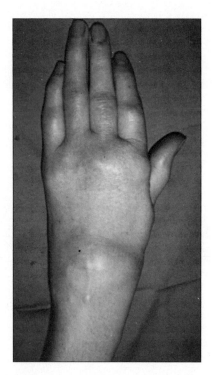

FIGURE 36-3

Dorsal view of the same wrist as in Figure 36-2.

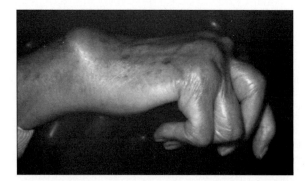

FIGURE 36-4

Lateral view of a rheumatoid arthritis wrist with "caput distal ulna" (i.e., dorsal prominence, perhaps ulnar or distal as well) due to loosening of the ligamentous supports in the radioulnocarpal area, permitting the radius and carpus to fall away from the ulna ("carpal supination").

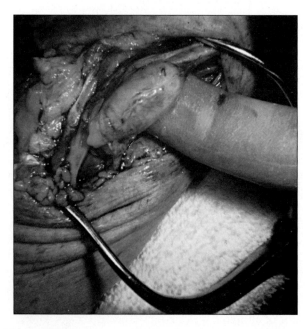

FIGURE 36-6

Dorsal surgical exposure of the ulnar area of a rheumatoid wrist demonstrates a "pseudocaput ulna" caused by a large fibrinous "loose body" in the dorsal portion of the distal radioulnar joint.

collapse deformities (carpal instability dissociative, carpal instability nondissociative, or carpal instability combined types) or cartilage and bone destruction.

4. End-point deformities in which the patient presents with subluxation (Fig. 36-7), dislocation (Fig. 36-8), or ankylosis of the wrist, usually in near-neutral position or with a lack of extension of the wrist, sometimes with 90° flexion or severe ulnar deviation stance (Fig. 36-9), indicate rupture of wrist extensors and possibly of digit extensor tendons.[11,41]

5. Digit stance deformities (Fig. 36-4),* particularly extension or flexion stance alterations during cascade testing (observation of digit stance during gravity-induced extension-flexion of the wrist) and inability to actively extend or flex a given digit: loss

of digit stances usually represents rupture of a digit extensor or flexor[39] and most (but not all) such ruptures occur at the wrist level in the carpal tunnel for flexors, over the distal radioulnar joint, or in the extensor compartments over various joint margins for the extensors.

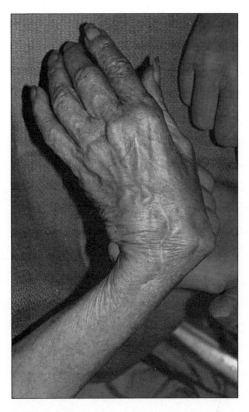

FIGURE 36-8
Dorsal view of a rheumatoid arthritis wrist that has dislocated ulnarward, leaving a prominent radius, radial styloid, and base of the thumb.

* References 3,25,36,38,41,42.

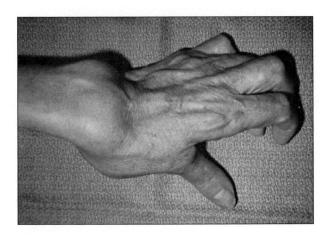

FIGURE 36-7
Radial-lateral view of a rheumatoid arthritis wrist, which has translated palmarward as a result of rupture of the wrist extensors (finger extensors have not yet ruptured).

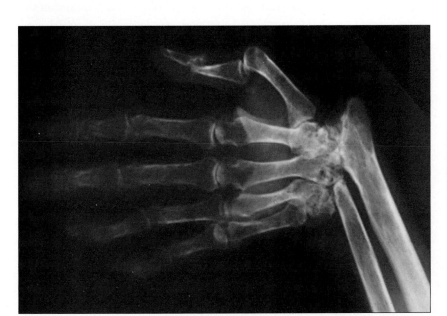

FIGURE 36-9
Rheumatoid arthritis with the severe ulnar translation and angulation of the wrist. Resorption of distal ulna and entire carpus (proximal and distal rows).

6. Signs of neurovascular alterations from normal may occur, such as the hyperemic or sweaty palm, Raynaud's phenomenon, and altered hair growth.

CONTACT (PALPATION AND MANUAL TESTING) CLUES OF RHEUMATOID INVOLVEMENT

1. Sensations are produced by fluid-filled tendon sheaths (tension and smoothness), synovial proliferation tendon sheaths (Figs. 36-10, 36-11, and 36-12) (tension and irregularities or thickenings), and "entrapped excursion" tendon sheaths (catching, triggering, or locking).

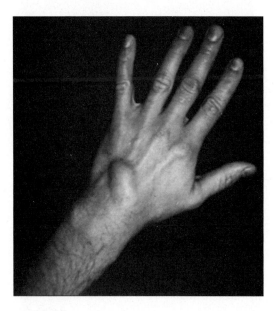

FIGURE 36-10

Dorsal view of a rheumatoid arthritis wrist with a prominent bulge of extensor tenosynovitis at the distal extensor digitorum communis compartment.

2. Perception of pain (tenderness) is produced by the probing finger or instrument. There is no more important and ubiquitous examination finding than tenderness. It can be localized to small areas (fingertip or ballpoint pen cap size), at the wrist it can be related extremely accurately to the underlying anatomic structures, the effect of motion or position can be tested, the degree of tenderness can be graded, the number of sites can be listed, and the reproduction by the palpation of the patient's principal or most typical pain(s) can be noted.
3. Bony or periarticular masses, irregularities, and displacements may be palpated during static and dynamic wrist configurations.
4. Both the active and passive ranges of motion can be tested. Passive motion testing should include maximizing or exceeding the active range of motion, traction, and compression of the wrist. Translation (ulnar, radial, dorsal, and ventral in supination and pronation) of the carpus is important to determine loss of stability. Similar testing of the distal ulna and the carpometacarpal joints should be performed.
5. Because all structures bypassing the wrist for functional needs in the hand are compartmentally disciplined as they pass this narrow node of access, they may be affected by the changes in and around the wrist, and the usual tests for vascular, neural, and musculotendinous function are indicated (Fig. 36-13). Vasculitis from the disease is more likely than vascular compression, but nerve compression at wrist level (carpal tunnel syndrome) (Figs. 36-13 and 36-14) is not unusual and tendon attenuation to rupture is quite common, usually beginning with the dorsal ulnar extensor tendons but not excluding the finger flexor tendons.
6. Strength, coordination, endurance, muscle atrophy, activities of daily living, and special function activities are also tested to observe the overall function of the

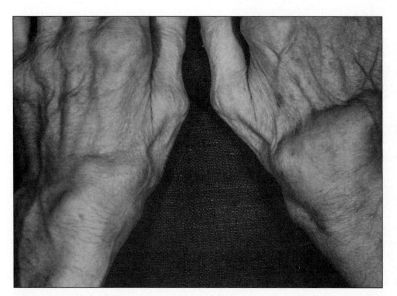

FIGURE 36-11

Dorsal view of paired rheumatoid arthritis wrists shows diffuse extensor tenosynovitis on the right, and mild synovitis involving the dorsal radial extensor compartment of the left wrist; note radial greater than ulnar involvement on the left wrist.

forces can be used to explain most of the deformities seen. Except for the cartilage loss and areas of bony erosions or resorption, these deformities are quite similar to post-traumatic ligamentous disruptions at the wrist. The commonly seen deformities, as visualized by imaging, are as follows.

1. Symmetric, soft-tissue swelling and thickening at the wrist
2. Effusion or synovitis of the wrist joints and of tenosynovial compartments
3. Osteopenia and joint space narrowing, usually seen earliest at the ulnocarpal, distal radioulnar, and scapholunate areas
4. Dorsal, ulnar, and distal subluxation of the distal ulna
5. Various collapse deformities of the carpus may occur, such as ulnar translation, either of the whole carpus (carpal instability nondissociative-type collapse) or whole carpus except the scaphoid (carpal instability combined-type) and scapholunate dissociation (rotary subluxation of scaphoid) with a flexed (vertical) alignment of the scaphoid (Fig. 36-23) and a carpal instability dissociative-dorsal intercalated segment instability or dorsiflexed posture of the rest of the proximal carpal row. Carpal instability nondissociative-dorsal intercalated segment instability patterns are also seen, but rarely. Palmar subluxation of the entire carpus or palmar subluxation plus supination of the ulnar carpus usually is associated with distal ulna subluxation. Carpal instability nondissociative-palmar intercalated segment instability or dorsally translated and flexed posture of the entire proximal carpal row and carpal instability dissociative-palmar intercalated segment instability patterns are also seen.
6. Various ankylosing to fusion patterns are also seen (Fig. 36-24). At the radiocarpal level, the entire radiocarpal joint or only one portion of it may be involved. For instance, radiolunate fusion spontaneously from the disease is not uncommon in rheumatoid arthritis and has proved so successful at maintaining wrist alignment and balance that the concept has been adopted as a surgical treatment. Midcarpal ankylosis to fusion may occur with or without the radiocarpal changes just described. Thus, radiocarpal, midcarpal, and total carpal ankylosis to fusion are the usual patterns; single joint ankylosis, except for the radiolunate joint, is uncommon in rheumatoid arthritis.
7. Erosion to resorption patterns is fairly common in arthritis, particularly in the more florid rheumatoid arthritis and in the arthritis mutilans-type erosive arthritis. Bones may shrink to shards or may disappear completely either solo, as a row, or as a column (Fig. 36-24). For instance, the thumb may come to rest on the radial styloid as a result of disappearance of the intervening trapezium and distal scaphoid. Some of the resorptions in the central carpus may resemble a proximal row carpectomy. Patients who have scleroderma (Fig. 36-25), dermatomyositis (Fig. 36-26), and psoriasis (Fig. 36-27) present with variations on the theme of bone resorption, loss of carpal height, and ulnar translation of the carpus.

In addition to the joint and capsuloligamentous damage as direct causes of the above-noted deformity patterns, there are numerous indirect causes, particularly damage to tendons. The extensor carpi ulnaris tendon may be attenuated, ruptured, or simply displaced anterior to the axis of rotation of the carpus. In any case, its effect as a strong ulnar deviator and sustaining extensor and pronator of the carpus is lost. Similarly, either or both of the radial wrist extensors may become ineffective, with profound effects on wrist extension or radial deviation. Damage to the palmar wrist flexors or to the extrinsic tendons to the digits affects wrist function also, but not so profoundly as loss of wrist and finger extensor tendons.

CLINICAL GUIDES TO TREATMENT DECISIONS

CONFIRMING THE DIAGNOSIS

Medical management and therapeutic measures of treatment are often initiated without a definite diagnosis and may be sufficiently effective that surgical

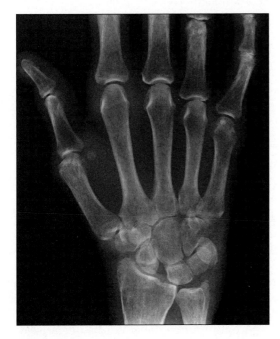

FIGURE 36-23

Posteroanterior view of a rheumatoid wrist, thumb, and metacarpal area shows early changes, including a scapholunate dissociation with dorsal intercalated segment instability.

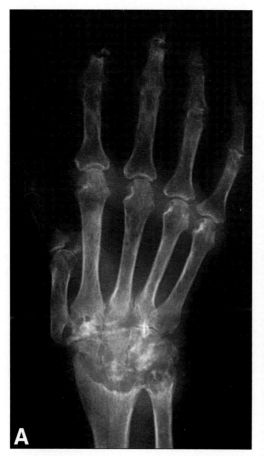
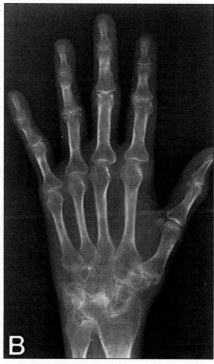

FIGURE 36–24

A, Posteroanterior view of "egg cup" ankylosis of the carpus, associated with a subluxation of the thumb carpometacarpal joint in rheumatoid arthritis of the right wrist. **B,** Posteroanterior view of a rheumatoid left wrist with severe carpal destruction but minimal deformity because of a spontaneous radiolunate fusion. There are many different spontaneous fusion patterns from the disease, but this one has been so successful in stabilizing the damaged carpus, yet retaining some mobility, that it has become a favored surgical treatment. It may be coupled with the Kapandji fusion of the distal radius and ulna.

intervention does not become necessary.* Confirmation of the diagnosis is attempted at various intervals and certainly should be demonstrated, if possible, before surgical intervention. However, diagnosis may remain on a presumptive basis even through a prolonged course of the usual rheumatoid arthritis medications: salicylates and nonsteroidal anti-inflammatory drugs for the first 3 to 6 months; hydroxychloroquine, penicillamine, gold, corticosteroids, methotrexate, azathioprine, and sulfasalazine as second-line drugs; and cyclosporine and monoclonal anti-CDr antibodies as investigational drugs. Locally active medications are often of great assistance in controlling pain, swelling, inflammation, and even damage, if the systemic medication is slow in affecting certain localized areas. Most such injectable medications are one form or another of local steroid,

although thiotepa, various gold compounds, and nitrogen mustard have also been used.

EVALUATING THE PATHOLOGIC FEATURES

Transient synovitis with pain and weakness but without instability or deformity usually responds to the medication treatments and adherence to rest, support splints, and adaptive measures. However, persistent synovitis despite treatment, the development of tendon entrapment, and increasing wrist deformity or destruction as well as nerve compression all suggest that permanent damage is being done and that surgical treatment is now worth considering. On the other hand, if pain and inflammation are reasonably controlled, the patient may do quite well with conservative treatment despite radiographic evidence of damage. There is a lack of correlation between the Steinbrocker staging of hand

---

* References 5-7,10,13,17,33,37,42.

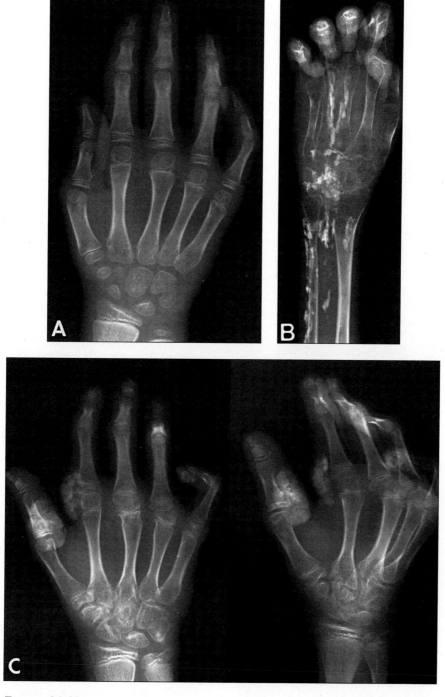

FIGURE 36-25

A, Posteroanterior view of a right wrist in juvenile scleroderma with diffuse loss of mineralization, particularly in the periarticular areas. **B,** Posteroanterior view of scleroderma in another wrist and hand shows severe osteopenia along with calcium deposits in the hand, wrist, and forearm. **C,** Posteroanterior and oblique views of scleroderma show calcifications at the thumb and index metacarpophalangeal joint; mild carpal collapse (ulnar translation and loss of carpal height).

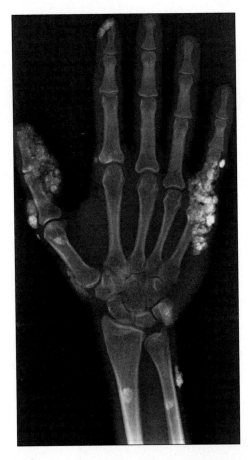

FIGURE 36-26

Posteroanterior view of a right wrist and hand in dermatomyositis, with little demineralization but with much calcification.

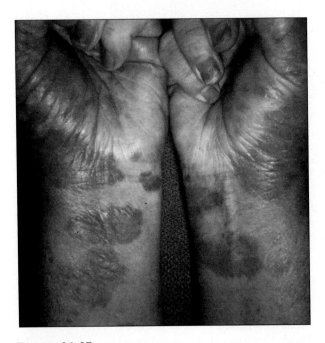

FIGURE 36-27

Psoriatic arthritis. Skin changes on the palmar aspect of the hand and wrist (erythema).

radiographs and the functional status of the rheumatoid patients.[30] If in doubt as to the functional status of the patient, an upper extremity functional assessment should be done.[12]

BALANCING THE PRIORITIES OF PERSON, DISEASE, AND TREATMENT

Reasonable life expectancy, vigor sufficient to cope with the surgical stress and the equivalent stress of rehabilitation, and an understanding of the need and limitations of the planned surgery or rehabilitation are the minimum requirements for the rheumatoid patient for whom operation is being considered.

A definite or strongly probable diagnosis and some indication that the combination of patient immune response plus medication is exerting some control of the disease process are also requirements for disease management when surgery is being considered. The patient should know that the operation may not influence the course of the disease and that disease "burnout" while possible is unlikely; more likely is a steady mild progression, a cyclic pattern of flare and remission, or a severe initial flare followed by a fairly steady state with minimal but some progression. This discussion, of course, is not just between patient and surgeon, but strongly involves the medical management group.

The patient should have a good understanding of the surgical treatments usually practiced, their values, their effects, and their disadvantages. These treatments, in order of their usual utility at the wrist, are as follows.

1. Synovectomy, which may involve both extensor and flexor tendons on radiocarpal and distal radioulnar joints, is common early in the rheumatoid process. Although open surgery has been the norm for this treatment, arthroscopic synovectomy may prove less disabling.[1]
2. Tendon repair, tenodesis, replacement, or transfer, if damaged beyond salvage, often accompanies synovectomy. Tendon transfer to balance the wrist may also need consideration.
3. Nerve decompression of the median nerve in the carpal tunnel, ulnar nerve in Guyon's canal, or the dorsal sensory nerves over bony or soft-tissue protrusions may be required.
4. Stabilization of the distal ulna soft tissues with or without excision of the head of the ulna may be done. If the head of the ulna is retained, bony stabilization by radioulnar fusion (the Kapandji procedure) may be safer than excision alone for long-term maintenance. If the head of the ulna is removed, retention or reconstruction of an intact soft-tissue column from distal stump of ulna to proximal carpus is important for stabilization of the stump and the carpus.

5. Stabilization of the carpus may be done. The common problem of palmar carpal subluxation and supination of the ulnar side of the carpus may be managed by static reconstruction or repair of the ulnocarpal support system with or without augmentation or replacement of the function of the extensor carpi ulnaris tendon, which seems to provide support in ulnar deviation, pronation, and extension. Ulnar deviation instability of the arthritic carpus may be stabilized by repositioning, followed by radiolunate fusion. Extension of this fusion to a radioscapholunate fusion or to a radiolunate-head of ulna fusion is commonly done. Less commonly, midcarpal instability and damage may be present with a relatively intact radiocarpal joint, and midcarpal fusion is then appropriate for the localized instability. Still popular for stabilizing the extensively involved arthritic wrist is stabilization of most joints of the wrist by ankylosis (permitting a few degrees of adaptive motion) or by bony fusion (radius to distal carpus or to metacarpus). Positioning of the stiffened wrist depends on the specific function requirements.

6. When joint cartilage damage is more of a problem than instability and retention of joint motion is considered a priority, there are several possible arthroplasties. These include partial fusion with interposition arthroplasty, excisional arthroplasty with soft-tissue or silicone interposition, or total joint arthroplasties. The last are more popular for the arthritic wrist than the higher-demand wrists.

SUMMARY

Although laboratory confirmation of the specific type of arthritis is desired and is nearly always available, sooner or later, most diagnoses can enter the "highly probable" category via history, imaging studies, and clinical course. In more than 90% of rheumatoid problems that affect the wrist, initial conservative treatment is proper and useful and augmented by operation only if there is early and critical damage. Surgical assistance at some stage of wrist disease is often useful and necessary. Its selection depends on:

1. the physiologic and psychologic tolerance required by the operation and available from the patient;
2. the average functional and cosmetic effectiveness of the surgical procedures;
3. the stress, risk, and permanence level of the operation; and
4. the cost-effectiveness of the operation.

REFERENCES

1. Adolfsson L, Nylander G: Arthroscopic synovectomy of the rheumatoid wrist, *J Hand Surg [Br]* 18:92-96, 1993.
2. Arkless R: Rheumatoid wrists: cineradiography, *Radiology* 88:543-549, 1967.
3. Backdahl M: Hand surgery in rheumatoid arthritis, *Mod Trends Plast Surg* 2:195-213, 1996.
4. Backhouse KM: The mechanics of normal digital control in the hand and an analysis of the ulnar drift of rheumatoid arthritis, *Ann R Coll Surg Engl* 43:154-173, 1968.
5. Barr WG, Blair SJ: Carpal tunnel syndrome as the initial manifestation of scleroderma, *J Hand Surg [Am]* 13:366-368, 1988.
6. Dray GJ: The hand in systemic lupus erythematosus, *Hand Clin* 5:145-155, 1989.
7. Drugs for rheumatoid arthritis, *Med Lett* 33:65-70, 1991.
8. Eberhardt K, Johnson PM, Rydgren L: The occurrence and significance of hand deformities in early rheumatoid arthritis, *Br J Rheumatol* 30:211-213, 1991.
9. Ertel AN: Flexor tendon ruptures in rheumatoid arthritis, *Hand Clin* 5:177-190, 1989.
10. Evans DM, Ansell BM, Hall MA: The wrist in juvenile arthritis, *J Hand Surg [Br]* 16:293-304, 1991.
11. Ferlic DC, Clayton ML: Tendon transfer for radial rotation in the rheumatoid wrist (abstract), *J Bone Joint Surg Am* 55:880-881, 1973.
12. Fess EE: *Documentation: Essential elements of an upper extremity assessment battery.* In Hunter JM, Schneider LH, Mackin EJ, et al., editors: *Rehabilitation of the hand,* ed 2, St. Louis, 1984, CV Mosby.
13. Flatt AE: *The care of the rheumatoid hand,* ed 4, St. Louis, 1984, CV Mosby.
14. Gordon SL: Lyme disease in children, *Pediatr Nurs* 20:415-418, 1994.
15. Hastings DE, Evans JA: Rheumatoid wrist deformities and their relation to ulnar drift, *J Bone Joint Surg Am* 57:930-934, 1975.
16. Hogh J, Ludlam CA, Macnicol MF: Hemophilic arthropathy of the upper limb, *Clin Orthop* 218:225-231, 1987.
17. Hollander JL: *Arthritis and allied conditions,* ed 8, Philadelphia, 1972, Lea & Febiger.

18. Jonsson B, Larsson SE: Hand function and total locomotion status in rheumatoid arthritis. An epidemiologic study, *Acta Orthop Scand* 61:339-343, 1990.

19. Kallman DA, Wigley FM, Scott WW Jr, et al.: The longitudinal course of hand osteoarthritis in a male population, *Arthritis Rheum* 33:1323-1332, 1990.

20. Kirchheimer JC, Wanivenhaus A: Declines in the range of motion and malalignment in hands of patients with juvenile rheumatoid arthritis studied over 6 years, *J Rheumatol* 17:1653-1656, 1990.

21. Leslie BM: Rheumatoid extensor tendon ruptures, *Hand Clin* 5:191-202, 1989.

22. Linscheid RL, Dobyns JH: Rheumatoid arthritis of the wrist, *Orthop Clin North Am* 2:649-665, 1971.

23. Moyer RA, Bush DC, Harrington TM: Acute calcific tendinitis of the hand and wrist: a report of 12 cases and a review of the literature, *J Rheumatol* 16:198-202, 1989.

24. Nalebuff EA, Feldon P, Millender LH: *Rheumatoid arthritis in the hand and wrist*. In Green DP, editor: *Operative hand surgery*, ed 3, New York, 1993, Churchill Livingstone.

25. Nalebuff EA, Potter TA: Rheumatoid involvement of tendon and tendon sheaths in the hand, *Clin Orthop* 59:147-159, 1968.

26. Pagliei A, Leclercq C, Goddard N, et al.: Palmar subluxation of the carpus in rheumatoid disease: a radiological evaluation, *Ann Chir Main Memb Super* 10:541-555, 1991.

27. Pahle JA, Raunio P: The influence of wrist position on finger deviation in the rheumatoid hand. A clinical and radiological study, *J Bone Joint Surg Br* 51:664-676, 1969.

28. Paparone PW: Polymyalgia rheumatica or Lyme disease? How to avoid misdiagnosis in older patients, *Postgrad Med* 97:161-164; 167-170, 1995.

29. Pirela-Cruz MA, Firoozbakhsh K, Moneim MS: Ulnar translation of the carpus in rheumatoid arthritis: an analysis of five determination methods, *J Hand Surg [Am]* 18:299-306, 1993.

30. Regan-Smith MG, O'Connor GT, Kwoh CK, et al.: Lack of correlation between the Steinbrocker staging of hand radiographs and the functional health status of individuals with rheumatoid arthritis, *Arthritis Rheum* 32:128-133, 1989.

31. Rose JH, Belsky MR: Psoriatic arthritis in the hand, *Hand Clin* 5:137-144, 1989.

32. Savelberg HH, Kooloos JG, Huiskes R, et al.: Stiffness of the ligaments of the human wrist joint, *J Biomech* 25:369-376, 1992.

33. Schneller S: Medical considerations and perioperative care for rheumatoid surgery, *Hand Clin* 5:115-126, 1989.

34. Schumacher HR Jr: *Primer on the rheumatic diseases*, ed 9, Atlanta, GA, 1988, Arthritis Foundation.

35. Shapiro JS: A new factor in the etiology of ulnar drift, *Clin Orthop* 68:32-43, 1970.

36. Shapiro JS: Wrist involvement in rheumatoid swan-neck deformity, *J Hand Surg [Am]* 7:484-491, 1982.

37. Simmons BP, Nutting JT: Juvenile rheumatoid arthritis, *Hand Clin* 5:157-168, 1989.

38. Stack HG, Vaughan-Jackson OJ: The zig-zag deformity in the rheumatoid hand, *Hand* 3:62-67, 1971.

39. Swanson AB, de Groot Swanson G: *Flexible implant resection arthroplasty in the upper extremity*. In Jupiter JB, editor: *Flynn's hand surgery*, ed 4, Baltimore, 1991, Williams & Wilkins, pp 342-386.

40. Swanson AB, de Groot Swanson G: Osteoarthritis in the hand, *Clin Rheum Dis* 11:393-420, 1985.

41. Taleisnik J: *Rheumatoid arthritis in the wrist. Surgery for rheumatoid arthritis in the wrist. Evaluation of the rheumatoid wrist*. In *The wrist*, New York, 1985, Churchill Livingstone.

42. Zancolli E: *Structural and dynamic bases of hand surgery*, ed 2, Philadelphia, 1979, JB Lippincott.

37

SOFT-TISSUE RECONSTRUCTION

Michael B. Wood, M.D.

ETIOLOGY
DIAGNOSIS
CLASSIFICATION
  TENOSYNOVITIS
    EXTENSOR TENOSYNOVITIS
    FLEXOR TENOSYNOVITIS
  WRIST SYNOVITIS
    ISOLATED WRIST SYNOVITIS WITH PRESERVED
    JOINT CONGRUITY
    WRIST SYNOVITIS WITH JOINT SUBLUXATION
    BUT WITH PRESERVED ARTICULAR SURFACES
      PALMAR RADIOCARPAL
      ULNAR RADIOCARPAL
      MIDCARPAL
      DISTAL RADIOULNAR
    WRIST SYNOVITIS WITH ARTICULAR
    DESTRUCTION
  TENDON RUPTURES
TREATMENT: OPTIONS AND RECOMMENDATIONS
  TENOSYNOVITIS
    EXTENSOR TENDONS OF THE WRIST
      FIRST TENDON COMPARTMENT OF WRIST

      SECOND TENDON COMPARTMENT OF WRIST
      THIRD TENDON COMPARTMENT OF WRIST
      FOURTH AND FIFTH TENDON
        COMPARTMENTS OF WRIST
      SIXTH TENDON COMPARTMENT OF WRIST
    FLEXOR TENDONS OF THE WRIST
  WRIST SYNOVITIS
    WITH PRESERVED JOINT CONGRUITY
    WITH JOINT SUBLUXATION BUT WITH
      PRESERVED ARTICULAR SURFACES
    WITH ARTICULAR CARTILAGE DESTRUCTION
  TENDON RUPTURE
    FINGER EXTENSOR TENDON RUPTURES AT THE
      WRIST
    EXTENSOR POLLICIS LONGUS TENDON
      RUPTURE AT THE WRIST
    FLEXOR POLLICIS LONGUS TENDON RUPTURE
      AT THE THUMB
    FINGER FLEXOR TENDON RUPTURES AT THE
      WRIST
SPECIAL PROBLEMS AND COMPLICATIONS
SUMMARY

Soft-tissue reconstruction is an important facet in the management of the wrist affected by rheumatoid arthritis. In rheumatoid arthritis of the wrist, there are preventive, corrective, and salvage surgical procedures. Frequently, timely recognition of persistent tenosynovitis or synovitis and appropriate surgical treatment can prevent or delay progression to fixed deformity, loss of joint motion, or articular destruction requiring salvage procedures of implant arthroplasty or arthrodesis. Soft-tissue reconstructive procedures should always be considered and assessed for their efficacy in the patient with rheumatoid-related wrist pathology before selecting more destructive surgical options.

However, in all instances surgical treatment should be avoided or delayed until an adequate course of nonoperative management of wrist synovitis or tenosynovitis has been attempted. Such nonoperative treatments include appropriate splinting of the wrist, selective intra-articular or tenosynovial corticosteroid injections, and optimal management of the systemic aspects of the disease process. The last treatment recommendations may best be directed by a rheumatologist or other experienced physician because they may include a trial of multiple drugs including various nonsteroidal anti-inflammatory agents, gold, penicillamine, methotrexate, sulfasalazine, hydroxychloroquine, and steroids. Moreover, these pharmacologic agents should be combined with appropriate rest, a selected exercise program, and optimal management of additional medical conditions. Splinting of the wrist (and usually the hand) is a mandatory component of the nonoperative treatment of wrist synovitis or tenosynovitis. For limited periods of up to 1 month, splinting may be required on a full-time basis (except for bathing and local skin care) during flares of local disease activity. However, splinting of the wrist on a part-time basis (at night during sleep and while at rest during the day) should not be overlooked even for the patient with a chronic and indolent inflammatory course affecting the wrist. Intra-articular corticosteroid injections should be reserved for well-localized and compartmentalized foci of synovitis or tenosynovitis that persist after a trial period for several weeks of the noninvasive treatment modalities.

ETIOLOGY

The basic cause of rheumatoid-related wrist pathology is, of course, rheumatoid arthritis—a collagen vascular disease of uncertain etiology. However, from the perspective of the pathomechanics leading to the development of rheumatoid-induced wrist changes requiring operation, persistent synovitis or tenosynovitis is the usual cause. Synovitis results in direct articular cartilage destruction, ligamentous laxity leading to joint subluxation and dislocation, and in some instances, secondary tendon ruptures.[9] Soft-tissue reconstructive surgical treatment for the wrist may be applicable for any of these stages of pathogenesis. Often indications and urgency for intervention are dictated by the magnitude of the patient's symptoms, which may include pain,

instability, limited motion, or weakness. However, in cases of persistent tenosynovitis and particularly extensor tenosynovitis associated with palmar carpal subluxation or dorsal ulnar subluxation, surgical intervention should be considered even with a paucity of symptoms because of the risk of tendon rupture.[8]

DIAGNOSIS

The diagnosis of rheumatoid involvement of the wrist is not difficult and is addressed in the preceding chapter. In a patient without a known history of rheumatoid arthritis, the diagnosis may depend on positive results of serologic studies or a synovial biopsy. In patients with known rheumatoid arthritis, the diagnosis of wrist involvement is typically by clinical examination. Occasionally, significant radiographic deterioration of the wrist may occur in the absence of clinical findings. The clinical features of the wrist affected by rheumatoid arthritis include swelling, increased local warmth over the affected joint, deformity, and limited joint range of motion. The localization and character of the swelling depend on the extent and localization of synovitis. If the swelling is diffuse and circumferential, synovitis of the radiocarpal joint is likely (Fig. 37-1). If the synovitis is localized over the dorsal aspect of the wrist and particularly if the soft-tissue swelling appears in a dumbbell-like configuration, then extensor tenosynovitis is likely.[12] In such an instance, the intact extensor retinaculum produces an apparent depression between the swollen extensor tenosynovium proximal and distal to the retinaculum. Except in patients with rather indolent synovitis or tenosynovitis, swelling is usually accompanied by locally increased warmth of the skin over the affected area.

Deformity unrelated to soft-tissue swelling may take many forms. If palmar subluxation of the carpus

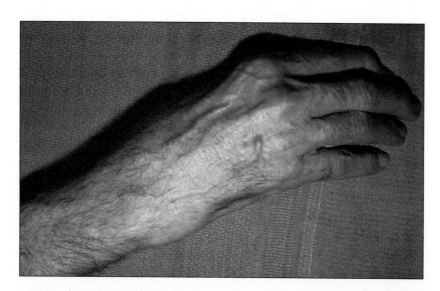

FIGURE 37-1

Photograph depicts diffuse, circumferential soft-tissue swelling of the wrist of a patient with radiocarpal synovitis.

is present, a step-off deformity with a prominence of the distal radius and ulna on the dorsal aspect may be obvious. The ulnar aspect of the carpus is particularly prone to a palmar subluxation with supination (Fig. 37-2).[14] This may lead to a somewhat erroneous conclusion of dorsal subluxation of the distal ulna. Although less common, true dorsal subluxation of the distal ulna relative to the radius may also be seen. With a marked degree of ulnar shift of the carpus relative to the radius, the wrist may appear radially angulated, usually with a concomitant ulnar drift deformity of the fingers, giving a zigzag-type appearance (Fig. 37-3). Limited joint range of motion invariably accompanies synovitis, with or without joint subluxation. However, this may be difficult to assess in a given patient because of the frequent bilaterality of the condition. The measured loss of joint range of motion by serial examinations over time may be an important clue to the extent of disease progression.

In most patients the diagnosis from clinical findings should be supported by radiographic studies. For all practical purposes, routine posteroanterior and lateral radiographs of the wrist are the only imaging studies required in most patients. With these images, the loss of height of the joint space, the presence or absence of joint subluxation or dislocation, and the degree of bony destructive changes can be accurately assessed (Fig. 37-4). In unusual circumstances, more sophisticated imaging techniques may be required. For accurate delineation of joint surface destruction, particularly when one is contemplating preservation of either radiocarpal or midcarpal articulations, trispiral tomography or computed tomography may be useful.[17] Computed axial tomography is particularly helpful for evaluating the degree of the distal radioulnar joint instability (subluxation), particularly when one is contemplating distal ulnar resection or fusion versus joint preservation. Only in unusual circumstances would additional imaging techniques such as radionuclide scanning, arthrography, ultrasound imaging, or magnetic resonance imaging be indicated. The role of arthroscopy in evaluating the rheumatoid wrist is not clear. It has been recommended for biopsy of synovium and to assess differences in joint cartilage deterioration between the midcarpal and radiocarpal joints.

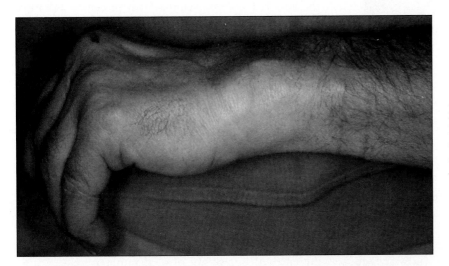

FIGURE 37-2

Photograph depicts ulnar aspect of hand and carpus palmarly subluxed and supinated relative to forearm bones.

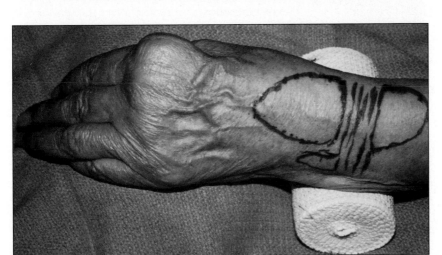

FIGURE 37-3

Photograph depicts apparent radial deviation of wrist as a result of ulnar translation of the carpus relative to radius. Outlined area illustrates soft-tissue swelling characterizing extensor tenosynovitis.

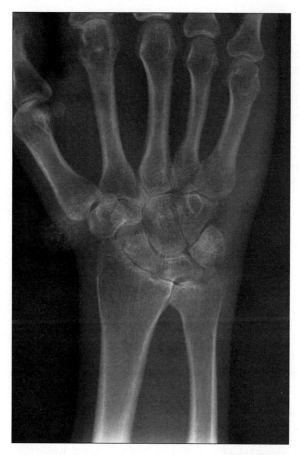

FIGURE 37-4

Posteroanterior radiograph of wrist demonstrates loss of articular joint space, subchondral bone erosions, and slight ulnar translation of the carpus relative to the radius.

CLASSIFICATION

For the purposes of this chapter, a comprehensive classification of conditions affecting the rheumatoid wrist is beyond the intended scope of discussion. However, the spectrum of conditions affecting the wrist that result from rheumatoid arthritis for which soft-tissue surgical procedures are applicable can be classified into three broad categories as follows.

TENOSYNOVITIS

Although many tissues and organ systems may be affected by rheumatoid arthritis, synovium, whether articular or tendon related, is a prime site of pathologic changes. Thus, virtually any site of tenosynovium may be involved with the disease process. About the wrist, this includes the extensor or flexor tendons (or both) and the wrist joint proper.

Extensor Tenosynovitis. Extensor tenosynovitis is common about the wrist, and because of the thin dorsal skin, it is usually obvious. It may be seen as an isolated

condition or in association with wrist synovitis. Moreover, it may be restricted to a single compartment or generalized to involve any or all dorsal extensor tendon compartments. As a single compartment entity, involvement of the first (abductor pollicis longus + extensor pollicis brevis) and sixth (extensor carpi ulnaris) compartments is well known. Both of these compartments share a similar structure of a relatively deep bony canal covered by an unyielding fibrous roof.[11] This anatomic arrangement may explain, in part, the prevalence of these tenosynovial syndromes. Perhaps the most common extensor compartments affected by rheumatoid tenosynovitis, however, are the fourth and fifth, usually in association with each other or with other compartments. The presenting symptoms with extensor tenosynovitis are usually localized to the affected compartments. These may or may not be tender, are usually associated with an increased warmth of the overlying skin, and may limit the patient's ability to perform a full range of finger motion. A characteristic of the swelling associated with involvement of the fourth dorsal compartment is an obvious movement of the tenosynovial mass with excursion of the finger extensor tendons. Moreover, as previously mentioned, the involved tenosynovial mass may present as a dumbbell shape because of a central indentation by the unyielding extensor retinaculum.

Flexor Tenosynovitis. The presence of flexor tenosynovitis may be less obvious because the patient does not typically present with a readily apparent mass. However, this condition is common about the wrist in rheumatoid arthritis.[7] It usually involves the digital flexor tendons in the digits or the wrist. When the finger or thumb flexor tendons are involved, there may be limited active finger flexion in the presence of a greater passive finger flexion or there may be triggering and crepitus. At the level of the wrist or carpal tunnel, digital flexor tenosynovitis may produce crepitus or limited range of motion and patients often present with symptoms of median neuropathy.

Flexor tenosynovitis may also affect the tendons of the flexor carpi radialis or flexor carpi ulnaris. These two sites may be characterized by fusiform swelling along the course of the involved tendon at the wrist, often associated with pain or tenderness.

WRIST SYNOVITIS

Synovitis typically involves both the proximal radiocarpal and the midcarpal articulations. With persistent synovitis, articular surface destruction leading to loss of the joint space and osteolysis leading to loss of bone height may occur. Moreover, capsular distension and gradual attenuation of capsular and extracapsular ligaments occur. The combined effects of all three of these events lead to joint subluxation and articular surface incongruity. Thus, depending on the stage of progression, wrist synovitis may be accompanied by varying degrees of joint subluxation and articular cartilage destruction.

Isolated Wrist Synovitis With Preserved Joint Congruity.

It is important to recognize these patients who have a wrist joint with persistent synovitis but with preservation of articular congruity because of the implications for the role of synovectomy as a prophylactic rather than a palliative treatment procedure (to be discussed). Such patients typically are characterized as complaining of loss of wrist motion, with or without pain, and exhibit fusiform circumferential swelling about the wrist. Radiographs may demonstrate a normal or slightly decreased joint space but with maintenance of a normal articulation relationship between the carpal bones and radius (Fig. 37-5). There may be a slight loss of the colinearity of the radius-lunate-capitate axis and most often this tends to be a palmar flexed intercalated segment instability pattern.

Wrist Synovitis With Joint Subluxation but With Preserved Articular Surfaces.

This pattern of synovitis with preserved articular surfaces but with subluxation is usually regarded as an intermediate stage of wrist synovitis disease progression. Such patients usually have significant thinning of articular cartilage but without osteolysis. Thus, although radiographs may suggest a relatively normal-appearing bone surface, the joint space is narrowed. Several patterns of subluxation may occur, often in combination.

PALMAR RADIOCARPAL. The proximal carpal row is displaced palmar to the distal radius and ulna. In such instances, the scaphoid and lunate appear to articulate with the palmar lip of the distal radius.

ULNAR RADIOCARPAL. The proximal carpal row is displaced in an ulnar direction. The scaphoid proximal pole appears to articulate with the scapholunate ridge of the distal radius and a gap exists between the radial styloid and scaphoid (Fig. 37-6). The lunate may be totally uncovered by the radius and appear to articulate with the distal ulna. Typically, the whole carpus assumes a radially deviated but ulnarly translated position.

MIDCARPAL. The most common midcarpal subluxation is a palmar intercalated segment instability deformity. In such a case, the lunocapitate axis demonstrates the distal articular surface of the lunate facing in a palmar direction by more than 15°. Occasionally, the opposite intercarpal collapse deformity may be seen—dorsiflexed intercalated segment instability. The midcarpal subluxation patterns may be seen without significant radiocarpal subluxation, but most often there is some degree of concomitant ulnar translation of the proximal carpal row.

DISTAL RADIOULNAR. The distal ulna typically is displaced in a dorsal direction relative to the distal radius

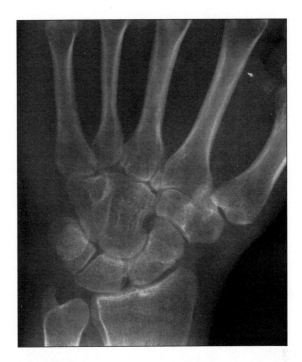

FIGURE 37-5

Posteroanterior radiograph of wrist with synovitis but with well-preserved bony architecture and no evidence of significant joint subluxation.

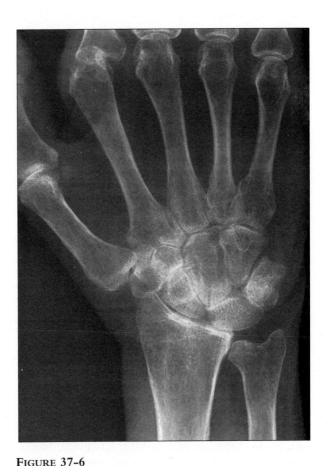

FIGURE 37-6

Posteroanterior radiograph of wrist demonstrates ulnar translation of carpus relative to radius.

and the ulnar side of the carpus. Usually some incongruity or overlap of the sigmoid notch–ulnar head articulation is apparent on radiographs.

In addition to fusiform circumferential swelling about the wrist, patients with accompanying joint subluxation may exhibit various degrees of deformity. Most commonly the distal radius is prominent dorsally with an apparent palmar step-off of the carpus. If there is significant ulnar translation, the wrist deviates in a radial direction, at times with an accompanying ulnar deviation of the fingers. In patients with distal radioulnar joint subluxation, the distal ulna appears prominent. The distal ulna may be reducible by direct pressure applied in a palmar direction but redisplaces on release of the pressure—the so-called piano key sign.[2]

Wrist Synovitis With Articular Destruction. Wrist synovitis with articular destruction represents the end stage of persistent synovitis, joint subluxation, and osteolysis. The extent of symptoms and treatment options varies greatly among patients. Usually patients in this category have symptoms of pain on attempted wrist motion, fixed deformity, or limitation of motion. However, some patients at this stage may have surprisingly little pain or deformity with relatively modest limitation of motion. The extent of articular destruction usually includes the entire wrist, but there may be partial sparing of one component or another—i.e., distal radioulnar joint, radiocarpal articulation, or midcarpal articulation.

TENDON RUPTURES

Tendon ruptures about the wrist are usually a consequence of persistent tenosynovitis leading to attritional loss of tendon substance or joint subluxation with articular destruction causing a mechanically abrasive attenuation of the tendon as it rubs across an irregular bone surface. Occasionally, a rupture of tendons may be related to an attritional tear from adjacent internal fixation hardware used for prior wrist reconstruction. The most commonly affected tendons for rupture are the common finger extensor tendons, particularly of the ulnar fingers. The extensor digiti quinti tendon is particularly vulnerable to rupture when the distal ulna is dorsally subluxed and the articular surface is destroyed.[15] Rupture may also affect the remaining extensor tendons to fingers or thumb or the flexor tendons to the digits.

The diagnosis of tendon rupture is usually not difficult if the patient has sufficient prerupture function to the thumb or fingers. Typically, a rather precipitous inability to extend or flex the affected digit or joint is noted, often without any obvious pain or specific trauma. The patient may erroneously attribute the

sudden loss of function to a flare of synovitis in a distal joint, i.e., metacarpophalangeal joints. However, the presence of preserved passive motion with the sudden loss of active motion should provide a clue to the diagnosis of tendon rupture. Occasionally, an acutely subluxed extensor tendon in the region of the metacarpal head may mimic the loss of finger extension seen with rupture of the extensor tendons at the level of the wrist. The two can usually be differentiated, however, by simple observation and palpation.

TREATMENT: OPTIONS AND RECOMMENDATIONS

The selection of surgical treatment options should be individualized based on the level of present symptoms, the patient's ability to functionally adapt to the disability, and the future risks to the patient regarding progressive loss of function if treatment is withheld. Moreover, in almost all instances surgical treatment considerations should follow a careful assessment regarding nonoperative and preferably noninvasive treatment options.

TENOSYNOVITIS

Extensor Tendons of the Wrist. A nonoperative treatment trial of optimal medical management and full-time splint use eventually weaning to part-time splinting is indicated in virtually all patients. The only exception would be a patient with marked deformity of the underlying bony surface who presents a risk of imminent tendon rupture. If a response is not evident within the first month, then intratenosynovial corticosteroid injection is warranted. Persistent symptoms beyond a 6-month period of appropriate nonoperative treatment in a patient with otherwise low rupture risk are an indication for surgical tenosynovectomy. If the extensor tenosynovitis is restricted to a specific compartment, the tenosynovectomy procedure should be limited to the affected tendons. There are some differences and peculiarities for each compartment.

First Tendon Compartment of Wrist. Adequate decompression of the first compartment is important at the time of tenosynovectomy because stenosis of the compartment may contribute to the etiology and persistence of the condition. Therefore, the dorsal roof of this compartment should be left unrepaired at operation.

Second Tendon Compartment of Wrist. Bowstringing of the radial wrist extensor tendons may be a problem after direct exposure of the second dorsal compartment for tenosynovectomy. Therefore, a generous portion of extensor retinaculum (greater than 1.5 cm) should be left in situ at tenosynovectomy. By approaching the extensor carpi radialis longus and brevis tendons proximal and distal to this preserved strip of extensor retinaculum, adequate débridement of the inflamed tenosynovial tissue can be achieved.

THIRD TENDON COMPARTMENT OF WRIST. The risk of rupture of the long extensor tendon of the thumb is appreciable, particularly if the bony bed of this compartment and Lister's tubercle is roughened and irregular. Thus, complete release of the extensor retinaculum over the third dorsal compartment and excision of Lister's tubercle is recommended. The extensor retinaculum may be directly repaired deep to the extensor pollicis longus tendon, leaving the tendon in a subcutaneous position.

FOURTH AND FIFTH TENDON COMPARTMENTS OF WRIST. The extensor digitorum communis, extensor indicis proprius, and extensor digiti quinti tendons should be exposed widely for adequate removal of invading tenosynovial tissue among these multiple tendons. Either a small strip (about 1 cm) of extensor retinaculum should be retained or repair after complete division of the extensor retinaculum is indicated to minimize bowstringing of these tendons. There is no need to retain the septum separating the fourth and fifth compartments.

SIXTH TENDON COMPARTMENT OF WRIST. The extensor carpi ulnaris tendon is frequently displaced in a palmar direction, thus negating its role as a dorsal stabilizer on the ulnar side of the wrist. Therefore, after tenosynovectomy, if the tendon is displaced, an effort to restore it to its dorsal position is indicated. Usually this can be done by a tight repair of the extensor retinaculum as well as creating a check-rein radially based loop about the tendon from a slip of extensor retinaculum (see Chapter 50).[5]

Regardless of which compartment is affected at tenosynovectomy, as much diseased tissue as possible should be excised. Tenosynovium about and between tendons should be aggressively resected. Intertendinous invading tenosynovium should be excised to an extent that does not jeopardize the tensile strength of the tendon.

Flexor Tendons of the Wrist. In general, the same preoperative management principles as outlined for extensor tendons are applicable to the flexor tendons at the wrist. A 6-month nonoperative trial may, however, be an inappropriate delay if there is a significant restriction of active digit flexion compared with patients who have passive finger range of motion and if median nerve function is significantly impaired. At flexor tenosynovectomy, it is advisable to release the transverse carpal ligament if there are any symptoms suggesting carpal tunnel syndrome. Moreover, if the flexor carpi radialis tendon is affected, decompression of the roof of the fibro-osseous canal of the flexor carpi radialis tendon is warranted.

WRIST SYNOVITIS

With Preserved Joint Congruity. In almost all patients with wrist synovitis and otherwise relatively normal radiographic appearance, a trial of nonoperative management is warranted. Intra-articular corticosteroid injection is indicated after 1 month if noninvasive pharmacologic management and splinting are ineffective.

Persistent synovitis after 6 months of nonoperative treatment is an indication for surgical synovectomy. The wrist should be approached through an extensile straight or undulating incision centered over the fourth dorsal compartment. Care should be taken to preserve the radiocapitate and radiotriquetral extracapsular ligaments. Excision of all hypertrophic synovium between radius and proximal carpal row, within the midcarpal articulation and about the triangular fibrocartilage, should be done using a fine-tipped synovectomy rongeur (Fig. 37-7). Distraction of the wrist by an assistant permits adequate access to the palmar aspect of all but the midcarpal and scaphotrapezial regions. If the distal radioulnar joint is affected, access to this region should be gained through the floor of the fifth dorsal compartment. It is important, however, when exposing the distal radioulnar joint to preserve the dorsal distal radioulnar ligament. Thus, joint exposure should be through an access point proximal to this ligament. At the conclusion of synovectomy, the wrist joint capsule and extensor retinaculum should be anatomically

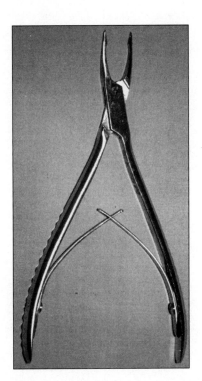

FIGURE 37-7

Photograph of rongeur used for synovectomy.

repaired. The wrist should be immobilized for at least 3 weeks in a slightly extended position. Thereafter, a part-time splinting and progressive mobilization program for the wrist may be initiated.

With Joint Subluxation but With Preserved Articular Surfaces. The same preoperative management principles outlined in the preceding section are applicable to this group of patients. In the presence of persistent synovitis, synovectomy is indicated. However, in addition to synovectomy, reduction of the subluxation, temporary internal fixation with transarticular Kirschner wires, and an attempt to restore longer-term stability by capsulodesis or tendon transfer is warranted. Usually, dorsal wrist capsulodesis can be accomplished by a "pants over vest"-type repair using proximally and distally based flaps of the attenuated dorsal wrist capsule and dorsal extra-articular ligaments. However, if the extensor retinaculum is markedly thinned, a portion of the extensor carpi radialis longus tendons can be used to augment the dorsal capsulodesis. If there is significant ulnar translational instability of the carpus, transfer of the extensor carpi radialis longus tendon to the extensor carpi ulnaris tendon is warranted (see Fig. 48-9).[3] This transfer also helps replace the extensor carpi ulnaris tendon over the dorsal aspect of the distal ulna. It is important at the time of capsulodesis or tendon transfer (or both) to ensure correct reduction of the subluxed articulations. This reduced position should be secured by one or more transarticular Kirschner wires. The wrist should be immobilized for 6 weeks, after which gradual mobilization with part-time splint support is initiated.

With Articular Cartilage Destruction. Most often the recommended treatment for patients with persistent wrist synovitis in the presence of articular destruction after an adequate attempt at nonoperative treatment involves some form of arthrodesis.[6] Arthrodesis for the articulations of the wrist including the distal radioulnar joint is addressed elsewhere in this text (see Chapters 25 and 38). Occasionally, some patients exhibit persistent wrist synovitis and the presence of articular destruction; they may be candidates for selective limited arthrodesis supplemented with synovectomy. Such may be the case in patients with advanced radiocarpal destruction but reasonable preservation of the midcarpal articulation or selective involvement or sparing of the distal radioulnar joint. These patients may benefit from fusion of the most involved articulation with synovectomy of the less involved levels where a reasonable articular congruity may exist (Fig. 37-8). The occasional patient with advanced wrist

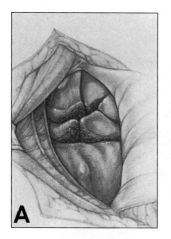
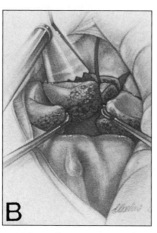
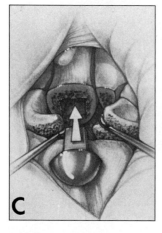
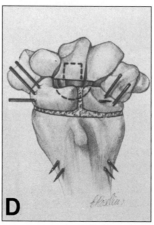

FIGURE 37-8

Surgical technique for combined radiocarpal arthrodesis and midcarpal arthroplasty. **A,** Radiocarpal and midcarpal joints are exposed. Erosive changes of the articular surfaces are depicted. **B,** Dissociation between the scaphoid and lunate facilitates exposure; excision of head of capitate and proximal pole of hamate. **C,** Body of capitate is prepared to receive the shortened stem of a condylar implant. **D,** Appearance after arthrodesis between radius, scaphoid, and lunate is completed. The assembled scapholunate unit should rotate enough to cover most of the condylar implant. *(From Taleisnik J: Combined radiocarpal arthrodesis and midcarpal (lunocapitate) arthroplasty for treatment of rheumatoid arthritis of the wrist,* J Hand Surg [Am] *12:1-8, 1987. Copyright, American Society for Surgery of the Hand, by permission of Churchill Livingstone.)*

articular destruction may be a candidate for limited or complete resection with soft-tissue interposition arthroplasty (Figs. 37-9 and 37-10).[1] Theoretically, these procedures may permit motion and correct wrist alignment. In most patients complete resection arthroplasty is plagued by complications related to instability, making arthrodesis or implant arthroplasty preferable alternatives. Moreover, resection arthroplasty in a patient with rheumatoid arthritis usually requires extensive bone resection to correct deformity. One should consider this procedure only in the patient in whom deformity can be overcome by excising only part or all of the proximal carpal row. Unfortunately, this is rarely the case in the wrist destroyed by rheumatoid arthritis.

A final treatment option for patients with articular destruction and pain in the presence of useful function

and acceptable alignment is a localized denervation procedure.[4] In contrast to patients with degenerative joint disease, this combination of symptoms is relatively unusual in rheumatoid arthritis. However, if present, denervation is a relatively simple technique that may palliate pain complaints and preserve motion. The technique of wrist articular denervation is well described in the literature.

TENDON RUPTURE

Recommended treatment for patients presenting with rupture of tendons about the wrist depends on the degree of perceived impairment to the upper limb as well as the specific tendon(s) involved. Some patients adapt well to a ruptured tendon and do not perceive this problem to add significantly to their overall disability. In

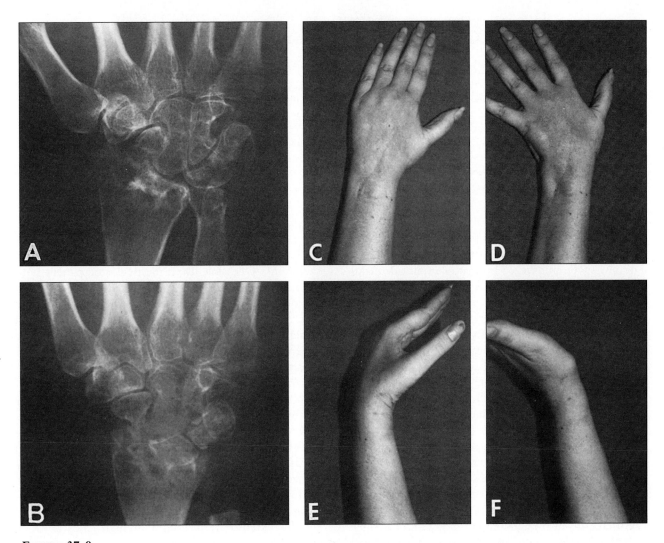

FIGURE 37-9

Appearance of the wrist before and after radiocarpal fusion and silicone condylar implant. **A,** Preoperative radiograph with proximal row collapse but fair midcarpal joint. **B,** Postoperative radiograph of fusion-arthroplasty combined with Darrach resection. **C, D, E,** and **F,** Range of wrist motion. *(From Taleisnik J: Combined radiocarpal arthrodesis and midcarpal (lunocapitate) arthroplasty for treatment of rheumatoid arthritis of the wrist,* J Hand Surg [Am] *12:1-8, 1987. Copyright, American Society for Surgery of the Hand, by permission of Churchill Livingstone.)*

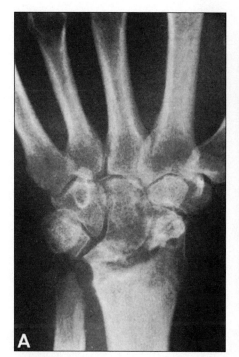 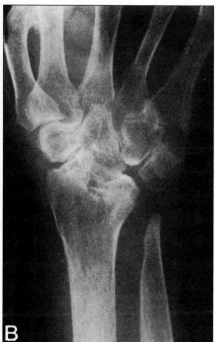

FIGURE 37–10

Rheumatoid wrist reconstruction, fibrous nonunion, and radiocarpal arthrodesis. **A,** Fibrous nonunion at the radiocarpal joint allows motion at this level and provides support for less affected midcarpal joint. Good cartilage maintenance is present between capitate and scapholunate cup. Wrist flexion was 30° and extension was 35° at 2-year follow-up. **B,** Fusion of radius to scaphoid and lunate with motion at the well-preserved midcarpal joint. Extension 45° and flexion 30°. *(From Ryu J, Watson HK, Burgess RC: Rheumatoid wrist reconstruction utilizing a fibrous nonunion and radiocarpal arthrodesis, J Hand Surg [Am] 10:830-836, 1985. Copyright, American Society for Surgery of the Hand, by permission of Churchill Livingstone.)*

such cases neglect of the problem may be warranted. Problems related to rupture of the thumb long flexor tendon may be minimized by a simple splint to maintain the thumb interphalangeal joint in 10° to 20° of flexion. Likewise, difficulties resulting from rupture of the finger extensor tendons with stiff and destroyed metacarpophalangeal joints may be decreased by the prolonged use of the splint to support the fingers in a moderately extended position and allow them to partially ankylose in this position. If, by contrast, tendon rupture occurs in a patient with a functional hand who is acutely aware of the resulting disability, surgical treatment is warranted.

Finger Extensor Tendon Ruptures at the Wrist.

Rupture of the extensor tendons to the fingers is a consequence of mechanical and tenosynovial infiltrative attritional substance loss of the tendons. Thus, the ruptured ends of the tendons are frayed and damaged over an extended length and are not suitable for direct end-to-end repair. Repair of the extensor tendons to the fingers at the wrist is most reliably accomplished by a side-to-side tenorrhaphy. This statement assumes there are intact remaining finger extensor tendons. If

no adjacent extensor tendons are available for side-to-side repair, intercalated tendon graft reconstruction is advised.[13] Occasionally, in the neglected patient with fixed contractures of the muscle belly to the ruptured tendon, tendon transfer is advised. The tendon selected for this purpose should provide a tendon length that reaches well distal to the level of the wrist. Thus the flexor digitorum superficialis tendon to the third or fourth finger is preferred.

Any surgical repair or reconstruction of the extensor tendons must also address the underlying bony pathology. Most often this is characterized by a dorsally displaced distal ulna or a dorsally prominent distal radius as a result of palmar carpal subluxation. In such patients, the distal ulna must be reduced and stabilized or excised or the carpus must be reduced with either concomitant wrist fusion or osteoplastic revision of the dorsal rim of the distal radius. At least half of the extensor retinaculum in such cases must be passed deep to the tendons. After any of these reconstruction techniques, the fingers and wrist should be immobilized in a moderately extended position for 4 weeks followed by a gradual mobilization program with part-time splinting.

Extensor Pollicis Longus Tendon Rupture at the Wrist. Rupture of the thumb long extensor at the wrist is usually associated with an abrasive effect from Lister's tubercle. In such patients, Lister's tubercle should be resected and the bony bed covered with a strip of extensor retinaculum. Reconstruction may be by a short intercalated tendon graft if the rupture is treated within a few weeks after the event. If treatment is delayed, the most reliable treatment is by transfer of the extensor indicis proprius tendon.[10] Aftercare is similar to that described for the fingers. However, in contrast to the fingers, immobilization must include the interphalangeal joint of the thumb.

Flexor Pollicis Longus Tendon Rupture at the Thumb. Rupture of the flexor pollicis longus tendon is characterized by a loss of flexion of the interphalangeal joint of the thumb without any obvious loss of metacarpophalangeal joint flexion. Repair options for this rupture can include a short tendon graft or a flexor digitorum superficialis transfer. A similar and equally reliable technique is simply interphalangeal joint tenodesis in a position of 10° to 20° of flexion. If the thumb interphalangeal joint is stable and congruent without any significant articular destruction, the tenodesis of the joint can be accomplished by coapting the distal stump of the flexor pollicis longus tendon into a bony bed in the palmar portion of the proximal phalanx combined with palmar capsulodesis of the interphalangeal joint. However, in patients with significant rheumatoid arthritis involvement of the thumb interphalangeal joint, arthrodesis of the joint in 10° to 20° of flexion with Kirschner wires or a Herbert screw is preferred. Aftercare follows that dictated for tendon graft or transfer or for joint arthrodesis. Obviously, postoperative treatment and rehabilitation are considerably less obtrusive to the patient when simple joint stabilization is done.

Finger Flexor Tendon Ruptures at the Wrist. Rupture of the finger flexor tendons at the wrist is uncommon and usually involves the flexor digitorum profundus tendons because of their position adjacent to the bones of the wrist. Isolated rupture of the flexor digitorum profundus tendon in the presence of a functioning superficialis tendon is often unrecognized, particularly in the patient with significant finger involvement by rheumatoid arthritis. Thus, treatment is rarely required. If treatment is required as a result of significant loss of active finger flexion for required activities, side-to-side tenorrhaphy is advised to either adjacent flexor digitorum profundus tendons or the flexor digitorum superficialis tendon to the same finger. In either case, attention is required to coapt the tendons under appropriate tension to avoid a quadriga effect in the case of side-to-side flexor digitorum profundus tenorrhaphy.[16] Moreover, when transferring the ruptured distal end of the flexor digitorum profundus to the intact superficialis tendon of the same finger, the flexor digitorum profundus stump should be sutured under greater tension to produce the desired flexion of the distal interphalangeal joint before that of the proximal interphalangeal joint. As in the case of the thumb interphalangeal joint, in the presence of a functioning superficialis tendon and concomitant normal active proximal interphalangeal joint range of motion, tenodesis of the finger distal interphalangeal joint or arthrodesis is also a treatment option.

SPECIAL PROBLEMS AND COMPLICATIONS

The major issues regarding special problems and complications for soft-tissue reconstruction of the rheumatoid wrist relate to persistence of the disease process and recurrence of synovitis or tenosynovitis. Untreated tenosynovitis, particularly in the face of joint subluxations about the wrist, may be associated with otherwise avoidable tendon ruptures. Thus, vigilance in this regard is important. There may be patients with recurrent synovitis or tenosynovitis who remain candidates for a repeat synovectomy or tenosynovectomy. This judgment is based on the clinical findings in a specific patient. Recurrent joint subluxation, however, after an attempt at reduction with or without capsulodesis or tendon transfer, should prompt consideration for joint stabilization by arthrodesis as a more reliable option. The usual problems with tendon repair or tendon transfer related to limited excursion are accentuated in the patient with rheumatoid arthritis. Thus, an aggressive postsurgical mobilization program is required after adequate healing time for the tendons. Such patients may require secondary tenolysis procedures.

SUMMARY

Soft-tissue reconstruction of the wrist affected by rheumatoid arthritis represents important treatment modalities. These procedures should be considered in the early stages as prophylactic measures for the patient in whom nonoperative attempts at controlling persistent synovitis or tenosynovitis have failed. Determination of the role of synovectomy with or without joint subluxation or with or without articular destruction is important for making rational and logical treatment recommendations and for ensuring more predictable results. These procedures should always be assessed for efficacy before considering more destructive salvage procedures. The judicious application of soft-tissue reconstruction about the wrist may avoid or at least not prolong the need for salvage surgical treatment methods.

REFERENCES

1. Albright JA, Chase RA: Palmar-shelf arthroplasty of the wrist in rheumatoid arthritis. A report of nine cases, *J Bone Joint Surg Am* 52:896-906, 1970.

2. Bäckdahl M: The caput ulnae syndrome in rheumatoid arthritis: a study of the morphology, abnormal anatomy and clinical picture, *Acta Rheumatol Scand Suppl* 5:1-75, 1963.

3. Boyce T, Youm Y, Sprague BL, et al.: Clinical and experimental studies on the effect of extensor carpi radialis longus transfer in the rheumatoid hand, *J Hand Surg [Am]* 3:390-394, 1978.

4. Buck-Gramcko D: Wrist denervation procedures in the treatment of Kienböck's disease, *Hand Clin* 9:517-520, 1993.

5. Burkhart SS, Wood MB, Linscheid RL: Posttraumatic recurrent subluxation of the extensor carpi ulnaris tendon, *J Hand Surg [Am]* 7:1-3, 1982.

6. Clayton ML, Ferlic DC: Arthrodesis of the arthritic wrist, *Clin Orthop* 187:89-93, 1984.

7. Ertel AN, Millender LH: *Flexor tendon involvement in rheumatoid arthritis.* In Hunter JM, Schneider LH, Mackin EJ, editors: *Tendon surgery in the hand,* St. Louis, 1987, CV Mosby, pp 370-384.

8. Ferlic DC: *Inflammatory and rheumatoid arthritis.* In Lichtman DM, editor: *The wrist and its disorders,* Philadelphia, 1988, WB Saunders, pp 344-364.

9. Flatt AE: *The care of the rheumatoid hand,* ed 3, St. Louis, 1974, CV Mosby, pp 78-138.

10. Goldner JL: Tendon transfers in rheumatoid arthritis, *Orthop Clin North Am* 5:425-444, 1974.

11. Hajj AA, Wood MB: Stenosing tenosynovitis of the extensor carpi ulnaris, *J Hand Surg [Am]* 11:519-520, 1986.

12. Millender LH, Nalebuff EA: Preventive surgery—tenosynovectomy and synovectomy, *Orthop Clin North Am* 6:765-792, 1975.

13. Shannon FT, Barton NJ: Surgery for rupture of extensor tendons in rheumatoid arthritis, *Hand* 8:279-286, 1976.

14. Taleisnik J: Rheumatoid synovitis of the volar compartment of the wrist joint: its radiological signs and its contribution to wrist and hand deformity, *J Hand Surg [Am]* 4:526-535, 1979.

15. Vaughan-Jackson OJ: Rupture of extensor tendons by attrition at inferior radio-ulnar joint: report of 2 cases, *J Bone Joint Surg Br* 30:528-530, 1948.

16. Verdan C: Syndrome of the quadriga, *Surg Clin North Am* 40:425-426, 1960.

17. Wood MB, Berquist TH: *The hand and wrist.* In Berquist TH, editor: *Imaging of orthopedic trauma and surgery,* Philadelphia, 1986, WB Saunders, pp 641-730.

38

WRIST FUSION: PARTIAL AND COMPLETE

John M. Rayhack, M.D.
Michael B. Wood, M.D.

PATHOPHYSIOLOGY
RADIOGRAPHIC FINDINGS
NONSURGICAL TREATMENT
SYNOVECTOMY
LIMITED WRIST ARTHRODESIS
RADIOLUNATE ARTHRODESIS
SURGICAL RADIOLUNATE ARTHRODESIS
  POSTOPERATIVE PROTECTION
  RESULTS OF RADIOLUNATE ARTHRODESES
RADIOSCAPHOLUNATE FUSION
RADIOSCAPHOLUNATE ARTHRODESIS WITH
  MIDCARPAL ARTHROPLASTY
SAUVÉ-KAPANDJI FUSION

COMPLETE WRIST ARTHRODESIS
  INDICATIONS
  SURGICAL APPROACH FOR COMPLETE FUSION
  INTERNAL FIXATION
  POSITION OF FUSION
  TWO-PIN FIXATION
  SURGICAL CLOSURE
  POSTOPERATIVE IMMOBILIZATION
  PIN REMOVAL
BILATERAL WRIST FUSION
COMPLICATIONS
ARTHRODESIS AFTER A FAILED ARTHROPLASTY
SUMMARY

Treatment of the rheumatoid wrist is a prodigious challenge to hand surgeons. Referred to as the "keystone of the hand," it is not surprising that pain, instability, and a fixed wrist deformity so commonly seen in an untreated rheumatoid patient culminate in finger deformity.[13,21,36] Due to the overwhelming importance of a stable, balanced, and painless wrist to hand and finger function, wrist treatment must frequently precede or be performed concurrently with treatment of hand deformities.[7,10]

In general, a total arthrodesis of the wrist has been considered a reliable and gratifying procedure. Despite this clinical success, a great deal of interest has been shown in limited wrist arthrodeses. By decreasing pain and preventing further deterioration of carpal position relative to the radius, limited wrist arthrodeses are playing an increasing role in the treatment of the rheumatoid wrist.

PATHOPHYSIOLOGY

Although early involvement of the wrist in rheumatoid arthritis is not as frequently seen as involvement of the hand, it is known that synovitis of the wrist may be the initial presentation of a patient with undiagnosed rheumatoid arthritis.[7] The destructive synovitis so prevalent in the rheumatoid wrist is intimately associated with the location of the supporting ligamentous structures.[22] With the concentration of proximal radiocarpal and ulnocarpal ligaments, it is no surprise that the ulnar styloid, ulnar head, and midscaphoid are the earliest areas of involvement.[6,14,22] These areas correspond to the ulnolunate and ulnar collateral ligament in the prestyloid recess and the radioscapholunate ligament on the palmar aspect of the scaphoid, respectively. With cartilaginous destruction, narrowing of the intercarpal and radiocarpal joint spaces occurs under the destructive influence of the highly inflammatory synovium. Weakening of the ligaments and capsules occurs through attenuation due to invasion or distension by the proliferating synovial tissue.[14] Secondary maladaptive changes occur as a result of the loss of these important supporting structures.

Interestingly, the midcarpal joint, which is relatively devoid of ligamentous attachments, remains relatively uninvolved by the destructive synovitis,[35] and involvement of the midcarpal joint is conspicuously absent. This fact permits limited arthrodeses to be considered as a therapeutic option despite the presence of advanced destruction of the radiocarpal articulation.

RADIOGRAPHIC FINDINGS

As the disease progresses unchecked, radiographic erosions proportional to the amount of diseased synovium are first seen in the ulnar head and ulnar styloid and then about the radial and palmar aspects of the scaphoid. Subsequently, erosions in the scaphotrapezial joint appear, and pseudocysts of the distal subchondral margin of the radius may be seen.[36]

With the progressive synovial involvement beneath the radioscaphocapitate (sling) ligament, rotatory subluxation of the scaphoid often occurs. Along with this collapse is an accompanying loss of carpal height,[6,22] radial tilting,[24,29,30] and supination of the carpus.[24,33] With time, scapholunate dissociation occurs (Fig. 38-1, A),[14] often associated with a palmar intercalated segment instability deformity (Fig. 38-1, B). A dorsal intercalated segment instability deformity and progressive palmar subluxation of the carpus may also be seen (Fig. 38-1, C).[14] As a result of the orientation of the radial articular surface, various degrees of ulnar translation of the carpus frequently occur (Fig. 38-1, D)[18,36] along with complete palmar dislocation of the wrist (Fig. 38-1, E).[3] This progressive collapse is hastened by the changes occurring along the ulnar side of the wrist.

With involvement of the prestyloid recess and invasion of the dorsal radioulnar ligament and the triangular fibrocartilage complex, the caput ulnae syndrome frequently occurs.[1] Dorsal subluxation or dislocation of the ulna occurs in association with supination of the carpus (Fig. 38-1, C). This blocks further dorsiflexion of the wrist. The extensor carpi ulnaris tends to progressively sublux palmarly as the ulna displaces dorsally.[32] With the palmar subluxation of the extensor carpi ulnaris, the wrist radially deviates, setting up possible attritional ruptures of the extensors[37] and setting in motion the longitudinal zigzag collapse of ulnar deviation or drift of the fingers at the metacarpophalangeal joint. This maladaptive change can become a difficult therapeutic challenge.[30]

NONSURGICAL TREATMENT

Most patients with early wrist involvement are initially treated by their primary care physician or rheumatologist, rather than by a hand surgeon. In its earliest stages, it is appropriate to consider medical treatment consisting of orally administered anti-inflammatory medications, judicious use of corticosteroid injections, and various splinting modalities.[7,14] Once it becomes clear that medical management is not successful in halting the progression of the disease, the role of hand surgeon takes on increasing importance. Because the hand surgeon must intervene at the earliest possible moment to prevent or to minimize destruction of ligaments, capsule, and bone, the determination of the presence of destructive articular synovium is of paramount importance.[36] To this end, wrist arthrography has been mentioned as a means of determining the early presence of articular synovitis, which may not be clinically evident.[26]

SYNOVECTOMY

Failure of medical management or the evidence of a proliferative synovitis without evidence of a major carpal collapse deformity coupled with persistent pain favors early synovectomy of the extensor tendons and wrist joint (see Chapters 37 and 47).

The benefits of early surgical intervention at this point have been known since the work of Smith-Petersen and co-workers[31] in the early 1940s. Yet, 50 years later, the benefits of early intervention are often overlooked, to the chagrin of the hand surgeon and often to the detriment of the patient. In addition to an early synovectomy of the extensor tendons and often the carpal canal,[11] a transfer of the extensor carpi radialis longus to the extensor carpi ulnaris is frequently beneficial to prevent early or impending radial deviation of the hand on the wrist, subsequent ulnar translation of the carpus, and ulnar deviation of the fingers.

LIMITED WRIST ARTHRODESIS

With the evidence of early destruction of the radiolunate and radioscaphoid joint, and often despite synovectomy, further conservative care may no longer be beneficial to the patient. Armed with the knowledge of the progressive carpal collapse that awaits the rheumatoid patient, it becomes apparent that aggressive surgical intervention is needed to maintain those structures that remain uninvolved in the rheumatoid wrist. Rather than proceeding with a complete wrist fusion or total wrist arthroplasty at this point, there is

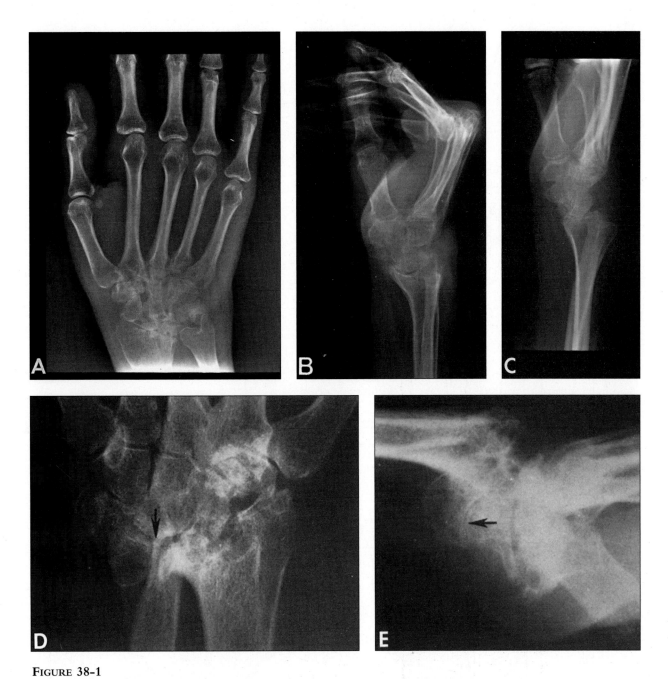

FIGURE 38-1

Progressive deterioration of wrist. **A,** Radiographic changes of erosive rheumatoid arthritis demonstrate subluxation of radiocarpal joint, prominent distal ulna with loss of carpal height, supination of the carpus, and radial tilting (loss of radial length and alignment). **B,** Palmar subluxation of the carpus; palmar instability of the wrist. **C,** Dorsal intercalated segment instability deformity and progressive palmar subluxation of the carpus and dorsal ulnar instability. **D,** Severe ulnar translocation of the carpus. **E,** Palmar dislocation of the carpus. Arrow shows location of midcarpal joint.

increasing interest in the concept of limited wrist arthrodeses (Fig. 38-2).[6,12,15,20,21]

The goals of limited wrist arthrodeses are to decrease pain and to increase function by restoring relative carpal alignment and to prevent further maladaptive carpal repositioning. Ulnar translation of the carpus down the inclined plane of the radius is further accelerated by supination of the carpus, an ulna minus deformity, and reabsorption of the triangular fibrocartilage complex.[15] By maintaining the metacarpals in alignment with the wrist, ulnar drift of the fingers can be prevented or at least minimized. Limited carpal fusions can be beneficial in not only treating wrist disease but also decreasing further deformity in the hand. Four limited arthrodeses are currently recommended in the rheumatoid wrist: the radiolunate fusion, the

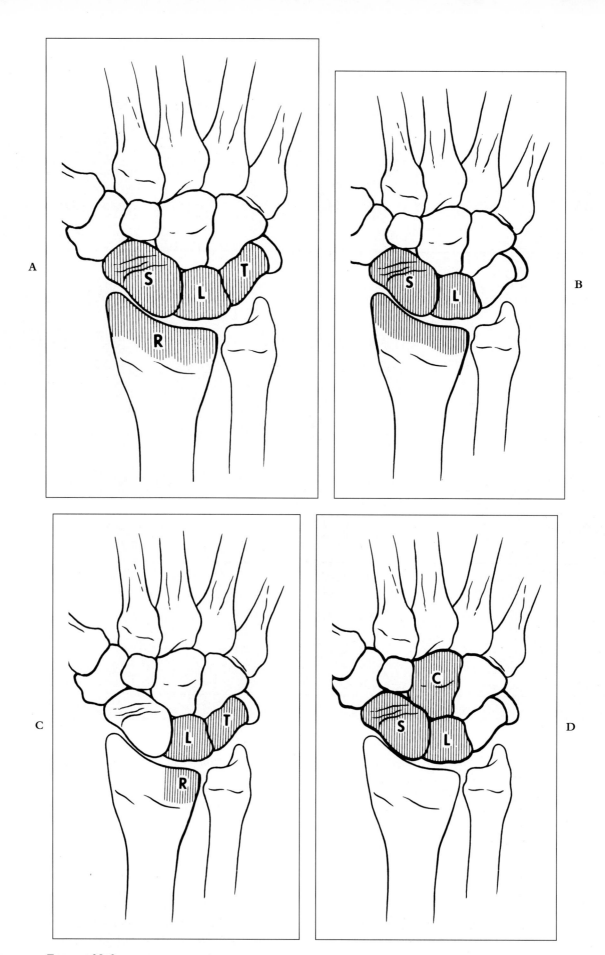

FIGURE 38-2

Limited wrist arthrodesis. **A,** Radius (*R*) to proximal carpal row (scaphoid [*S*], lunate [*L*], triquetrum [*T*]). **B,** Radio-scaphoid lunate fusion. **C,** Radiolunate (or combined radiolunotriquetral) fusion. **D,** Midcarpal fusion (scaphoid, lunate, capitate [*C*]).

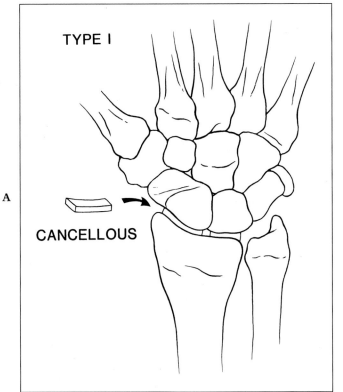

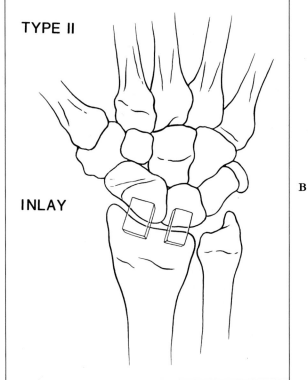

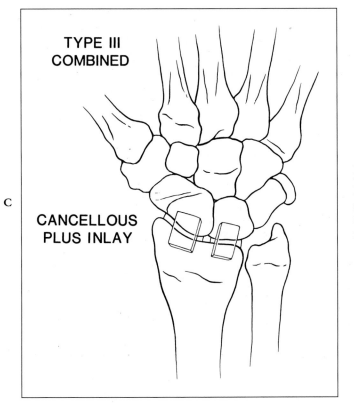

FIGURE 38-3

Limited wrist arthrodesis. Types of fusion. **A,** Cancellous bone graft interposition fusion (Type I). **B,** Cortical bone graft inlay fusion (Type II). **C,** Combined cancellous graft and cortical inlay between radius and scaphoid and radius and lunate.

radioscapholunate fusion with and without midcarpal arthroplasty, and the distal radioulnar arthrodesis (the Sauvé-Kapandji procedure). These fusions can be performed by cancellous interposition grafting or cortical inlay grafts (Fig. 38-3).

RADIOLUNATE ARTHRODESIS

The rheumatoid wrist demonstrates two intrinsic compensatory mechanisms that are frequently capable of blocking further ulnar migration of the carpus.

First, the articular surface of the radius undergoes a little-recognized and often subtle remodeling to form an osteophyte-like projection that can provide ulnar support under the lunate.[6] The second mechanism is a spontaneous radiolunate arthrodesis.[6,33]

Spontaneous radiolunate arthrodesis can result from progressive cartilaginous destruction or from arthrofibrosis with a fixed position of the wrist.[14] As noted by Linscheid and Dobyns,[14] this spontaneous arthrodesis of the radiolunate articulation may proceed to a complete wrist arthrodesis with progressive involvement of the midcarpal joint. Some patients have the arthritic process limited to the radiocarpal joint, with little to no involvement of the midcarpal joint. When spontaneous radiolunate fusion occurs, further subluxation of the carpus stops and reasonable motion can often occur.[14,35]

With spontaneous arthrodesis, the wrist usually settles in a stable position, although persistent deformity may be present despite the solid arthrodesis.[15] Chamay et al.[6] reported the follow-up results of nine spontaneous radiolunate arthrodeses and an additional three cases after ulnar head resection, which may not be considered to be true "spontaneous" arthrodeses. The range of motion was quite limited after spontaneous radiolunate arthrodeses, and after the surgical radiolunate arthrodesis it decreased early and to an equal degree (Table 38-1). Loss of range of motion postoperatively compared with preoperative values was also observed by Linscheid and Dobyns[15] and Ishikawa et al.[12] Therefore, despite relief of pain and an apparent loss of motion related to the arthritis, further reduction in motion can be expected after radiolunate fusion.

Despite the decrease in the wrist range of motion, the impetus for considering a surgical radiolunate arthrodesis can be attributed to the observation that the spontaneous arthrodesis was often successful in limiting progressive ulnar migration of the carpus and stabilizing wrist involvement.

The indications for radiolunate arthrodesis are a painful wrist with radiocarpal instability, progressive

ulnar shift of the carpus, or palmar subluxation of the carpus. Additionally, an absence of destructive changes in the proximal scaphoid pole is necessary to exclude this bone from the arthrodesis site.[21] The radiolunate fusion is preferred because it preserves more motion than the more encompassing radioscapholunate fusion yet solves the problem of carpal instability. Another prerequisite is minimal bony deformity and destruction limited to the radiocarpal joint.[12,15,20,21]

Contraindications to limited arthrodesis are a rapidly progressive destructive rheumatoid process, nonfunctioning or ruptured wrist extensors, or the intraoperative discovery of a significant arthritic process in the midcarpal joints.[20,21]

SURGICAL RADIOLUNATE ARTHRODESIS

The surgical approach for a radiocarpal fusion can be a longitudinal oblique dorsal skin incision, preferably angled from the radius distally to the ulna proximally (Fig. 38-4, *A*).[20,21] Alternatively, a straight middorsal longitudinal incision can be used and, in our opinion, is preferred. Chamay et al.[6] used two surgical approaches in seven surgical radiolunate arthrodeses. In three cases a dorsoulnar approach was used, and in four a dorsal midline approach was preferred. Interestingly, transverse incisions have been advocated in rheumatoid patients to avoid hematoma, delayed skin healing, and wound slough, yet most authorities recommend against a transverse incision because it limits exposure and compromises further exposure if additional operations are needed.[27]

Regardless of the surgical approach chosen, care must always be taken to protect the skin, subcutaneous tissue, and sensory nerves. This protection is facilitated by carrying the incision directly down to the extensor retinaculum and then reflecting the soft tissues radially and ulnarly (Fig. 38-4, *B*) (see Chapter 7). Vessels perforating the extensor retinaculum should be cauterized as the soft-tissue flaps are elevated. A synovectomy of the extensor tendons is performed if needed after the extensor retinaculum is reflected as radial- and ulnar-based flaps. Division of the terminal portion of the posterior interosseous nerve proximal to the radiocarpal joint diminishes postoperative joint pain.[9] The dorsal capsule is then divided transversely and distally in a T-shaped fashion, reflected, and maintained as two distally based flaps (Fig. 38-4, *B*).

The distal ulna may be resected through a separate capsular incision if it is a source of pain or if it is unstable (see Chapter 34). Care must be taken to preserve the ulnocarpal ligaments for later reconstruction of the ulnar supporting structures.[20,21]

Turning to the radiocarpal joint, the articular cartilage and subchondral bone are removed down to the level of cancellous bone. Exposure of this area is

| | Range of Motion (°) | | |
| Type | Spontaneous | Surgical | |
		Preop	Postop
Flexion	23 (25–50)	38 (10–40)	22 (10–35)
Extension	35 (0–45)	53 (35–65)	34 (20–48)

Table 38-1. Range of Motion After Radiolunate Arthrodesis

Postop, postoperative; *preop*, preoperative.

facilitated by acute wrist flexion. We prefer use of a rongeur and osteotomes to shape the proximal carpal row and distal radius rather than a bur, although the latter can be used with low speed and adequate irrigation. The midcarpal joint must be opened to check for signs of destructive arthritis at this time. Limit the decortication to a narrow area of the radius and the lunate if only a radiolunate arthrodesis is desired (Fig. 38-4, *C*). By trying to avoid violating the articular cartilage of the scaphoid and triquetrum, the surgeon may be impressed by the relatively small transverse surface area available for the arthrodesis. The orientation of the major surface area is thus dorsal-palmar and care must be taken to decorticate the palmar lunate and radial surface. Use of Kirschner wires as bone positioners may facilitate this exposure and assist in the correct subsequent placement of the lunate relative to the radius.

With the decortication completed, the ulnarly translated carpus is repositioned radially so that the lunate is seated in apposition to the lunate fossa of the radius. The lunate should be maintained in neutral position. Dorsal or palmar angulation of the lunate should be corrected. Failure to internally fix the lunate in neutral rotation may result in a flexion deformity with subsequent anterior dislocation of the capitate.[6]

Fixation of the lunate to the radius is achieved either through multiple Kirschner wires placed from the dorsal radius into the palmar lunate or through the dorsal lunate into the radius (Fig. 38-4, *C*).[20,21] Fixation may also be achieved through the use of small cancellous screws.[6] Kirschner wires and staples may also be combined.[12] Alternatively, a specialized plate may be used to effect this fixation. The Stanley-Shelley plate (Fig. 38-5),[34] specifically made for the radiolunate arthrodesis, uses two prongs inserted from the ulnar side into the lunate. A cam effect allows compression of the fusion surfaces with tightening of the screw into the radius. Although we have not had an opportunity to

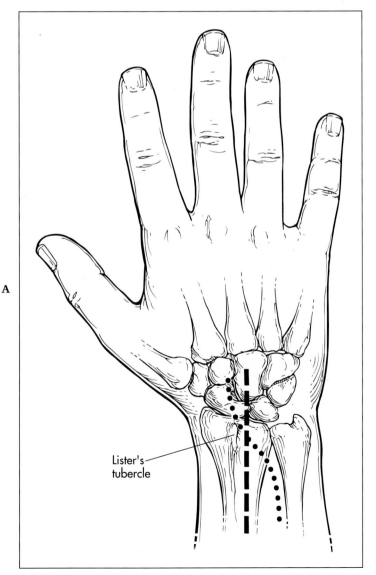

A

Lister's tubercle

FIGURE 38-4

Surgical technique for limited radiolunate fusion. **A,** Surgical incisions: Straight (*dashed line*) incision recommended for most rheumatoid patients. Curvilinear (*dotted line*) incision for cosmetic reasons and better access to the distal radioulnar joint.   *Continued.*

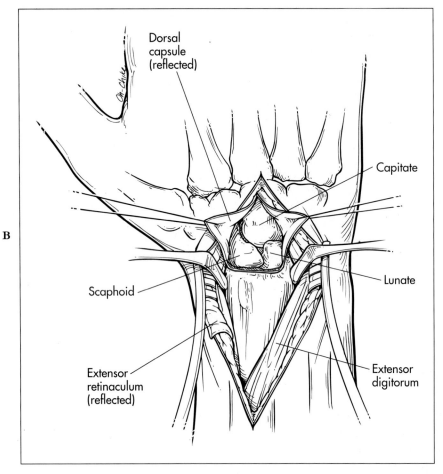

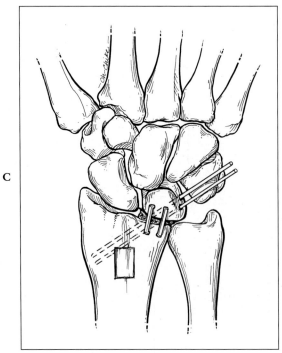

FIGURE 38-4, CONT'D.

B, Extensor retinaculum can be divided between the first and second extensor compartments and reflected ulnarly or it can be divided between the 5-6 extensor compartments and reflected radially; the joint capsule is incised with an inverted T-shaped arthrotomy. **C,** Cancellous bone graft is harvested from the distal radius; interposition graft; and internal fixation with Kirschner wires and staples.

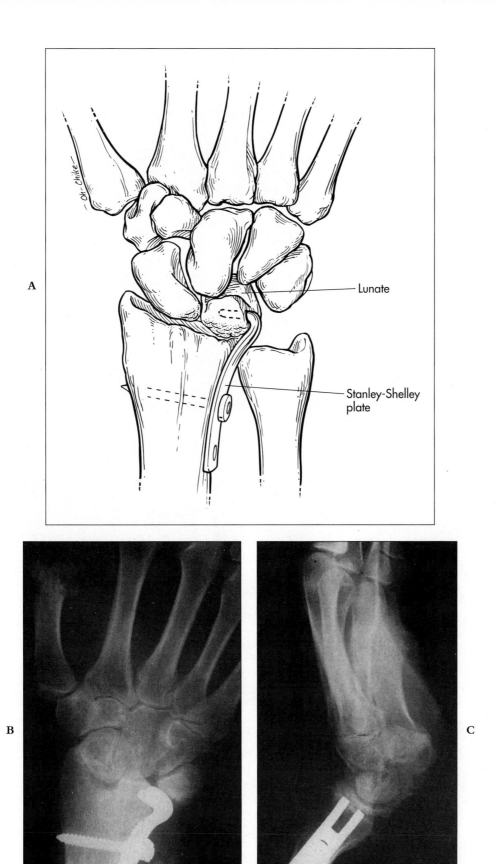

Lunate

Stanley-Shelley plate

A

B

C

FIGURE 38-5

A, Internal fixation with the Stanley-Shelley plate for radiolunate fusion. **B** and **C,** Radiolunate fusion consolidation after bone graft and application of the Stanley-Shelley plate. *(From Stanley JK, Boot DA.[34] By permission of the British Society for Surgery of the Hand.)*

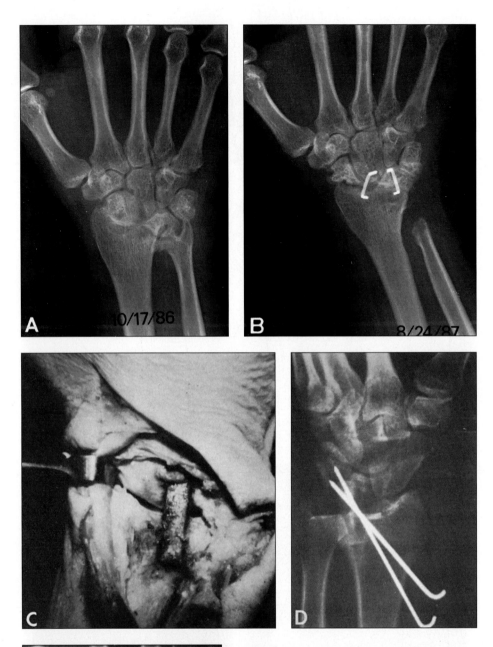

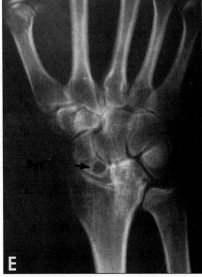

FIGURE 38-6

Radiolunate fusion performed with iliac crest graft inlayed or placed in a slot between distal radius and lunate. **A,** Preoperative radiograph of wrist shows resorption and destruction of the radio-carpal joint and radioulnar joint. **B,** Postoperative radiolunate fusion with inlay graft and two staples; distal ulna resection. **C,** Surgical approach shows key-slot cortical graft (corticocancellous) between distal radius and lunate. **D,** Intraoperative radio-graph shows lunate secured to lunate fossa of distal radius slot bone graft and fixation with two oblique Kirschner wires. *(**C** and **D**, From Linscheid RL, Dobyns JH.[15] Copyright, American Society for Surgery of the Hand, by permission of Churchill Livingstone.)* **E,** Final appearance of radiolunate fusion in rheumatoid arthritis; cystic change in proximal scaphoid *(arrow)*. Five-year follow-up.

use this plate, it would seem that one must be cautious to avoid involvement of the lunotriquetral joint while applying this specialized plate.

Bone graft may be added from the distal radius or from the distal ulna if it has been resected. Linscheid and Dobyns[15] used an iliac crest graft wedged into slots created in the radius and lunate and filled the interstices with additional cancellous bone graft (Fig. 38-6). Such a slotted graft may also be taken from the radius if desired. By slightly distracting the arthrodesis there is less chance of settling during the healing process, thus avoiding compressive forces on the scaphoid and the subsequent development of arthrosis.[15]

In four of the cases from Chamay et al.[6] and four of the cases from Linscheid and Dobyns,[15] a Sauvé-Kapandji or Lauenstein procedure broadened the radiolunate fusion to include the distal radioulnar joint with the radiolunate fusion. As seen in Figures 38-7, *A* through 38-7, *C*, the radiolunate arthrodesis is bolstered by such a fusion. This increases the healing surface of the radiolunate arthrodesis; however, it may add time to the surgical procedure. As noted in Figure 38-7, *C*, there can be a substantial amount of resorption of the ulna, suggesting that perhaps a smaller resection of the remaining ulna is needed compared with a non-rheumatoid patient. In the three cases from Chamay et al.,[6] a Darrach resection of the ulna was performed rather than radioulnar arthrodesis. This is certainly the most common treatment today for the caput ulnae syndrome in conjunction with the radiolunate arthrodesis. With the diminished physical demands placed on this articulation by the rheumatoid patient, the Darrach resection seems to be a quite successful alternative.

POSTOPERATIVE PROTECTION

After the surgical procedure, it is generally recommended that a short arm cast be worn for at least 6 weeks.[6,20,21] This may then be followed by a removable splint for an additional 4 to 6 weeks until the arthrodesis is solid.[20,21] Removal of the Kirschner wires is performed between 6 and 8 weeks after the fusion. The cancellous screws or surgical staples are often secure and nonbothersome and usually do not require removal.

RESULTS OF RADIOLUNATE ARTHRODESES

Critical analysis of the results of radiolunate arthrodeses in the published series demonstrates that a perfect end result can be expected in 75% to 80% of patients. In the series by Chamay et al.,[6] internal fixation was lost in two patients and a nonunion developed in one patient. The series by Linscheid and Dobyns[15] also demonstrated one nonunion. Three fibrous unions and one nonunion occurred in the series by Ishikawa et al.[12] In the series by Stanley and Boot,[34] of 16 patients, for

example, there were three poor results and one fair result. Interestingly, but perhaps not unexpectedly, no improvement occurred in the range of motion compared with the preoperative status. In Linscheid and Dobyns'[15] series of 13 cases, there were one poor result and one fair result (15%). Grip strength was unchanged by operation. Linscheid and Dobyns'[15] series demonstrated only a modest improvement in grip strength in a few instances. This finding should not come as a surprise to the operating surgeon because it is difficult for the rheumatoid patient to gain strength once it has been lost.[15]

A successful radiolunate arthrodesis does not always guarantee proper alignment of the rest of the carpus. Stanley and Boot[34] demonstrated one patient who had bowstringing of the extensor tendons after radiolunate joint fusion and developed a late ulnar deviation stance. This indicates the importance of anatomic repair of the extensor retinaculum, and wrist extensor tendon transfer may be necessary at operation.

Successful radiolunate arthrodesis coupled with a midcarpal synovectomy does not always succeed in halting the development of further articular destruction.[6,15] In the series by Chamay et al.,[6] radiographic follow-up demonstrated further deterioration of the wrist, which was severe in four wrists and slight in eight. Linscheid and Dobyns[15] demonstrated mild progressive deterioration of the midcarpal joint in three patients. Ishikawa et al.[12] demonstrated further midcarpal narrowing in seven wrists. Because midcarpal deterioration was severe in each of these series, it is probably wisest to perform a complete wrist arthrodesis in a patient with rapidly progressive disease. Unfortunately, it is not always possible for the surgeon to know if the disease process is "rapidly progressive"; thus, close follow-up is indicated in any limited arthrodesis patient.

RADIOSCAPHOLUNATE FUSION

With concurrent destruction of the scaphoid and lunate articular surfaces, it is still possible to preserve the midcarpal joint by performing a radioscapholunate arthrodesis (Fig. 38-8). Because restriction of wrist motion was seen in radiolunate arthrodeses, it is generally agreed that wrist motion in a radioscapholunate arthrodesis will be even further reduced (Fig. 38-9). Nalebuff et al.[21] stated that only 25% to 50% of wrist motion can be preserved through such a fusion. Interestingly, Ryu et al.,[27] in their attempt to perform a soft-tissue arthroplasty (pseudofusion) at the radiocarpal joint, ended up with a radioscapholunate arthrodesis in 59.4% of their 32 wrists. In this series, range of motion was 44° of extension and 25.3° of flexion. Seven of these patients had "mild pain that did not limit any wrist loading." In the 10 patients in whom the desired

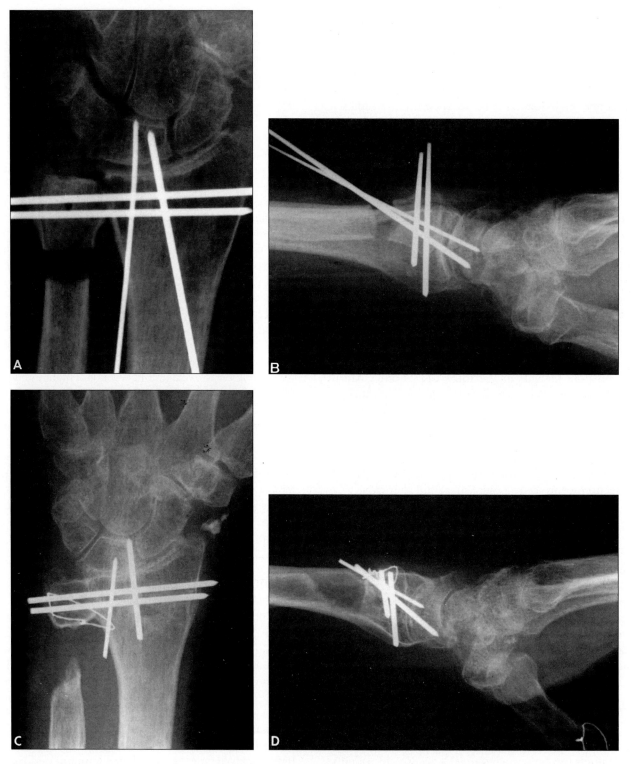

FIGURE 38-7

A, Anteroposterior radiographic view of a combined radiolunate and distal ulna–radius fusion with Kirschner wires. **B,** Lateral view of combined radiolunate and distal radioulnar fusion (Sauvé-Kapandji procedure). **C,** Healed radiolunate fusion and distal radioulnar fusion (Sauvé-Kapandji). Note aligned midcarpal joint. **D,** Lateral view of healed fusions. Note alignment of lunate with lunate fossa of distal radius.

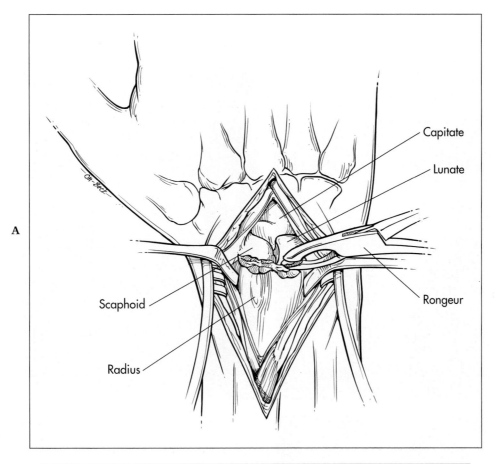

Capitate

Lunate

Rongeur

Scaphoid

Radius

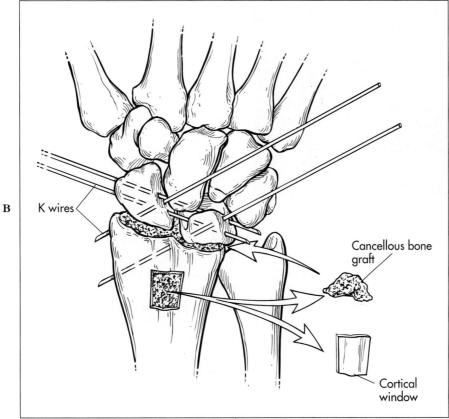

K wires

Cancellous bone
graft

Cortical
window

Figure 38-8

Radioscapholunate fusion. **A,** Operative decortication of articular surface of distal radius, proximal lunate, and scaphoid. **B,** Radioscapholunate fusion with bone graft from the distal radius (cancellous graft) and internal fixation with Kirschner (*K*) wires (iliac crest bone graft is suitable alternative).

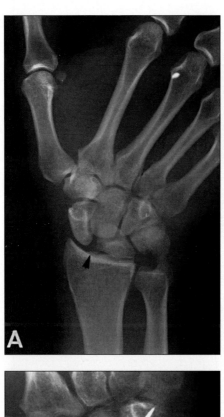

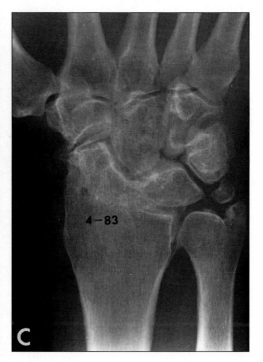

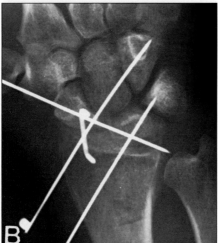

FIGURE 38–9

A, Advanced scapholunate dissociation (*arrowhead*) with painful radiocarpal joint motion in a patient with post-traumatic arthritis. **B,** Radioscapholunate fusion. Internal fixation with Kirschner wires and compression 3M bone staple. **C,** Example of solid radiocarpal fusion with preservation of midcarpal joint.

soft-tissue arthroplasty was achieved, there was extension averaging 68° and flexion averaging 37.5°. Remarkably, no patient in this fibrous arthroplasty group had any pain at follow-up. It is intriguing that 36% of patients with the radioscapholunate arthrodesis had pain yet none of the arthroplasty patients had any pain. The hypothesis to explain this finding has been that the fibrous nonunion tends to "give," thus protecting the midcarpal joints.[27]

RADIOSCAPHOLUNATE ARTHRODESIS WITH MIDCARPAL ARTHROPLASTY

Taleisnik[35] was among the first to champion the use of limited wrist arthrodesis in rheumatoid arthritis despite the presence of destructive changes of the midcarpal joint. Realizing that a radiolunate or radioscapholunate fusion coupled with midcarpal destruction was likely to fail, Taleisnik advocated the use of silicone replacement arthroplasty of the lunocapitate joint and radioscapholunate arthrodesis.

The surgical technique included a radioscapholunate arthrodesis performed through a straight dorsal incision obliquely placed between the base of the third metacarpal and the distal ulna. At the midcarpal joint, the proximal pole of the capitate and a portion of the hamate were removed with an osteotome or bone saw. A size 11 to 13 condylar implant was then implanted in the capitate (Fig. 38-10). The scapholunate joint was decorticated, grafted, and pinned. The scapholunate unit was then

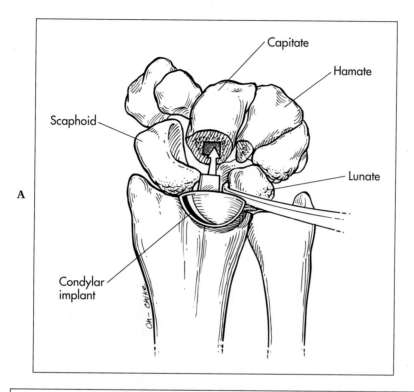

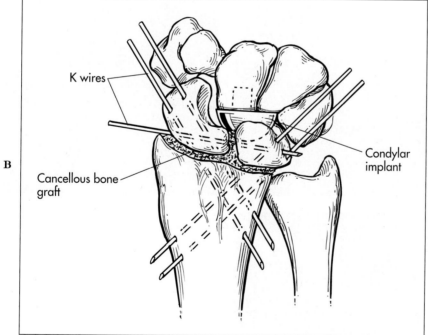

FIGURE 38-10

Radioscapholunate fusion combined with proximal capitate silicone condylar replacement (after Taleisnik). **A,** Condylar implant inserted into proximal capitate. **B,** Radiocarpal fusion with cancellous bone graft, Kirschner-wire fixation, and midcarpal joint replacement with a condylar implant.

pinned to the radius with 0.045- or 0.054-in. Kirschner wires (Fig. 38-10, *B*).

The follow-up of this technique averaged a relatively short time (18.9 months). All patients experienced relief of pain. Preoperative and postoperative range of motion are noted in Table 38-2. One complication, a radioscapholunate pseudoarthrodesis, occurred; however, this patient had no pain.

Despite these encouraging results, Taleisnik[35] cautioned that "the procedure may not be durable enough for the younger and more vigorous patients, as well as for those in need of walking aids." As recognized by Taleisnik, such a procedure risks the potential development of silicone synovitis. A soft-tissue interposition has been suggested as a possible alternative to avoid this potential complication. As with other limited arthrodeses, the ultimate long-term results of this procedure must be evaluated over an extended time (Fig. 38-11).

SAUVÉ-KAPANDJI FUSION

While considering limited wrist arthrodeses, it is appropriate to mention the concept of distal radioulnar arthrodesis with the creation of a pseudarthrosis in the distal ulna (the so-called Sauvé-Kapandji or Lauenstein fusion) (see Chapter 34). This procedure was originally described in 1936[28] and is frequently performed in association with a radiolunate arthrodesis (Fig. 38-7). According to Taleisnik, the Sauvé-Kapandji arthrodesis is indicated when ulnar translocation "is impending, but not severe enough to justify stabilization by radiolunate fusion."[36] In practice, it is difficult for the hand surgeon to make this determination, and the choice between a radiolunate arthrodesis and a Sauvé-Kapandji arthrodesis may be difficult to make. The Sauvé-Kapandji arthrodesis appears to be necessary for cases in which a proximal row carpectomy or soft-tissue arthroplasty is

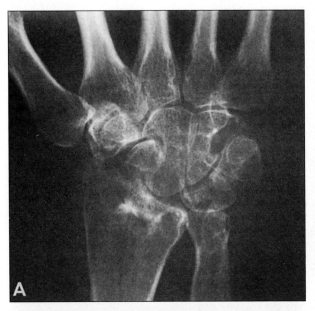

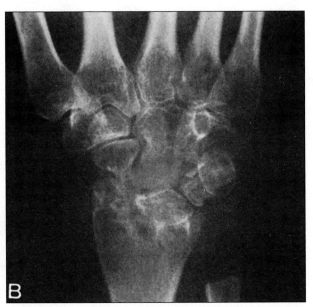

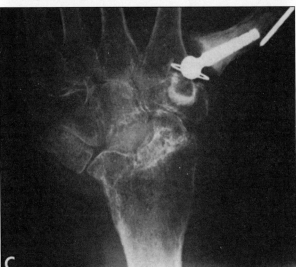

FIGURE 38-11

A, Preoperative radiograph of advancing radiocarpal arthritis. Note preservation of midcarpal joint. **B,** Excellent postoperative result of radioscapholunate fusion and preserved midcarpal joint. **C,** Successful radioscapholunate fusion and midcarpal arthroplasty. Thumb trapeziometacarpal joint stabilization with ball-socket joint implant. *(From Taleisnik J: Treatment of rheumatoid arthritis of the wrist,* J Hand Surg [Am] *12:1-8, 1987. Copyright, American Society for Surgery of the Hand, by permission of Churchill Livingstone.)*

being considered and further ulnar-sided support is needed.

To treat dorsal subluxation of the ulna with a Darrach resection in cases with early ulnar translation of the wrist risks loss of ulnar-sided support and potentially hastens ulnar translation of the carpus. We prefer the Sauvé-Kapandji procedure with this presentation of ulnar carpal translation. With a stable carpus, Darrach resection or other semiarthroplasties of the distal radioulnar joint are sufficient. Armed with this knowledge, the surgeon can decide how to best stabilize the carpus based on the findings of the individual case. Instability of the ulnar stump may be seen after the Sauvé-Kapandji procedure at the pseudarthrosis site and this may require stabilization by the pronator quadratus (see Chapter 34).[36] As with other limited arthrodeses, constant follow-up is necessary to determine if further progression of wrist deformity occurs. One should view the rheumatoid wrist as a continuum rather than as an end result, even with a successful limited arthrodesis. Only through long-term follow-up will we be able to determine the ultimate fate of limited arthrodesis in the rheumatoid patient.

COMPLETE WRIST ARTHRODESIS

INDICATIONS

For patients with a rather severe wrist deformity (Figs. 38-12, *A* and *B*) and pain, a complete wrist arthrodesis may be the only viable surgical option. In those wrists with severe deformity, poor bone stock, or poor soft-tissue support, arthrodesis is the treatment of choice. History of a wrist infection or the need for permanent crutch use precludes wrist arthroplasty and also supports a total wrist arthrodesis. Failed wrist arthroplasties are also candidates for such a fusion.[14]

SURGICAL APPROACH FOR COMPLETE FUSION

Several operative skin incisions have been recommended for complete wrist arthrodesis. Most surgeons prefer a straight dorsal incision for rheumatoid patients as the least risk for increasing tension at the suture site in the postsurgical period (see Chapter 7).[21] The ulnar, Smith-Petersen approach, resecting the distal ulna and using it as a graft, is rarely used today. Skin slough has been noted with the dorsal lazy S incision, and it is not recommended.[19] A gentle semicircular incision has been preferred by Millender and Nalebuff.[19]

Once the skin is incised and taken down to the extensor retinaculum, the same approach is used as in the limited wrist arthrodesis (Figs. 38-4, *B* and *C*). A distal-based capsule flap is created.[21] A synovectomy is performed, and the radial and ulnar capsule and triangular fibrocartilage are preserved if they are still functionally

intact. Release of the ligaments, if necessary, is performed to allow proper positioning of the carpus relative to the radius. The distal radioulnar joint may be approached at the same time to permit a concurrent Sauvé-Kapandji arthrodesis or Darrach resection, as indicated. Decortication of the articular surfaces is performed, and an effort is made to preserve the palmar radial shelf to avoid median nerve compression and to preserve length.

INTERNAL FIXATION

Several options are available to the surgeon once the surgical exposure has been made. To provide stability until the arthrodesis has healed, the fixation options include the use of a large, rigid Steinmann pin,[21] a flexible Rush rod,[7,13,17,19] and two flexible Rush rods.[21] The AO plate fixation has been described in the performance of rheumatoid wrist arthrodesis[4] and is gaining popularity compared with other techniques. The two remaining options to be decided are the use of bone graft (inlay or onlay) and the decision to place the metal fixation inside or outside the metacarpal canal.

Nalebuff, Millender, and colleagues[19-21] popularized the intermetacarpal technique using a large Steinmann pin (Fig. 38-12). In this technique the largest Steinmann pin that will fit into the radial medullary canal is drilled between the index-long or long-ring metacarpal space. It is countersunk proximal to the metacarpal heads by 2 to 3 cm.[20,21] The addition of a staple or additional Kirschner wire is often necessary to improve the stability of the fixation. If severe bone loss exists, e.g., arthritis mutilans, Nalebuff et al.[20,21] strongly recommend use of the intramedullary canal technique. It is contraindicated in the case of an excessively small intramedullary canal.

With the intramedullary technique, the possibility of concurrent or subsequent metacarpophalangeal arthroplasty should be considered. If performed at the same time, one should place the 3/32-in. pin down the

---

Table 38-2. Range of Motion After Radioscapholunate Arthrodesis

Type	Range of Motion (°)	
	Preop	Postop
Wrist extension	42.78	42.23
Wrist flexion	37.50	23.07
Ulnar deviation	21.50	20.76
Radial deviation	6.42	12.87

Postop, postoperative; *preop*, preoperative.
Data from Taleisnik J.[35]

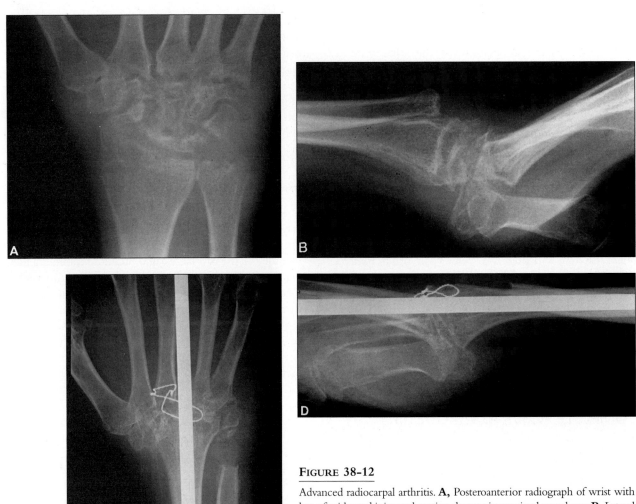

FIGURE 38-12

Advanced radiocarpal arthritis. **A,** Posteroanterior radiograph of wrist with loss of midcarpal joint and erosive changes in proximal carpal row. **B,** Lateral radiograph shows dorsal displacement of distal ulna and significant collapse of the radiocarpal joint. **C,** Wrist fusion with intramedullary rod, dorsal bone graft, and tension band wire. **D,** Lateral radiograph of wrist fusion with intramedullary rod; neutral position of wrist flexion-extension.

medullary canal from the resected neck level. If not, a dorsal hole is drilled into the metacarpal and the pin is placed into the medullary canal.

The use of cancellous iliac crest graft or a cortico-cancellous onlay graft in wrist fusion is recommended by most authors, with Kirschner wire or Steinmann pin internal fixation (Fig. 38-13). Bone grafting appears to improve the overall healing rate for arthrodeses of the rheumatoid wrist. The disadvantages of the iliac crest grafts are that a general anesthetic is required which may increase the risks, especially with potential cervical spine instability. Only 1 of 15 arthrodeses performed without bone graft by Koka and D'Arcy[13] developed a nonunion. This becomes more remarkable given the fact that no postoperative immobilization was used. A 4-mm Rush nail was placed in the medullary canal of the long finger metacarpal. Other surgeons have not been as fortunate. This technique, as originally recommended by Mannerfelt and Malmsten,[17] has been criticized for not providing sufficiently rigid fixation.[20,21] In fact, some surgeons prefer an onlay slotted graft technique (Fig. 38-14) or a reversed distal radius onlay graft (Fig. 38-15) to improve fixation, graft apposition, and union rates. For the slotted graft, the graft is placed between a slot in the radius and a slot in the second and third metacarpal bases. For the onlay graft, cancellous bone from the radius is placed across the radius and carpus to the base of the metacarpals and held with a tension band wire. In both series, the authors[8,39] reported high union rates without the risk or problems of retained internal fixation.

POSITION OF FUSION

Palmer and co-workers[25] have shown that most activities of daily living are performed between 5° of

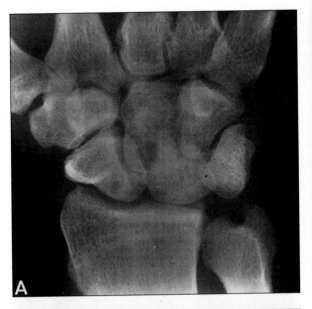

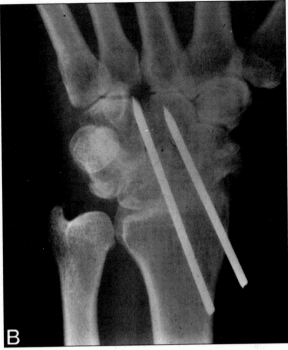

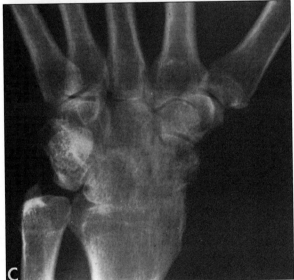

FIGURE 38-13

A, Rheumatoid arthritis with loss of cartilage midcarpal joint and palmar rotation of scaphoid and lunate. **B,** Cancellous bone graft to radiocarpal and midcarpal joints; internal fixation with two Steinmann pins (Ruby technique). **C,** Complete radiocarpal fusion. Healed, with preservation of carpometacarpal joint and distal radioulnar joint.

flexion and 30° of extension and between 10° of radial deviation and 15° of ulnar deviation. Therefore, it is not surprising that the rheumatoid wrist functions quite well in neutral flexion-extension and slight ulnar deviation. This position has been advocated by Nalebuff[22] as the ideal position for wrist arthrodesis. Studies from Beaton et al.[2] and O'Driscoll et al.[23] demonstrated that maximum grip strength is present on wrist extension (30°) and ulnar deviation (8°). This position maximizes the tendon-muscle length-tension relationship for grip strength. This may not be as important a consideration in rheumatoid patients who are generally weaker. In addition, fusion techniques may not allow positioning the wrist in extension unless precontoured plates are

selected (Fig. 38-16). Arthrodesis of the wrist in slight ulnar deviation is associated with less ulnar deviation of the metacarpophalangeal joints. This allows the extensor carpi ulnaris to be used as a tendon transfer if needed.[14] Radial deviation of the rheumatoid wrist should be avoided because it may tend to augment ulnar drift of the fingers.[30]

TWO-PIN FIXATION

Nalebuff and colleagues[21] advocated the use of 5/64- or 7/64-in. diameter pins in an intermetacarpal fixation technique. This "stacked pin effect" gives increased rotational stability. Another advantage of this technique

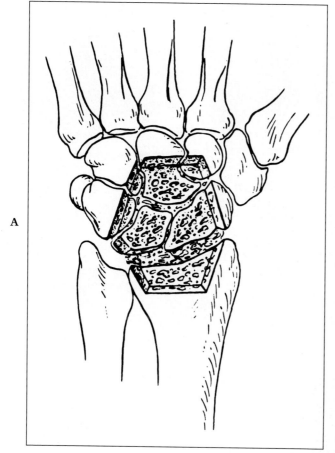

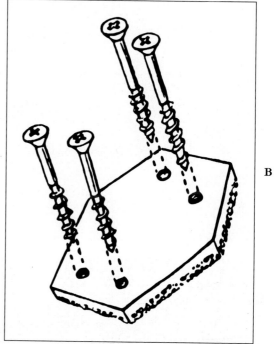

FIGURE 38-14

Dorsal "bone" plate technique (after Rayan). **A,** The articular cartilage of the radiocarpal and intercarpal joints is removed. A cancellous bone graft bed is made by removing the dorsal cortex of the radius and carpal bones. **B,** Inner table of iliac crest corticocancellous graft shaped to the decorticated bed, drilled, and tapped for interfragmenting screw fixation. *(From Rayan GM: Wrist arthrodesis,* J Hand Surg [Am] *11:356-364, 1986. Copyright, American Society for Surgery of the Hand, by permission of Churchill Livingstone.)*

is that these pins may be bent to allow for more wrist extension (or flexion) if desired. Additionally, the smaller caliber pins minimize compression of the musculi interossei, which may be a problem in techniques using large caliber pins. However, care must be taken to place these in the dorsal interosseous space to avoid the neurovascular bundles.

SURGICAL CLOSURE

In the surgical closure, it is recommended that the surgeon place the dorsal retinaculum under the extensor tendons to protect against abrasion from bone edges.[7] Because the wrist is no longer capable of motion, the extensor tendons no longer need the entire extensor retinaculum to avoid bowstringing during extension. We recommend using the distal two-thirds of the extensor retinaculum as interposition beneath the extensor tendons since it can be used to greater advantage by preventing tendon rupture. Often a drain

is inserted after extensor retinaculum transfer. The proximal one-third of the extensor retinaculum can be maintained to minimize bowstringing if the wrist is fixed in extension. A loose closure of subcutaneous tissue and skin should be performed. Interrupted sutures are preferred and should be left in longer than 2 weeks if any doubt arises about the tissue integrity.

POSTOPERATIVE IMMOBILIZATION

Immobilization in the postsurgical period is usually provided for the comfort of the patient and to promote healing of the arthrodesis. The recommendations for postoperative protection run the gamut from no immobilization[13] to cast immobilization for up to 4 months.[16] In some instances, it may be necessary to apply a sugar-tong splint for 2 to 3 weeks in supination to protect the distal radioulnar joint.[7] In general, several weeks of cast immobilization[20,21] may be followed by a removable plastic orthosis for a total of 8 to 12 weeks of

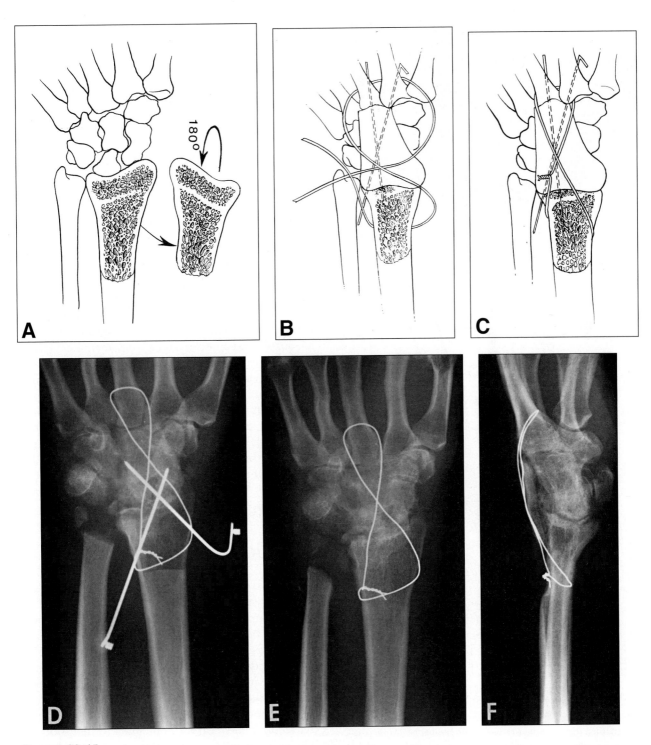

FIGURE 38-15

Wrist arthrodesis with dorsal radial bone graft (modified Gill technique). **A,** Preparation and excision of dorsal radial bone graft after wrist joint exposed through a straight dorsal incision; dorsal cortical surface of radius undergoes an osteotomy 5 cm proximal to radiocarpal joint. **B,** Articular surfaces removed from scaphoid, lunate, capitate, and distal radius as well as base of third metacarpal. Distal radius graft rotated 180°; narrow end (proximal) placed over third metacarpal base. Internal fixation with Kirschner (K) wires and 20-gauge figure-of-eight tension band wire. **C,** Completed fusion shows tightened tension band wire; K wire between metacarpals and distal radius. **D,** Clinical case demonstrates early result of wrist arthrodesis; K wires placed retrogradely across distal radius and carpal bones. **E** and **F,** Completed fusion of radiocarpal joint. (Anteroposterior and lateral radiographs.)

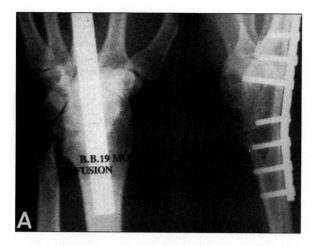

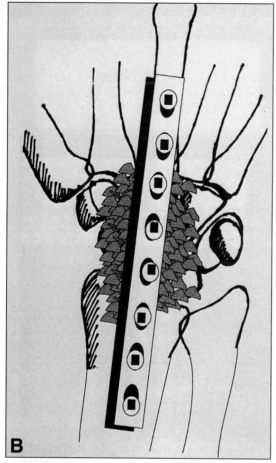

FIGURE 38-16

A, Arthrodesis technique. AO compression plate. **B,** Cancellous bone grafting. *(From Bolano LE, Green DP: Wrist arthrodesis in post-traumatic arthritis: a comparison of two methods,* J Hand Surg [Am] *18:786-791, 1993. Copyright, American Society for Surgery of the Hand, by permission of Churchill Livingstone.)*

immobilization until the arthrodesis has healed. It is important to find a balance between protection of the arthrodesis site and the need to minimally inhibit the patient's activities of daily living. As in limited arthrodeses, each surgical case must be individualized based on the needs of the patient and the confidence of the surgeon in the operative technique used.

PIN REMOVAL

The Steinmann pin can be removed as early as 4 months after the procedure if discomfort so dictates.[20,21] In the single-pin technique, rarely does the pin need to be removed. Once in a while, a pin migrates distally, and it needs to be removed. Hardware removal is considered easier with the use of small caliber pins. Screws, plates, or staples rarely need removal in rheumatoid patients. The bone onlay technique (Figs. 38-14 and 38-17) does not require screw removal and is not associated with problems of extensor tendon rupture.

BILATERAL WRIST FUSION

It is well known that rheumatoid patients can function with an arthrodesis of both wrists. However, many patients with wrist deformity, good bone stock, adequate wrist muscles, and a spontaneous or surgical wrist fusion of one wrist prefer a mobile second wrist. Such individuals are candidates for either a Swanson flexible implant arthroplasty or total joint implant arthroplasty (see Chapter 39).[20,38] In the situation in which an arthroplasty is contraindicated in a patient whose other wrist has been arthrodesed in neutral position, the second wrist should be positioned in slight flexion (5°-15°). It is generally accepted that the position of 15° of palmar flexion aids the patient with personal hygiene.[10,14]

COMPLICATIONS

There seems to be general agreement that a successful wrist arthrodesis is easy to achieve in a patient with rheumatoid arthritis. Although 100% union rates have been described,[21] nonunions do occur.[5,8,13] This is especially true in the "loose or wet type" of rheumatoid arthritis with unstable joints and extensive synovitis. Nonunions are also more frequently found in the patient with arthritis mutilans in which there is poor bone stock. Nonunion has prompted the recommendation for bone graft at the fusion site. The intramedullary pin fixation technique has also led to fracture of the third metacarpal.[13] Fortunately, the presence of a nonunion does not preclude a good clinical result in all cases. A radiocarpal pseudarthrosis has also been intentionally created in the hopes of providing some motion yet maintaining wrist stability.[27] Unfortunately, a 59% rate of unintentional radiocarpal arthrodesis in this report suggests that the procedure is somewhat unreliable in obtaining the intended results.

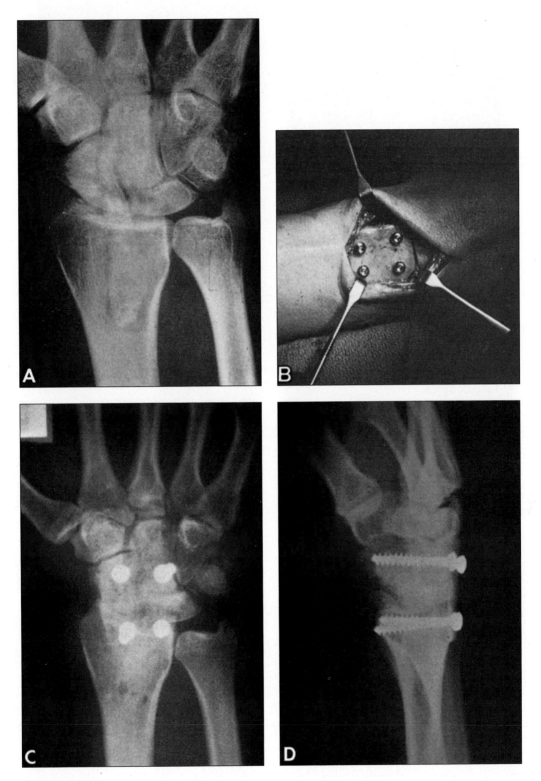

FIGURE 38-17

A, Post-traumatic arthritis of the wrist in a 29-year-old manual worker. **B,** Interoperative photograph after fixation of the graft in its bed. **C** and **D,** Posteroanterior and lateral radiographs 12 weeks postoperatively; solid fusion is evident. *(From Rayan GM: Wrist arthrodesis,* J Hand Surg [Am] *11:356-364, 1986. Copyright, American Society for Surgery of the Hand, by permission of Churchill Livingstone.)*

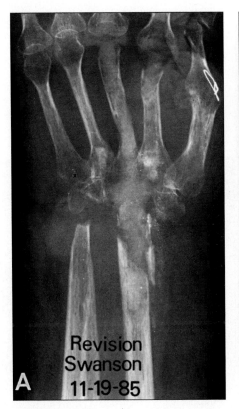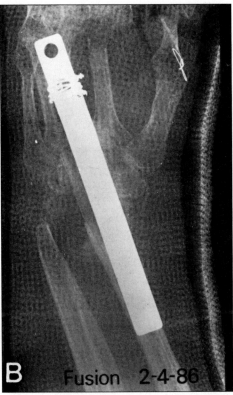

FIGURE 38-18

Dorsal compression plate (after failed total wrist arthroplasty). **A,** Failed Swanson wrist arthroplasty with revision of previous Swanson implant in a patient with rheumatoid resorptive arthropathy. **B,** Successful fusion with a standard AO neutralization plate.

ARTHRODESIS AFTER A FAILED ARTHROPLASTY

Arthrodesis after a failed wrist arthroplasty is a special circumstance needing individualized surgical techniques. Wrist fusion after a failed arthroplasty requires an extensible surgical débridement of reactive synovium exposure and the addition of substantial bone graft due to the loss of bone stock. In the case of a cemented arthroplasty, bone graft is needed within the distal radius and carpus after complete removal of bone cement from both the metacarpals and the distal radius. In some cases, removal of bone cement requires that a channel is cut in the dorsal cortex of the distal radius and that bone grafting is performed using a cortical bone strut across the distal radius and the carpus and coapting the distal carpal row to the metacarpal bases. Special techniques including combined internal fixation and external fixation have been recommended.[16] In the rheumatoid patient with a bone defect created by the silicone spacer, bone graft is also needed if a successful arthrodesis is to be obtained. Despite the need for additional bone graft, total wrist arthrodesis is a reasonable approach after a failed arthroplasty (Fig. 38-18). This potential salvage procedure should be discussed with the patient before the performance of a total wrist arthroplasty.

SUMMARY

The main challenge of treating a rheumatoid wrist deformity is determining which procedure is best for the patient given the patient's functional needs and present physiologic state. Many variables need to be evaluated in making the decisions involved in limited and total wrist arthrodeses. Occasionally, these decisions are made for the surgeon, e.g., ruptured wrist extensor tendons. However, new problems arise that deserve renewed attention, e.g., the development of midcarpal arthritis despite a previously successful radiolunate arthrodesis. Only the continued evaluation of the rheumatoid patient in the postoperative period will optimize treatment of this usually progressive disease. This continued evaluation will also help to delineate the long-term results of some of the newer procedures and guide surgeons regarding the indications for and the expected results from these therapeutic modalities in the future.

REFERENCES

1. Backdahl M: The caput ulnae syndrome in rheumatoid arthritis. A study of the morphology, abnormal anatomy and clinical picture, *Acta Rheum Scand Suppl* 5:1-75, 1963.

2. Beaton DE, O'Driscoll SW, Richards RR: Grip strength testing using the BTE work simulator and the Jamar dynamometer: a comparative study. Baltimore Therapeutic Equipment, *J Hand Surg [Am]* 20:293-298, 1995.

3. Black RM, Boswick JA Jr, Wiedel J: Dislocation of the wrist in rheumatoid arthritis. The relationship to distal ulna resection, *Clin Orthop* 124:184-188, 1977.

4. Bracy DJ, McMurtry RY, Walton D: Arthrodesis in the rheumatoid hand using the AO technique, *Orthop Rev* 9:65, 1980.

5. Brumfield RH Jr, Conaty JP, Mays JD: Surgery of the wrist in rheumatoid arthritis, *Clin Orthop* 142:159-163, 1979.

6. Chamay A, Della Santa D, Vilaseca A: Radiolunate arthrodesis. Factor of stability for the rheumatoid wrist (French), *Ann Chir Main* 2:5-17, 1983.

7. Clayton ML: Surgical treatment at the wrist in rheumatoid arthritis: a review of thirty-seven patients, *J Bone Joint Surg Am* 47:741-750, 1965.

8. Clendenin MB, Green DP: Arthrodesis of the wrist—complications and their management, *J Hand Surg [Am]* 6:253-257, 1981.

9. Dellon AL, Seif SS: Anatomic dissections relating the posterior interosseous nerve to the carpus, and the etiology of dorsal wrist ganglion pain, *J Hand Surg [Am]* 3:326-332, 1978.

10. Ferlic DC: Implant arthroplasty of the rheumatoid wrist, *Hand Clin* 3:169-179, 1987.

11. Henderson ED, Lipscomb PR: Surgical treatment of rheumatoid hand, *JAMA* 175:431-436, 1961.

12. Ishikawa H, Hanyu T, Saito H, et al.: Limited arthrodesis for the rheumatoid wrist, *J Hand Surg [Am]* 17:1103-1109, 1992.

13. Koka R, D'Arcy JC: Stabilisation of the wrist in rheumatoid disease, *J Hand Surg [Br]* 14:288-290, 1989.

14. Linscheid RL, Dobyns JH: Rheumatoid arthritis of the wrist, *Orthop Clin North Am* 2:649-665, 1971.

15. Linscheid RL, Dobyns JH: Radiolunate arthrodesis, *J Hand Surg [Am]* 10:821-829, 1985.

16. Louis DS, Hankin FM: Arthrodesis of the wrist: past and present, *J Hand Surg [Am]* 11:787-789, 1986.

17. Mannerfelt L, Malmsten M: Arthrodesis of the wrist in rheumatoid arthritis. A technique without external fixation, *Scand J Plast Reconstr Surg* 5:124-130, 1971.

18. McMurtry RY, Youm Y, Flatt AE, et al.: Kinematics of the wrist. II. Clinical applications, *J Bone Joint Surg Am* 60:955-961, 1978.

19. Millender LH, Nalebuff EA: Arthrodesis of the rheumatoid wrist. An evaluation of sixty patients and a description of a different surgical technique, *J Bone Joint Surg Am* 55:1026-1034, 1973.

20. Nalebuff EA, Fatti JF, Weil CE: *Arthrodesis of the rheumatoid wrist: indications and surgical technique.* In Lichtman DM, editor: *The wrist and its disorders,* Philadelphia, 1988, WB Saunders, pp 365-372.

21. Nalebuff EA, Feldon PG, Millender LH: *Rheumatoid arthritis in the hand and wrist.* In Green DP, editor: *Operative hand surgery,* ed 2, vol 3, New York, 1988, Churchill Livingstone, pp 1655-1766.

22. Nalebuff EA, Garrod KJ: Present approach to the severely involved rheumatoid wrist, *Orthop Clin North Am* 15:369-380, 1984.

23. O'Driscoll SW, Horii E, Ness R, et al.: The relationship between wrist position, grasp size, and grip strength, *J Hand Surg [Am]* 17:169-177, 1992.

24. Pahle JA, Raunio P: The influence of wrist position on finger deviation in the rheumatoid hand. A clinical and radiological study, *J Bone Joint Surg Br* 51:664-676, 1969.

25. Palmer AK, Werner FW, Murphy D, et al.: Functional wrist motion: a biomechanical study, *J Hand Surg [Am]* 10:39-46, 1985.

26. Ranawat CS, Harrison MO, Jordan LR: Arthrography of the wrist joint, *Clin Orthop* 83:6-12, 1972.

27. Ryu J, Watson HK, Burgess RC: Rheumatoid wrist reconstruction utilizing a fibrous nonunion and radiocarpal arthrodesis, *J Hand Surg [Am]* 10:830-836, 1985.

28. Sauvé and Kapandji: Nouvelle technique de traitement chirurgical des luxations récidivantes isolées de l'extrémité inférieure du cubitus, *J Chir* 47:589-594, 1936.

29. Shapiro JS: A new factor in the etiology of ulnar drift, *Clin Orthop* 68:32-43, 1970.

30. Shapiro JS, Heijna W, Nasatir S, et al.: The relationship of wrist motion to ulnar phalangeal drift in the rheumatoid patient, *Hand* 3:68-75, 1971.

31. Smith-Petersen MN, Aufranc OE, Larson CB: Useful surgical procedures for rheumatoid arthritis involving joints of upper extremity, *Arch Surg* 46:764-770, 1943.

32. Spinner M, Kaplan EB: Extensor carpi ulnaris. Its relationship to the stability of the distal radio-ulnar joint, *Clin Orthop* 68:124-129, 1970.

33. Stack HG, Vaughan-Jackson OJ: The zig-zag deformity in the rheumatoid hand, *Hand* 3:62-67, 1971.

34. Stanley JK, Boot DA: Radio-lunate arthrodesis, *J Hand Surg [Br]* 14:283-287, 1989.

35. Taleisnik J: Combined radiocarpal arthrodesis and midcarpal (lunocapitate) arthroplasty for treatment of rheumatoid arthritis of the wrist, *J Hand Surg [Am]* 12:1-8, 1987.

36. Taleisnik J: Rheumatoid arthritis of the wrist, *Hand Clin* 5:257-278, 1989.

37. Vaughan-Jackson OJ: Rupture of extensor tendons by attrition at the inferior radio-ulnar joint, *J Bone Joint Surg Br* 30:528-530, 1948.

38. Vicar AJ, Burton RI: Surgical management of the rheumatoid wrist—fusion or arthroplasty, *J Hand Surg [Am]* 11:790-797, 1986.

39. Wood MB: Wrist arthrodesis using dorsal radial bone graft, *J Hand Surg [Am]* 12:208-212, 1987.

TOTAL WRIST ARTHROPLASTY

Robert D. Beckenbaugh, M.D.

History
  Indications and Contraindications
  Design Development of Total Wrist
    Arthroplasty
  Surgical Technique
  Postoperative Care
    Loose Fit
    Normal Fit
    Tight Fit
Revision Surgery and Salvage After Total
  Wrist Arthroplasty

Alternative Total Wrist Arthroplasty
  Devices
    Meuli Total Wrist Arthroplasty
    Trispherical Total Wrist Arthroplasty
    Clayton, Ferlic, Volz Total Wrist
      Arthroplasty
    GUEPAR Total Wrist Arthroplasty
    Menon Total Wrist Arthroplasty
Summary

HISTORY

The concept of performing fixed total joint arthroplasties of the wrist emerged quickly after the early dramatic success seen with total hip arthroplasty. Several designs of prostheses developed in the early 1970s used the same principles of plastic and metal articulation with cement fixation (Fig. 39-1).[26,28,38] Initial results demonstrating that pain relief and mobility were obtainable have encouraged continued development in the field of fixed-fulcrum total joint arthroplasty of the wrist. Unlike the experience with the hip, however, the longevity of the initial good results was reduced, and the number of complications and need for reoperations were higher.[3,9,12] Because of the early failures, continued development and utilization of total wrist arthroplasties have been slower than in some joints.

Other factors have restricted the use of total wrist arthroplasties, including relative success with: 1) limited soft-tissue procedures (synovectomy and stabilization), 2) arthrodesis, and 3) silicone interposition arthroplasty.*

---

* References 7,9,10,14,20,21,23,30,36,38-40.

All of these procedures are more conservative than total wrist replacement with a metal and plastic device because they require less bone resection, are more easily salvaged after failure, and have no inherent risk of loosening or adverse effect from a large foreign body (allergy, infection). The surgeon and patient must compare the increased benefits of total wrist arthroplasty and its complications with the benefits and complications of the other more conservative procedures.

The advantages of wrist arthrodesis are obvious. The procedure is durable, provides pain relief, and, in many instances, is functional.[29,41,42,45]

The disadvantages of wrist arthrodesis are also obvious but often not emphasized. For example, it has been stated that arthrodesis provides for more power as a result of stabilization and relief of pain, and this is correct. However, eliminating wrist motion *decreases* power grip, removing the mechanical advantage and excursion available to the finger flexors with wrist dorsiflexion. Stabilizing the wrist in a neutral fashion may help prevent ulnar deviation of the fingers secondary to radial deviation of the wrist. However, eliminating the shock absorption of ulnar wrist motion

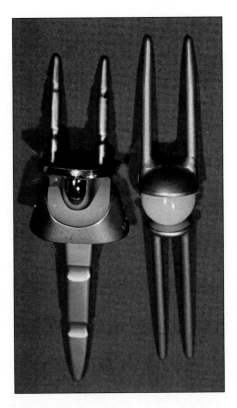

FIGURE 39-1

Volz (*left*) and Meuli (*right*) initial wrist prostheses. Note both original prostheses were designed for insertion into the index and long metacarpals, and their proximal stems were structured over the prosthetic central axis. *(From Beckenbaugh RD:* Arthroplasty of the wrist. *In Morrey BF, editor:* Joint replacement arthroplasty, *vol 1, New York, 1991, Churchill Livingstone, pp 195-215. By permission of Mayo Foundation.)*

increases the external ulnar deviation forces applied to the digits.

Absence of wrist motion in patients with rheumatoid arthritis can be functionally disabling.[31] In those patients with severe shoulder and elbow disease, eliminating wrist motion can make functional tasks of eating, hair care, and personal hygiene more difficult. Total wrist arthroplasty has many practical and theoretical advantages compared with wrist arthrodesis. In selecting a procedure for an individual patient, the potential benefits, complications, and need for reoperations must be compared with the relative ease and permanency of arthrodesis, and the patient must assist the surgeon in making the proper choice.

In 1973 Swanson[39] reported on the development of a silicone rubber interpositional arthroplasty similar to the design of his finger implant. Conceptually, it is a true total wrist replacement in that both the radial carpal and midcarpal joint functions are replaced. The use of a pliable spacer, however, is different mechanically and functionally from a solid metal and plastic prosthetic wrist arthroplasty. With silicone devices, the

forces across the prosthesis are dampened, greatly diminishing the chances of loosening—a common problem in most total wrist arthroplasties. There are potentials for prosthetic fracture, however, as well as subsidence of the prosthesis within bone.[8,11,34,37] In addition, with total wrist arthroplasty, restoration of wrist length is possible, whereas some shortening occurs with silicone arthroplasty and this may be associated with potential adverse effects on the contractile potential of the extrinsic finger musculotendinous units.

Silicone wrist arthroplasty is easily salvaged (by replacement or fusion), is associated with a small amount of foreign body, and has not been associated with significant silicone synovitis seen with individual carpal implants.[16,32,35] It is therefore a relatively conservative way to remove the diseased joint and provide for wrist motion. The durability and longevity of the procedure, however, are limited and probably equivalent to fixed-fulcrum solid prostheses, which are clinically superior in function. The use of silicone implants is generally restricted at this time. The use of metal grommets and stronger silicone has not resolved the problems of implant fracture and subsidence.

INDICATIONS AND CONTRAINDICATIONS

The basic indication for total wrist arthroplasty is pain, deformity, and limited motion in rheumatoid arthritis patients in whom multiple upper extremity joints are involved and there is a distinct need for motion. Degenerative and post-traumatic arthritis of the wrist are frequently unilateral and most often associated with normal shoulder, elbow, and hand function. In these patients, the more conservative approaches such as arthrodesis (limited or total) are generally indicated. If there are special needs or desires for motion in these candidates, total wrist arthroplasty may be indicated. Patients in this category must be strongly advised of the limited use that is allowed postoperatively. For example, the patient may feel good enough and function well enough after total wrist arthroplasty with isolated wrist disease that the patient would wish to participate in sports such as golf or tennis and perform heavy labor such as carpentry. The devices and fixation available will not, however, allow these heavy impact activities without anticipated failure by loosening. A musician, however, with special needs for motion, anticipated light activities, and isolated wrist disease may be an excellent candidate for the procedure.

The paradox of treatment in these conditions is that in the traumatic and degenerative conditions the bone stock and quality are better than in rheumatoid arthritis and the potential results and longevity are superior. The quality of bone in rheumatoid arthritis varies. In general, the disease results in decreased bone density and strength. The addition of steroid therapy or some of the newer immunologic-oriented drugs may significantly

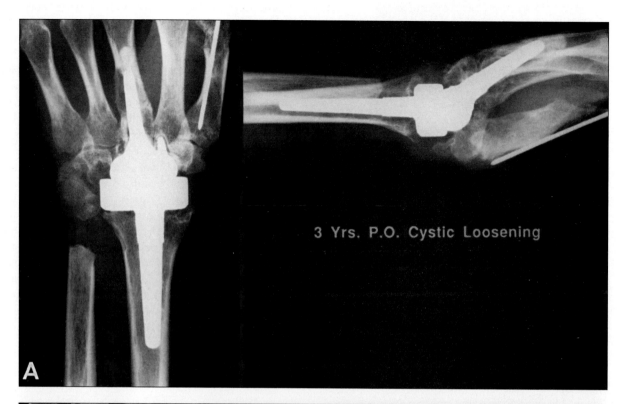

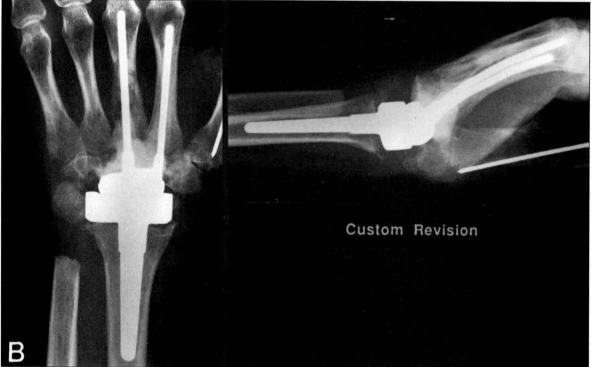

FIGURE 39-2

A, Anteroposterior and lateral views 3 years after biaxial (DePuy) arthroplasty with cystic resorption and loosening of distal component. **B,** Four months after revision arthroplasty with custom two-prong distal component. *P.O.,* postoperative. *(From Beckenbaugh RD: Arthroplasty of the wrist. In Morrey BF, editor: Joint replacement arthroplasty, vol 1, New York, 1991, Churchill Livingstone, pp 195-215. By permission of Mayo Foundation.)*

weaken the bone. If deficient bone stock is present (medullary canals with soft fatty marrow), the procedure of total wrist arthroplasty may be contraindicated or require special custom implants (Fig. 39-2).

A history of sepsis is a relative contraindication to total wrist arthroplasty. However, aggressive débridement and antibiotic therapy may allow the procedure in certain instances.

The absence of functioning radial wrist extensors is a contraindication to total wrist arthroplasty. This condition is actually rare, even in rheumatoid arthritis, but it should be suspected if the wrist has a significant flexion (not subluxation) deformity preoperatively. If the radial wrist extensors cannot be repaired surgically, the procedure must be abandoned. Absence of the extensor carpi ulnaris (primarily an ulnar deviator of the wrist) is not a contraindication to total wrist arthroplasty, and likewise its presence is not sufficient to substitute for absent radial wrist extensors.

Excessive bone loss is not a contraindication to total wrist arthroplasty, and the procedure can be performed by direct implantation in the metacarpals distally. Use of double- or long-stemmed implants is preferred in this situation. Retention of some portion of the distal carpal row improves fixation. Previous wrist procedures, including resection of the distal ulna or synovectomy, do not have adverse effects on wrist arthroplasty unless certain techniques have been used. Deficiency of the extensor retinaculum can allow palmar subluxation of the wrist extensors radially or of the digital extensors ulnarly and this leads to deformity. Therefore, the extensor retinaculum or a part of it must be present or be reconstructed for total wrist arthroplasty to be successful.

Previous wrist arthrodesis does not preclude total wrist arthroplasty if the wrist extensors are intact. The primary indication to take down a wrist arthrodesis is to improve function in a patient who has a need for motion as a result of increasing shoulder, elbow, or digit rheumatoid disease and loss of function. An example might be a person with bilateral wrist fusions who can no longer care for the perineum because of absence of wrist flexion.

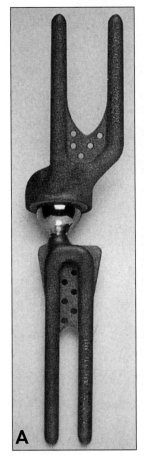
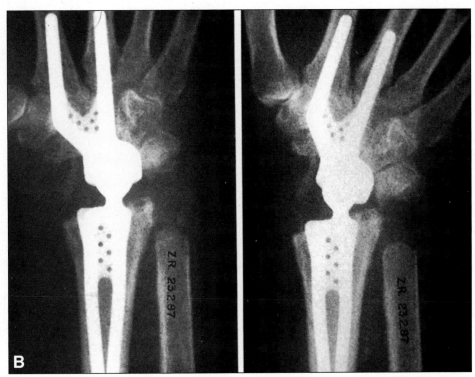

FIGURE 39-3

A, Meuli prosthesis designed for insertion without cement fixation. **B,** Postoperative radiographs of Meuli prosthesis in a patient with rheumatoid arthritis. *(From Beckenbaugh RD: Arthroplasty of the wrist. In Morrey BF, editor: Joint replacement arthroplasty, ed 2, vol 1, New York, 1996, Churchill Livingstone, pp 387-409. By permission of Mayo Foundation.)*

DESIGN DEVELOPMENT OF TOTAL WRIST ARTHROPLASTY

Fixed-fulcrum arthroplasties became available in the United States in the early 1970s. The original devices implanted were of the design by Meuli[26] or by Volz[43] (Fig. 39-1).

The Meuli prosthesis was a ball and socket trunnion design with two malleable stems made of Protosul. The design allowed a range of motion in excess of normal and theoretically had minimal internal constraints. It was, however, difficult to balance wrist motion because the intrinsic center of motion was not the same as that of the wrist.[22,24,46,47] As a result, the device allowed the wrist to develop an ulnar deviation deformity.[4] To correct this problem, the prosthetic distal component was soon modified in several ways with some success.[4,22] The major long-term problem with the ball and socket design was loosening of the distal component.[12] This occurs because in the functional mode the device is constrained; when one pushes up from a chair or pushes open a door with the wrist in a fixed position, all forces are transmitted to the distal component, resulting in loosening. The current Meuli design incorporates a small capsular ball articulation and does not use cement (Fig. 39-3).

The Volz design used a minimally constrained concept with a curved anterior posterior, grooved flexion extension track (Fig. 39-1). The device functions nicely but has a small contact point, increasing the radial-ulnar "teeter-totter" effect and therefore was also associated with problems of balance. Like Meuli, Volz redesigned the distal component to better balance the wrist, but the problem was not completely solved. The Volz design, because of its semiconstrained feature, was associated with an acceptable rate of loosening and longevity.[6] However, because of persistent balance problems the implant is not commonly used today.[13,27,44]

Both the Volz and Meuli devices were used with cement fixation, as was suggested in the 1970s. The early clinical results were encouraging with pain relief, preservation of motion, and improved function. During this period several other types of devices were developed. The various devices were associated with limited success, however, and were never extensively used. The concept of total wrist arthroplasty, however, was successful, and in the 1980s a second generation of prostheses was developed.

I have designed an ellipsoidal articulating wrist device with porous-coated stems for consideration of enhancement of cement fixation and possible biologic fixation without cement (Fig. 39-4). This device was first conceived in 1978 and developed through the early 1980s. It has undergone early clinical trials with moderate levels of success.[5] The design provides for offsetting of the radial component stem in both the dorsal and radial directions with regard to the articular surface to more properly palmarly and ulnarly displace the center of rotation of the wrist. The porous surface on the stem and base of the radial component achieves excellent fixation without the need for methyl methacrylate cement (Fig. 39-5). The distal component contains a single stem and small trapezoidal fixation stump, with porous coating applied to the stem and base area for enhancement of cement fixation. Early results and evaluations have indicated that fixation of the distal component is the primary problem in this form of total wrist arthroplasty, and for those patients with deficient bone stock, new designs have been developed to enhance fixation, including the development of double-pronged and long, single-pronged components (Fig. 39-6). It is anticipated that, in those patients who have previous failed operations such as silicone arthroplasty and in those patients with deficient bone stock or soft bone, the two-pronged or long-pronged distal components will be used.

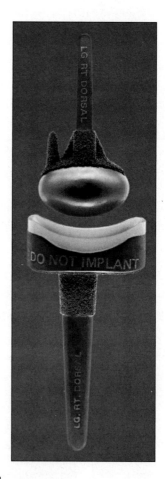

FIGURE 39-4

Biaxial prosthesis (DePuy). Porous coating adjacent to proximal and distal articulating surfaces for enhancement of cement fixation or possible eventual bone ingrowth. Offset stem on radial component (see text). *(From Beckenbaugh RD: Arthroplasty of the wrist. In Morrey BF, editor: Joint replacement arthroplasty, vol 1, New York, 1991, Churchill Livingstone, pp 195-215. By permission of Mayo Foundation.)*

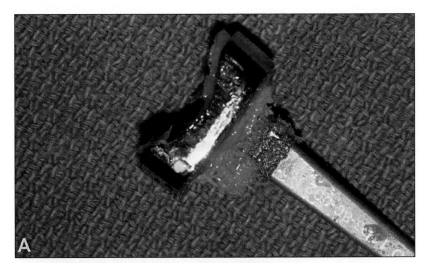

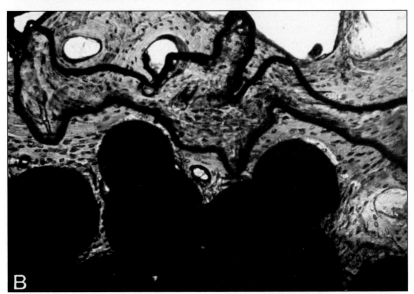

Figure 39-5

A, Biaxial prosthesis, proximal component removed during revision surgery. Note bony ingrowth adjacent to porous-coated stem. **B,** Photomicrograph of histologic section shows bony and fibrous ingrowth leading to the porous-coated radial stem.

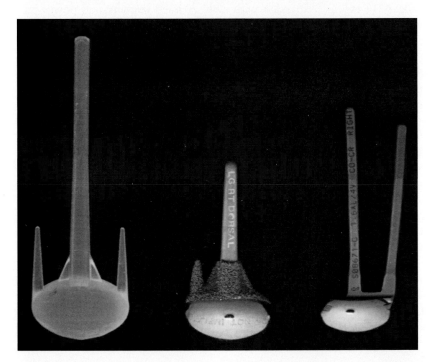

Figure 39-6

Prototypes of custom and double-pronged metacarpal component models designed for use in bone-deficient patients and revision procedures.

SURGICAL TECHNIQUE

The surgical technique for total wrist arthroplasty is basically the same, regardless of the device used. Individual variations in the techniques are limited to specific design features. The technique for biaxial wrist arthroplasty is described.

Radiographic templates with 6% magnification are used to determine the appropriate prosthetic size: small, medium, or large. In general, the largest prosthesis possible should be used. The templates are also useful in estimating the amount of bone to be resected.

The incision is made straight longitudinally and centered over the dorsum of the wrist (Fig. 39-7, *A*). A curved or angled incision is not necessary and may result in necrosis of skin edges. The skin and subcutaneous flaps are sharply elevated from the underlying extensor retinaculum. A longitudinal incision is made through the midportion of the fourth dorsal compartment (Fig. 39-7, *A*). With scissors, the compartment of the extensor pollicis longus is opened ulnarly and the tendon is retracted as the retinaculum is sharply incised radially to unroof the second dorsal compartment. Dissection is carried further radially in a *subperiosteal* manner to expose the tendons of the first dorsal compartment from their course adjacent to the radial styloid. These tendons must be visualized and carefully protected during the bony resection of the distal radius; otherwise they may be easily damaged by the saw. An extensor tenosynovectomy is then performed as appropriate.

Dissection is carried ulnarly to the fifth dorsal compartment, which is, however, not opened unless it is necessary to perform a synovectomy. The common digital extensors are retracted radially and an incision is made in the distal radioulnar joint capsule. A 1- to 2-mm rim of capsule is preserved on the radius and later used for repair. The capsule is subperiosteally dissected ulnarly, leaving the fifth and sixth dorsal compartments intact and exposing the distal ulna. The ulna is resected with the sagittal saw just proximal to the sigmoid notch of the radius (Fig. 39-7, *B*). The distal ulna is *always* resected in biaxial total wrist arthroplasty because disruption of the distal radioulnar joint or ulnar abutment against the prosthesis will occur after resecting the distal radius.

A T-shaped incision is made in the dorsal wrist capsule, based transversely across the radiocarpal joint and extending longitudinally in the axis of the third metacarpal (Fig. 39-7, *C*). The capsule is sharply dissected distally in two triangular flaps to the base of the metacarpals. Some synovium may be left during this portion of the procedure; this tissue is used to cover the prosthesis during closure.

The wrist is sharply flexed and the distal end of the radius is exposed. With a power sagittal saw, the radius is resected in a plane perpendicular to the long axis of the radius. The amount of bone removed will vary to achieve proper tension, but the initial cut should be the minimum width to allow a perpendicular distal surface of the radius and is generally at the level of the middle of the sigmoid notch (Fig. 39-7, *D*). The wrist is extended and the sagittal saw is used to prepare a slightly concave (apex distal) resection of the carpus through the distal carpal row. In general, a 2.5-cm-wide space should be left for the prosthesis and the palmar capsule should be preserved if possible (not mandatory). After making the radius and carpal saw cuts, it is easiest to remove the distal radius by sharp dissection from the adjacent soft tissues. By flexing the wrist, the deformed carpal bones can be removed easily from the palmar capsule or radius with a knife or rongeur.

The preparation of the medullary canals for the prosthetic stems involves a longitudinal incision made along the periosteum of the third metacarpal. The periosteum is elevated just distal to the metaphyseal plane to allow two Hohman retractors to be placed. This maneuver aids immensely in the accurate identification and preparation of the medullary canal of the third metacarpal (Fig. 39-7, *E*). The wrist is flexed, and using a small sharp awl, a canal is developed from the midportion of the neck of the capitate through to the third metacarpal medullary canal. A blunt awl is passed down the canal until it strikes the distal, firm end of the metacarpal head. The depth is noted with a finger and the awl is withdrawn. The length to the metacarpal head end point can be checked along the dorsal metacarpal shaft to confirm the intramedullary position of the awl. Failure to reach an end point indicates that there may have been perforation of the metacarpal shaft.

Once identified, the medullary canal is gradually expanded with awls, presized reamers, and power burs to accept the stem of the prosthesis (Fig. 39-7, *F*). With an awl, a separate hole is placed in the trapezoid or index metacarpal for the small prosthetic base stud. Medial and lateral burring are performed with the side-cutting power reamers to accept the wings of the prosthetic base and carefully adjusted to allow a snug fit. Care is taken to orient the distal component in a plane parallel to the plane of the hand, avoiding any rotation. The distal component trial is inserted and, if seating is satisfactory, attention is turned to the radial medullary canal. Further work to the distal bones is not necessary after fitting the trial, except in the trapezoidal stud. Here, the canal must be enlarged 1 mm in diameter to accept the increased dimension of the porous-coated stem. The softer bone on the third metacarpal-capitate axis does not require overreaming.

The trial prosthesis is removed and attention is turned proximally to the distal radius. With an awl, a channel is prepared starting at the midportion of the medullary canal of the radius. The radial reamers are inserted using

Text continued on p. 936.

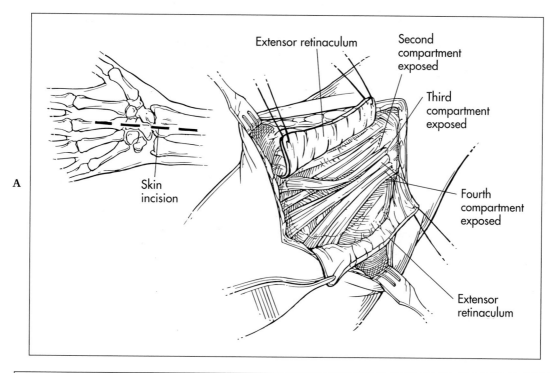

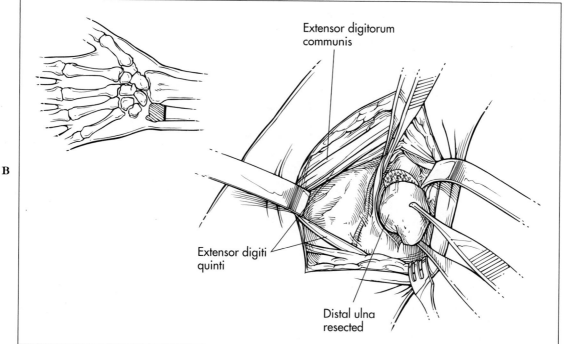

FIGURE 39-7

A, The tendons of the second through fourth compartments are exposed through a longitudinal incision in the dorsal retinaculum. **B,** After subperiosteal exposure, enough distal ulna is resected to be just proximal to the level of the sigmoid notch or the level of the transverse excision of the radius.

Continued.

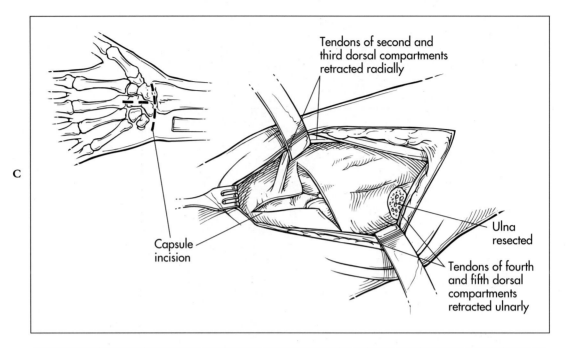

C

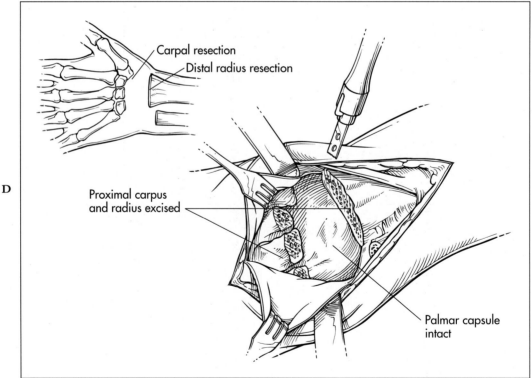

D

FIGURE 39-7, CONT'D.

C, The capsular incision in a T-shaped manner is elevated distally by sharp dissection, preserving capsular flaps for later closure over the prosthesis. **D,** Enough carpus is sharply excised to allow the proper space for the prosthesis. It is desirable to leave the distal one-half of the distal carpal row intact if this bone stock is present.

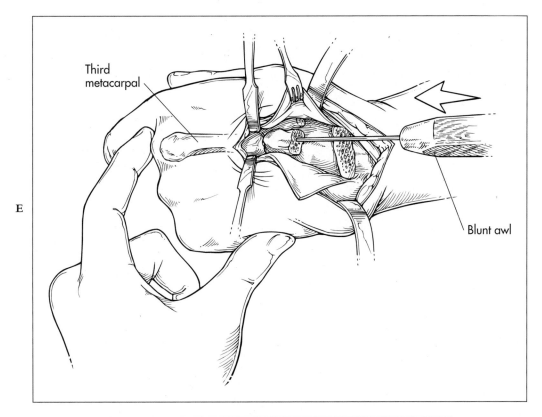

E

Third
metacarpal

Blunt awl

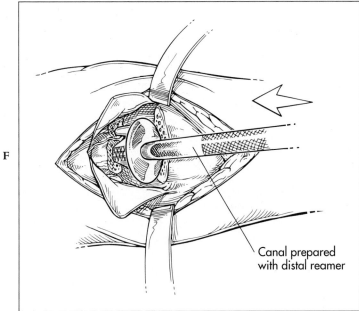

F

Canal prepared
with distal reamer

FIGURE 39-7, CONT'D.

E, Extending the incision periosteally along the third metacarpal and exposing it with two Hohman retractors greatly increase ease of identifying and preparing the canal of the third metacarpal. **F,** The impactor-reamer can be used to develop the proper shape for seating of the distal component, but usually some bone removal with a rongeur and power bur is necessary.   *Continued.*

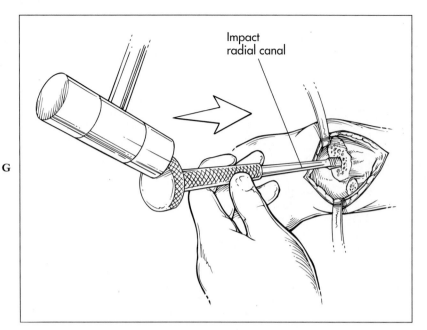

Impact radial canal

G

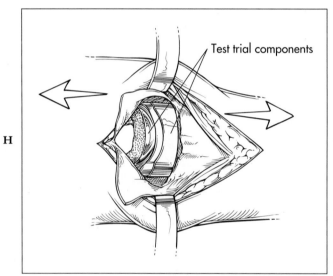

Test trial components

H

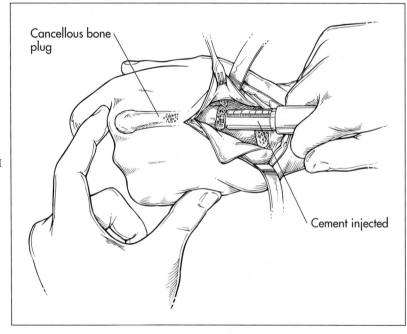

Cancellous bone plug

I

Cement injected

FIGURE 39-7, CONT'D.

G, The proximal medullary canal bone is impacted rather than removed to increase the potential for fixation without cement. **H,** The hand is distracted to identify the amount of tension in the wrist. With the trial implants (proximal and distal) in place, it should not be possible to distract the distal component beyond the polyethylene edge of the proximal component. **I,** Cancellous bone may be used as a plug in the midportion of the metacarpal. The cement is injected in a semiliquid state under pressure.

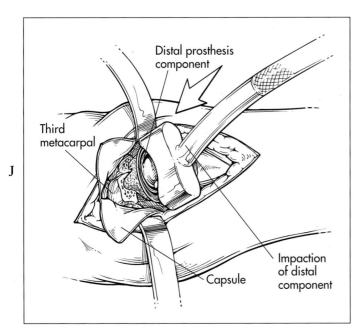

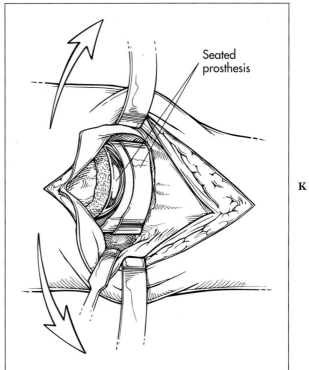

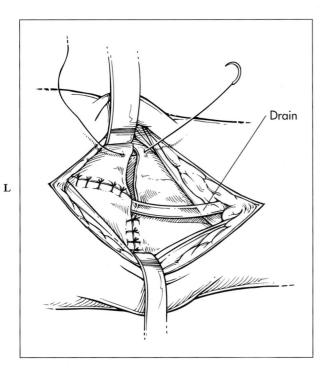

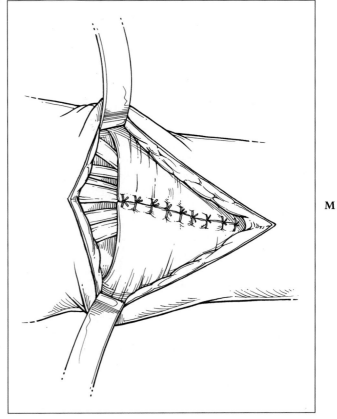

FIGURE 39-7, CONT'D.

J, The distal component is inserted and firmly impacted into the third metacarpal. Excess cement is removed. **K,** After seating the proximal and distal prosthetic components, the wrist is put through a range of motion and any abutting bone is resected. **L,** Capsular repair is important. It is accomplished with interrupted sutures over a deep suction drain. **M,** Retinacular tissues are closed as a single layer over the second through fourth dorsal compartments. It is important to repair the retinaculum to prevent subluxation of the extensor tendons palmar to the prosthesis during wrist palmar flexion.

Continued.

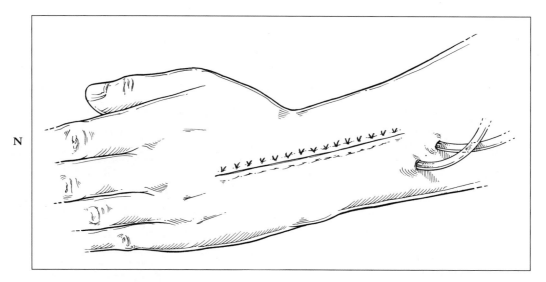

FIGURE 39-7, CONT'D.

N, A second subcutaneous drain is used and long arm compression dressings are applied.

a mallet to impact the medullary bone, not remove it. It is easiest to start with the small-sized reamer and progressively enlarge it to the proper size. The reamer is placed to make the transverse plane parallel to the transverse plane of the radius. The reamer normally self-centers as it is driven proximally in the medullary canal unless the canal is exceptionally large. In these cases, the radial shaft is palpated proximally and the stem position is confirmed radiographically (Fig. 39-7, G).

The proximal trial component is inserted and the end of the radius is trimmed to allow a flat surface-to-surface contact fit. The distal trial is inserted and the wrist is put through a range of passive motion and a test for tension. The trial prosthesis is slightly looser than the real prosthesis, which has a 1-mm porous surface and slightly thicker polyethylene bearing. Ideal or moderate tension is such that the prosthesis can just be distracted approximately 1 mm after reduction. Tight tension is present if seating (location) of the joint is just barely possible and no distraction is present (Fig. 39-7, H). The fit is considered loose if the distal component can be distracted beyond the distal margins of the polyethylene on the sides of the proximal component. If the fit is too tight, more bone can be resected from the radius. If the fit is loose, increased attention is paid to capsular reconstruction with longer periods of immobilization. It is not advisable to increase the tension by incompletely seating the components. At this point, a survey radiograph (biplanar imaging) may be taken to assess the correct position and alignment of the components.

A decision is made as to whether methyl methacrylate cement should be used to supplement the fixation. In all situations except those involving previous medullary canal implants or excessive osteoporosis, the proximal component does not require cement and cement is not desirable because of excessive stress shielding and resorption of the distal radius. In revising silicone prostheses with moderate resorption in the canal, it may be necessary to use bone cement for fixation of the proximal component. However, because the silicone prosthesis stem narrows quite rapidly, the proximal stem of the radial component of the biaxial replacement frequently centers and has firm fixation in the proximal radial shaft. If this is the case, the excess space available about the stem of the biaxial prostheses and the medullary canal of the radius where the previous silicone implant was present can be filled with local bone graft, eliminating the need for cement fixation, even in these revision cases.

The distal component is nearly always cemented. In patients with normal bone stock and hardness, this may not be necessary. In revision surgery when double-pronged or long single-stemmed prostheses are used, methyl methacrylate fixation is generally necessary.

The methyl methacrylate cement is mixed in a standard fashion (one-half batch is enough), and when it becomes pasty it is placed in a 12-mL plastic syringe, the tip of which has been widened by an awl or straight hemostat. A metallic syringe holder (available from a standard glass syringe) is necessary to provide adequate pressure to fill the medullary canal with cement (Fig. 39-7, I). Before injection of the cement in a liquid state a small amount of cancellous bone is impacted distally in the medullary canal of the third metacarpal to act as a plug. Cement (2 to 4 mL) is injected distally and the prosthesis is impacted (Fig. 39-7, J). Excess cement is trimmed, and the cement is allowed to cure with distal pressure maintained on the metacarpal component.

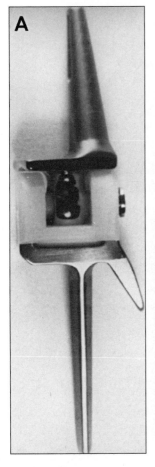
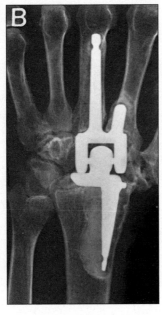
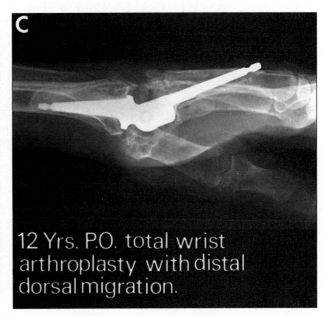

FIGURE 39-11

Trispherical total wrist device. **A,** The device is semiconstrained with a central axis pin. Anteroposterior **(B)** and lateral **(C)** radiographs of a patient 12 years after insertion. The patient has minimal motion but only slight pain and has had progressive loosening of the distal component, which has remained stable over the last several years. P.O., postoperatively. *(From Beckenbaugh RD:* Arthroplasty of the wrist. *In Morrey BF, editor:* Joint replacement arthroplasty, *vol 1, New York, 1991, Churchill Livingstone, pp 195-215. By permission of Mayo Foundation.)*

TRISPHERICAL TOTAL WRIST ARTHROPLASTY

This device is the only fixed articulating device with significant use. The constraints inherent in the hinge limit excess deformity and prevent dislocation, but the inherent constraint could increase chances of failure at the bone-cement interface. Some reports,[18,19] however, suggest satisfactory clinical function with few complications. Some loosening and subsidence have occurred but have not necessarily required revision (Fig. 39-11).

CLAYTON, FERLIC, VOLZ TOTAL WRIST ARTHROPLASTY

Clayton, Ferlic, and Volz have developed an ellipsoidal prosthesis for fixation without cement which is similar in concept to the biaxial design with ellipsoidal articulating surfaces (Fig. 39-12, *A*).[15,17] The device has had early success but has also been associated with problems of loosening and imbalance and is currently under reevaluation and not available for general use.

GUEPAR TOTAL WRIST ARTHROPLASTY

Alnot[1,2] has described a new ellipsoidal wrist device for fixation with bone cement using a polyethylene proximal component and a distal component fixed with screws. The early results have been inconclusive, but the ellipsoidal surfaces have been reported to provide for satisfactory function in preliminary reports. The device is currently being used to a limited degree in France (Fig. 39-12, *B*).

MENON TOTAL WRIST ARTHROPLASTY

Menon[25] has also developed an ellipsoidal wrist arthroplasty device incorporating a concept of resurfacing of the distal radius and the carpus with porous

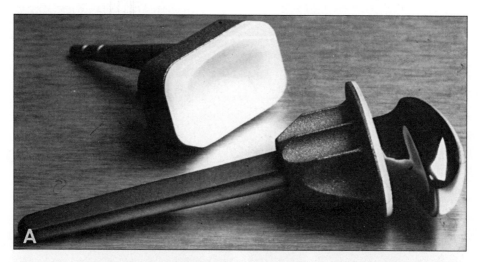

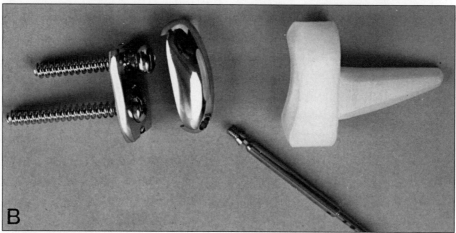

FIGURE 39-12

A, Clayton, Ferlic, and Volz (CFV) prosthesis. The proximal component is ellipsoidal with variable-sized articular surfaces and a distal concave metal-backed polyethylene component. **B,** The GUEPAR wrist. The distal component is a metal ellipsoid and is inserted on the index and long metacarpals with screws. Proximal polyethylene component is offset similar to the biaxial design and is a polyethylene nonmetal-backed component. *(From Beckenbaugh RD: Arthroplasty of the wrist. In Morrey BF, editor: Joint replacement arthroplasty, vol 1, New York, 1991, Churchill Livingstone, pp 195-215. By permission of Mayo Foundation.)*

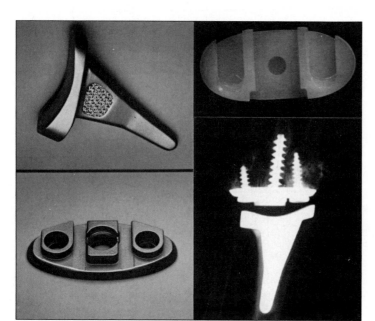

FIGURE 39-13

Menon prosthesis, designed with a physiologic articular interface and screw fixation of the distal component. *(From Beckenbaugh RD: Arthroplasty of the wrist. In Morrey BF, editor: Joint replacement arthroplasty, ed 2, vol 1, New York, 1996, Churchill Livingstone, pp 387-409. By permission of Mayo Foundation.)*

fixation of the proximal metallic base to the distal radius and the incorporation of a polyethylene surface, distal concave ellipsoidal component that is metal-backed and fixed to the carpus with screws. He has had excellent results from a few preliminary cases and is in the process of developing the prosthetic devices and instruments for more general use (Fig. 39-13).

SUMMARY

Total wrist arthroplasty is a continually evolving procedure which is now offering patients with deforming wrist arthrosis an option of providing for pain relief with a mobile stable wrist as opposed to the more traditional procedure of arthrodesis. The procedures are associated with a higher rate of potential failure, and each individual patient must contribute to the decision as to whether the traditional motion-limiting procedures of arthrodeses will be used to relieve pain and provide for permanent solutions to the problems or whether the more aggressive procedure of wrist arthroplasty with attempts to provide for motion in addition to pain relief and stability is undertaken. It is anticipated that, with the increased technologic improvements that are occurring in the development and refinement of the current and newly expected designs, the procedure of wrist arthroplasty will be able to offer greater potential for success and experience greater utilization in the near future.

REFERENCES

1. Alnot JY: L'arthroplastie totale Guepar de poignet dans la polyarthrite rhumatoïde, *Acta Orthop Belg* 54:178-184, 1988.
2. Alnot JY: Report to the Implant Committee, International Federation of the Society for Surgery of the Hand, Paris, France, May 1992.
3. Beckenbaugh RD: Implant arthroplasty in the rheumatoid hand and wrist. Current state of the art in the United States, *J Hand Surg* 8:675-678, 1983.
4. Beckenbaugh RD: Total joint arthroplasty. The wrist, *Mayo Clin Proc* 54:513-515, 1979.
5. Beckenbaugh RD, Brown ML: Early experience with biaxial total wrist arthroplasty. Presented at the 45th Annual Meeting of the American Society for Surgery of the Hand, Toronto, Canada, September 24 to 27, 1990.
6. Bosco JA III, Bynum DK, Bowers WH: Long-term outcome of Volz total wrist arthroplasties, *J Arthroplasty* 9:25-31, 1994.
7. Bracey DJ, McMurtry RY, Wallow D: Arthrodesis of the wrist using the AO technique, *Orthop Rev* 9:65-70, 1980.
8. Brase DW, Millender LH: Failure of silicone rubber wrist arthroplasty in rheumatoid arthritis, *J Hand Surg [Am]* 11:175-183, 1986.
9. Clayton ML: Surgical treatment at the wrist in rheumatoid arthritis: a review of thirty-seven patients, *J Bone Joint Surg Am* 47:741-750, 1965.
10. Clayton ML, Ferlic DC: Tendon transfer for radial rotation of the wrist in rheumatoid arthritis, *Clin Orthop* 100:176-185, 1974.
11. Comstock CP, Louis DS, Eckenrode JF: Silicone wrist implant: long-term follow-up study, *J Hand Surg [Am]* 13:201-205, 1988.
12. Cooney WP III, Beckenbaugh RD, Linscheid RL: Total wrist arthroplasty. Problems with implant failures, *Clin Orthop* 187:121-128, 1984.
13. Dennis DA, Ferlic DC, Clayton ML: Volz total wrist arthroplasty in rheumatoid arthritis: a long-term review, *J Hand Surg [Am]* 11:483-490, 1986.
14. Fatti JF, Palmer AK, Mosher JF: The long-term results of Swanson silicone rubber interpositional wrist arthroplasty, *J Hand Surg [Am]* 11:166-175, 1986.
15. Ferlic DC: Results and changes. ASSH Newsletter on Total Wrist Arthroplasty, January 1992.
16. Ferlic DC, Jolly SN, Clayton ML: Salvage for failed implant arthroplasty of the wrist, *J Hand Surg [Am]* 17:917-923, 1992.
17. Ferlic DC, Menon J, Meuli HC: Indications and techniques for total wrist arthroplasty. Presented at the 47th Annual Meeting of the American Society for Surgery of the Hand, Phoenix, Arizona, 1992.
18. Figgie HE III, Ranawat CS, Inglis AE, et al.: Preliminary results of total wrist arthroplasty in rheumatoid arthritis using the trispherical total wrist arthroplasty, *J Arthroplasty* 3:9-15, 1988.
19. Figgie MP, Ranawat CS, Inglis AE, et al.: Trispherical total wrist arthroplasty in rheumatoid arthritis, *J Hand Surg [Am]* 15:217-223, 1990.
20. Gellman H, Rankin G, Brumfield R Jr, et al.: Palmar shelf arthroplasty in the rheumatoid wrist. Results of long-term follow-up, *J Bone Joint Surg Am* 71:223-227, 1989.
21. Goodman MJ, Millender LH, Nalebuff EA, et al.: Arthroplasty of the rheumatoid wrist with silicone rubber: an early evaluation, *J Hand Surg [Am]* 5:114-121, 1980.
22. Hamas RS: A quantitative approach to total wrist arthroplasty: development of a precentered wrist prosthesis, *Orthopedics* 2:245-255, 1979.

23. Linscheid RL, Dobyns JH: Radiolunate arthrodesis, *J Hand Surg [Am]* 10:821-829, 1985.

24. McMurtry RY, Youm Y, Flatt AE, et al.: Kinematics of the wrist. II. Clinical applications, *J Bone Joint Surg Am* 60:955-961, 1978.

25. Menon J: Total wrist replacement using the modified Volz prosthesis, *J Bone Joint Surg Am* 69:998-1006, 1987.

26. Meuli HC: Arthroplastie du poignet, *Ann Chir* 27:527-530, 1973.

27. Meuli HC: Arthroplasty of the wrist, *Clin Orthop* 149:118-125, 1980.

28. Meuli HC, Fernandez DL: Uncemented total wrist arthroplasty, *J Hand Surg [Am]* 20:115-122, 1995.

29. Mikkelsen OA: Arthrodesis of the wrist joint in rheumatoid arthritis, *Hand* 12:149-153, 1980.

30. Millender LH, Nalebuff EA: Preventive surgery—tenosynovectomy and synovectomy, *Orthop Clin North Am* 6:765-792, 1975.

31. Palmer AK, Werner FW, Murphy D, et al.: Functional wrist motion: a biomechanical study, *J Hand Surg [Am]* 10:39-46, 1985.

32. Peimer CA, Medige J, Eckert BS, et al.: Reactive synovitis after silicone arthroplasty, *J Hand Surg [Am]* 11:624-638, 1986.

33. Rettig ME, Beckenbaugh RD: Revision total wrist arthroplasty, *J Hand Surg [Am]* 18:798-804, 1993.

34. Simmen BR, Gschwend N: Swanson silicone rubber interpositional arthroplasty of the wrist and of the metacarpophalangeal joints in rheumatoid arthritis, *Acta Orthop Belg* 54:196-209, 1988.

35. Smith RJ, Atkinson RE, Jupiter JB: Silicone synovitis of the wrist, *J Hand Surg [Am]* 10:47-60, 1985.

36. Stanley JK, Boot DA: Radio-lunate arthrodesis, *J Hand Surg [Br]* 14:283-287, 1989.

37. Stanley JK, Tolat AR: Long-term results of Swanson Silastic arthroplasty in the rheumatoid wrist, *J Hand Surg [Br]* 18:381-388, 1993.

38. Straub LR, Ranawat CS: The wrist in rheumatoid arthritis. Surgical treatment and results, *J Bone Joint Surg Am* 51:1-20, 1969.

39. Swanson AB: Flexible implant arthroplasty for arthritic disabilities of the radiocarpal joint. A silicone rubber intramedullary stemmed flexible hinge implant for the wrist joint, *Orthop Clin North Am* 4:383-394, 1973.

40. Taleisnik J: Rheumatoid arthritis of the wrist, *Hand Clin* 5:257-278, 1989.

41. Vicar AJ, Burton RI: Surgical management of the rheumatoid wrist—fusion or arthroplasty, *J Hand Surg [Am]* 11:790-797, 1986.

42. Viegas SF, Rimoldi R, Patterson R: Modified technique of intramedullary fixation for wrist arthrodesis, *J Hand Surg [Am]* 14:618-623, 1989.

43. Volz RG: The development of a total wrist arthroplasty, *Clin Orthop* 116:209-214, 1976.

44. Volz RG: Total wrist arthroplasty. A clinical review, *Clin Orthop* 187:112-120, 1984.

45. Wood MB: Wrist arthrodesis using dorsal radial bone graft, *J Hand Surg [Am]* 12:208-212, 1987.

46. Youm Y, Flatt AE: Design of a total wrist prosthesis, *Ann Biomed Eng* 12:247-262, 1984.

47. Youm Y, McMurtry RY, Flatt AE, et al.: Kinematics of the wrist. I. An experimental study of radial-ulnar deviation and flexion-extension, *J Bone Joint Surg Am* 60:423-431, 1978.

40

VARIANT FORMS OF ARTHRITIS: JUVENILE RHEUMATOID ARTHRITIS, SYSTEMIC LUPUS ERYTHEMATOSUS, AND PSORIATIC ARTHRITIS

Spencer A. Rowland, M.D.
Julio Taleisnik, M.D.

JUVENILE RHEUMATOID ARTHRITIS
  SUBGROUPS OF JUVENILE RHEUMATOID ARTHRITIS
    SYSTEMIC JUVENILE RHEUMATOID ARTHRITIS
    POLYARTICULAR JUVENILE RHEUMATOID ARTHRITIS
    PAUCIARTICULAR JUVENILE RHEUMATOID ARTHRITIS
  DIAGNOSTIC STUDIES
    LABORATORY ABNORMALITIES
    PATHOLOGIC FEATURES
    CLINICAL AND RADIOLOGIC FINDINGS IN THE WRIST
  TREATMENT
    SPLINTING AND PHYSIOTHERAPY
    INTRA-ARTICULAR STEROID INJECTION
    SYNOVECTOMY

OTHER SURGICAL PROCEDURES
SUMMARY
SYSTEMIC LUPUS ERYTHEMATOSUS
  DIAGNOSTIC STUDIES
    CLINICAL MANIFESTATIONS
    LABORATORY ABNORMALITIES
    PATHOLOGIC FEATURES
    RADIOLOGIC FINDINGS
    DIAGNOSIS
  SUMMARY
PSORIATIC ARTHRITIS
  ETIOLOGY
  DIAGNOSTIC STUDIES
    CLINICAL MANIFESTATIONS
    RADIOLOGIC FINDINGS
  SURGICAL TREATMENT
  SUMMARY

JUVENILE RHEUMATOID ARTHRITIS

Chronic arthritis in children comprises a heterogeneous group of conditions that are different from those in adult seropositive rheumatoid arthritis[3] and continue to present diagnostic problems. For this reason, a brief review of the history and classification follows.

Childhood inflammatory arthritis was first cited in 1864 by Cornil.[18] In 1896, George Fredrick Still presented 22 cases that became the classic early description of arthritis in children.[54] The systemic variety is frequently referred to as Still's disease. In 1972, the first publication of classification criteria in the United States appeared in the *Bulletin on Rheumatic Diseases*,[2] and there is now a general acceptance of the term "juvenile arthritis" to encompass all of the rheumatoid diseases in children that are associated with the development of peripheral or axial arthritis of either an inflammatory or noninflammatory nature[15] (Table 40-1). In 1989, criteria were developed for the diagnosis and classification of children with juvenile rheumatoid arthritis (JRA).[16] In addition, three subgroups of JRA were defined that had

Table 40-1. Diagnostic Classification of Juvenile Arthritis

A. Connective tissue diseases
   1. Juvenile rheumatoid arthritis
   2. Systemic lupus erythematosus
   3. Dermatomyositis
   4. Vasculitis
   5. Scleroderma
B. Seronegative spondyloarthropathies
   1. Juvenile ankylosing spondylitis
   2. Psoriatic spondyloarthritis
   3. Reiter's syndrome
   4. Inflammatory bowel disease (regional enteritis, ulcerative colitis)
C. Infectious arthritis
   1. Bacterial arthritis (including staphylococcal infection, gonorrhea, tuberculosis)
   2. Viral arthritis
   3. Fungal arthritis
   4. Lyme disease
D. Reactive arthritis
   1. Rheumatic fever
   2. Yersinial arthritis
E. Rheumatic diseases associated with immunodeficiency
F. Congenital anomalies and genetically determined abnormalities of the musculoskeletal system
   1. Constitutional diseases of bone
   2. Lysosomal storage diseases
   3. Heritable disorders of collagen and fibrous connective tissue
   4. Amyloidosis
G. Nonrheumatic conditions of bones and joints
   1. Traumatic arthritis
   2. Reflex neurovascular dystrophy
   3. Legg-Calvé-Perthes disease
   4. Slipped capital femoral epiphysis
   5. Toxic synovitis of the hip
   6. Osteochondritis dissecans
   7. Chondromalacia patellae
   8. Plant-thorn synovitis
H. Hematologic diseases
   1. Sickle cell anemia
   2. Hemophilia
   3. Leukemia and lymphoma
I. Neoplastic diseases
   1. Neuroblastoma
   2. Malignant and benign tumors of cartilage, bone, and synovium
   3. Histiocytosis
J. Arthromyalgia
   1. Growing pains
   2. Psychogenic rheumatism

From Cassidy JT, Levinson JE, Brewer EJ Jr.[16] By permission of the Arthritis Foundation.

different prognostic implications. These subdivisions are systemic disease, polyarthritis, and pauciarticular disease (oligoarthritis).[9,10,15,30]

To diagnose JRA, the following criteria must be met[16] (Table 40-2):

1) The age at onset must be younger than 16 years. Most acknowledge that this is an arbitrary cutoff point having no biologic significance.
2) Arthritis is present in one or more joints. Arthritis is defined as *swelling* or *joint effusion* or the presence of two or more of the following: pain on joint motion, limitation of joint motion, joint tenderness, or increased heat in the joint.
3) The duration of the disease must be greater than 6 weeks.
4) Other forms of juvenile arthritis must be excluded.

SUBGROUPS OF JUVENILE RHEUMATOID ARTHRITIS

JRA is divided into three subgroups according to the number of joints involved and whether or not systemic disease is present. The subgroup is determined by the clinical picture in the first 6 months after the disease onset (Table 40-3). *Polyarthritis* involves five or more joints; *pauciarticular disease* (oligoarthritis), four or fewer joints; and *systemic disease*, arthritis with documentation of intermittent fever of at least 39°C for 2 weeks.[10]

The subgroups of JRA differ not only in their clinical manifestations but also in prognosis, joint

Table 40-2. Diagnostic Criteria for the Classification of Juvenile Rheumatoid Arthritis

1. Age at onset younger than 16 years
2. Arthritis in one or more joints, defined as swelling or effusion, or by the presence of two or more of the following signs: limitation of range of motion, tenderness or pain on motion, and increased heat
3. Duration of disease of 6 weeks to 3 months
4. Type of onset of disease during the first 4 to 6 months classified as:
   a. Polyarthritis: five or more joints
   b. Pauciarthritis: four or fewer joints
   c. Systemic disease: intermittent fever, rheumatoid rash, arthritis, visceral disease (hepatosplenomegaly, lymphadenopathy)
5. Exclusion of other rheumatic diseases

From Cassidy JT: *Juvenile rheumatoid arthritis*. In Kelly WN, Harris ED Jr, Ruddy S, Sledge CB, editors: *Textbook of rheumatology*, ed 3, vol 2, Philadelphia, 1981, WB Saunders. By permission of the publisher.

disability, types of extra-articular complications, serologic findings, and sex distribution.[11,12,50]

Systemic Juvenile Rheumatoid Arthritis. Systemic juvenile rheumatoid arthritis accounts for 20% to 26% of all cases of JRA[17,50] and has a predilection for boys. By definition, all the patients have high intermittent fevers for more than 2 weeks and usually have a typical rheumatoid rash characterized by small red macules with a central clearing.[50] Of the many manifestations, fever and rash have the greatest diagnostic value.[17] Hepatosplenomegaly, generalized lymphadenopathy, pericarditis, myocarditis, and pneumonitis[17,50] may be present in various degrees. In the series of 32 patients reported by Schaller and Wedgwood,[52] 29 had overt arthritis the first 6 months of the disease, and polyarthritis ultimately developed in all. The arthritis in 19 of the 32 patients became chronic, persisting after remission of systemic syndromes.

Polyarticular Juvenile Rheumatoid Arthritis. This subgroup involves five or more joints, accounts for approximately 40%[17,50] of the onsets of arthritis, and is seen predominantly in girls.[17] These patients may have a low-grade fever[17] but they do not have a rash.[50] The onset resembles adult arthritis in that the arthritis is symmetrical, involving the metacarpophalangeal and proximal interphalangeal joints of the hand, and may have associated rheumatoid nodules. Knees, wrists, ankles, and elbows are the most frequent sites of initial involvement.[17] The morbidity of this type is from arthritis.[50]

Pauciarticular Juvenile Rheumatoid Arthritis. By definition, this subgroup has disease limited to four or fewer joints. Monarticular arthritis, once described in a separate category, is now considered a part of this subgroup.[17,50] Pauciarticular arthritis affects primarily girls. The initial joint most often affected is the knee and it is usually unilateral. In the report by Schaller

Table 40-3. Modes of Onset of Juvenile Rheumatoid Arthritis

Feature	Systemic	Polyarticular		Pauciarticular	
Presentation	Extra-articular manifestations (fever, rash, organomegaly, serositis, myalgia, hematologic changes)	Symmetric arthritis involving large and small joints		Asymmetric arthritis involving few joints, usually large	
	Arthritis	Five or more joints affected		Fewer than four joints affected, frequently only one joint	
		RF Negative	RF Positive	Type I	Type II
Patients (%)	20	25–30	10	25	15–20
Age at onset (median) (yr)	5	3	> 8	2	10
Sex distribution	M > F	F > M	F > M	F > M	M > F
Rheumatoid factor	Generally negative	Negative	Positive	Generally negative	Generally negative
Antinuclear antibodies	Generally negative	Positive in 25%	Positive in 75%	Positive in 50%	Generally negative
Course	Systemic manifestations are self-limited; arthritis may become chronic, with severe destructive arthritis developing in 25%	Majority do well, severe sequelae develop in 10%, particularly hip and temporomandibular joint problems	Resembles adult rheumatoid disease; severe destructive arthritis in 50% of cases	Arthritis mild; morbidity associated with ocular problems (i.e., iridocyclitis)	Course variable; ankylosing spondylitis pattern may develop

RF, rheumatoid factor.
From Jay S, Helm S, Wray BB: Juvenile rheumatoid arthritis, *Am Fam Phys* 26:139-147, 1982. By permission of the American Academy of Family Physicians.

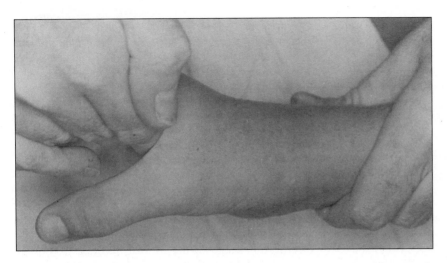

FIGURE 40-1

Loss of wrist extension, one of the earliest clinical signs of rheumatoid arthritis in the child. This finding may be present before palpable wrist synovitis. *(From Granberry WM and Mangum GL: The hand in the child with juvenile rheumatoid arthritis, J Hand Surg 5:105-113, 1980. Copyright, American Society for Surgery of the Hand, by permission of Churchill Livingstone.)*

and Wedgwood[52] of 98 joints involved in 46 children with pauciarticular arthritis, 4 involved the wrist. Joint destruction was uncommon in this group. When a single joint is involved, arthrocentesis followed by cultures and sensitivities and synovial fluid analysis should be done to eliminate the possibility of a septic joint.[17]

The most devastating condition that can occur with pauciarticular arthritis is iridocyclitis, which, if undetected and untreated, can lead to complete blindness.[13] For that reason slit-lamp examinations have been recommended every 4 months with pauciarticular disease in patients positive for antinuclear antibody and at least once each year in all other JRA patients.

DIAGNOSTIC STUDIES

Laboratory Abnormalities. Except in the pauciarticular subgroup, increased erythrocyte sedimentation rate, low-grade anemia, and thrombocytosis are frequently present.[17] Neutrophilic leukocytosis may be high in the *systemic* disease onset, moderate in the *polyarticular* disease onset, and normal in the *pauciarticular* disease onset. A positive result of the latex-fixation test is seen in 10% to 20% of children with JRA[17]; however, it is usually seen when the disease onset is late in childhood.[50] Severe erosive joint disease is seen in the polyarticular type of onset.[17,50,52] Increased antinuclear antibody titers are found in as many as 50% of patients and correlate with early onset (younger than age 6 years), pauciarticular type of onset, and chronic iridocyclitis.[17]

Pathologic Features. The pathologic manifestations of JRA are different than those in the adult[1,17] because of the characteristics of the growing skeleton. Narrowing of joints and bone erosion from the invading pannus may not be seen until late in the disease because of the amount of articular cartilage present in the immature

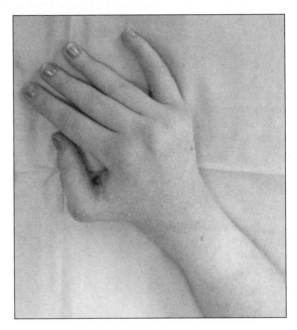

FIGURE 40-2

Ulnar deviation of the wrist is common in juvenile rheumatoid arthritis. It is associated with radial deviation of the fingers.

skeleton.[1] Enlargement of the epiphyses, accelerated maturation, and premature closure of the physeal line are often seen. Therefore, cylindrical bones can be shorter or longer depending on the stage of the physeal involvement, and periosteal new bone may be seen in the vicinity of the involved joint.[1]

Clinical and Radiologic Findings in the Wrist. The wrist is the most frequently involved joint in the upper extremity in JRA, with the majority of the patients having wrist involvement at some point in the course of the disease.[23,51] In the review by Chaplin et al.,[17] of 828 wrists with JRA, 487 (59%) showed radiologic evidence of wrist involvement and, in long-term follow-up, wrist

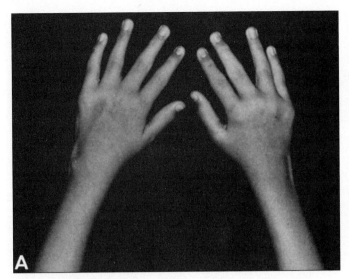
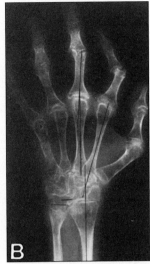
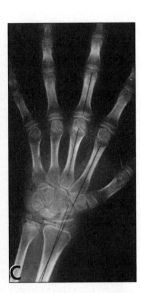

FIGURE 40-3

A, Juvenile rheumatoid arthritis in an 11-year-old girl shows various degrees of radial deviation of the metacarpophalangeal joints. **B** and **C,** Radiographs show the lines for measurement of **(B)** the metacarpophalangeal degree of radial deviation measured as the angle of the third metacarpal to the proximal phalanx and **(C)** wrist deviation measured along the center of the radius and second metacarpal. *(From Granberry WM and Mangum GL: The hand in the child with juvenile rheumatoid arthritis,* J Hand Surg *5:105-113, 1980. Copyright, American Society for Surgery of the Hand, by permission of Churchill Livingstone.)*

involvement was as high as 95%. In the series by Weinberger et al.,[57] wrist involvement occurred in 54% of the children with JRA 1 year after the onset of the disease. Severe wrist changes were reported by Nalebuff et al.[47,48] to be directly related to the time since the onset of arthritis. Weinberger et al.[57] found radiologic evidence of wrist abnormalities in 59% of children with JRA 1 year after onset of disease and in 93% of 73 patients 5 years after onset of the disease. They also found spontaneous fusion of the carpal bones in 54%.

Granberry and Mangum[27] made the observation that one of the earliest clinical signs of rheumatoid arthritis in a child is the loss of complete extension of the wrist (Fig. 40-1), which may be present before the onset of any palpable wrist synovitis and usually precedes radiologic changes by several months. This loss of wrist extension is associated with varied degrees of pain and swelling. Unlike findings in adults with rheumatoid arthritis, Granberry and Mangum found in their clinical study of 100 wrists that ulnar deviation of the wrist rather than radial deviation is the rule in JRA (Fig. 40-2). Some degree of ulnar deviation as measured on radiographs was also present in all of their patients and was associated with radial rather than ulnar deviation of the fingers (Fig. 40-3).[27] Vanio and Oka[56] found a definite correlation among ulnar shortening, ulnar deviation of the wrist, and radial deviation of the fingers at the metacarpophalangeal joint.

The first bony radiologic changes are extra-articular osteoporosis followed by premature ossification of the carpal bones that has been accelerated by chronic hyperemia (Fig. 40-4).[4,20,44] Narrowing of the intercarpal and carpometacarpal spaces gives the overall appearance of crowding of the carpal bones (Fig. 40-5).[25] The carpal bones become somewhat irregular in shape and their trabeculations become coarse.[4] Erosions appear around the carpus and distal radial and ulnar epiphysis (Fig. 40-6). Early closure of the ulnar epiphysis may occur, and this frequently causes an obliquity of the distal ulna, resulting in the ulnar styloid side being longer than the radial side (Fig. 40-6). The ulna then becomes progressively shorter in relation to the radius (Fig. 40-7).[27,31] Palmar subluxation[27] and ulnar translocation of the carpus on the radius may be seen in various degrees and rarely in the extreme situation may lead to bayonet deformity, as described by Chaplin et al.[17] Spontaneous fusion may occur between some or all of the carpal or carpometacarpal joints (or both).[43] Any part or all of the above bone changes may occur to some degree.

In the study by Weinberger et al.,[57] the most common radiographic finding was intercarpal joint space narrowing, followed in frequency by narrowing of the radiocarpal and carpometacarpal joints. Bony fusion of the carpal bones was seen in 52% of the patients to some degree. Carpometacarpal fusion was present in 54% of the patients. Changes in carpal bone shape were frequent, and this was associated with overgrowth of carpal epiphyses, coarse trabeculation, and bony erosion.

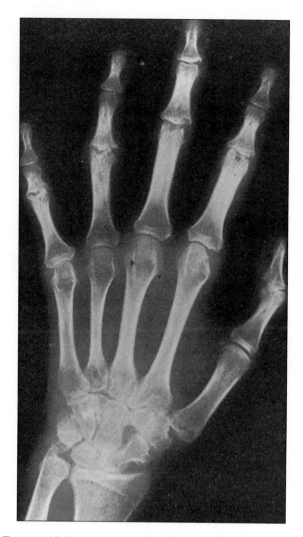

FIGURE 40-4

Early carpal changes in juvenile rheumatoid arthritis. Erosions, early carpal bone fusion, closure of the ulnar physis, and narrowing of the radiocarpal and carpometacarpal joints. *(Courtesy of Dr. Robert Persellin.)*

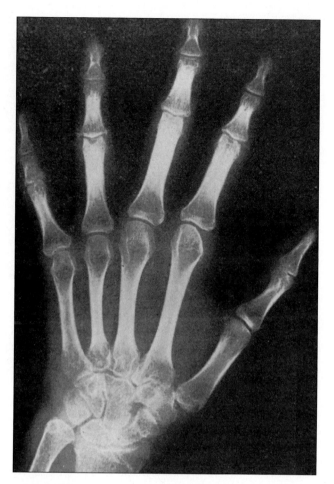

FIGURE 40-5

Narrowing of the intercarpal and carpometacarpal spaces gives the overall appearance of crowding of the carpal bones. *(Courtesy of Dr. Robert Persellin.)*

TREATMENT

Various modalities have been used in the treatment of JRA. The best approach is the use of a pediatric-rheumatology team consisting of a pediatric rheumatologist for medical management; an occupational therapist for splinting; a physical therapist for exercises and pain control; a nurse for patient and parent education; a social worker to help schoolteachers and nurses understand the child's illness and assist with financial forms and home problems; and orthopedic and hand surgeons.

Splinting and Physiotherapy. The child with JRA should have an intense program of physical and occupational therapy, with the involved wrist put through its maximum range of motion at least twice a day. Use of

the wrist is encouraged when possible. Night splints to maintain a functional position are essential (Fig. 40-8).[17]

Findley et al.[23] reported that their preferred management of the JRA wrist used splinting, heat, range of motion, rest, and exercise according to the phase of wrist inflammation. When severe wrist pain is present, a resting day splint is indicated. When the pain becomes milder, some form of wrist-support splinting with the fingers free is used in an attempt to correct any flexion or ulnar deviation. A dynamic splint such as a palmar pneumatic bag, as suggested by Findley et al.,[23] or a spring-loaded brace used by Miller (personal communication) may also be indicated (Fig. 40-9). Miller has the patient wear a spring splint night and day except for two 30-min periods, at which time vigorous range of motion exercises are done.

Intra-Articular Steroid Injection. Evans et al.[20] reported their results after the injection of 20 to 30 mg of triamcinolone into the radiocarpal joint in 10 wrists of 10 patients during general anesthesia. Nine

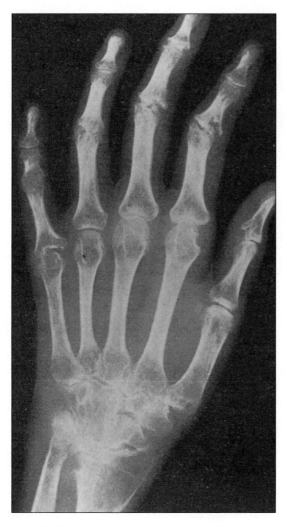

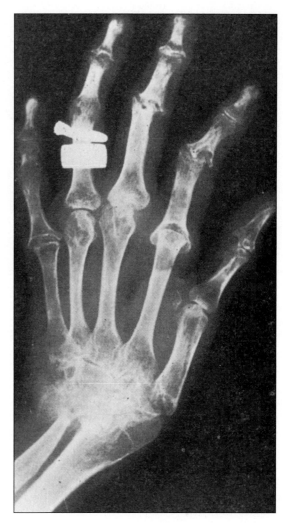

FIGURE 40-6

Erosions around the carpus with narrowing of the radiocarpal joint, loss of carpal height, positive ulna variance, and early closure of the ulnar physis. Note elongated ulnar styloid. *(Courtesy of Dr. Robert Persellin.)*

FIGURE 40-7

Advanced disease of juvenile rheumatoid arthritis shows progressive ulnar translation of the carpus and resorption of the distal ulna. *(Courtesy of Dr. Robert Persellin.)*

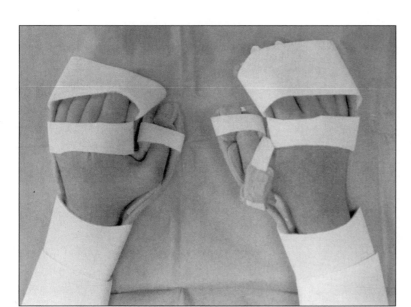

FIGURE 40-8

Rheumatoid hand splints. Wearing night splints is mandatory to help prevent progression of deformity, especially during the growth-spurt years. *(Courtesy of Dr. Malcolm Granberry.)*

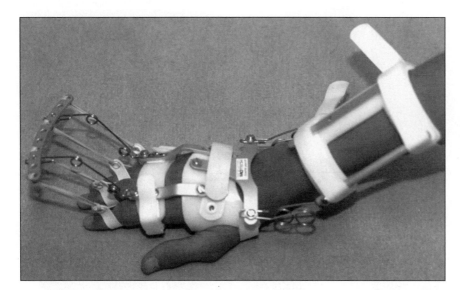

FIGURE 40-9

Dynamic splint for correction of wrist and finger deformities in juvenile rheumatoid arthritis. Note spring-loaded wrist splint and dynamic, rubber-band finger extension. *(Courtesy of Dr. Michael Miller.)*

patients were in the pauciarticular subgroup and one was in the polyarticular subgroup. Soft-tissue swelling was decreased in eight, two patients became pain free, and seven patients had improved range of motion.

Synovectomy. The literature regarding wrist synovectomy is scant, but the benefit appears to be quite real (Fig. 40-10). Fink et al.[24] reported improvement in the range of wrist motion in three of five patients after synovectomy. Eyring et al.[21] reported on 48 multiple joint synovectomies, 10 of which were of the wrist, and the patients were followed an average of 24 months. The wrist improved in eight patients. Two patients, however, lost motion and one required manipulation. In two cases, erosions in the radius and carpus had apparently healed. Kampner and Ferguson[37] reported wrist synovectomy in two patients and both wrists became ankylosed. Granberry and Mangum[27] reported wrist synovectomy in three patients; two wrists became ankylosed. Jacobsen et al.[35] reported late results after synovectomy in four wrists. Synovectomy produced little benefit in relieving pain and it did not stop radiographic deterioration.

We generally prefer synovectomy of the wrist extensor tendons and wrist joint through a dorsal incision (longitudinal). The extensor retinaculum should be preserved for late transfer deep to the finger extensor tendons (Fig. 40-10). One of us (J.T.) prefers a more oblique incision (Fig. 40-11) to provide good exposure without excessive skin penetration. The incision should be kept ulnar to Lister's tubercle and the path of the extensor pollicis longus tendon because the area directly over the finger extensor tendons is subjected to skin necrosis and dehiscence. Skin flaps are kept full thickness and must be handled with care, avoiding rough retraction and unnecessary dissection. In all cases, the extensor pollicis longus is released from the extensor retinaculum and retracted to expose the extensor surface of the wrist capsule when synovectomy of the wrist only (and not the extensor tendons) is anticipated (Figs. 40-11, *A* through *C*). In most patients, an extensor tenosynovectomy is needed and here the entire dorsal retinaculum must be reflected for adequate exposure (Figs. 40-11, *D* through *I*). This retinacular flap is started ulnarly over the extensor carpi ulnaris and is reflected radially (radial-based flap). Proximal and distal transverse incisions are used to delineate the width of the retinacular flap. Preservation of deep antebrachial and distal pretendinous fascia is important along with reconstruction of part of the retinaculum to prevent bowstringing when wrist motion is close to normal. If wrist motion is limited, the entire extensor retinaculum can be passed deep to the extensor tendons. Sharp dissection is suggested for the dorsal tenosynovectomy (Fig. 40-12). In some cases, reconstruction of the extensor carpi ulnaris sheath and transfer of the extensor carpi radialis longus to balance the wrist may be indicated (Fig. 40-11, *I*).

Other Surgical Procedures. Various other surgical procedures have been used in the JRA patient in an attempt to prevent or to correct wrist deformity, but the number of procedures and the follow-up are too small to be meaningful and they are mentioned only for completeness. Procedures include proximal row carpectomy with Silastic sheet interposition, distraction lengthening of the ulna, and soft-tissue release of the palmar wrist capsule to correct flexion contracture.[20]

SUMMARY

From the information gleaned from the literature, the authors' personal experience, and the experience of others,[26,29,47] the key to managing the wrist in JRA is conservation, gradually allowing intercarpal and radiocarpal fusion to take place naturally while maintaining the wrist in a functional position.[33] The use of

causes laxity of the supporting ligaments of joints and results in deformities similar to rheumatoid arthritis. These deformities are usually passively correctable, but they can become fixed with time.[34] Histologic examination of the synovium reveals a fibrous villous synovitis, typically without the pannus formation that destroys cartilage.[19] Joint aspirations usually reveal clear fluid with a leukocyte count less than 4×10^9/L, and most cells are lymphocytes.[22]

Radiologic Findings. Generalized osteoporosis may be present; however, the major radiologic changes of the wrist are secondary to ligamentous laxity. The distal ulna can dislocate dorsally. Various degrees of carpal translocation may occur, and intercarpal ligament laxity can result in scapholunate dissociation and carpal collapse of various degrees. The joint spaces between the carpal articular spaces appear normal, but their relationship to each other may be altered because of ligamentous laxity. Aseptic necrosis of carpal bones has been reported by a few authors.[28,39,53] Urman et al.[55] reviewed the literature in 1977 and found 140 patients in whom aseptic necrosis developed and five cases involved carpal bones. Almost all of the 140 patients had been treated with systemic administration of cortisone. Green and Osmer[28] attributed the aseptic necrosis to vasculitis. Because most SLE patients are treated with systemic administration of cortisone, it is difficult to be sure whether the necrosis

is due to vasculitis, cortisone, or both. It is important to have an awareness that necrosis can occur and can be a source of pain.[53]

Diagnosis. Joint symptoms are the most frequent clinical manifestation of SLE, occurring in approximately 90% of patients at some time during the course of their disease.[39] Joint symptoms preceded the onset of the disease in 64% of the patients in one study.[39] Pain with joint motion, stiffness, joint effusion, and periarticular swelling may be present. The joint pain is usually mild.[8] Raynaud's phenomenon has been reported in as many as 50% of SLE patients and was the primary cause of disability in that it does not respond to cortisone.

Ligamentous laxity is the most common physical finding in the hands.[20] Laxity of the ligaments about the wrist joint does not cause a problem in most instances.[8,39] Bleifeld and Inglis[8] reported that 22% of their patients' wrists could be displaced palmarward because of ligamentous laxity. Dray et al.[19] reported their findings and surgical experience in 10 patients with deformities associated with SLE. Dorsal subluxation of the distal ulna was present in 14 wrists, two resulting in extensor tendon attrition rupture and four requiring excision. Various degrees of carpal instability were present in 12. The average postoperative follow-up was 62 months, with satisfactory results. Ten patients showed mild ulnar translocation of the carpus on the radius. Twelve patients demonstrated mild intercarpal dissociation; 5 of the 12 had an abnormal gap between the scaphoid and lunate. Nine patients had apparent radiographic evidence of shortening of the scaphoid, and four patients had rotation of the lunate. Severe carpal collapse was reported in six patients, two of whom had open reduction and Steinmann pin fixation. In one of these patients the deformity recurred, and the other patient was lost to follow-up. The authors concluded that most patients with SLE had some evidence of wrist involvement but that symptoms were infrequent and operative indications, therefore, limited. In cases of painful intercarpal collapse, attempts at soft-tissue reconstruction will not be adequate and arthroplasty should be considered.

SUMMARY

SLE is a systemic disease that results in arthralgia and joint instability in the majority of patients. The arthralgia responds to medical management, and because there is no destructive synovitis, synovectomies are not indicated. Instability as a result of ligamentous laxity is a problem that frequently needs to be resolved surgically when the thumb and fingers are involved but rarely with involvement of the wrist joint. Because there is a propensity for ulnar translocation of the carpus on the radius to occur, it is the authors' opinion that a Sauvé-Kapandji procedure or a limited radiocarpal arthrodesis should be performed rather than excision of the distal

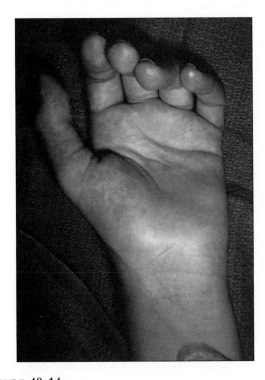

FIGURE 40-14

Juvenile systemic lupus erythematosus. Palmar erythema involving the thenar eminence, thumb, and palmar radial aspect of the hand and wrist.

Table 40-4. The 1982 Revised Criteria for Classification of Systemic Lupus Erythematosus

Criterion*	Definition
1. Malar rash	Fixed erythema, flat or raised, over the malar eminences, tending to spare the nasolabial folds.
2. Discoid rash	Erythematous raised patches with adherent keratotic scaling or follicular plugging (or both); atrophic scarring may occur in older lesions.
3. Photosensitivity	Skin rash as a result of unusual reaction to sunlight, by patient history or physician observation.
4. Oral ulcers	Oral or nasopharyngeal ulceration, usually painless, observed by a physician.
5. Arthritis	Nonerosive arthritis involving two or more peripheral joints, characterized by tenderness, swelling, or effusion.
6. Serositis	a) Pleuritis—convincing history of pleuritic pain or rub heard by a physician or evidence of pleural effusion. or b) Pericarditis—documented by electrocardiogram or rub or evidence of pericardial effusion.
7. Renal disorder	a) Persistent proteinuria greater than 0.5 g per day or greater than 3+ if quantitation not performed. or b) Cellular casts—may be red cell, hemoglobulin, granular, tabular, or mixed.
8. Neurologic disorder	a) Seizures—in the absence of offending drugs or known metabolic derangements; e.g., uremia, ketoacidosis, or electrolyte imbalance. or b) Psychosis—in the absence of offending drugs or known metabolic derangements; e.g., uremia, ketoacidosis, or electrolyte imbalance.
9. Hematologic disorder	a) Hemolytic anemia—with reticulocytosis. or b) Leukopenia—less than 4,000 leukocytes/mm^3 total on two or more occasions. or c) Lymphopenia—less than 1,500 lymphocytes/mm^3 on two or more occasions. or d) Thrombocytopenia—less than 100,000 platelets/mm^3 in the absence of offending drugs.
10. Immunologic disorder	a) Positive LE cell preparation. or b) Anti-DNA: Antibody to native DNA in abnormal titer. or c) Anti-SM: Presence of antibody to Sm nuclear antigen. or d) False-positive serologic test result for syphilis known to be positive for at least 6 months and confirmed by *Treponema pallidum* immobilization or fluorescent treponemal antibody absorption test.
11. Antinuclear antibody	An abnormal titer of antinuclear antibody by immunofluorescence or an equivalent assay at any time and in the absence of drugs known to be associated with "drug-induced lupus syndrome."

* The proposed classification is based on 11 criteria. For the purpose of identifying patients in clinical studies, a person shall be said to have systemic lupus erythematosus if any 4 or more of the 11 criteria are present, serially or simultaneously, during any interval of observation. From Rothfield NF.[50] By permission of the publisher.

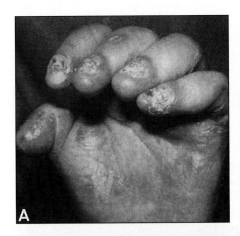
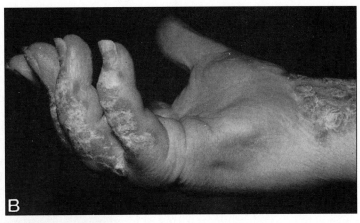
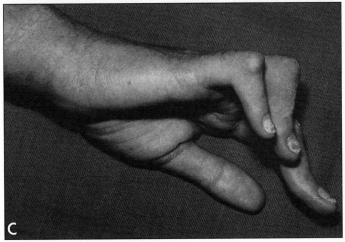

FIGURE 40-15

Psoriatic arthritis. **A** and **B,** Scales and plaques evident on the dorsal aspect of the fingers and palmar aspect of the wrist. **C,** Psoriatic arthritis produced flexion deformities of the finger proximal interphalangeal joints and hyperextension of the distal interphalangeal joints. Limited wrist motion (near ankylosis). *(From Rose JH, Belsky MR: Psoriatic arthritis in the hand,* Hand Clin *5:137-144, 1989. By permission of WB Saunders.)*

ulna for painful subluxation of the distal ulna. For severe carpal collapse with palmar subluxation, a wrist arthrodesis is the authors' preference.

PSORIATIC ARTHRITIS

The association of psoriasis with inflammatory polyarthritis was first described in 1818 by Baron Jean Alibert.[6] In 1948, with the demonstration of rheumatoid factor separating inflammatory arthritis into seropositive and seronegative subgroups and with the development of criteria for the diagnosis of rheumatoid arthritis, the concept of psoriatic arthritis as a distinct disease entity was developed.[6]

ETIOLOGY

Psoriatic arthritis is an inflammatory polyarthritis, usually seronegative,[46] that differs from rheumatoid arthritis in that the inflammation causes an intraarticular fibrosis and osteoneogenesis with final stiffness or spontaneous fusion of the joint (or both).[46,58] The exact pathologic process is somewhat confusing in the literature. The inflammatory process takes place without a predominance of hypertrophic synovitis,

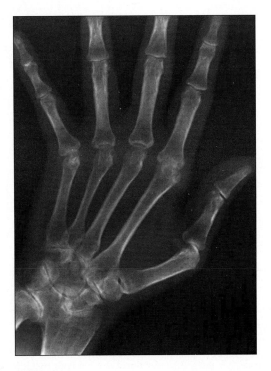

FIGURE 40-16

Acute ankylosis of the wrist in psoriatic arthritis. Fusion of proximal carpal row to the distal radius. Deformity at the distal radioulnar joint (asymptomatic).

and yet microscopically the synovium cannot be differentiated from rheumatoid synovium.[6]

The osteonecrosis has been described as subchondral by some,[5] yet by others the erosions are said to be in the bare area of joints,[45] which is the same as in rheumatoid arthritis.

DIAGNOSTIC STUDIES

Clinical Manifestations. Clinically, the patient with psoriatic arthritis presents with one of five clinical patterns.[6,46]

Group 1: Classic psoriatic arthritis with predominant involvement of the distal interphalangeal joints and nail lesions.

Group 2: Arthritis mutilans due to osteolysis of the phalanges and metacarpals.

Group 3: Symmetric polyarthritis with a predilection for bony ankylosis of the proximal and distal interphalangeal joints.

Group 4: Oligoarticular arthritis with asymmetrical involvement of the distal and proximal interphalangeal and metacarpophalangeal joints and at times a flexor tenosynovitis producing the "sausage digit."

Group 5: Sacroiliitis and spondylitis associated with psoriatic arthritis.

Although skin lesions usually precede arthritic involvement (Fig. 40-15), in some patients arthritic symptoms occur first, making early diagnosis difficult. In the series by Leonard et al.[41] of 30 patients with psoriatic arthritis, the initial diagnosis was incorrect in two-thirds of the patients. Nail dystrophy in some form occurs in 80% of the patients with psoriatic arthritis (Fig. 40-15, *A*).[56] There are no laboratory tests

A

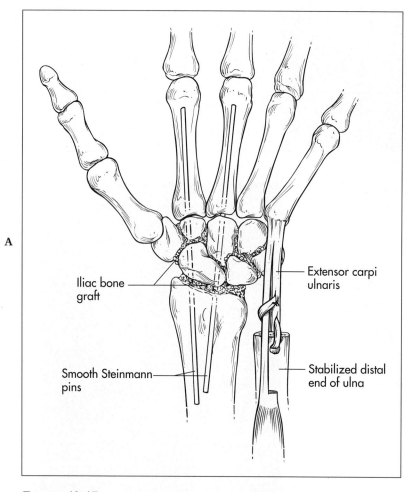

Iliac bone graft

Extensor carpi ulnaris

Smooth Steinmann pins

Stabilized distal end of ulna

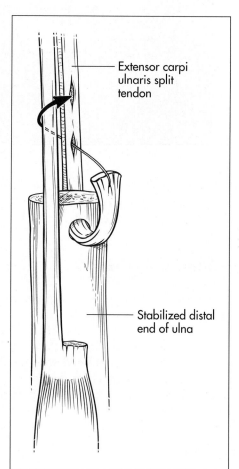

B

Extensor carpi ulnaris split tendon

Stabilized distal end of ulna

FIGURE 40-17

Fusion of the wrist with excision of the distal ulna. **A,** Fusion of the wrist is performed with resection of the joint articular cartilage, cancellous bone graft, and internal fixation with two intramedullary Steinmann pins. The distal ulna is stabilized by using one-half of the extensor carpi ulnaris tendon placed through the distal ulna. **B,** View of the technique for interweaving the ulnar half of the extensor carpi ulnaris through the distal end of the resected ulna and back through and around the radial half of the extensor carpi ulnaris and back again within the tendon itself.

that aid in the diagnosis of psoriatic arthritis. An increased erythrocyte sedimentation rate, anemia, and transient leukocytosis may be present.[6] Belsky et al.,[5] in reviewing 50 wrists in 25 patients with psoriatic arthritis, reported that 16 patients had minimal or no wrist involvement, whereas 33 had moderate or severe wrist involvement, 17 of whom had spontaneous fusion (Figs. 40-15, C and 40-16). No palmar subluxation of the carpus occurred in any of these patients. In this series, 26 wrists became progressively stiff in a satisfactory functional position without pain. Only eight surgical procedures were performed: arthroplasties, osteotomies, fusions, and ulnar resections. Blair and Kilpatrick[7] treated a severe wrist flexion contracture with proximal row carpectomy, but the wrist fused spontaneously postoperatively.

Belsky et al.[5] found a higher incidence of postoperative infection in psoriatic arthritic patients than in rheumatoid patients and suggested that patients with significant skin involvement be hospitalized several days before operation for dermatologic management. This is in contrast to Lynfield et al.[42] who stated that psoriatic skin plaques rapidly pick up hospital pathogens and elective surgery should be done soon after hospital admission. They demonstrated that standard presurgical skin preparation can sterilize psoriatic plaques and the psoriatic sites heal as fast as normal skin.

Radiologic Findings. The radiologic findings vary according to the amount of joint destruction. They can be minimal, with periarticular reactive bone formation, or they can demonstrate severe destruction, with marked bone erosions, spontaneous fusions, and proximal row collapse.[5,45]

SURGICAL TREATMENT

Surgical treatment of the psoriatic wrist may be necessary occasionally, although it is not the primary

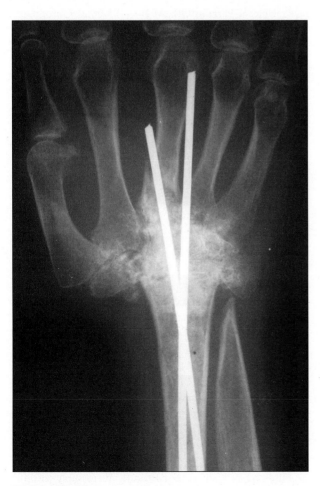

FIGURE 40-18

Fusion of a wrist with psoriatic arthritis. The two Steinmann pins have a "clothespin" grasp on the base of the third metacarpal, resisting rotation of the wrist.

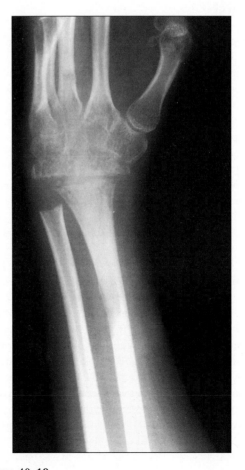

FIGURE 40-19

Psoriatic arthritis. Subsidence of a silicone implant within the intramedullary canal of the distal radius. Note bone-bone contact. Fusion is recommended for the psoriatic wrist. (*Courtesy of Dr. Donald Ferbe.*)

site for the disease, and when it does affect the wrist, spontaneous fusion usually occurs. The wrist should be splinted in a functional position. If the wrist is painful despite splints, formal radiocarpal fusion is recommended (Fig. 40-17), either alone or with excising the distal ulna. Techniques of fusion may vary, but Carroll and Dick[14] have had excellent success with a dorsal inlay graft whereas others prefer Steinmann pins, Rush rods, tension band wiring, and cancellous grafts (Fig. 40-18). In the younger patient, an internal fixation plate (fusion or reconstruction plate) can be used along with cancellous bone grafts. Silicone joint replacement is contraindicated in the wrist with destructive changes from psoriatic arthritis (Fig. 40-19). Our preference is the inlay graft technique in which a sliding graft from the distal radius is placed distally over the carpus and held in place with a tension band figure-of-eight technique (see Chapter 38).

SUMMARY

Psoriatic arthritis is a variant of rheumatoid arthritis that can affect the wrist. The inflammatory synovitis can occur before the development of skin conditions. Joint space narrowing can occur to the significant degree of requiring surgical intervention. Joint fusion is the treatment of choice; synovectomy is not indicated in psoriatic arthritis.

REFERENCES

1. Aegerter EE, Kirkpatrick JA Jr: *Orthopedic diseases,* ed 4, Philadelphia, 1975, WB Saunders, p 167.
2. Anonymous: Criteria for the classification of juvenile rheumatoid arthritis, *Bull Rheum Dis* 23:712-719, 1972.
3. Ansell BM: Juvenile chronic arthritis, juvenile rheumatoid arthritis, and inflammatory arthropathies of childhood, *Curr Opin Rheumatol* 2:799-803, 1990.
4. Ansell BM, Kent PA: Radiological changes in juvenile chronic polyarthritis, *Skel Radiol* 1:129-144, 1977.
5. Belsky MR, Feldon P, Millender LH, et al.: Hand involvement in psoriatic arthritis, *J Hand Surg [Am]* 7:203-207, 1982.
6. Bennett RM: *Psoriatic arthritis.* In McCarty DJ, editors: *Arthritis and allied conditions: a textbook of rheumatology,* ed 11, Philadelphia, 1989, Lea & Febiger, pp 954-971.
7. Blair WF, Kilpatrick WC Jr: Proximal row carpectomy: an unusual indication, *Clin Orthop* 153:223-225, 1980.
8. Bleifeld CJ, Inglis AE: The hand in systemic lupus erythematosus, *J Bone Joint Surg Am* 56:1207-1215, 1974.
9. Brewer EJ Jr, Bass J, Baum J, et al.: Current proposed revision of JRA criteria. JRA Criteria Subcommittee of the Diagnostic and Therapeutic Criteria Committee of the American Rheumatism Section of The Arthritis Foundation, *Arthritis Rheum* 20(suppl 2):195-199, 1977.
10. Bywaters EG, Ansell BM: Monoarticular arthritis in children, *Ann Rheum Dis* 24:116-122, 1965.
11. Calabro JJ: *Juvenile rheumatoid arthritis.* In McCarty DJ, editors: *Arthritis and allied conditions: a textbook of rheumatology,* ed 11, Philadelphia, 1989, Lea & Febiger, pp 913-925.
12. Calabro JJ, Holgerson WB, Sonpal GM, et al.: Juvenile rheumatoid arthritis: a general review and report of 100 patients observed for 15 years, *Semin Arthritis Rheum* 5:257-298, 1976.
13. Calabro JJ, Parrino GR, Atchoo PD, et al.: Chronic iridocyclitis in juvenile rheumatoid arthritis, *Arthritis Rheum* 13:406-413, 1970.
14. Carroll RE, Dick HM: Arthrodesis of the wrist for rheumatoid arthritis, *J Bone Joint Surg Am* 53:1365-1369, 1971.
15. Cassidy JT, Brody GL, Martel W: Monarticular juvenile rheumatoid arthritis, *J Pediatr* 70:867-875, 1967.
16. Cassidy JT, Levinson JE, Brewer EJ Jr: The development of classification criteria for children with juvenile rheumatoid arthritis, *Bull Rheum Dis* 38:1-7, 1989.
17. Chaplin D, Pulkki T, Saarimaa A, et al.: Wrist and finger deformities in juvenile rheumatoid arthritis, *Acta Rheumatol Scand* 15:206-223, 1969.
18. Cornil V: Memoire sur les coincidence patholoqiqies du rhumatisme articulaive chronique, *C R Soc Biol (Paris)* 4:2-25, 1864.
19. Dray GJ, Millender LH, Nalebuff EA, et al.: The surgical treatment of hand deformities in systemic lupus erythematosus, *J Hand Surg [Am]* 6:339-345, 1981.
20. Evans DM, Ansell BM, Hall MA: The wrist in juvenile arthritis, *J Hand Surg [Br]* 16:293-304, 1991.
21. Eyring EJ, Longert A, Bass JC: Synovectomy in juvenile rheumatoid arthritis. Indications and short-term results, *J Bone Joint Surg Am* 53:638-651, 1971.
22. Fessel WJ: Systemic lupus erythematosus in the community. Incidence, prevalence, outcome, and first symptoms; the high prevalence in black women, *Arch Intern Med* 134:1027-1035, 1974.
23. Findley TW, Halpern D, Easton JK: Wrist subluxation in juvenile rheumatoid arthritis: pathophysiology and management, *Arch Phys Med Rehabil* 64:69-74, 1983.
24. Fink CW, Baum J, Paradies LH, et al.: Synovectomy in juvenile rheumatoid arthritis, *Ann Rheum Dis* 28:612-616, 1969.

25. Fischman AS, Abeles M, Zanetti M, et al.: The coexistence of rheumatoid arthritis and systemic lupus erythematosus: a case report and review of the literature, *J Rheumatol* 8:405-415, 1981.

26. Granberry WM, Brewer EJ Jr: Results of synovectomy in children with rheumatoid arthritis, *Clin Orthop* 101:120-126, 1974.

27. Granberry WM, Mangum GL: The hand in the child with juvenile rheumatoid arthritis, *J Hand Surg [Am]* 5:105-113, 1980.

28. Green N, Osmer JC: Small bone changes secondary to systemic lupus erythematosus, *Radiology* 90:118-120, 1968.

29. Griffin PP, Tachdjian MO, Green WT: Pauciarticular arthritis in children, *JAMA* 184:23-28, 1963.

30. Gristina AG, Kelsey WM, Green DL, et al.: Pauciarticular juvenile arthritis, *South Med J* 69:440-441, 1976.

31. Hafner R, Poznanski AK, Donovan JM: Ulnar variance in children—standard measurements for evaluation of ulnar shortening in juvenile rheumatoid arthritis, hereditary multiple exostosis and other bone or joint disorders in childhood, *Skel Radiol* 18:513-516, 1989.

32. Hargraves MM, Richmond H, Morton R: Presentation of two bone marrow elements: the "tart" cell and the "L.E." cell, *Proc Staff Meet Mayo Clin* 23:25-28, 1948.

33. Harrison SH: *Wrist and hand problems and their management.* In Arden GP, Ansell BM, editors: *Surgical management of juvenile chronic polyarthritis,* New York, 1978, Grune & Stratton, p 161.

34. Hastings DE, Evans JA: The lupus hand: a new surgical approach, *J Hand Surg [Am]* 3:179-183, 1978.

35. Jacobsen ST, Levinson JE, Crawford AH: Late results of synovectomy in juvenile rheumatoid arthritis, *J Bone Joint Surg Am* 67:8-15, 1985.

36. Jungers P, Dougados M, Pelissier C, et al.: Influence of oral contraceptive therapy on the activity of systemic lupus erythematosus, *Arthritis Rheum* 25:618-623, 1982.

37. Kampner SL, Ferguson AB Jr: Efficacy of synovectomy in juvenile rheumatoid arthritis, *Clin Orthop* 88:94-109, 1972.

38. Kaposi MK: Neue beitrage zur kenntniss des lupus erythematosus, *Arch Dermatol Syph* 48:36-78, 1872.

39. Labowitz R, Schumacher HR Jr: Articular manifestations of systemic lupus erythematosus, *Ann Intern Med* 74:911-921, 1971.

40. Lahita RG, Bradlow HL, Kunkel HG, et al.: Increased 16 alpha-hydroxylation of estradiol in systemic lupus erythematosus, *J Clin Endocrinol Metab* 53:174-178, 1981.

41. Leonard DG, O'Duffy JD, Rogers RS: Prospective analysis of psoriatic arthritis in patients hospitalized for psoriasis, *Mayo Clin Proc* 53:511-518, 1978.

42. Lynfield YL, Ostroff G, Abraham J: Bacteria, skin sterilization, and wound healing in psoriasis, *NY State J Med* 72:1247-1250, 1972.

43. Maldonado-Cocco JA, Garcia-Morteo O, Spindler AJ, et al.: Carpal ankylosis in juvenile rheumatoid arthritis, *Arthritis Rheum* 23:1251-1255, 1980.

44. Martel W, Holt JF, Cassidy JT: Roentgenologic manifestations of juvenile rheumatoid arthritis, *Am J Roentgenol* 88:400-423, 1962.

45. Martel W, Stuck KJ, Dworin AM, et al.: Erosive osteoarthritis and psoriatic arthritis: a radiologic comparison in the hand, wrist, and foot, *AJR* 134:125-135, 1980.

46. Moll JM, Wright V: Psoriatic arthritis, *Semin Arthritis Rheum* 3:55-78, 1973.

47. Nalebuff EA, Feldon PG, Millender LH: *Rheumatoid arthritis in the hand and wrist.* In Green DP, editor: *Operative hand surgery,* ed 2, vol 3, New York, 1988, Churchill Livingstone, pp 1655-1766.

48. Nalebuff EA, Yerid G, Millender L: The incidence and severity of wrist involvement in juvenile rheumatoid arthritis (abstract), *J Bone Joint Surg Am* 54:905, 1972.

49. Osler W: On the visceral complications of erythema exudativum multiforme, *Am J Med Sci* 110:629-646, 1895.

50. Rothfield NF: *Systemic lupus erythematosus: clinical aspects and treatment.* In McCarty JD, editor: *Arthritis and allied conditions: a textbook of rheumatology,* ed 11, Philadelphia, 1989, Lea & Febiger, pp 1022-1048.

51. Rowland SA: Stabilization of the ulnar side of the rheumatoid wrist, following radiocarpal Swanson's implant arthroplasty and resection of the distal ulna, *Bull Hosp Jt Dis Orthop Inst* 44:442-448, 1984.

52. Schaller J, Wedgwood RJ: Juvenile rheumatoid arthritis: a review, *Pediatrics* 50:940-953, 1972.

53. Simmons BP, Nutting JT: Juvenile rheumatoid arthritis, *Hand Clin* 5:157-168, 1989.

54. Still GF: On a form of chronic joint disease in children, *Proc Roy M Chir Soc Lond* 9:10-15, 1896-1897.

55. Urman JD, Abeles M, Houghton AN, et al.: Aseptic necrosis presenting as wrist pain in SLE, *Arthritis Rheum* 20:825-828, 1977.

56. Vanio K, Oka M: Ulnar deviation of the fingers, *Ann Rheum Dis* 12:122-124, 1963.

57. Weinberger A, Evans D, Ansell BM: Wrist involvement in juvenile chronic arthritis five years after onset of disease, *Isr J Med Sci* 18:653-654, 1982.

58. Wright V: Psoriatic arthritis: a comparative study of rheumatoid arthritis, psoriasis, and arthritis associated with psoriasis, *Arch Dermatol* 80:27-35, 1959.

XI

DEVELOPMENTAL DISORDERS

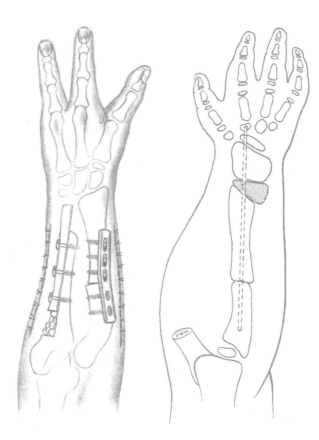

41

MADELUNG'S DEFORMITY

David Vickers, M.B.B.S.

ETIOLOGY AND CLINICAL APPEARANCE
PATHOLOGY AND NATURAL HISTORY
CLINICAL MANIFESTATIONS
MANAGEMENT
    PREFERRED TREATMENT
    SURGICAL TECHNIQUE

DISCUSSION AND CLINICAL EXAMPLES
ESTABLISHED LATE MADELUNG'S DEFORMITY
    PREFERRED APPROACH
    TECHNIQUE
SUMMARY

ETIOLOGY AND CLINICAL APPEARANCE

Madelung's deformity, a classic deformity at the wrist, is the result of dysplasia of bone and soft tissues. In 1878, before x-rays were discovered, Madelung, without any knowledge of its etiology, gave an elegant clinical description of the spontaneous subluxation of the hand that now bears his name.[7] In 1929 Léri and Weill[6] described a familial deformity at the wrist termed "dyschondrosteosis," and subsequently Langer[5] proposed that Madelung's disease and the familial variety were the same condition. The gene is dominant with incomplete penetrance. Sporadic cases occur less frequently. In overt Madelung's deformity (Fig. 41-1), the general appearance is the reverse of the silver (dinner) fork deformity of Colles' fracture. The head of the ulna is prominent dorsoulnarly because the hand has displaced radiopalmarly with the tilting and bowing of the distal radius. There is a variable degree of shortening of the forearm. An unequal deformity of both wrists is usual, and the condition is more common in females. A further manifestation of the familial dysplasia is sometimes seen in a generalized hypoplasia of the radius and mesomelic dwarfism.

Reverse Madelung's deformity (Fig. 41-2) is similar to the silver (dinner) fork deformity of a distal radius fracture. The head of the ulna is palmar with the wrist arched dorsally. Madelung's deformity and reverse Madelung's deformity have been observed to coexist in opposite wrists of the same patient and in twins. A similar deformity at the wrist can follow fracture, repetitive injury from gymnastics, sepsis, or osteochondroma, but these are not the conditions referred to by Madelung. Madelung's deformity may be a feature of various syndromes, but these cases are quite rare.

PATHOLOGY AND NATURAL HISTORY

"Bony" (epiphyseal and physeal) and soft-tissue anomalies have been described that are responsible for Madelung's deformity.[10] The bony lesion termed "dyschondrosteosis" is a dysplasia that histologically resembles achondroplasia. Langenskiöld et al.[4] verified the theory of Ranvier that the cells of the cambium layer of the periosteum progressively stream from the periphery of the physis at the zone of Ranvier. They suggested that disorders of this process might be a factor in the pathogenesis of osteochondroma, enchondroma, achondroplasia, and dyschondrosteosis.

In the most extreme case, there is generalized hypoplasia of the whole radius with underdevelopment of the radial head as well as the wrist deformity. In some cases, the radius is markedly bowed, indicating early aberrant growth. In very young children, however, the forearm appears normal; the only sign of disease is a

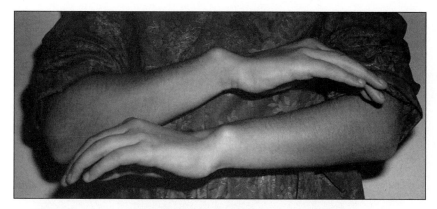

FIGURE 41-1

Advanced painful Madelung's deformity in an 11-year-old girl. Dorsal prominent distal ulna; supinated carpus.

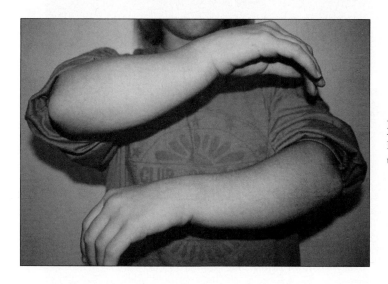

FIGURE 41-2

Reverse Madelung's deformity. Extension deformity of the wrist. Palmar prominent distal ulna.

change in the radiologic appearance of the distal radius. About midway through childhood, a localized lesion in the ulnopalmar zone of the distal radius becomes more apparent and causes a distortion of growth. The bony lesion acts as a tether to growth, pulling the radial epiphysis off line as the remaining normal physis proliferates. The physeal lesion is always located in the ulnar zone of the distal radius, but its focus varies in the anteroposterior plane (Fig. 41-3). In classic Madelung's deformity, the lesion is essentially palmar. Meanwhile the ulna grows straight. The ulnar head then becomes prominent as the hand drops away, with signs of radial deformity appearing at the wrist. In a reverse Madelung's deformity, the lesion is essentially dorsal. All degrees of variation between these two extremes occur. The deformity that results from a bony lesion midway between the two is sufficiently specific to deserve a separate title and has been termed "chevron carpus."[10] In a pure example of this lesion, clinical deformity is not apparent but the radiograph shows triangulation of the carpus wedged between the radius and ulna.

In all dyschondrosteosis lesions, the radiograph reveals a paucity of growth in the affected area. Over a period of years a conical lucent zone develops, the apex of which dates the onset of the dysplasia. The ulnar zone

of the distal radius "trails" in the anteroposterior radiograph, often terminating in a groove and bony spike where the metaphysis joins the diaphysis (Fig. 41-4). Nielsen and I[10] believe that this groove and spike are evidence of an abnormal ligamentous tether—the radiolunate ligament—that is attached to the proximal pole of the lunate (the apex of a chevron carpus) and the radial groove. This structure is histologically a ligament, frequently more than 5 mm in diameter, and very strong (Fig. 41-5). It is always a palmar structure, unlike the bony dysplastic lesion which can vary its location in the anteroposterior plane. The bony lesion determines the direction of tilt of the radial epiphysis, whereas the ligament tethers the carpus, resisting normal carpal migration with growth. The radial attachment of the triangular fibrocartilage complex also fails to advance, so instead of this structure having a transverse direction it becomes quite oblique.

CLINICAL MANIFESTATIONS

The three main reasons for consultation in the patient with Madelung's deformity have been pain, deformity, and more recently the monitoring of children of an

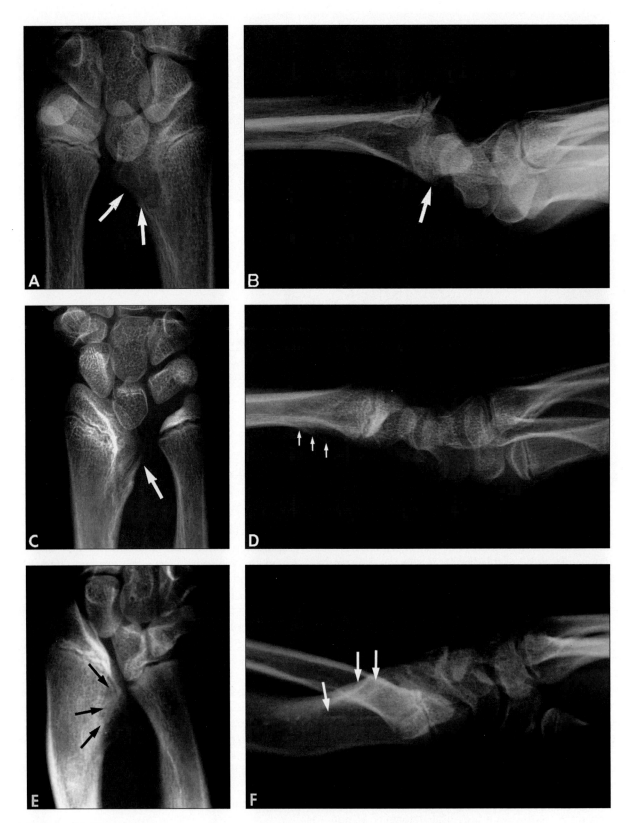

FIGURE 41-3

A and **B,** Madelung's deformity after ulnar palmar dyschondrosteosis of the radius. The clear zone in the metaphysis is palmar. A radiolunate ligament (metaphyseal groove and spike) (*arrows*) is present. **C** and **D,** Chevron carpus. The dyschondrosteosis lesion is in the midulnar zone. A radiolunate ligament is present (note metaphyseal bone spike) (*arrows*). **E** and **F,** Reverse Madelung's deformity. An ulnar dorsal lesion is accompanied by a dorsal clear zone in the metaphysis (*arrows*). Evidence of a radiolunate ligament is present (note palmar displacement of distal ulna).

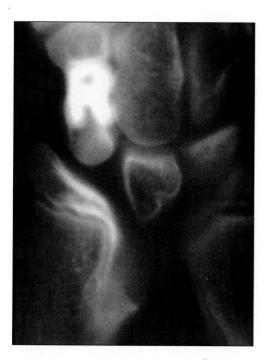

FIGURE 41-4

This tomogram of advanced dyschondrosteosis exhibits total lack of support for the lunate because the physis has "turned the corner" and is left behind. The metaphyseal groove and spike are evidence of a radiolunate ligament attachment at the site of growth retardation.

affected parent. Patients treated up to 17 years ago are now bringing their children at a young age because they are aware of the natural inheritance of Madelung's deformity. Colleagues now are also informed regarding early referral.

There is no general agreement about the origin of *pain* or its significance in management of Madelung's deformity. Previous authors[1,5,6] have regarded pain as intermittent and of only moderate severity usually insufficient to warrant surgery. This opinion was reasonable when salvage surgery after maturity was the only available treatment. Now the opportunity to intervene during childhood and eliminate the deforming process has significantly changed the indications for surgery. Moderate pain and deformity are sufficient indications now for patient and parents to request surgical treatment during childhood.

Pain may originate from distortion of the distal radioulnar joint or from deformity at the radiocarpal or midcarpal joints. Pain can be the result of impaction or abrasion of joint surfaces or of ligament or capsular fatigue. The distal radioulnar joint is malformed and unstable but may only come in contact with the carpus at the extremes of rotation, especially supination. The wrist joint is malformed and unstable and the carpus assumes a triangular appearance. In the most extreme

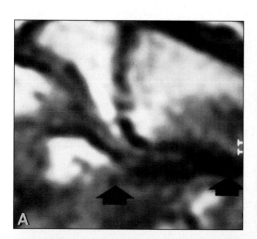

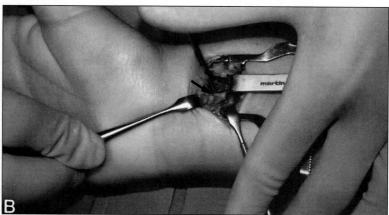

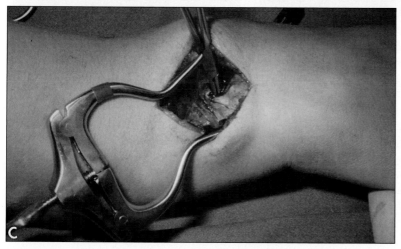

FIGURE 41-5

A, Magnetic resonance image clearly demonstrates the thick ligament linking the lunate well proximal to the radial physis (*between arrows*).
B, The radiolunate ligament is a palmar structure streaming from the proximal pole of the lunate to the radius well proximal to the wrist (palmar approach to the distal radius) (*arrow*).
C, Dorsal approach to reverse Madelung's deformity. The radiolunate ligament still occupies a palmar location (end of needle holder).

examples of Madelung's and reverse Madelung's deformity, the wrist joint is subluxed. Impaction of carpal bones against the radius or ulna is unlikely, except at the extremes of motion. Deformity of the carpal bones and the distal radius restricts the usual kinematic behavior of the joint. Ligament and capsular fatigue arise from instability. Fagg[1] mentioned the importance of the soft tissues as a source of pain in the younger patient but noted that there was no correlation between the severity of symptoms and the radiologic appearance. The midcarpal joint is also involved because of the triangular development of the carpal bones. The chevron carpus is in a different category, as the lunate fixed by the radiolunate ligament is trapped between the radius and ulna. The bony anomaly becomes a fossa for the lunate and impaction is maximum in this variety of wrist dysplasia. The lunate is incapable of motion when the wrist is flexed or extended, requiring this motion to occur at a more distal level within the midcarpal joint.

The *deformity* or appearance of the wrist is quite variable and clearly depends on the underlying pathology (Fig. 41-3). The shortness of the forearm likewise is variable. At the end stage of Madelung's deformity, the distal radius has turned in an ulnar and palmar direction, taking the hand with it, while the ulna has proceeded straight to become prominent dorsoulnarly. The hand otherwise normally rotates into a slightly supinated position relative to the forearm beneath the ulnar head (Fig. 41-1).

The *ranges of motion* are decreased in all directions except the direction of the deformity. The loss of supination is often the most significant functional problem.

MANAGEMENT

There has been argument in the past regarding indications for and efficacy of osteotomy in Madelung's deformity. At least one group of surgeons has stated that salvage surgery is rarely justifiable.[12] But my experience and that of others[8] suggest that this opinion is incorrect. In previous reviews on the subject, reverse Madelung's deformity was not mentioned and the intermediate chevron carpus was not recognized. Osteotomy can improve the profile of the wrist, but scarring is quite visible and functional gain may be small. This is a difficult procedure that requires correction of the palmar and ulnar tilt of the radius, rotation, malalignment, and radioulna variance. Shortness of the radius can be minimized by an open wedge osteotomy, as advocated by Murphy et al.[8] This procedure has the further advantage of a palmar approach, which is more cosmetic. The most recent approach to salvage surgery is a gradual distraction and realignment technique, which may be superior but is still being evaluated.

PREFERRED TREATMENT

I believe the best opportunity to control all varieties of deformity at the wrist secondary to distal radial dyschondrosteosis is to intervene during childhood. Excision of the bony and soft-tissue tethers (physiolysis) prevents further deformity as the bones grow and may result in general functional and cosmetic improvement. There is significant reduction in pain and improved range of motion.[10] Ideally, this should be performed early before the deformity is unacceptable. Even in late presentations with only a few years of growth remaining, physiolysis will produce a worthwhile benefit. Osteotomy in adulthood may be avoidable if the results of early surgery are successful. Although the deforming process is still reversible in advanced dysplasia, early surgery is advised because there is only a limited capacity for correction to occur or for the process to be corrected in the remaining years of growth. Another advantage of growth restoration is allowance for joint surfaces to remodel. This is not possible following an osteotomy after skeletal maturity. The radioulnar joint is rarely involved enough in this disease to exhibit significant change after growth restoration; however, the radioulna variance improves.

The procedure to resect a bone bridge formed prematurely across the physis, and its replacement with fat graft, has been named "physiolysis." Some centers use the term "epiphysiolysis" for the same procedure, but this term has various meanings. Other interposition materials, especially cranioplast, have been used in a large number of traumatic cases.[9] The author favors the use of fat, as recommended by Langenskiöld.[3]

SURGICAL TECHNIQUE

The operative procedure is performed during general anesthesia in a bloodless field. The principle of physeal surgery is to remove the bone lesion (or block) connecting the epiphysis across the physis to the metaphysis. In classic Madelung's deformity, a palmar approach is made through a transverse incision 1 to 2 cm proximal to the most proximal wrist crease. The approach then passes on either side of the flexor carpi radialis (whichever seems the more direct approach) and radial to the digital flexor tendons, which are displaced ulnarly to expose the pronator quadratus muscle. The median nerve and radial artery should be protected, especially from self-retaining retractors. The distal edge of the pronator quadratus is reflected sufficiently for the palmar surface of the distal radius to be exposed. With passive motion of the wrist and palpation of the region of the radiocarpal joint, one can usually determine the level of the joint. When there is clinical, radiologic, or magnetic resonance imaging evidence of a radiolunate ligament, the lunate may be fixed and can be confused with the distal radius. At this time the radiolunate ligament can be sought and excised, or this step can be taken after the osteotomy is performed.

A longitudinal osteotomy directing the osteotome from proximal to distal is done in the metaphyseal region of the distal radius about 5 mm into the bone from the radioulnar joint (Fig. 41-6). In cases of advanced deformity, the lunate is overlying the radius and is fixed. There is a possibility that it can be mistaken for the distal radius and cut with an osteotome. Care must be taken to avoid this injury to the lunate. Imaging is suggested. After the longitudinal radial osteotomy is performed, the small piece of the ulnar zone which is still attached by soft tissues is turned aside with the osteotome and the cavity between the two components of the radius is inspected. The small piece of radius (ulnar metaphyseal portion) that is reflected should be retained if possible. The wrist joint is not widely opened, if at all. One now inspects the cut edge of the radius for some evidence of physeal tissue. Because the physis "turns the corner" and runs more longitudinally

in dyschondrosteosis, it is sometimes difficult to locate. If the first osteotomy cut is too shallow, one might see only a sheet of white tissue, which may be physis or abnormal fibrous tissue. In this case, a further osteotomy is done a few millimeters more radial, and the wafer of bone thus produced is removed. One then inspects the radius again, and often in the more distal portion physeal tissue becomes apparent. More bone is removed then from the metaphysis to further define the physeal line. A small gouge is useful for taking away larger pieces of bone, but this is replaced by a motorized bur to do the final definition of the physeal line.

In physeal surgery of the distal radius, magnification with an operating loupe or operating microscope is recommended and experience with or knowledge of physeal surgery is essential. At the end of the dissection, one should observe that the cartilage of the physis is continuous from the dorsal periosteum to the palmar periosteum, with no untidy margins. The tourniquet is now deflated to allow hemostasis after some minutes of elevation. Persistent bleeding points may be sealed with

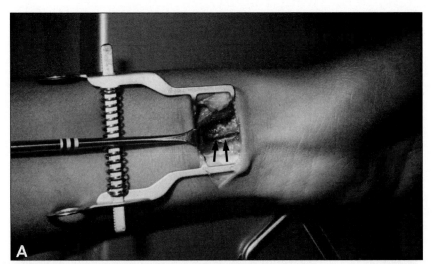

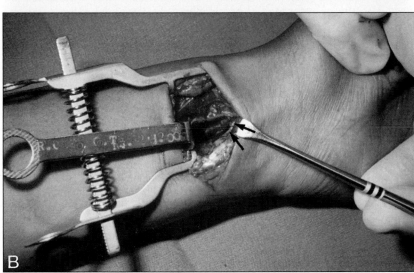

FIGURE 41-6

A, Palmar transverse incision, with flexor carpi radialis and digital flexors retracted to the ulnar side. The flat surface of radius is visible in the floor of the wound after reflection of the pronator quadratus. The initial longitudinal osteotomy has been performed and is visible opposite the retractor (banded) (*arrows*). **B,** At the completion of the resection of abnormal bone, the wavy physeal line (*arrows*) is visible in the depth of the cavity, running obliquely up to the palmar cortex distally.

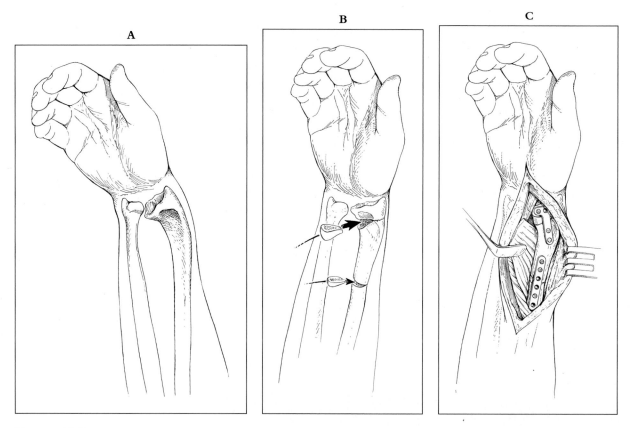

FIGURE 41-7

Corrective open wedge osteotomy. **A,** Ulnopalmar bowing with shortening of the distal radius. Dorsolateral subluxation, ulnar head. **B,** Oblique osteotomy under lunate fossa compartment of epiphysis carried to physis beneath scaphoid fossa, then wedged open to accept a trapezoidal bone graft. Further correction of curvature and length by a more proximal osteotomy. **C,** Small T plates may be used to fix graft distally and a stronger cortical plate, proximally.

small quantities of bone wax. After hemostasis has been achieved, the tourniquet is reinflated and a generous piece of fat is obtained from the ulnar aspect of the proximal forearm. The surgical cavity in the radius is washed out with isotonic saline and the fat is immediately inserted to completely fill the cavity. It is most important that the fat make intimate contact with the physeal tissue. The best way to achieve this objective is to use a slightly oversized piece of fat that is held in place after the release of retraction by the flexor tendons. It has usually been unnecessary to use sutures to stabilize the fat. After skin closure, a short arm plaster splint is applied palmarly to assist in stabilization of the fat graft and to improve comfort. The splint is removed at approximately 2 weeks.

In the older patient or one with little remaining growth potential, the osteotomized epiphysis, which also represents the lunate fossa, may be elevated and a wedge-shaped bone graft inserted. Additional correction may also be achieved with a secondary open wedge osteotomy more proximally (Fig. 41-7).

In *reverse Madelung's deformity* the principles of the procedure are the same; however, a dorsal longitudinal incision is used because the bony lesion is dorsally located in the ulnar zone of the distal radius. The incision extends proximally from Lister's tubercle for 6 cm. A limited incision is made in the extensor retinaculum, and the approach then passes between the extensor pollicis longus and the wrist extensors. Longitudinal osteotomies in the radius are made on the ulnar side through the metaphysis of the distal radius, and the physis is located. Metaphyseal bone is removed as the physis becomes prominent in the floor of the cavity. If the radiolunate ligament is present and can be clearly observed, it is excised. Because it is a palmar structure even in reverse Madelung's deformity, it is usually visualized only after the osteotomy has been performed. Once again a generous fat graft is inserted into the surgical cavity, and in these cases the extensor retinaculum and the extensor pollicis longus tendon are used to stabilize the fat graft.

In the case of *chevron carpus* where there is little bony deformity, or after maturity when one is not planning an osteotomy and restoration of growth is not a possibility, a simple excision of the palmar radiolunate ligament is performed to relieve pain. A transverse palmar incision is used, but this is usually at a slightly more distal level than that of the classic Madelung's deformity in the child requiring a physiolysis. Once again, the approach passes ulnar to the flexor carpi radialis and radial to the digital flexor tendons, with care taken not to exert pressure on the median nerve. After the palmar surface of the distal radius is located, the lunate is palpated. It may be quite prominent and fixed, even when the hand is moved. If the capsule of the wrist joint is incised on either side of the prominence, one can then be certain that this is the lunate. The palmar radiolunate ligament is easily identified extending from the lunate to the metaphyseal region of the radius. This ligament should not be confused with the abnormal obliquely oriented triangular fibrocartilage, which is not attached to the lunate. The ligament is detached from the proximal pole of the lunate and a reasonable length is excised. It is not necessary to excise the whole ligament. No fat graft is required in these cases. After excision of the ligament, lunate compression is relieved. One can see into the radiocarpal joint, and by moving the hand one can observe that proper motion has been restored in the radiocarpal joint. The wound is closed as before. Splintage is not mandatory.

DISCUSSION AND CLINICAL EXAMPLES

Since 1979, I have performed the physiolysis procedure on 31 wrists (22 patients). All of these patients are now mature. Excision of the radiolunate ligament alone for painful chevron carpus after maturity has been performed on four wrists. A preliminary report was made in 1980[11] and a more detailed analysis presented in 1992.[10] There have been no poor outcomes or any dissatisfied patients or relatives. Early in the series some patients requested a physiolysis procedure on the lesser affected wrist, but frequently this request was denied because at the time the physiolysis procedure was still under evaluation. One temporary median nerve palsy from retraction recovered quickly, and in one case the lunate was mistaken for the distal radius and partly osteotomized, fortunately with no ill effect. No patient who presented early has required an osteotomy after the physiolysis procedure.

In advanced dyschondrosteosis causing any variety of Madelung's deformity, a normal wrist is not possible with any surgical treatment. This situation, as illustrated in Figure 41-4, exhibits such a large defect that even growth restoration cannot possibly fill this void or correct the substantial angular deformity. Two patients who presented late with advanced deformity (Figs. 41-1 and 41-2) achieved some benefit from the physiolysis procedure but still required osteotomy. One other patient with total radial dysplasia and incomplete response to physiolysis was offered a fusion at the distal radioulnar joint (Sauvé-Kapandji procedure) but declined. Excision of the prominent ulnar head is not recommended. After surgical treatment, all patients

experienced significantly less pain and some were completely pain free. Denervation might be an incidental factor, but it was not an objective of the procedure. The anterior and posterior interosseous nerves were not selectively observed or dissected during the procedure. All patients had an increased range of motion, especially in supination—in one case an increase of 70° (Fig. 41-8). The stability of the distal radioulnar joint appears to be unaffected by the operation.

In cases of generalized radial dysplasia, the head of the radius is hypoplastic and bowing of the radius is evidence of long-standing asymmetric growth; the ulna hypertrophies to take more of the load at the wrist. To a degree, this situation can be reversed if growth is restored in the distal radius with a physiolysis procedure (Fig. 41-9).

The hallmark of the *chevron carpus* is pain, which is frequent and quite disabling. A constant feeling of "tension" in the wrist is described. An example is the case of a 20-year-old woman who consulted several orthopedic surgeons for wrist pain. She had become emotionally disturbed because nobody believed her complaint was significant. After an excision of the palmar radiolunate ligament, her pain and feeling of tension immediately ceased and have not returned. Her family reports that her personality has been transformed. A patient not treated (Fig. 41-10, *B*) appears to represent the end result of a lifetime affliction with a painful chevron carpus. We believe that this late deformity may be preventable.

The prophylactic potential of physiolysis if performed early enough is demonstrated by two 12-year-old girls with a similar family history and similar radiographs who had quite different outcomes (Fig. 41-11). The patient treated with physiolysis had no more pain and her clinical deformity decreased. No osteotomy or other treatment has been necessary. The wrist of the second girl (Figs. 41-11, *D* through *F*) continued to deteriorate with further growth, necessitating a radial osteotomy and ulna shortening. Her wrist remains painful.

The most exciting and challenging decision regarding prophylaxis is when to perform physiolysis in a child with the potential to develop Madelung's deformity. The children of parents with Madelung's deformity are now presenting for assessment. Because the gene is dominant with incomplete penetrance, it is likely that some children in the family, especially females, will be affected. Radiographs provide the earliest evidence of the malady (Fig. 41-12). The radial epiphysis assumes a "teardrop" shape because the ulnar component is slow to develop. Truncation of the ulnar metaphysis of the radius becomes progressively more evident with growth and subsequent radiographic examination. The development of the carpus is delayed to a lesser extent than that of the radius. The published standards in Greulich and Pyle[2] fortunately illustrate the wrist, so these are

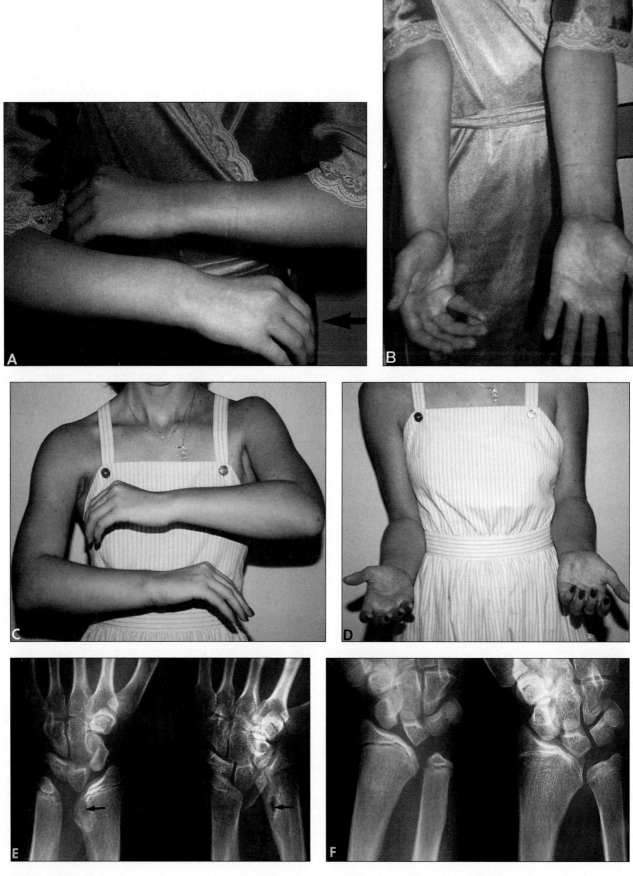

FIGURE 41-8

A, A 12-year-old girl had the physiolysis procedure on the right side only, which was painful and exhibited no supination **(A** and **B)**. At maturity, she had a barely visible deformity and 70° supination **(C** and **D)**. **E,** The radiograph revealed significant growth in the right radius, with a more rounded lunate. **F,** The unoperated left side showed no change in the radius or the lunate during the same period.

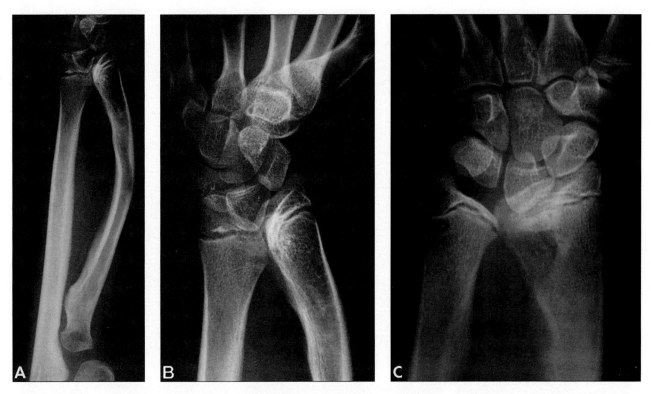

FIGURE 41-9

A and **B,** Generalized radial dysplasia with changes in the radial head, radial bowing, and Madelung's deformity. The ulna is expanded in response to its loading. **C,** Two years after physiolysis, the radius has grown to assume its proper role at the wrist.

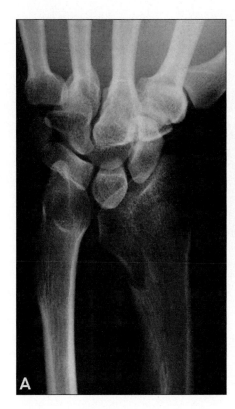

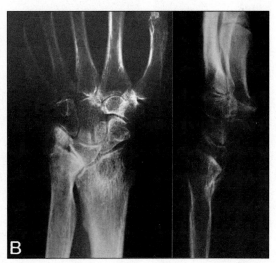

FIGURE 41-10

A, Young adult patient with a painful chevron carpus with clear radiologic evidence of the radiolunate ligament. **B,** End-stage chevron carpus in an elderly woman. The notch of the radiolunate ligament is still clearly visible.

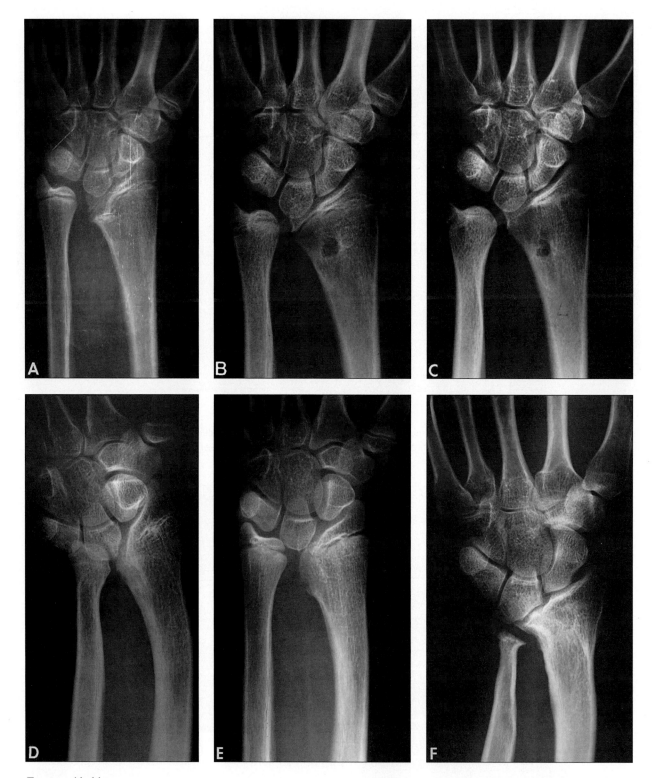

FIGURE 41-11

Two girls of a similar age with a family history and similar radiographs of Madelung's deformity were treated with physiolysis and osteotomy. **A,** The first girl with the physiolysis procedure presented with typical Madelung's deformity of the left wrist. **B** and **C,** Radiographic appearance after physiolysis; early appearance **(B)** and late appearance **(C)**. In the second girl of similar age, the radial osteotomy and ulna shortening produced an inferior result that remained painful. **D,** Preoperative appearance of right wrist. **E,** After osteotomy. **F,** Late treatment result.

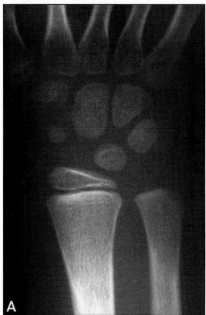
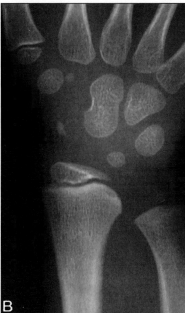
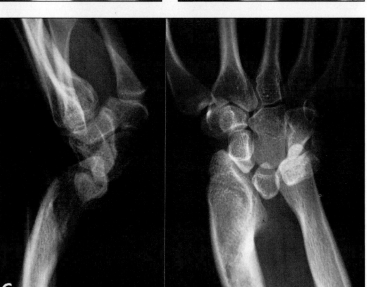

FIGURE 41-12

A, Normal radiograph of a 5-year-old girl. **B,** Radiograph of the left wrist of a 5-year-old girl with a strong family history of overt Madelung's deformity (mother and maternal aunt). The "teardrop" radial epiphysis is under-developed in the ulnar zone and the ulnar metaphysis is truncated. The distal radial epiphysis is 2 years behind the standard; the carpus is 1 year behind, and the metacarpals are equal to the standard, indicating that the focus of the dysplasia is the distal radius. **C,** Radio-graphs of maternal aunt with advanced symp-tomatic Madelung's deformity.

most useful in assessing wrist development in dyschon-drosteosis. A lucent notch or groove and spike in the junction between the metaphysis and the diaphysis is clear evidence of a radiolunate ligament. Magnetic res-onance imaging of the wrist can quite clearly demon-strate the presence of the ligament, knowledge of which may help the surgeon during the operative approach. Biplanar magnetic resonance imaging may also be help-ful in visualizing the physeal bar location and direction. In young children, the only clinical deformity may be prominence of the head of the ulna. They are otherwise asymptomatic. The changing clinical appearance, how-ever, reinforced by the radiologic signs, assists in the decision to intervene. The development of pain is a most important indication to suggest that surgical inter-vention of a prophylactic nature is warranted.

ESTABLISHED LATE MADELUNG'S DEFORMITY

PREFERRED APPROACH

In the patient with an established Madelung's defor-mity who presents with pain and limited motion after the physes have closed, a different operative approach is recommended from that preferred by the author.[8] This surgical management can be a formidable problem because the deformity of the distal radius is well estab-lished and the carpal bones have undergone adaptive changes during growth. Treatments based on ulna shortening or resection of the distal ulna are the tradi-tional forms of treatment but do not address the under-lying problem. The experience at the Mayo Clinic reflects the outcome in 11 patients treated by biplanar corrective opening wedge osteotomy of the radius.[8] In three patients, the operative procedure also included ulna recession. The authors reported pain relief in all of the patients without adversely affecting wrist or forearm motion. Although reduction of the distal radioulnar joint was improved, it remained incongruous in a number of patients. Because Madelung's deformity is a hereditary disorder transmitted by autosomal dominance trait, the early recognition of this in families should provide the opportunity for the corrective surgery proposed earlier in this chapter rather than the salvage procedure described here.

In the operative approach for established chronic Madelung's deformity, the purpose of surgical intervention is to correct the abnormal radiocarpal relationship, improve radial length, and reduce the instability and loss of rotation related to the distal radioulnar joint. The rationale for the corrective osteotomy (Fig. 41-7) is based on the premise that an ulnopalmar approach to the distal radius allows a biplanar osteotomy to restore the lunate fossa articular surface to a position where it can provide increased lunate support. It also allows one to resect the soft-tissue tether and to inspect and restore alignment to the distal radioulnar joint.

TECHNIQUE

Exposure is performed through a longitudinal palmar incision (Figs. 41-13, *A* and *B*) at the interval between the flexor carpi radialis and the radial artery (or between the ulnar neurovascular bundle and the finger flexor tendons). The pronator quadratus will need to be reflected either radial to ulnar or ulnar to radial, depending on which approach is chosen (Fig. 41-13, *B*). The ulnar approach allows one to reflect the pronator quadratus from the distal ulna and to expose the ulnopalmar aspect of the distal radius. The appearance of a stout fibrous cord from the lunate fossa proximally may tether the ulnar palmar aspects of the physis of the distal radius. This fibrous cord should be excised. The metaphyseal area of the distal radius is cleared to a midpoint on the radius, and the physeal line, if present, should be identified. An osteotome is then placed parallel and 1 cm proximal to the rim of the lunate fossa and angled dorsodistally at the lunate fossa under radiographic control. A Kirschner wire can be drilled into the approximate spot for confirmation under image intensification if doubt exists as to position. The osteotomy is then performed under image control and the epiphysis is gently wedged open to produce a biplanar correction. If needed, external fixation (which was used in 6 of 11 patients in the Mayo series) can be used to provide radiocarpal distraction and facilitate graft insertion (Figs. 41-14, *A* through *G*). A corticocancellous trapezoidal

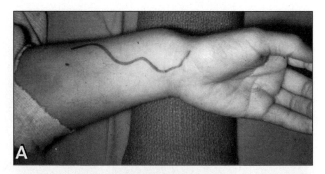

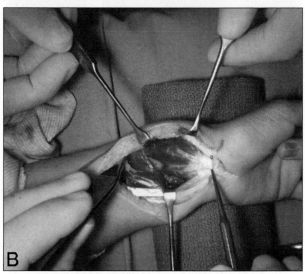

FIGURE 41-13

A, Surgical approach for corrective osteotomy is made palmar and radial between the radial artery and the flexor carpi radialis, started distally and brought proximally in a curvilinear fashion. **B,** Exposure of the pronator quadratus, which has an abnormal insertion onto the ulnopalmar corner of the radial epiphysis. Together with a thick fibrous band, the pronator quadratus appeared to be tethering the ulnar palmar corner of the epiphysis. *(From Murphy MS et al.[8] Copyright, American Society for Surgery of the Hand, by permission of Churchill Livingstone.)*

bone graft is then fashioned from the iliac crest and inserted at the osteotomy site. Imaging is used to check correction of the radioulnar inclination and palmar tilt of the radius. Kirschner wires and an AO fixation plate (miniplate) can be used for fixation (Figs. 41-14, *C* and *D*). If necessary, ulna recession can be performed to correct excessive positive ulna variance. This can help correct dorsal overriding of the ulnar head on the carpus and subluxation of the distal radioulnar joint.

In the Mayo series, three patients had sufficient bowing of the ulna to justify a second more proximal osteotomy of the radius. In two patients with an open physis, the osteotomy was placed under the rim of the radius with resection of the physeal bar as described earlier in this chapter. Silicone block rather than fat

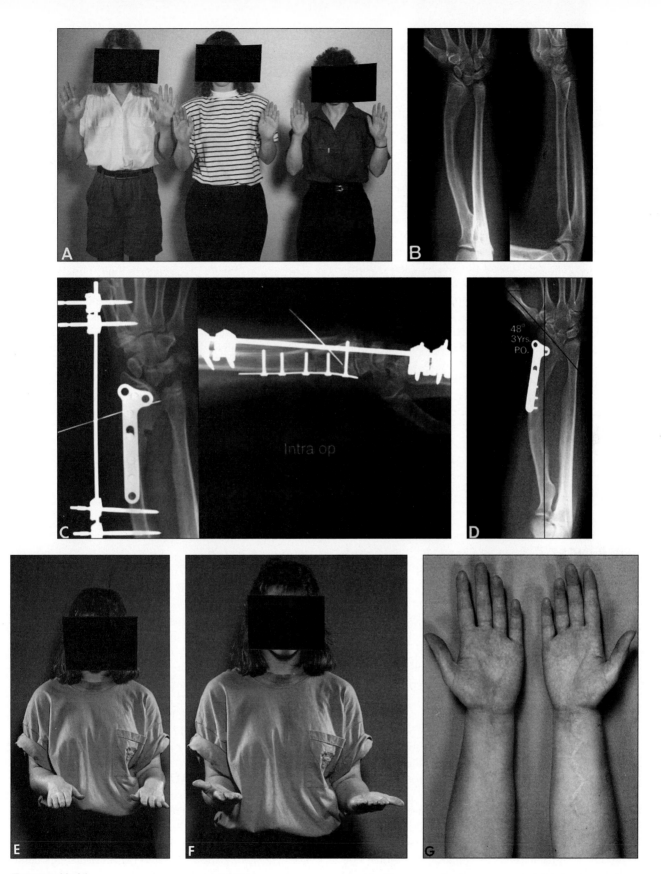

Figure 41-14

A, Preoperative clinical appearance of a 15-year-old student, her 11-year-old sister, and 39-year-old mother. Discomfort increased in the wrist with supination and strenuous activities. **B,** Preoperative radiographs show closure (epiphysiodesis) of the ulnar aspect of the radial physis, ulna plus deformity, radial shortening, and forearm bowing. The radiolunate angle is 50°. **C,** A double osteotomy was performed with distraction by an external fixator and internal fixation with a buttress plate and Kirschner wire. **D,** Radiograph at 3 years after surgery shows residual forearm bowing, ulna plus variance, 48° radioulnar angle, and carpal deformity. The radioulnar joint has, however, remained reduced, the carpus is stable on the forearm, and there is a full range of motion. There is little or no discomfort with activities at 5 years after surgery. **E,** Forearm pronation. **F,** Forearm supination. **G,** Comparative appearance with improvement on the right, with decreased bowing and less prominence of the ulnar head. Nearly equal forearm length. *(From Murphy MS et al.[8] Copyright, American Society for Surgery of the Hand, by permission of Churchill Livingstone.)*

was chosen as the interposition material to prevent re-formation of the bar.

The results of corrective osteotomy showed improved pain and functional activities of daily living (Figs. 41-14, *E* through *G*). The prominence of the ulna head was reduced and a majority of patients had improved forearm pronation and supination. Full congruity of the distal radioulnar joint was not achieved because of the developmental distortion of the ulnar head and the dysplasia of the sigmoid notch. Wrist extension averaged 47°; wrist flexion, 54°; and radioulnar deviation combined, 51°. Pronation increased to 56° (range, 10°-85°) and supination averaged 66° (range, 10°-75°). Radiographic assessment demonstrated improved radioulnar inclination and radiolunate contact with less evidence of ulnar carpal translation. Complications of the procedure were few, with no deep infections or nonunions. Two patients had secondary corrective osteotomy; one patient had an ulnar fracture after plate removal, requiring further open reduction, bone grafting, and repeat plating; one patient required radioulnar arthrodesis as a salvage procedure.

SUMMARY

Madelung's deformity is a progressive lesion involving the physeal region of the distal radius. In symptomatic patients seen early, physiolysis is strongly recommended. Clarification of *classic Madelung's, reverse Madelung's,* and *chevron carpus* is important in surgical decision making. Corrective osteotomy for late deformity helps to restore forearm length and decrease pain at both radiocarpal and radioulnar joints, but it does not restore a normal wrist for either motion or strength. Prophylactic physiolysis in a patient with a positive family history is currently being investigated. Better imaging techniques (including magnetic resonance imaging) may improve early diagnosis and afford the opportunity for corrective surgical intervention.

REFERENCES

1. Fagg PS: Wrist pain in the Madelung's deformity of dyschondrosteosis, *J Hand Surg [Br]* 13:11-15, 1988.
2. Greulich WW, Pyle SI: *Radiographic atlas of skeletal development of the hand and wrist,* ed 2, Stanford, California, 1959, Stanford University Press.
3. Langenskiöld A: An operation for partial closure of an epiphysial plate in children, and its experimental basis, *J Bone Joint Surg Br* 57:325-330, 1975.
4. Langenskiöld A, Elima K, Vuorio E: Specific collagen mRNAs elucidate the histogenetic relationship between the growth plate, the tissue in the ossification groove of Ranvier, and the cambium layer of the adjacent periosteum. A preliminary report, *Clin Orthop* 297:51-54, 1993.
5. Langer LO: Dyschondrosteosis, a hereditable bone dysplasia with characteristic roentgenographic features, *Am J Roentgenol* 95:178-188, 1965.
6. Léri A, Weill J: Une affection congénitale et symétrique du développement osseux: la dyschondrostéose, *Bull et mem Soc Med Hôp de Paris* 53:1491-1494, 1929.
7. Madelung O: Die spontane Subluxation der Hand nach vorne, *Verhandl d deutsch. Gesellsch f Chir, Berl* 7:259-276, 1878.
8. Murphy MS, Linscheid RL, Dobyns JH, et al.: Radial opening wedge osteotomy in Madelung's deformity, *J Hand Surg [Am]* 21:1035-1044, 1996.
9. Peterson HA: *Partial growth arrest.* In Morrissy RT, editor: *Lovell and Winter's pediatric orthopedics,* ed 3, vol 2, Philadelphia, 1990, JB Lippincott.
10. Vickers D, Nielsen G: Madelung deformity: surgical prophylaxis (physiolysis) during the late growth period by resection of the dyschondrosteosis lesion, *J Hand Surg [Br]* 17:401-407, 1992.
11. Vickers DW: Premature incomplete fusion of the growth plate: causes and treatment by resection (physiolysis) in fifteen cases, *Aust N Z J Surg* 50:393-401, 1980.
12. Watson HK, Pitts EC, Herber S: Madelung's deformity: a surgical technique, *J Hand Surg [Br]* 18:601-605, 1993.

ADDITIONAL READING

Beals RK, Lovrien EW: Dyschondrosteosis and Madelung's deformity: report of three kindreds and review of the literature, *Clin Orthop* 116:24-28, 1976.

Dannenberg M, Anton JI, Spiegel MB: Madelung's deformity: consideration of its roentgenological diagnostic criteria, *AJR* 42:671-676, 1939.

Dobyns JH, Wood VE, Bayne LG: *Congenital hand deformities.* In Green DP, Hotchkiss RN, editors: *Operative hand surgery,* ed 3, vol 1, New York, 1993, Churchill Livingstone, pp 515-520.

Gelberman RH, Bauman T: Madelung's deformity and dyschondrosteosis, *J Hand Surg* 5:338-340, 1980.

Golding JS, Blackburne JS: Madelung's disease of the wrist and dyschondrosteosis, *J Bone Joint Surg Br* 58:350-352, 1976.

Nielsen JB: Madelung's deformity: a follow-up study of 26 cases and a review of the literature, *Acta Orthop Scand* 48:379-384, 1977.

Ranawat CS, DeFiore J, Straub LR: Madelung's deformity: an end-result study of surgical treatment, *J Bone Joint Surg Am* 57:772-775, 1975.

Scheffer MM, Peterson HA: Opening-wedge osteotomy for angular deformities of long bones in children, *J Bone Joint Surg Am* 76:325-334, 1994.

42

GROWTH-PLATE INJURIES

David Vickers, M.B.B.S.

Injuries of the Growth Plates (Physes) at the
  Wrist
Classification
Clinical Investigations
Physeal Arrest
Injury Management
Treatment of Physeal Arrest
Personal Experience
Summary

INJURIES OF THE GROWTH PLATES (PHYSES) AT THE WRIST

Injuries of the physes (epiphyseal plate, growth plate) at the wrist are common but rarely produce deformity or complications of growth. Sepsis produces a more serious injury of the physis and is more difficult to treat because it is often extensive and multifocal. Burn injuries involving the physis likewise are difficult to treat, especially because of the loss of overlying integument.

Injury to the immature skeleton tends to produce a fracture or physeal separation rather than a dislocation or ligament injury because the ligaments are relatively strong. The deep components of the radiocarpal ligaments attach to the perichondrial ring, so an angular force produces a fracture proximal to this level. When the physis is involved, the fracture mainly propagates through the weakest zone: the hypertrophic-precalcific zone. The force may, however, digress through other zones or into bone, especially if the physis is undulating, as is the case in the older child. Metaphyseal fracture is much more common than epiphyseal fracture. The epiphysis is involved only in compressive or high-energy injuries.

CLASSIFICATION

Numerous classifications have been proposed during almost 100 years. The Salter-Harris classification of five types is the most widely used.[7] *Type I* injury traverses horizontally across the physis and is usually only seen in the very young when the physis is thick and straight. A *type II* injury includes separation of a triangular piece of metaphyseal bone at one boundary of the physeal fracture. More than 50% of physeal fractures are type II. Type I and type II injuries are generally responsible for the clinical diagnosis of slipped epiphysis. A *type III* injury traverses the physis incompletely and then extends through the epiphysis into the joint. This fracture is rare except in the phalanges and requires accurate reduction and fixation if displaced. A *type IV* injury involves physis, metaphysis, and epiphysis in a straight line or a Z pattern. Accurate reduction and fixation is required. The common varieties of this type are the lateral condyle fracture of the humerus and the triplane fracture of the distal tibia. A *type V* injury involves crushing of the physis without a bony fracture and is rare. Some orthopedists dispute its existence as a solitary lesion.

Crushing is common with any type of physeal fracture in high-energy injuries. This has led to other classifications that include subgroups for comminution; total loss of bony tissue; and perichondrial ring, periosteal, or vascular injury. The most recent classification by Peterson[6] has a rational grouping based on a clinical study with relevance to epidemiology and increasing severity of injury to the physis. Vickers[8] has reported that patients treated for premature fusion of the physis exhibit a high incidence of multiple fractures, with a significant proportion being of the compound or complicated variety. These have been termed "supertrauma" to stress the point that the amount of energy dissipated in creating the fracture may be more significant in prognosis than the classification alone. Any element of compression is especially dangerous to the physis. Apophyses which are traction centers of ossification can pull off, producing instability, but they cannot produce a significant growth disturbance and are clearly different from physeal injuries.

A vascular insult will further interfere with the sequence of growth. If the nutrient vessel to the epiphysis and the adjacent germinal zone of the physis is breached, there will be growth arrest downstream in the area of ischemia. This complication is most likely when the nutrient vessel is intracapsular, which is not the case in the distal radius but could affect growth in the distal ulna. Ischemia of the calcifying zone of the physis will not cause growth arrest but will inhibit calcification, producing a progressive radiolucent zone in the metaphysis.

CLINICAL INVESTIGATIONS

Careful detective work using plain radiographs in conjunction with a history of injury and a detailed study of the clinical deformity is sufficient for diagnosis in most cases. Apart from obvious bony sclerosis across the cartilaginous physis, the interpretation of the Harris growth arrest lines[2] and the symmetry of the zone of new growth in the metaphysis usually indicate the presence and location of a partial physeal fusion. Often the zone of new growth is of a different density, usually greater, that I refer to as the "opalescent zone." Triangularization of the opalescent zone indicates partial growth arrest at the apex of the triangle (Fig. 42–1).

For many years hypocycloidal and trispiral tomograms have been used in complex cases of physeal injury. More recently, spiral computed tomography and magnetic resonance imaging have shown the pathologic features more clearly. Ordinary computed tomography has been disappointing in some cases, giving the impression of a greater percentage of fusion than actually exists. Magnetic resonance imaging has been used in a limited number of cases, and although clear contrast images are produced, the cuts, which are 0.7 to 3 mm,

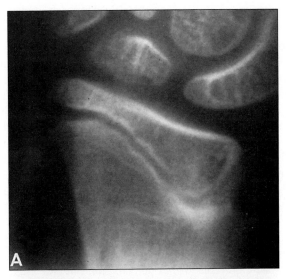

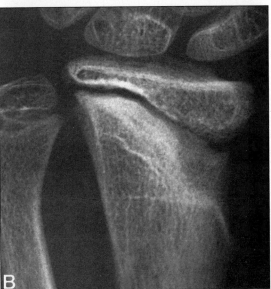

FIGURE 42–1

A, Tomogram of premature partial fusion of the distal radius with faint Harris lines converging to point of fusion. **B,** One year later this line is more visible and an opalescent zone of new growth is forming distal to this, the asymmetry of which indicates early correction.

may not be thin enough. T2-weighted images demonstrate the cartilage most accurately. With current technology, I favor spiral computed tomography whereas Peterson favors axial-directed magnetic resonance imaging.

PHYSEAL ARREST

When there is a bone bridge across the physis binding the epiphysis to the metaphysis, no growth is possible in this zone. The overall effect of this depends on the size of the bridge, its location, and the age of the child at the time of injury. Small or microscopic bridges may break down spontaneously, causing no long-term complications.

A peripheral bridge forms a pivot point causing angular deformity, with some real, but mostly apparent, shortening. Even small bridges persist. A central bridge causes tenting of the physis, real shortening, and joint deformity. Central bridges are usually large, because the forces of growth can break down smaller ones. Total fusion allows no growth, but it causes no angular deformity. Because the forearm is a duplex system, growth disturbance in one bone causes luxation of the adjacent joint as the other bone grows normally.

More than 20 years of personal experience have shown me that excision of a bone bridge across the physis (physiolysis) can restore natural growth, which not only prevents further deformation but also adds the capacity to decrease the current deformity. Although angular deformity and shortening can be corrected by traditional salvage procedures (such as osteotomy, limb lengthening, or contralateral physiodesis), re-formation of joint surfaces can only occur with growth restoration, and it should be emphasized that this is the most unique benefit of physiolysis. Spontaneous correction of deformity is superior to salvage surgery in every way, but there are limits beyond which natural processes are insufficient. Angular deformity of more than 20° or significant shortness close to maturity may require

supplemental osteotomy or lengthening. Rotatory deformity will not correct at any age. The generally accepted limit of fusion for a reasonable outcome after bridge resection from a lower limb bone is 50% of the physis. When more than 50% is involved, the remaining physis is inadequate, and the surgical void in the bone after excision produces significant mechanical weakness. In the upper limb, however, a fall on the outstretched hand after physiolysis could and often does cause collapse and failure (Fig. 42-2), so in the distal radius the upper limit for resection of a bone bridge may be closer to 30%. In cases in which the fusion of the physis is more than 50%, there is virtually no growth, and fusion will usually increase slowly with early closure of the entire physis. In these cases, or when a portion of the epiphysis was lost at the time of injury, radial lengthening using a cantilever apparatus has been helpful in restoring alignment of the hand. Premature fusion of the radius is much more common than in the ulna, because the radius is the load-bearing member at the wrist and is much more likely to be injured from a fall or compression injury.

INJURY MANAGEMENT

Before any treatment is undertaken, it is most important that the parents are informed that a growth

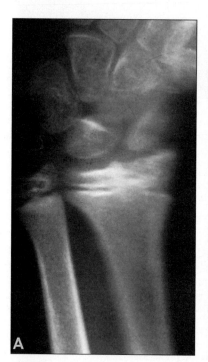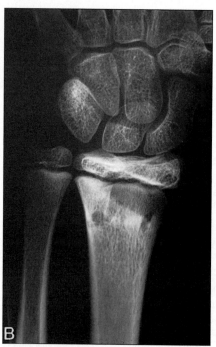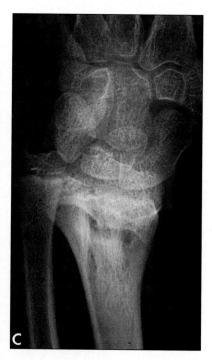

FIGURE 42-2

A, A 12-foot fall from a window caused a compressive fracture of the distal radial epiphysis. The tomogram shows a complex dorso-radial fusion with some flattening and ischemia of the epiphysis. The bone bridge traversed the bone and occupied 30% of the physis. **B,** Just over 2 years later, after excision of the physeal bar, new growth has kept pace with the ulna. **C,** After a heavy fall, the poorly supported epiphysis was crushed, necessitating an osteotomy.

disturbance might arise from the injury, especially in the case of "supertrauma." Treatment can minimize but not remove the risk. Follow-up will be required for several years in simple cases and until maturity in the more complex injuries. This process of close patient follow-up allows early detection of a premature fusion, which can be treated by physeal bar excision procedures.

Undisplaced fractures of the growing end of the bone involving the physis may be managed by immobilization and close observation. At the first sign of displacement, the treatment regimen is altered. Where there is a simple displacement of the epiphysis (type I or type II injury), its reduction should be achieved during general anesthesia and it should be maintained in the corrected position with casting. Generally, the epiphysis reduces easily and fully, but on occasion there is a small lateral displacement that is acceptable. A young child has a great capacity to remodel bones, so small imperfections of reduction are more acceptable than repeated manipulation, which could cause serious injury to the soft physeal cartilage. The reasoning is different in the older child because the capacity to remodel close to maturity is not as impressive and frequently injury to a physis late in childhood will go on to premature fusion in any case. A more accurate reduction is necessary and repeated manipulation is justifiable. An open reduction is rarely indicated in type II injuries except with major trauma when there is significant instability. Levers or elevators should not be used for displaced fractures with physeal involvement.

Open reduction will be more frequently indicated in type III and type IV injuries. A step off of the articular surface, or in the physis, is usually an indication for accurate open reduction. If internal fixation is required, *only smooth pins* should be used where the fixation crosses the physis. The pins should be passed through the central zone rather than the periphery, as close to right angles as possible. Only one or two pins should be used. If possible, the pins should be removed at or before 3 weeks. At the wrist, a threaded form of fixation may be used to fix a metaphyseal fragment to the diaphysis of the bone, but it must be well clear of the physis.

TREATMENT OF PHYSEAL ARREST

In the case in which a premature partial (less than 50%) physeal fusion (arrest) is proved, there may be specific indications to proceed with surgical excision. This operation is most beneficial in the younger child before too much deformity has developed. The indications for surgical treatment vary quite significantly in older children. I have used the Langenskiöld technique,[3] which involves a limited excision of the area that has fused, followed by implantation of a fat graft into the surgical cavity. Peterson[5] has extensive experience with the use of cranioplast as the interposition material. Before operation is attempted, the surgeon must have a clear three-dimensional impression of the location and extent of the bone bridge. Peripheral bone bridges are the easiest to approach and treat. A more central bridge within the bone must be approached through the metaphysis so the healthy surrounding physeal tissue is not disturbed. The portal of entry in the metaphysis is of no particular importance unless it creates a large metaphyseal defect that requires protection until bone remodeling occurs.

All physiolysis surgery should be performed during general anesthesia and with a tourniquet. If there is any doubt regarding the location of the bone bridge, Kirschner wires can be inserted into the bone so that the point of the wire will be adjacent to the area of interest. The bone is then screened radiologically in several views to assess the situation (Fig. 42-3). It is a good idea to place the Kirschner wires peripheral to the intended path of approach so that they can remain in place until the tips are exposed at the site of abnormality. The initial bony dissection is performed with a gouge or a rongeur. When the zone of the bone bridge is located, one is looking for any evidence of physeal cartilage. The area of bone forming the bridge is generally extremely hard compact bone. Once physeal cartilage is located, it can be followed to further define the physis in continuity. Magnification and good lighting are essential for accuracy. One must be careful not to remove too much healthy physis in the process of defining the limits of the bridge. On initial inspection, the physis may be thin, white, and wavy and can occur in patches. Ultimately, the cartilage becomes straighter and thicker and in younger children may have a slightly blue tinge. As one clears the bridging bone, the quality of the bone becomes more cancellous, which is an indicator of the adequacy of the resection. Eventually, the physis displayed is continuous in the floor of the cavity.

After excision of peripheral bridges, the exposed physis extends in a U shape from one edge of the bony cavity to the other. In more central bridges, as one looks through the metaphyseal portal, one sees a ring of physeal cartilage with the bone of the epiphysis in the center. It is important that the cavity be made tidy because loose pieces of periosteum, bone, or flaps of physeal cartilage can all cause failure. The metaphyseal side of the physis can be better defined by using a motorized bur so the cartilage is prominent and will make close contact with the interposition material. Once the excision is complete, the tourniquet is deflated long enough for hemostasis to occur. If bleeding points persist in part of the cavity, some bone wax may be used. Then, the tourniquet is reinflated and the cavity is washed with saline. It is then completely filled with a large piece of fat, which may be harvested from the wound edges or from a remote

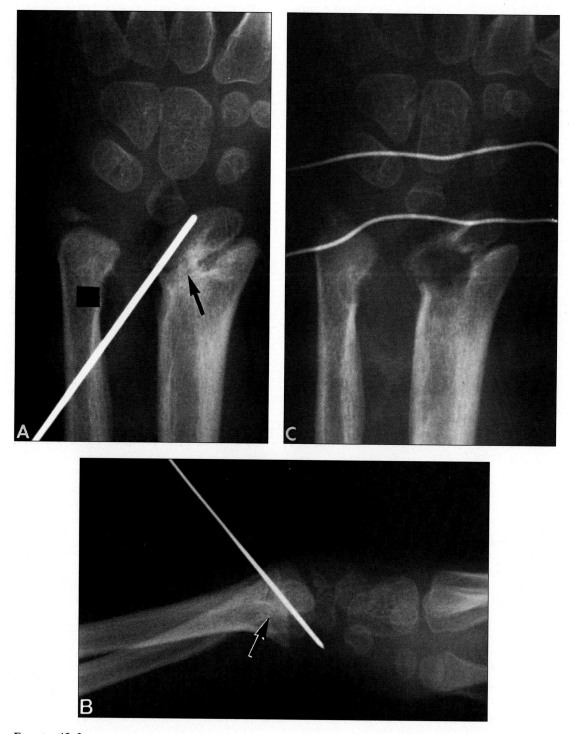

FIGURE 42–3

Intraoperative radiographs are sometimes useful in locating a bone bridge and, if necessary, to check the clearance at the end of the excision. This was a postsepsis fusion after a compound fracture. **A** and **B,** Location of ulnar physeal bar (*arrow*) with metal marker. (Black rectangle over artifact on film.) **C,** Postresection radiographic check of clearance and physeal response.

site if necessary. If the piece of fat is slightly bigger than the cavity, the soft tissues repaired over the surgical defect ensure that it is stable and in good contact with the floor of the cavity. If there is any doubt, absorbable sutures can be used to stabilize the fat. After skin closure, a splint is usually applied for the time required for wound healing, mainly for comfort.

PERSONAL EXPERIENCE

Since 1973 I have performed 153 physiolysis procedures. Twenty-four of these have followed upper limb trauma, mostly of the distal radius. Langenskiöld and Österman,[4] Bright,[1] Williamson and Staheli,[9] and Peterson[5] have also reported on several upper limb

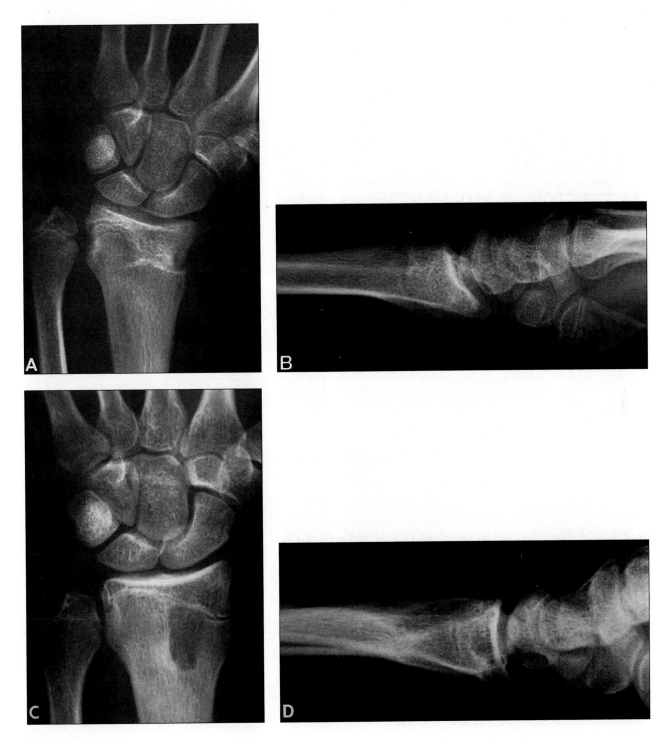

FIGURE 42-4

A and **B,** After a fall from a horse, a peripheral fusion developed in this girl and involved 25% of her physis, producing significant deformity. **C** and **D,** After physiolysis, the deformity corrected within a 2-year period.

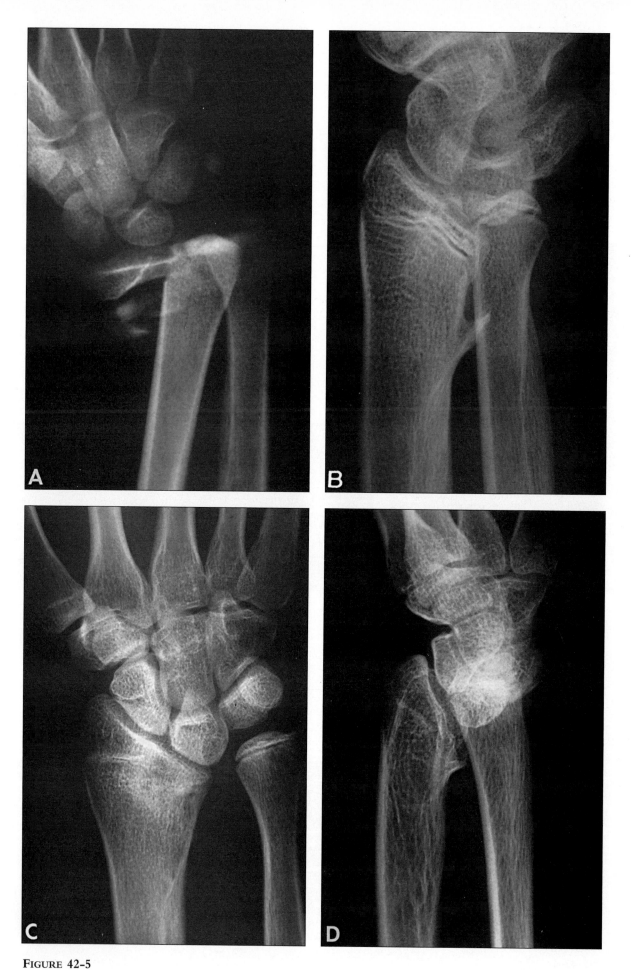

FIGURE 42-5

A, High-energy fracture of the distal radius. **B,** The ulnar zone fused and was successfully excised, preventing significant deformity. **C,** In contrast, a similar case was not treated during growth and required an osteotomy **(D).**

cases. The larger bones of the lower limb show a more vigorous response after physiolysis than the smaller bones in the upper limb. Dramatic recovery is often seen in the femur, but it is almost microscopic in the phalanges, causing frequent failure. The distal radius exhibits a satisfactory response in the majority of cases and physiolysis is worthwhile when the physeal fusion is peripheral or limited and when more than 1 year of growth is possible before maturity.

An example of a most satisfactory outcome is the case of an 11-year-old girl who fractured her distal radius in a fall from a horse (Fig. 42-4). She was examined at several centers before presenting at age 13.5 years with a 25% fusion of her dorsoradial physis. This lesion produced clinical and radiologic deformity. During a 2-year period after physiolysis, she recovered almost fully.

A second illustrative case is that of a boy who suffered a grossly displaced fracture of his distal radius at age 9.5 years (Fig. 42-5). A limited peripheral physeal fusion developed subsequently. The lesion was best seen in the 45° supinated view of his wrist taken 4 years later. Six months after physiolysis, his radius is almost mature and there has been sufficient remodeling of his joint surface to improve his prognosis.

Sepsis, especially septic arthritis, can produce the most serious fusion, many of which are untreatable. The child in Figure 42-6 gave a history of "abscess on the bone" earlier in childhood and presented with a central fusion right across the distal radius involving 50% of the physis. One year after physiolysis the radial epiphysis has advanced, but the surgical cavity did not repair itself but merely elongated with growth, causing significant structural weakness. Although the surgical cavity does become narrower with growth, this is an extremely slow process that takes many years.

SUMMARY

Physeal injury involving the distal radius is not uncommon. The majority of cases are Salter-Harris types I and II injuries that do not produce clinical deformity. Accurate reduction should be attempted

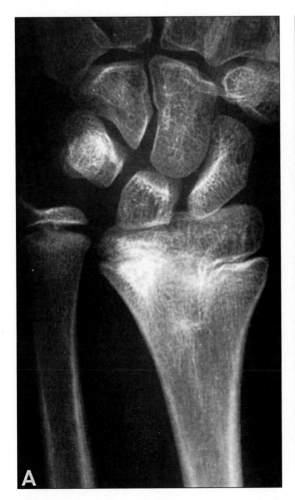 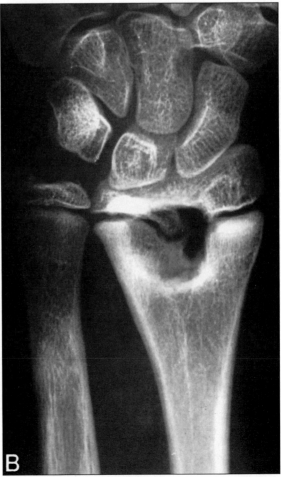

FIGURE 42-6

A, Sepsis can produce extensive fusion. **B,** The bone bridge 1 year after physiolysis is satisfactory.

during anesthesia with closed manipulation using traction. Salter-Harris types III and IV injuries are less common but have greater potential for lasting deformity. Accurate closed or open reduction is recommended. If Kirschner wires must cross the physis, they should be smooth, centrally placed, and cross the physis at as close to a right angle as possible. Fixation of the epiphysis to epiphysis or metaphysis to metaphysis is preferable.

If physeal fusion (physeal bar) occurs after trauma, excision and interposition of fat (or cranioplast) is recommended. The younger the patient, the better the result. Three-dimensional imaging with computed tomography or magnetic resonance imaging is recommended to accurately map the location of the fusion (physeal bar). Experience in physeal surgery improves the surgeon's ability to recognize the extent of the lesion and the most appropriate surgical approach.

After the successful excision of a physeal bar, restored growth prevents further deformity and may progressively correct a degree of established deformity. Improvement in the shape of joint surfaces is the most important benefit, not achievable with any other surgical procedure for these types of injuries.

REFERENCES

1. Bright RW: *Physeal injuries.* In Rockwood CA Jr, Wilkins KE, King RE, editors: *Fractures in children,* Philadelphia, 1984, JB Lippincott, pp 87-172.
2. Harris HA: Growth of long bones in childhood, with special reference to certain bony striations of metaphysis and to the role of vitamins, *Arch Intern Med* 38:785-806, 1926.
3. Langenskiöld A: An operation for partial closure of an epiphyseal plate in children, and its experimental basis, *J Bone Joint Surg Br* 57:325-330, 1975.
4. Langenskiöld A, Österman K: *Surgical elimination of post-traumatic partial fusion of the growth plate.* In Houghton GR, Thompson GH, editors: *Problematic musculoskeletal injuries in children,* London, 1983, Butterworths, pp 14-31.
5. Peterson HA: *Partial growth plate arrest.* In Morrissy RT, editor: *Lovell and Winter's pediatric orthopaedics,* ed 3, vol 2, Philadelphia, 1990, JB Lippincott, pp 1071-1089.
6. Peterson HA: Physeal fractures: part 3, classification, *J Pediatr Orthop Surg* 14:439-448, 1994.
7. Salter RB, Harris WR: Injuries involving the epiphyseal plate, *J Bone Joint Surg Am* 45:587-622, 1963.
8. Vickers DW: Premature incomplete fusion of the growth plate: causes and treatment by resection (physiolysis) in fifteen cases, *Aust N Z J Surg* 50:393-401, 1980.
9. Williamson RV, Staheli LT: Partial physeal growth arrest: treatment by bridge resection and fat interposition, *J Ped Orthop* 10:769-776, 1990.

43

DEFORMITIES AND PROBLEMS OF THE WRIST IN CHILDREN WITH MULTIPLE HEREDITARY OSTEOCHONDROMATA

Hamlet A. Peterson, M.D.

BACKGROUND AND PROBLEM
TREATMENT
    EXCISION OF OSTEOCHONDROMATA
    HEMIEPIPHYSEAL STAPLING OF DISTAL RADIUS
    LENGTHENING OF ULNA
    SURGICAL STRAIGHTENING OF ULNA
    OSTEOTOMY AND SHORTENING OF RADIUS

EXCISION OF DISTAL ULNA
RELATED PROBLEMS
    PROXIMAL RADIAL DISLOCATION
    MADELUNG'S DEFORMITY
    KIENBÖCK'S DISEASE
SUMMARY

BACKGROUND AND PROBLEM

Multiple hereditary osteochondromata (MHO), also called multiple exostoses or diaphyseal aclasis, is a disorder of enchondral bone growth manifested by abnormal metaphyseal bone prominences capped with cartilage and accompanied by defective metaphyseal remodeling and asymmetrical retardation of longitudinal bone growth. It is the most frequent benign bone tumor. Deformities of the forearm are seen in 30% to 60% of patients with the disorder.[5,14] The most common deformity is a combination of relative shortening of the ulna, bowing of either or both of the bones of the forearm, increased ulnar tilt of the distal epiphysis of the radius (radial articular angle [RAA]) (Fig. 43-1), ulnar deviation of the hand, progressive ulnarward translocation of the carpus (carpal slip) (Fig. 43-2), and dislocation of the proximal radial head.[5] Relative shortening of metacarpals frequently accompanies the forearm deformities.[3]

In a review of 98 forearms, Fogel et al.[5] found the most frequent location of lesions of the forearm and hand was the distal ulna, followed closely by the distal radius, metacarpals, and phalanges (Fig. 43-3). A feature common to all was bowing of the radius and relative shortening of the ulna. Twenty percent had carpal slip, 19% had an RAA greater than 30°, and 14% had a dislocated or subluxated proximal radius (Fig. 43-4).

Little has been written about the natural history of MHO.[6] The lesions are rarely noticed before age 1 year and often not until age 2 or 3 years. In general, the lesions continue to enlarge with growth. This enlargement causes the deformities to progress, leading to variable weakness, functional impairment, and cosmetic deformity.[5] Once growth ceases, the lesions stop enlarging.[3] The rate of enlargement of lesions varies but can be marked (Fig. 43-5, A through D).

Without treatment during the growth period, progressive relative ulna shortening, bowing, increased RAA, increasing carpal slip, and increasing subluxation or dislocation of the proximal radius occur often (Fig. 43-6). Most of the existing literature concentrates on the etiology, epidemiology, and treatment of the condition. More emphasis should be placed on preventing the deformities from occurring. This is best accomplished by the early excision of lesions primarily about the distal ulna and radius and proximal ulna and radius when lesions are present there. This allows optimal potential growth of the ulna and radius.[9,10]

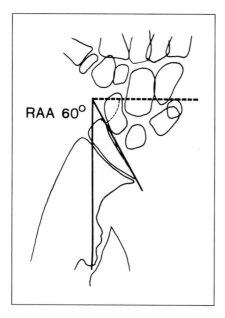

FIGURE 43-1

The radial articular angle (*RAA*) is the angle between two constructed lines: one along the articular surface of the radius and the other perpendicular to a line that bisects the head of the radius and passes through the radial edge of the distal radial epiphysis. The normal RAA is between 15° and 30°. *(From Fogel et al.[5] By permission of the journal.)*

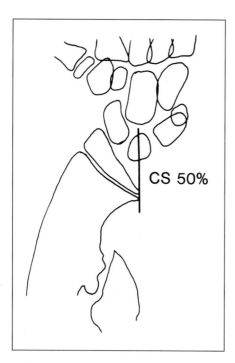

FIGURE 43-2

Ulnarward carpal slip (*CS*) or displacement of the lunate off the radius is measured as the percentage of contact of the lunate with the radius determined by an axial line drawn from the center of the olecranon through the ulnar edge of the radius. The line normally bisects the lunate. CS is considered abnormal when the lunate is displaced ulnarward by more than 50%. *(From Fogel et al.[5] By permission of the journal.)*

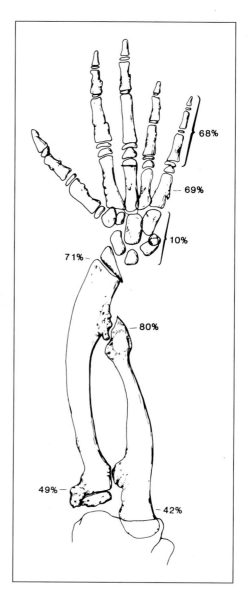

FIGURE 43-3

Incidence of osteochondromata in 98 forearms, according to location. *(From Fogel et al.[5] By permission of the journal.)*

TREATMENT

EXCISION OF OSTEOCHONDROMATA

Osteochondromata should be excised as soon as it becomes clear that growth patterns of the involved bones are being altered. Angular deformity is usually due to bowing of the ulna, the radius, or both. Increased ulnar deviation and decreased radial deviation of the wrist is a frequent accompanying deformity, which is rarely troublesome to the patient unless it is marked. The amount each of these angular deformities contributes to decreased forearm rotation is difficult to determine.

Length discrepancy is manifest by undergrowth of the ulna compared with the radius as well as undergrowth of both the radius and the ulna compared with

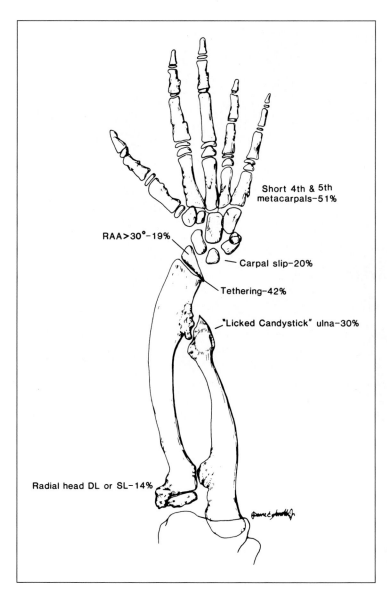

Short 4th & 5th
metacarpals–51%

RAA>30°–19%

Carpal slip–20%

Tethering–42%

"Licked Candystick" ulna–30%

Radial head DL or SL–14%

FIGURE 43-4

Incidence of deformities in 98 forearms. *RAA*, radial articular angle; *DL*, dislocation; and *SL*, subluxation. *(From Fogel et al.[5] By permission of the journal.)*

the opposite forearm. Excision of osteochondromata of the distal ulna will slow or stop the radial-ulnar growth differential[5,9] and allow the cortical bone to regenerate. Cortical bone is important if future lengthening is contemplated or becomes necessary.

Osteochondroma growth on the radial (lateral) side of the proximal ulna is an infrequent[3] but definite cause of radial head subluxation or dislocation from direct lateral pressure (Fig. 43-7). Proximal radial dislocation in this instance is best prevented by early excision of the ulnar osteochondroma. If there is an accompanying osteochondroma of the proximal radius, the two lesions should not be excised at the same time because this predisposes to postoperative synostosis. Osteochondromata of the distal radius and ulna can be excised at the same time if they are not opposing each other and if the excisions are done through separate incisions.

Other indications for early excision are pain from repeated external trauma to the prominences and rapid

enlargement or rapid radiographic changes suggestive of malignant transformation, an extremely rare occurrence in children.[10] Cosmesis can also be a concern of parents, especially of girls. When the parents and the patient are informed that removal of the bump results in minimal scar, the cosmetic concern is often lessened.[6]

When excision of an osteochondroma is undertaken, all of the cartilage cap must be removed while avoiding violation of the physis. The margins of the surgical incision should be palpated for adjacent bumps, which may be only cartilage and not visible on radiographs. If these adjacent lesions are not removed, they will enlarge in the future, causing the patient to surmise that the surgeon failed to remove the entire original lesion.

Lesions that are never excised can develop into situations that are difficult to manage (Fig. 43-8). Spontaneous synostosis of opposing lesions frequently occurs in the ankle (tibia and fibula)[13] and can occur in the wrist (radius and ulna). Opposing lesions of the

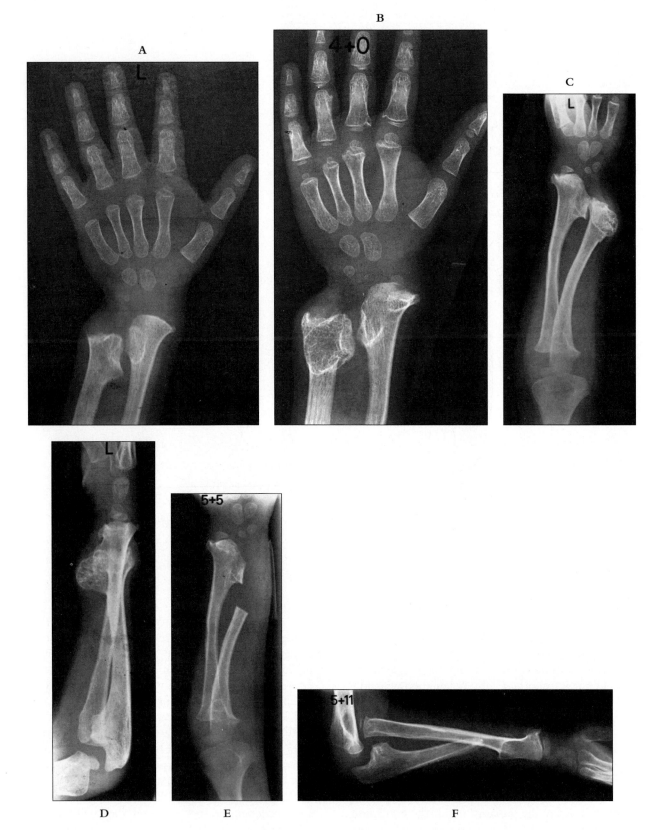

FIGURE 43-5

Multiple hereditary osteochondromata with rapid growth and consequences of excision of the distal ulna. **A,** Multiple bone osteochondromata in a young boy (approximately age 2 years). **B,** Age 4 years 0 months: rapid growth of lesions and increasing wrist deformity. **C,** Age 5 years 4 months: marked increase in carpal slip and loss of forearm rotation. **D,** Lateral view. Note maintenance of radial head location. **E,** Age 5 years 5 months: excision of distal ulna; immediate gain in full forearm rotation. **F,** Age 5 years 11 months: complete dislocation of proximal radius.

G   H

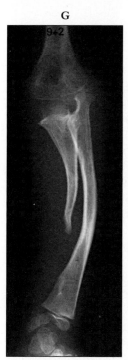
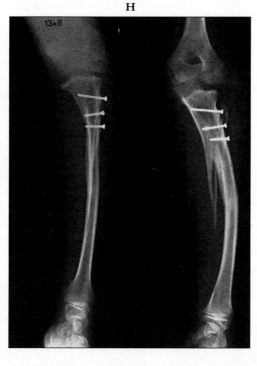

FIGURE 43-5, CONT'D.

G, Age 9 years 2 months: the proximal ulna has not grown. The radial bowing is unchanged (possibly due to absence of the ulna tether), the radial head remains dislocated anteriorly and has become painful, and the forearm rotation is reduced. The radial head was excised and the proximal radius fused to the proximal ulna (one-bone forearm). **H,** Four and a half years postoperatively there is full elbow motion with no pain or instability, normal wrist position and function, and no forearm rotation.

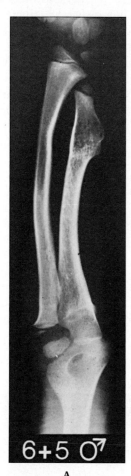
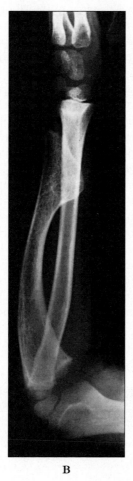
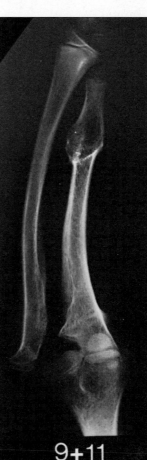
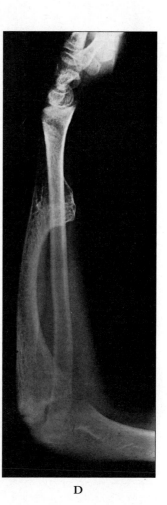

A   B   C   D

FIGURE 43-6

Dislocation of proximal radius associated with an osteochondroma of distal ulna in young boy. **A,** Age 6 years 5 months: large sessile osteochondroma of distal ulnar metaphysis, with relative shortening of the ulna, ulnar and radial bowing, and early subluxation of proximal radius with asymmetric ossification of the proximal radial epiphysis. **B,** Lateral view shows same features. Excision of the osteochondroma was advised but not accomplished at that time. **C,** Age 9 years 11 months: the distal ulnar epiphysis has grown away from the osteochondroma. Note that the relative radioulnar length discrepancy has increased, but that the relative distal ulna shortening is unchanged compared with **A.** This is because the proximal radius has completely dislocated and displaced proximally at the elbow. For the same reason, the radial articular angle appears to be less marked. **D,** The diminished ulnar bowing (compare with **B**) is unusual and possibly associated with the complete dislocation of the proximal radius.

distal radius and ulna cause less deformity than if only one bone is involved.[14]

HEMIEPIPHYSEAL STAPLING OF DISTAL RADIUS

Hemiepiphyseal stapling of the distal radius in the treatment of MHO was first described by Siffert and Levy.[12] Although this corrects the RAA and carpal slip,[5,10] it has less effect on the radioulnar length discrepancy or the bowing of the radius or the ulna (Fig. 43-9). It is a good adjunctive procedure to improve the radial-carpal relationships, but it is less effective if used alone.[6,14] Stapling makes prediction of the final radioulnar discrepancy more difficult.[9] It should be used with

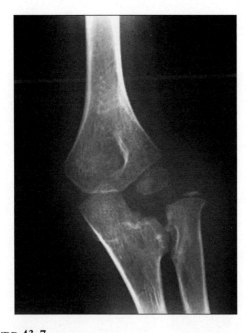

FIGURE 43-7

Boy, age 5 years 9 months: osteochondroma of proximal ulna pushes proximal radius radialward.

caution in children younger than age 10 years because staples are not easy to insert in small bones and because permanent physeal arrest beneath the staples could result in overcorrection of the RAA or in relative shortening of the radius. While the staples are in place the patient needs to be evaluated at least every 6 months. The staples should be removed when the deformity is corrected, usually in 18 months, if the child is growing rapidly. In older children (girls older than age 13 years and boys older than age 15 years) stapling has little application because there is limited growth remaining to correct the deformity.

LENGTHENING OF ULNA

The rationale for ulna lengthening is that the hypoplastic ulna, the keystone of the complex deformity, tethers the ulnar side of the radial physis, which increases the RAA and carpal slip and theoretically decreases ulnar support of the carpus and increases ulnar side pressure on the radial epiphysis.[5] Because of the inherent growth discrepancy between the ulna and the radius, some relative shortening of the ulna usually recurs after lengthening in the immature patient. This is particularly true if the procedure is not combined with another procedure such as excision of osteochondromata or straightening of the ulna. Therefore, slight overlengthening at the time of surgical lengthening is not detrimental if the child is still growing.[4,5,11] Ulna lengthening alone does not result in significant improvement of forearm rotation, RAA, or carpal slip.[5]

Many techniques of ulna lengthening are available. The lengthening can be a forceful, one-stage distraction in surgery by using a transverse,[2,4,5,9,11] oblique, or step-cut osteotomy[4,5,9,10,14] (Fig. 43-9, *C*). The length gained by this technique is limited to 10 to 20 mm. Greater length is usually not possible because of bowing of the radius, soft-tissue tightness, or local osteochondromata not previously removed. Lengthening

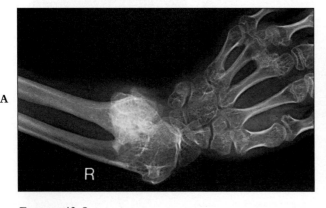
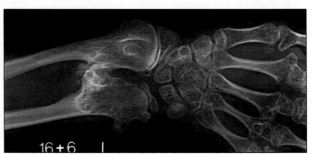

FIGURE 43-8

Boy, age 16 years 6 months: multiple hereditary osteochondromata were never treated. **A,** Right wrist is fixed in ulnar deviation and flexion and there is no forearm rotation. **B,** Left wrist radioulnar diastasis with no forearm rotation. Attempt to excise these lesions would predispose to postoperative synostosis.

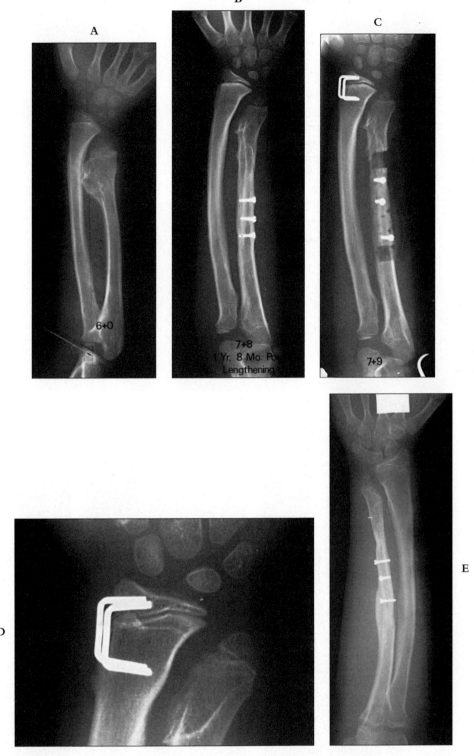

FIGURE 43-9

A, Six-year-old boy with osteochondromata of distal ulna and relative shortening of ulna, bowing of radius, increased radial articular angle, increased carpal slip, and ulnar deviation of the hand. At this time, osteochondromata of distal ulna were excised and one-stage, long step-cut osteotomy ulna lengthening of 10 mm was performed. **B,** Age 7 years 8 months: 1 year 8 months after lengthening, relative shortening of ulna has improved. There is no change in radial bowing, radial articular angle, or carpal slip. **C,** Age 7 years 9 months: repeat one-stage 10-mm lengthening of the ulna with insertion of two staples on the radial side of the distal radius. **D,** Age 8 years 7 months: 10 months after stapling, there is growth on ulnar side of distal radial epiphysis, decreased radial bowing, and improvement of both radial articular angle and carpal slip. Note growth arrest line documenting asymmetric growth since staple insertion. **E,** Age 8 years 9 months: staples have been removed, osteochondromata excised, and metal marker inserted in distal ulnar metaphysis to document future growth of distal ulna. *(From Peterson.[10] By permission of JB Lippincott.)*

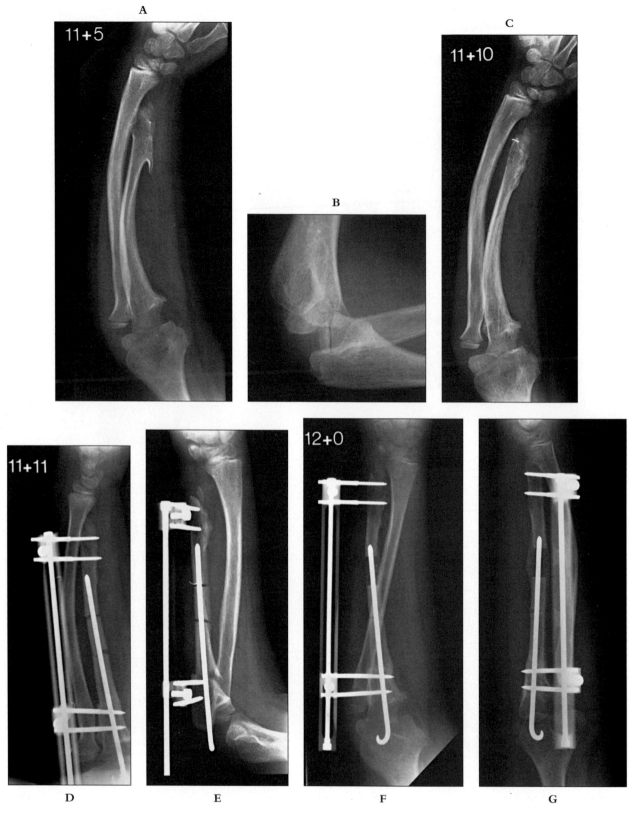

FIGURE 43–10

Boy, age 11 years 5 months. This case demonstrates ulna straightening and lengthening. **A,** Ulna bowing and shortening with radial bowing and proximal head subluxation. The cartilage caps over these osteochondromata are much larger than the osseous prominences. **B,** Lateral view: note radial head posterior subluxation. The distal ulnar osteochondromata were excised and a metal marker was inserted. **C,** Age 11 years 10 months: 5 months after excision of distal ulnar osteochondromata. Note no increased radial head subluxation. **D,** Age 11 years 11 months: multiple osteotomies were done and Rush pin was inserted after straightening the ulna. Lengthening was accomplished with Orthofix prototype lengthener (PTO 450). **E,** Ulna is straight. Head of radius is subluxated posteriorly. **F,** Age 12 years 0 months: lengthening was 0.75 mm/day in four increments over 25 days (total length gained, 17 mm). Lengthening stopped at this time to prevent distal ulna from pulling off the Rush pin. Note early bone formation in lengthened interval. **G,** Lengthening device was removed 58 days after application and osteotomies.

more than 20 mm has been reported when accompanied by division of the interosseous membrane.[9] Transverse osteotomies can be bone grafted and held at length with a plate,[2,4] whereas oblique and step-cut osteotomies can be fixed with two or three transverse screws.[5] These osteotomies heal rapidly without bone grafts (Figs. 43-9, *B* and *E*). More length can be gained by external distraction devices (e.g., Wagner or Orthofix) that use transverse corticotomy or osteotomy[1,4,9,11] (Fig. 43-10) or step-cut osteotomy.[6] These also heal rapidly with or without bone grafting and with or without internal fixation.[1,4,7] The lengthening process is currently done at the rate of 1 mm per day, usually ¼ mm four times a day.

Lengthening of the ulna with concomitant division of the ulnar collateral ligament and osteotomy of the radius has been reported.[14] I have had no experience with this.

Surgical Straightening of Ulna

The most recent advance in the treatment of these forearm deformities is surgical straightening of the ulna. This can be accomplished by multiple osteotomies and insertion of an intramedullary pin and may be accompanied by lengthening of the ulna (Figs. 43-10, *D* through *G*). This also will not improve forearm rotation, but when it is combined with other procedures, it can diminish future additional loss of forearm rotation.

Each of the operations mentioned above can be combined with others. Excision of large osteochondromata about the distal ulna, however, cannot easily be combined with lengthening of the ulna. Regardless of the type of lengthening performed, the increased longitudinal pressure results in compression or crushing of the distal metaphysis where the cortical bone has been removed along with the osteochondromata. Pin placement for attachment of lengthening devices in the distal ulna is also difficult because of weakening of the bone in this area. Thus, my preference at the present time is to excise all osteochondromata as early as possible and to proceed with lengthening as soon as the cortical bone has had time to regenerate (usually 6 to 12 months in older children). In younger children, delay between lesion excision and lengthening can be greater to allow the discrepancy to increase to proportions warranting lengthening, provided the proximal radius does not begin to subluxate. Close observation is imperative.

Osteotomy and Shortening of Radius

Osteotomy of the distal radius to correct the RAA and surgical shortening of the radius to equalize radioulnar length discrepancy are seldom used and probably should be considered only after growth is complete.[5,6] The RAA can be improved easily in the growing child by insertion of staples on the radial side of the physis, an operation that yields less morbidity than osteotomy. Multiple osteotomies of the radius to correct bowing are difficult to perform because of limited possibilities for surgical exposure. A single osteotomy of the radius corrects only one locus of a long bow deformity and usually requires internal fixation to maintain the desired rotation orientation.

Radial shortening is undesirable because the involved forearm is already usually shorter than the contralateral forearm.[4] Radial shortening also usually requires application of a plate and screws, which would need to be removed later. Radial shortening has been used in combination with ulna lengthening.[8] I have had no experience with this combination.

Excision of Distal Ulna

Excision of the distal ulna might be considered for large lesions associated with complete loss of forearm rotation. Excision of the distal ulna in a growing child results in dislocation of the proximal radius, with subsequent pain and loss of forearm rotation and elbow flexion-extension (Figs. 43-5, *E* through *G*). When this occurs, treatment by excision of the radial head and surgical osteosynthesis of the proximal radius and ulna (creation of a one-bone forearm) can result in excellent elbow and wrist function but no forearm rotation (Fig. 43-5, *H*). Thus, excision of the distal ulna should be considered only in cases in which a one-bone forearm is the best result expected from any treatment.

RELATED PROBLEMS

Proximal Radial Dislocation

The cause of dislocation of the proximal radius in any particular case is often difficult to determine. The contributing causes include relative shortening of the ulna, bowing of the radius, bowing of the ulna, and an osteochondroma of the proximal ulna or radius, causing proximal diastasis (Fig. 43-7). Usually there is a combination of factors. The best way to prevent proximal radial dislocation is early excision of osteochondromata from the distal ulna and from the proximal ulna, if such lesions are present.

A dislocated radial head in a growing child is difficult to treat, and if it is asymptomatic, it is frequently not treated.[14] If the radial head articular surface is still concave and if there is little or no angulation of the proximal radius, an attempt at reduction can be considered. Reduction can be accomplished by gradual lengthening of the ulna with an external lengthener (Wagner, Orthofix). Once the distal ulna is at proper length with respect to the distal radius, the distal radius can be incorporated onto the lengthener and the lengthening can be continued.[4,9] When the proximal radius has been distracted past the level of the capitellum, it can be reduced and the annular ligament can be repaired with a strip of triceps tendon.

Once growth is complete, a symptomatic dislocated radial head can be excised. This will relieve pain but not improve motion.

MADELUNG'S DEFORMITY

MHO has been described as similar to Madelung's deformity. In MHO, the distal ulna is shorter than the radius. In Madelung's deformity, the ulna is longer and subluxated dorsally (see Chapter 44). The anterior subluxation of the wrist and hand which is seen in Madelung's deformity is uncommon in MHO.[5]

Major osteochondroma involvement of the distal radius with relative overgrowth of a normal ulna (Fig. 43-11) resembles Madelung's deformity, but it is rare[3] and can always be distinguished by one or more osteochondromata.

KIENBÖCK'S DISEASE

An association between avascular necrosis of the carpal lunate (Kienböck's disease) and ulna minus variance has been noted.[2] There are no reports in the literature of an MHO patient with Kienböck's disease despite numerous MHO patients who have significant relative shortening (up to several centimeters) of the ulna at maturity.

SUMMARY

Management of forearm deformity due to MHO should be aggressive.[5,6,10] Osteochondromata about the distal ulna, or radius, or both should be excised at an early age to allow optimal growth of these bones. Once cortical bone has regenerated, the ulna can be lengthened. For a girl between 10 and 13 years old and a boy between 10 and 15 years old, staples across the physis of the radial side of the distal radius as a concurrent procedure improve the RAA and carpal slip. Straightening and lengthening the ulna over an

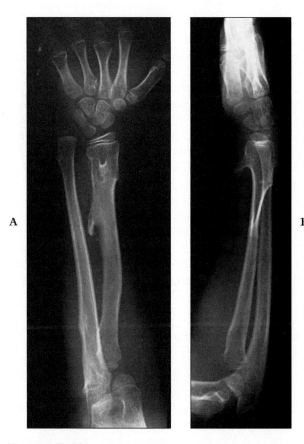

A   B

FIGURE 43-11

Girl, age 7 years 9 months who had major involvement of distal radius and minimal involvement of ulna. Note relative radial shortening and medial subluxation of proximal radius, both rare. **A,** Anteroposterior view. **B,** Lateral view.

intramedullary rod decreases forearm bowing and length discrepancy. This treatment greatly decreases the likelihood of proximal radial dislocation. It does not improve forearm rotation.

Generally, surgical treatment improves cosmetic appearance more than function. Reduction of progression of deformity and functional impairment and, in particular, prevention of radial head dislocation are the paramount goals of any operation for this complex disorder.

REFERENCES

1. Abe M: Lengthening of the ulna for the forearm deformity, *J Jpn Soc Surg Hand* 2:249-254, 1985.

2. Armistead RB, Linscheid RL, Dobyns JH, et al.: Ulnar lengthening in the treatment of Kienböck's disease, *J Bone Joint Surg Am* 64:170-178, 1982.

3. Bock GW, Reed MH: Forearm deformities in multiple cartilaginous exostoses, *Skeletal Radiol* 20:483-486, 1991.

4. Dal Monte A, Andrisano A, Capanna R: Lengthening of the radius or ulna in asymmetrical hypoplasia of the forearm (report on 7 cases), *Ital J Orthop Traumatol* 6:329-342, 1980.

5. Fogel GR, McElfresh EC, Peterson HA, et al.: Management of deformities of the forearm in multiple hereditary osteochondromas, *J Bone Joint Surg Am* 66:670-680, 1984.

6. Fogel GR, Peterson HA: Forearm deformity in multiple osteochondromata, *Orthop Consult* 5(7):7-12, 1984.

7. Irani RN, Ziegler RW, Petrucelli RC, et al.: Ulnar lengthening for negative ulnar variance in hereditary multiple exostoses (abstract), *Orthop Trans* 6:350, 1982.

8. Kameshita K, Itoh S, Wada J, et al.: Ulnar lengthening combined with radial shortening for the forearm deformity in multiple osteochondroma, *J Jpn Orthop Assoc* 59:501-502, 1985.

9. Masada K, Tsuyuguchi Y, Kawai H, et al.: Operations for forearm deformity caused by multiple osteochondromas, *J Bone Joint Surg Br* 71:24-29, 1989.

10. Peterson HA: Multiple hereditary osteochondromata, *Clin Orthop* 239:222-230, 1989.

11. Pritchett JW: Lengthening the ulna in patients with hereditary multiple exostosis, *J Bone Joint Surg Br* 68:561-565, 1986.

12. Siffert RS, Levy RN: Correction of wrist deformity in diaphyseal aclasis by stapling: report of a case, *J Bone Joint Surg Am* 47:1378-1380, 1965.

13. Snearly WN, Peterson HA: Management of ankle deformities in multiple hereditary osteochondromata, *J Ped Orthop* 9:427-432, 1989.

14. Wood VE, Sauser D, Mudge D: The treatment of hereditary multiple exostosis of the upper extremity, *J Hand Surg [Am]* 10:505-513, 1985.

44

THE CHILD'S WRIST: DIAGNOSTIC AND TREATMENT PROBLEMS

James H. Dobyns, M.D.
William P. Cooney, M.D.

DEVELOPMENTAL ANOMALIES OF THE WRIST
  SKELETON
    NORMAL PATTERN OF DEVELOPMENT
    COALITIONS, ACCESSORY CARPAL BONES, AND
      OTHER VARIATIONS
    CARPAL COALITIONS
    CONGENITAL OR DEVELOPMENTAL SYNDROMES
    (CARPAL CHANGES)
CONGENITAL ANOMALIES OF THE WRIST
  THE DISTAL RADIUS
    THE DEFICIENT RADIUS
    TREATMENT
    CENTRALIZATION
  THE DISTAL ULNA
PROCEDURES
  ULNA DEFICIENCY
    TYPE I
    TYPE II
    TYPE III
    TYPE IV
  THE DEFORMED DISTAL ULNA
THE CARPUS
  CARPAL ANOMALIES
  LIGAMENT LAXITY
  SKELETAL ABNORMALITIES OF THE CARPUS
  CARPAL DEFORMITIES AND DEVELOPMENTAL
    CONDITIONS

INJURIES TO THE IMMATURE WRIST
  THE DISTAL RADIUS
  THE DISTAL ULNA
  MADELUNG'S DEFORMITY
  CARPAL INJURY
  SCAPHOID FRACTURES IN CHILDREN
  PREISER'S DISEASE
DIFFERENTIAL DIAGNOSIS OF PROBLEMS OF THE
  IMMATURE WRIST
  1) TRAUMA
  2) CONGENITAL OR DEVELOPMENTAL
  3) ARTHROPATHY
  4) SKELETAL DYSPLASIA
  5) NUTRITIONAL DISORDERS
  6) TUMORS
  7) NEUROMUSCULAR DEFICITS
A DIAGNOSTIC METHODOLOGY FOR PROBLEMS OF
  THE IMMATURE WRIST
  HISTORY
  PHYSICAL EXAMINATION
  PROVOCATIVE MANEUVERS
  IMAGING
  INVASIVE METHODS
SUMMARY

The wrist is known as an area of prolific diagnostic and treatment problems.* This is even more true in the child or adolescent wrist where function is seldom stopped by pain or deformity, where ossifying structures are often in radiolucent stages, where body defenses may slow characteristic development, where deformity develops swiftly and intractably due to rapid growth and plasticity, and where developmental differences may result in biomechanical consequences.†

In this chapter, the differential diagnosis of problems of the juvenile wrist will be featured, with special attention to the effects of anomalies of the wrist area and to the effects of injury to the wrist area during the developmental period between gestation and closure of long bone physes.

DEVELOPMENTAL ANOMALIES OF THE WRIST SKELETON

NORMAL PATTERN OF DEVELOPMENT

Ontogenesis of the wrist area is well covered in Chapter 4 of this text. The ossification of various carpal bones is important in differential diagnosis of injuries or disease of the wrist (Table 44-1).

COALITIONS, ACCESSORY CARPAL BONES, AND OTHER VARIATIONS

Only the trapezium, trapezoid, and capitate originate in their definitive form; the other carpals change in form and relationships. The scaphoid represents a fusion of at least two cartilaginous elements. Failure of fusion of the usual two "centralia" elements is said to account for the "os centrale" in about 1.5% of the population (Fig. 44-1). Whether such failure of fusion can also account for the occasional bipartite or tripartite scaphoid has not been definitely determined, but most multisegment scaphoids in children are probably fracture residua.[69,100,104] A few multisegment scaphoids, associated with multiple other congenital anomalies of the forearm, carpus, and hand, appear to be bona fide congenital multipartite scaphoids, but even here it is difficult to eliminate the possibility of fractures, stress or otherwise, that may have occurred before ossification. The incidence of Preiser's disease, for instance, is alarmingly high in the wrist with a hypoplastic scaphoid.[32] The lunate has an extensive ossific nucleus, which may result in a proximal accessory called the "os triangulare," said to be present in 0.74% of the population. Again, this known pattern of development does not satisfactorily explain the occasional finding of a

Table 44-1. Ossification of Carpal Bones	
Histologic Visualization	**Gestation Period**
1. Upper limb bud appearance, opposite somites 8–12	26–28 days
2. Chondrification of wrist mesenchymal condensations	4–6 weeks
3. Interzones define wrist joints	7–8 weeks
4. Cellular condensations: flexor retinaculum and ligaments	51 days
5. Cellular condensations for triangular fibrocartilage	52 days
6. Carpal joint cavities develop	57 days
7. Carpals, distal forearm, proximal metacarpals are all present in cartilage but not ossified	At birth
8. Capitate	2.5–2.9 months
9. Hamate	3.1–4.2 months
10. Distal radius epiphysis	12 months
11. Triquetrum	2–2.5 years
12. Lunate	3–3.5 years
13. Scaphoid	3–5 years
14. Trapezoid	4 years–5 years 9 months
15. Trapezium	4 years 3 months–6 years
16. Pisiform	8–10 years
17. Distal ulna epiphysis	6 years

multisegment lunate in a young child.[3] The same hypotheses, noted previously regarding the scaphoid, are relevant here.

The ulnar styloid is a separate carpal element, which usually joins the rest of the ulna at about the 10th week of ontogenesis, but it may remain separate as the "accessory ulnare."[85] This must be distinguished from the ulna styloid nonunion, which is a fairly common residue of the Colles-type injury to the child's wrist. The styloid process of the radius also begins as a separate ossification center and may remain separate, the "accessory carpi radiale," or may be separate as a result of trauma.

Despite the likelihood that double ossification centers in carpal bones are associated with extensive other signs of anomalous development or are the residua of injuries, which may not have been detected, there are literature reports of double ossification centers in scaphoid, lunate, hamate, pisiform, trapezium, and triquetrum in individuals thought to be normal.[85,106] As many as 25 accessory bones have been reported about

---

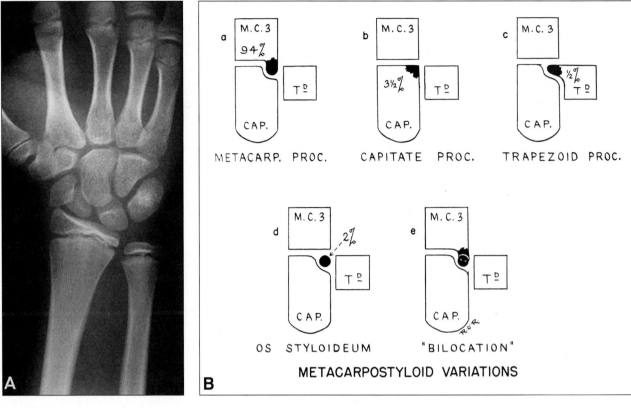

FIGURE 44-1

A, Os centrale secondary to failure of fusion of two scaphoid cartilaginous elements. This can be confused with nonunion of scaphoid. **B,** Variation in processus styloideus shows incidence of extra metacarpal (*M.C., METACARP.*) process (*PROC.*), capitate (*CAP.*) process, trapezoid (*T^D*) process (*top*) of styloideum. *(From O'Rahilly R.[85] By permission of the journal.)*

the carpus,[34,85] and we have seen several types that have not been reported. Carpal bone enlargement or large accessories occur, usually overlying more normal carpal elements. If there is any complaint, it is usually that of restriction of motion, but pain may also result.

One of the most common accessory bones, called the "os styloideum," is found dorsally and distally in the carpus, lying between the second and third metacarpal bases and the adjacent portions of the trapezoid and capitate. Whether fused to the third metacarpal base (its normal developmental pattern) or not, it may be enlarged (called a "carpal boss" or "carpe bossu" in such instances)[27] and may also be symptomatic. Because it lies within the fibers of the insertion of the extensor carpi radialis brevis, which can exert a strong or excessive pull on this cartilage-to-cartilage or cartilage-to-bone interface, there is speculation that at least some of these carpal boss conditions can be trauma related, either single incident or cumulative stress. Some of them are symptomatic and may require treatment, not unlike the similar condition of Osgood-Schlatter's disease at the tibial tubercle and patellar tendon insertion where rest and anti-inflammatory medication may be needed.

CARPAL COALITIONS

Coalitions have been described between all of the carpals adjacent to one another and may involve more than two carpal bones, radius and carpals, or carpals and metacarpals. It has been said that carpal coalitions involving more than two bones or coalitions bridging the two carpal rows are more likely to indicate a syndrome,[88] but not always. Lunatotriquetral coalitions, for instance, do not bridge the two rows (Fig. 44-2). It is one of the most common of the coalitions and often occurs as an isolated anomaly, yet there are sex, family, and race associations with this anomaly, which has been reported as 2:1 in females, more common in certain families, and much more common in certain black groups. Reported incidence has varied from 0.08% to 0.13% in the general population to as high as 61.5% bilaterally in certain Nigerian populations. It is common enough that radiologic categories have been described[30] that can be applied to any carpal coalition.

Carpal coalitions have been subdivided into four types. Category 1 is an incomplete fusion, resembling a pseudarthrosis; category 2 is a fusion with a "notch"

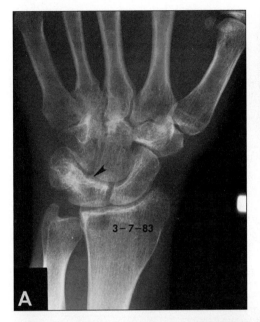

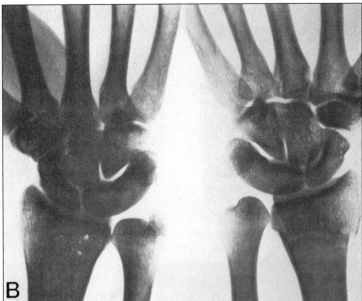

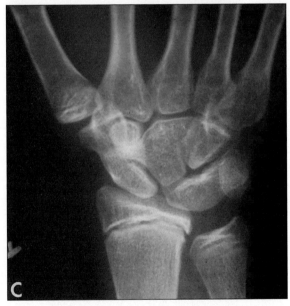

FIGURE 44-2

A, Lunotriquetral coalition (*arrowhead*) is most common carpal coalition, bringing bones of the proximal carpal row—Category 3. **B,** Bilateral lunotriquetral fusion in South African Bantu. *(B, From deVilliers Minnaar AB.[30] By permission of the British Editorial Society of Bone and Joint Surgery.)* **C,** Lunotriquetral coalition in association with scaphoid, trapezium-capitate coalition, and os centrale.

of variable depth; category 3 is a complete fusion; and category 4 is a complete fusion associated with other anomalies. Among isolated carpal coalitions, capitate-hamate is the second most common, followed by pisiform-triquetrum, trapezium-trapezoid, scaphoid-capitate, and triquetrum-hamate (Fig. 44-3). As noted previously, carpal coalitions are common in many different syndromes, including central deficiencies, hereditary symphalangia, fetal alcohol syndrome, Noonan's syndrome, arthrogryposis, diastrophic dwarfism, dyschondrosteosis, Ellis-van Creveld syndrome, hand-foot-uterus syndrome, otopalatodigital syndrome, Holt-Oram syndrome, Turner's syndrome, and ulnar hypoplasia.[22] Wrists may demonstrate combinations of accessory carpal bones and coalitions.[16,18]

Other congenital or developmental variants at the wrist include hypoplasia, hyperplasia, osteodensity, osteolysis, gigantism, shape differences, articular surface and facet differences, slope or angle differences, and length differences. The last two are particularly noticeable in the radius and ulna. Alterations of the slope and tilt of the distal radius are common (see Chapters 41 and 42); equivalence of length versus differences in length between radius and ulna is common, usually designated as ulna plus, neutral, or minus, depending on whether the ulna is longer, equal to, or shorter than the radius. Standards of normal at the carpus include ulna variance, carpal height ratio, radial inclination, radial tilt, carpal radial ratios, carpal ulna ratios, and the length of the third metacarpal. The age of the child

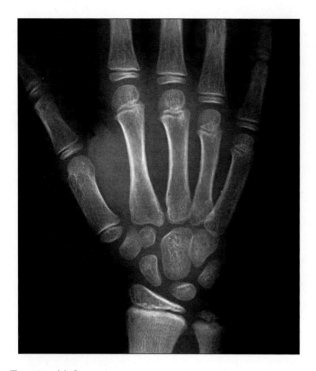

FIGURE 44-3

Capitate-hamate coalition (incomplete)—Category 1. Second in frequency and most common coalition of the distal carpal row.

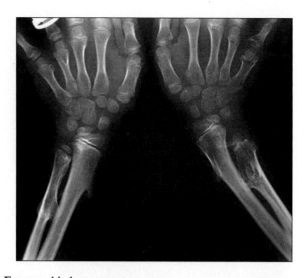

FIGURE 44-4

Osteochondroma of distal radius and distal ulna. Growth may be affected by pressure effects of osteochondroma or from influence of physeal growth center.

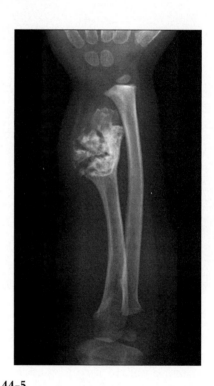

FIGURE 44-5

Maffucci's syndrome of enchondromatosis affects growth of the ulna and produces a large bone and soft-tissue mass. Tumor resection and bone graft recommended.

and the ossification of the carpus determine what measurements can be obtained. Some measurements cannot be done, and the normal standards are not yet available in the child. Carpal length, carpal angle, and ulna variance are probably most used for the immature carpus.[47,49,57,61,90]

CONGENITAL OR DEVELOPMENTAL SYNDROMES (CARPAL CHANGES)

Madelung's disease, osteochondromatosis (Fig. 44-4), and the syndromes with coalitions are developmental conditions, the treatment of which is mentioned later in this chapter and in other chapters. Other conditions or syndromes include enchondromatosis, with or without vascular anomalies (Maffucci's syndrome) (Fig. 44-5), and the various carpal osteolysis syndromes.[1,6,7,97] All of these are generalized systemic conditions, and the wrist problems, if any, are usually low on the priority list for treatment. There are other related angiogenesis conditions (Klippel-Trénaunay and related syndromes) (Fig. 44-6). The causes of the rare carpal osteolysis conditions,[6,50,97] usually associated with similar tarsal problems, have also been recognized (Table 44-2). Other syndromes* involving the wrist have also been observed but most are quite uncommon. Heritable and endocrine disorders of connective tissue metabolism

represent a large number of syndromes in this category.[55] Several of these have already been mentioned under other headings, and in none of them is the wrist problem of primary significance (Table 44-3).

Wynn-Davies[111] established criteria for generalized joint laxity, which can include the wrist.

---

* References 55,58,64,74,75,97,111.

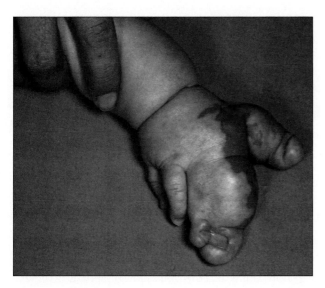

FIGURE 44-6

A patient with Klippel-Trénaunay syndrome presented with enlargement of thumb ray, complex syndactyly with gigantism of index and long fingers, and enlargement of forearm and wrist. Note partial congenital constriction band.

Table 44-2. Causes of Carpal Row Osteolysis

Farber's disease
Carpal and tarsal osteolysis (recessive)
Carpal and tarsal osteolysis (dominant)
Neurogenic acro-osteolysis
Acro-osteolysis of Joseph
Acro-osteolysis of Shinz
Arthrodento-osteodysplasia (Hadju–Cheney syndrome)
Lipodermatoarthritis
Massive osteolysis of Gorham

---

1. Hyperextension of the wrist.
2. Hyperextension of the carpometacarpal joint of the thumb.
3. Hyperextension of the metacarpophalangeal joints.
4. Excessive dorsiflexion of the ankle.
5. Hyperextension of the elbows and knees.

These conditions of hyperlaxity include 1) Marfan's syndrome and congenital contractural arachnodactyly; 2) homocystinuria (similar findings to Marfan's, but with more likelihood of carpal anomalies, specifically malformation of the capitate and a small lunate); and 3) osteogenesis imperfecta (the most common heritable form of osteoporosis, including at least four disease types). There are also systemic congenital or developmental syndromes whose effect on collagen and other soft tissues may result in significant joint deformity, including the wrist. Some of these are arthrogryposis, the pterygium syndromes, congenital contractural arachnodactyly, and melorheostoses.[40] The potential consequences of wrist deformities in these conditions are usually outweighed by other musculoskeletal or other systemic associations, although in some, such as the Madelung's deformity and arthrogryposis, patients may present with the wrist problem as a therapeutic need.

CONGENITAL ANOMALIES OF THE WRIST

THE DISTAL RADIUS

The Deficient Radius. Shortening or deformity of the radius from whatever cause constantly affects the carpus, which relies on the radius for its principal proximal support.* If the distal radius is simply not present, a condition referred to as radial aplasia, or radial

---

* References 35,39,42,87,105,110.

Table 44-3. Skeletal Dysplasia

Achondroplasia	Metatropic dysplasia
Pseudoachondroplasia	Chondrodysplasia punctata (Conradi's disease)
Acromelic dysplasia (Ellis-van Creveld syndrome)	De Lange's syndrome (Amsterdam dysplasia)
Diastrophic dysplasia	Focal dermal dysplasia (Goltz's syndrome)
Pyknodysostosis	Onycho-osteodysplasia (nail-patella syndrome)
Acrocephalosyndactyly (Apert's syndrome)	Mucopolysaccharide dysostoses
Holt-Oram syndrome	(Hurler, Scheie, Hunter, Sanfilippo, Morquio,
& other heart syndromes	Maroteaux-Lamy, Sly & DiFerrante syndromes)
Short trunk dysplasia (spondyloepiphyseal dysplasia	Cytogenetic diseases (trisomy syndromes:
congenita & Morquio's syndrome)	trisomy 21 or Down's syndrome; trisomy 18,
Mucolipid dysostoses	trisomy 13, trisomy 8; deletion syndromes:
Ehlers-Danlos syndromes	4p- syndrome, 5p- syndrome or cri du chat,
Hypochondroplasia	13q- syndrome, 18q- syndrome; sex chromosome
Mesomelic dysplasia (includes dyschondrosteosis)	syndromes: Turner's and Klinefelter's)

hemimelia, the carpus will usually have a contact but dislocation posture with the distal ulna, provided that there is a distal ulna.[35] If there are no forearm bones, the carpus will articulate with whatever proximal skeletal remnant there may be and will be displaced distally with the hand. The degree of radial deficiency has been classified into four types (Fig. 44-7).[5]

In the assessment of the child with a deficient radius, it is essential that a complete physical examination be performed to look for associated conditions. There are several blood disease syndromes (Fanconi's anemia, thrombocytopenia-absent radius); congenital heart disease syndromes (Holt-Oram); craniofacial abnormalities; congenital scoliosis syndromes (Klippel-Feil and Goldenhar); and chromosome abnormalities (trisomy 18, 21, and 13). The combined VATER (or VACTERL) syndromes are among the more frequent with ventricular septal defects, vertebral anomalies; atresia and tracheoesophageal fistula; and renal anomalies associated with more severe grades of radial aplasia (Bayne type III,

a partial proximal radius, and type IV, a total absence of the radius). Important functional considerations depend on the presence or absence of the thumb (usually absent) and the elbow (functional motion or no motion). Flatt[38] pointed out that the fully developed radial aplastic hand is a hideous deformity and functional liability. Functional use relates to mobility of digits, stability of the wrist, length of the extremity, and presence of an opposable thumb. Our experience demonstrates that the thumb is the key appendage for pinch and grip and that treatment of the thumb deficiency has more benefit than other procedures.

Treatment. The principles of treatment for radial aplasia involve both functional and cosmetic considerations. In the milder forms of this condition (Fig. 44-7) (stage I, a short radius and the distal radial epiphysis is present but delayed in appearance, and stage II in which the radius is present but hypoplastic), operations directed at restoring length to the radius and support for the

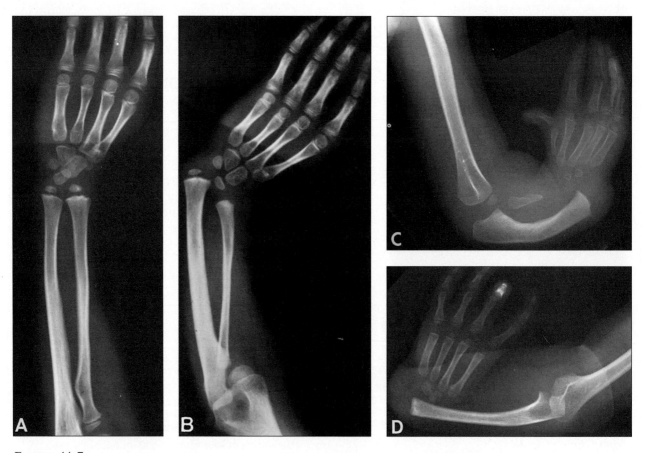

FIGURE 44-7

Classification of distal radius deficiency (radial aplasia). **A,** Bayne type I. The distal radius epiphysis is present but delayed in appearance; radius slightly shortened compared with the ulna. Carpal bones are hypoplastic. Lengthen radius if radial angulation is present, and correct for absent thumb. **B,** Bayne type II. Hypoplastic radius and thick hypertrophic ulna (bowing may be present). Lengthening of radius or centralization of the carpus on the ulna is recommended. **C,** Bayne type III. Partial to nearly complete absence of the radius; bowing of ulna is usually present. Ulna is short and the forearm is hypoplastic. Centralization of carpus on ulna is recommended. **D,** Bayne type IV. Complete absence of radius. Carpus is completely supported. Marked radial deviation. Minor ulna bowing. Staged distraction followed by centralization is recommended.

carpus are favored. Occasionally, manipulation and stretching of both the wrist and elbow can improve position or motion or both, clinical improvements which can be maintained by appropriate splinting. The need for persistent stretching of the elbow to gain 90° of motion can be effective if parents are taught to do it early and conscientiously. Serial casts or splints can likewise be helpful to correct the wrist deformity. The casts, to be effective, must be changed at biweekly intervals, extend above the elbow, and have good purchase on the radial side of the hand, yet exclude the thumb.

Surgical treatment in stages I and II is necessary when there is no improvement with stretching and serial casts. Steps to consider include release of tight radial structures (fibrous anlage and skin, joint capsule, contracted radial extensor and flexor tendons if present). Care in identifying and protecting the median nerve is stressed. We have found tendon transfer and tendon repositioning of the extensor ulnaris insertion and hypothenar muscles are important to improve their moment arm effect. If any part of the extensor or flexor carpi radialis is present, it must be either released or transferred. If the radial length is more than 2 cm shorter than the ulna, controlled radial lengthening with a Kessler frame (Figs. 44-8 and 44-9) (or other similar limb distractor) is recommended. We prefer a Z-cut lengthening of the radius with slow distraction of 1 to 2 mm/day. A transverse osteotomy for lengthening is also effective but may require a second operation for a bone graft if ossification does not follow the radial corticotomy. Slow distraction places the median nerve and other radial soft tissues (in tension) at less risk because the degree and speed of the lengthening

can be controlled. We prefer this approach to the one-stage, occasionally rough or forceful, single-stage lengthening of the radius. An alternative is to perform soft-tissue release as one stage and secondary lengthening in a second stage. Free tissue autografts (i.e., proximal fibula) to replace or lengthen the radius have not been demonstrated to be of practical value.

Treatment considerations for stages III and IV (Figs. 44-7, *C* and *D*) depend on experience and preferences of the surgeon, need for additional surgery (i.e., thumb), age of the child, and previous treatment already initiated. When the distal ulna is fully present and there is absence of the radius, stage III (partial absence of the radius, mild to proximal third) or stage IV (complete absence of the radius), the current treatment choices emphasize immediate placement of the carpus on the distal ulna. Initially, this procedure was called "centralization" of the hand. Some authors believe early manipulation and splinting to be helpful but not essential first steps before the centralization procedure. However, depending on patient age, preliminary manipulation, serial casts, and splints should not be discouraged because these techniques involve the parents early on in the treatment program. After the patient is age 7 to 9 months, it is not clear that these conservative maneuvers have any benefit.

Centralization. This procedure involves release of radial structures (anlage) (Fig. 44-9), excision of excessive ulnar skin, tendon release or transfer, and central placement of the carpus onto the ulnar epiphysis where it is held with a longitudinal Kirschner (K) wire, Steinmann pin, or intramedullary rod. The centralized

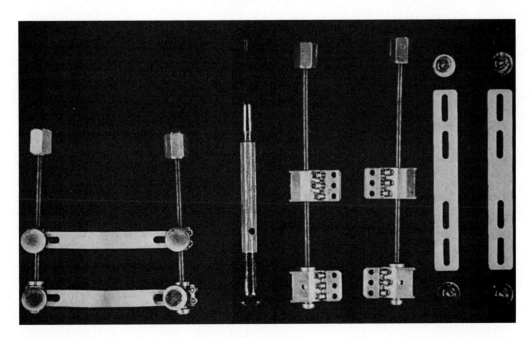

FIGURE 44-8

External distraction frame for repositioning of the radial angulated and shortened carpus (Kessler design).

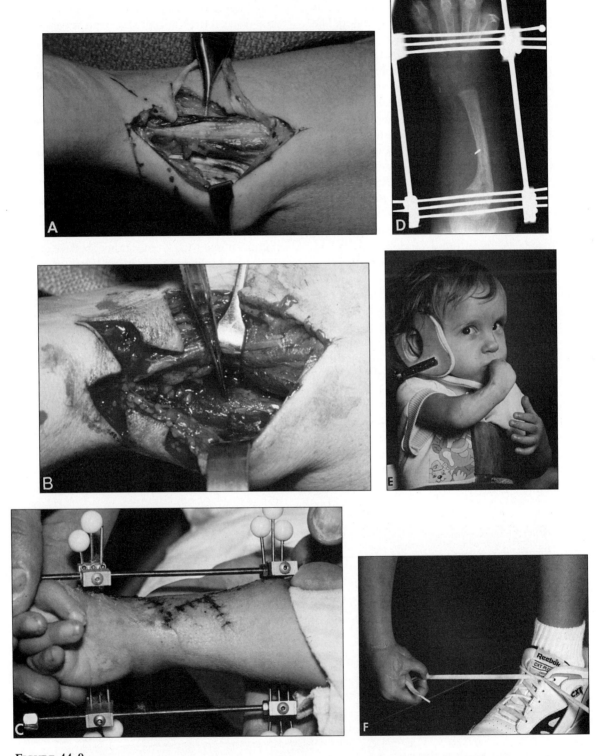

FIGURE 44-9

Radial aplasia. **A,** Skin Z-plasty release on the radial side of the wrist followed by excision of the radial anlage (hand to left and elbow to right). **B,** After excision of the anlage, the ulna can be identified for corrective osteotomy. Retracted extensor tendons are located under the retractor (*top*). **C,** Wound closure of Z-plasty. Distraction frame with transfixion pins placed through the carpus (*left*) and proximal forearm (*right*). **D,** Centralized carpus unit after gradual distraction lengthening. **E,** Function of hand and wrist unit after centralization, tendon transfer rebalance, and hand therapy. Cervical brace required to assist in correction of torticollis. **F,** Similar patient after distraction lengthening, centralization of carpus, and pollicization of index finger.

carpus can be fused to the ulna (chondrodesis or arthrodesis) or positioned onto the ulna and maintained by soft-tissue or bony support (or both). Bayne[5] favored release and soft-tissue support whereas Lamb[63] described arthrodesis (chondrodesis). Most authors agree that centralization should be done early (by 12 to 18 months) when possible. Flatt[38] and Manske et al.[71] favored an ulnar approach, identifying ulnar nerve, artery, and vein, separating out the ulnar extensor and flexor wrist tendons (extensor carpi ulnaris [ECU] < flexor carpi ulnaris [FCU]) and taking up the extra skin. Dobyns et al.,[33] Riordan,[94] and Buck-Gramcko[15] used a central (dorsal to dorsal-radial) incision, identifying the median nerve, tight radial tendons, and radial anlage.

For the arthrodesis (chondrodesis) procedure, the distal end of the ulna is squared off with a scalpel and placed either against or into a groove cut out of the carpus. Usually the side "slots" include excision of all of the lunate and part of the capitate and hamate. Lamb[63] stressed that the carpal slot is as long as is the width of the ulna. The third metacarpal is aligned with the ulna and an intramedullary rod (K wire) is placed from the third metacarpal distally across the carpus and into the distal ulna proximally. Position of the hand can be pronation or supination, but a midposition of rotation and neutral flexion-extension appears best. Capsule repair to support the carpus and tendon rebalancing are recommended to help maintain the balance achieved by the chondrodesis procedure. At a young age, sutures can be placed directly through cartilage to reattach capsule and tendons or to insert tendon transfers. The ECU is generally shortened and reattached to the base of metacarpal 5, and some authors[38] move the hypothenar muscles proximally onto the ulna and tighten the pisiform and FCU attachments in an effort to further rebalance the radial deviating tendency of the wrist.

Postoperative care includes a plaster splint from fingertips to the axilla of the shoulder and the elbow is bent at 90°. A moist Dobyns' dressing (fine mesh gauze-cotton and fine mesh gauze) is applied over skin flaps to help contour the soft tissues and assist drainage. We change dressings at 48 hours and 2 weeks, using a resorbable gut suture (5-0 chromic) for skin closure. A supportive splint is worn day and night for 6 weeks. A night splint is recommended for 6 to 12 months. The intramedullary wire or rod is removed when it comes loose.

A second option for centralization involves placement of the carpus onto the ulna but without arthrodesis. Buck-Gramcko[15] calls this radialization because he aligns the ulna with the index metacarpal, in effect positioning the ulna more radialward. In this technique, soft-tissue rebalancing and adequate soft tissues are necessary. The goal is to preserve some useful range of wrist motion (25° to 30°). This procedure is favored by Bayne,[5] Buck-Gramcko,[15] Bora et al.,[13] and Riordan[94]

but has the risk of recurrence of some degree of radial deviation. The procedure may require forceful reduction of the hand-carpal unit onto the distal ulna. It must be held in this position by K wires or intramedullary rods and maintained by appropriate tendon transfers. Two skin incisions (radial Z-plasty release and ulna skin resection) are preferred. Capsular flaps can be constructed to help support the carpus on the distal ulna.

Our preference is a staged procedure in which the hand unit is first released from radial contracture and then gradually lengthened (Kessler distractor). The first stage is followed by centralization of the hand (carpus) onto the distal ulna with appropriate soft-tissue tightening and tendon transfer. First we expose the carpus and distal ulna with a radial Z-plasty incision. We next identify and protect the median nerve (often the most radial structure) and release radial flexor or extensor tendons (if present) and resect any palpable anlage. The radial tendons usually are absent, but if they are present and demonstrate excursion of functional use, they are tagged for later transfer to the ulnar side of the wrist. After radial release, we apply the Kessler frame which is attached distally to the carpus into the metacarpals (two parallel 0.035-in. K wires) and proximally to the distal third of the ulna. Gradual lengthening of the soft tissues is performed, usually over 2 to 3 weeks (1 mm/day for 14-20 days) to allow ease of reduction of the carpus onto the distal ulna.

The second stage follows with the centralization procedure (of Bayne[5]) or the radialization described by Buck-Gramcko.[15] The carpus is centralized on the ulna by a K wire or small Steinmann pin placed through the index or long finger metacarpal across the carpus into the ulna. If the ulna is bowed, a corrective osteotomy and lengthening procedure can be performed (Fig. 44-10). On the radial side of the wrist, the flexor carpi radialis and extensor carpi radialis tendons (usually only extensor carpi radialis is available) are transferred to the base of metacarpal 5. The ECU is shortened and tightened and the FCU tendon is moved to a more ulnar and distal insertion. The hypothenar muscles are not touched because they may be needed later (e.g., for opponens transfer). Capsular flaps, especially ulnar and dorsal, are tightened to pull and hold the carpus and hand in an ulnar dorsal direction. Skin closure involves an ulnar dermadesis (to tighten ulnar skin) and the radial Z-plasty release. Cast immobilization is for 8 weeks (or longer) to allow for a fibrocapsule to tighten. The K wire (Steinmann pin) is not removed until 8 to 10 weeks. Support splints (night static) and day splints (static or dynamic emphasizing ulnar deviation) are applied. Thumb opposition, which should always be recommended, is performed 6 months later (age, 18 to 24 months).

We recently reviewed the treatment of radial aplasia at the Mayo Clinic.[24] Late results have demonstrated significant benefit to hand and wrist function with a

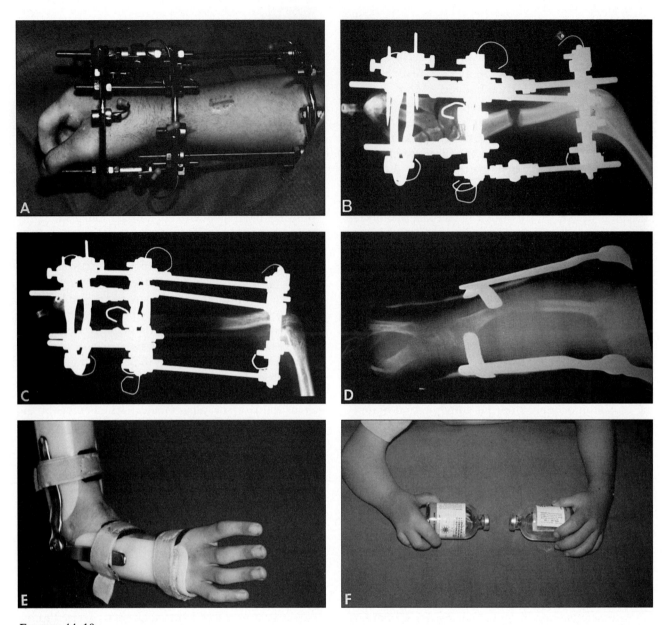

FIGURE 44-10

Radial aplasia. Secondary corrective ulna osteotomy and lengthening. **A,** Ilizarov frame application to carpal unit, distal ulna, and proximal ulna. Angulation can be achieved at the same time as repositioning of the carpal unit by differential lengthening of Ilizarov side bars. **B,** Radiographic view of ulna corticotomy and lengthening. **C,** After 4 weeks of gradual distraction, 5 cm in length is achieved along with carpal realignment. **D,** Twelve weeks after lengthening the bone rejuvenate has developed without bone grafting. Support brace. **E,** Lengthened and realigned forearm and wrist in protective brace before pollicization procedure. **F,** Hand-wrist-forearm appearance at the completion of treatment compared with uninvolved opposite extremity. Need elbow flexion contracture.

two-stage approach (three stage if you include thumb opposition transfer with Huber opponensplasty). While some degree of recurrence of radial drift is not uncommon, the functional use of the hand and wrist is improved and the presence of motion is preferred over the option of wrist chondrodesis or arthrodesis. It appears that a little radial angulation helps function (although not always appearance). The range of motion in our patients averaged 32°, which is quite similar to motion ranges from 28° (Bora et al.[13]) to 40° (Bayne[5])

previously reported. The ulna appears to broaden, grows better, and even resembles a radius in some cases. The advantage over arthrodesis, aside from the loss of motion, appears to be less damage to the ulnar growth plate (physes), a longer forearm, and the mild residual radial deviation that helps the hand get to the face, hair, or earrings.

Almost all authors agree that it is best to 1) operate on these children early, 2) provide long-term supportive splinting, and 3) follow them at yearly intervals.

Unfortunately, cardiac, renal, spinal, or gastrointestinal anomalies may take precedence, delaying hand and wrist surgery or leaving parents in frustration to protect the child from other operations until they are older and can make choices. In our experience, these delayed operations do not work as well and compromise long-term functional use.

In summary, in the treatment of radial aplasia, if the distal ulna is present, but not the distal radius, the current procedure of choice is to reduce the dislocated carpus onto the distal ulna epiphysis. To avoid compression damage to the ulna physis or the ulnocarpal articular surfaces, this maneuver is usually preceded by distraction lengthening at the ulnocarpal level or by skeletal, fascial, and tendon release or lengthening (radial) or shortening (ulnar) procedures. Unless preliminary distraction has resulted in sufficient stretching to provide easy reduction and positioning of carpus on distal ulna, such surgery usually involves release of all tight fascial bands or cartilage anlages, lengthening and transfer of tight musculotendinous units, tightening and transfer of elongated musculotendinous units, or shortening of the skeletal elements (usually by creating a cavity between the scaphoid and lunate or by excising part or all of the proximal carpal row). Treatment of radial aplasia and radial clubhand deformity is based on these principles. The radius, which is only mildly short but has a satisfactory articular relationship with the carpus, can be leveled with or elongated past the ulnar length and this can be repeated as necessary during the growth years.

THE DISTAL ULNA

The problems created by a severely short distal ulna may include palmar tilt of the wrist and hand from tight fascial tissues but more often radial head subluxation or dislocation as a consequence of stress loading from hand and wrist function along the axis of the radius. This can be a serious problem, whatever the cause of the deficient ulna, but one of the more common causes is due to osteochondromata in the wrist area. The usual surgical treatments for the problems of the moderately short ulna are discussed in Chapter 43. If surgery is needed for the severely short ulna, it is often the one-bone-forearm procedure. This procedure has the advantage of curtailing most of the supination-pronation movement available for the hand unit, which can only be compensated by some residue of rotation in the wrist or by shoulder rotation. One-bone-forearm procedures have specific advantages of: 1) immediate lengthening of the forearm unit with increased potential for growth-lengthening by providing two physes in the single forearm bone, 2) increase in stability of the forearm and the elbow, 3) usually an increase of elbow motion if the dislocated radial head can be reduced or prevented

from affecting elbow flexion or extension, and 4) an improved appearance of the forearm and elbow.

PROCEDURES

ULNA DEFICIENCY

Treatment of ulna deficiency depends on individualized patient needs and the classification of the deformity.

Type I. Distal ulna is present with only minimal shortening.

Type II. Proximal ulna is present with distal ulna anlage.

Type III. Complete absence of the ulna (quite rare).

Type IV. Fusion of radius to the humerus. Ulna anlage is present and produces bowing of the radius.

For many patients no surgical treatment is indicated. The classic concept of one-bone forearm may not be appropriate when there is minimal forearm or wrist instability because retaining some degree of forearm rotation greatly increases functional use.

To start, most authors[53,84,101,108] recommend supportive splinting or serial casting to correct the ulna deviation deformity of the wrist. This is particularly true for types I and III. Flatt[38] believed that, from birth to age 6 to 12 months, serial casting should always be applied from fingers to upper arm. Usually the ulnar angulation can be corrected early in types I and III because the ulna anlage is not a major factor. It is not clear that there is any value in persistence of cast or splints in types II and IV if initial attempts at realignment are unsuccessful.

When surgical treatment is considered, the controversy involves the importance of anlage excision and the need to form a one-bone forearm. In type I deformity (ulnar hypoplasia), ulna lengthening may be considered late (in midchildhood, years 3 to 6) either alone or with corrective osteotomy of the radius. Most type I hypoplastic cases, however, do not require any surgical treatment.

In type II deformities (partial aplasia ulna with ulnar anlage), surgical treatment is usually necessary (Fig. 44-11). The first step involves excision of the ulnar anlage. It is a tether to longitudinal growth and appears to be the main cause of ulnar bowing of the radius. Logic suggests that by excision of the anlage early, the limb growth would not be stunted and better limb function would be preserved.

Anlage excision from the wrist proximal to the midforearm is generally recommended.[95,108] Ulnar carpal bones may be deficient. The anlage extends to

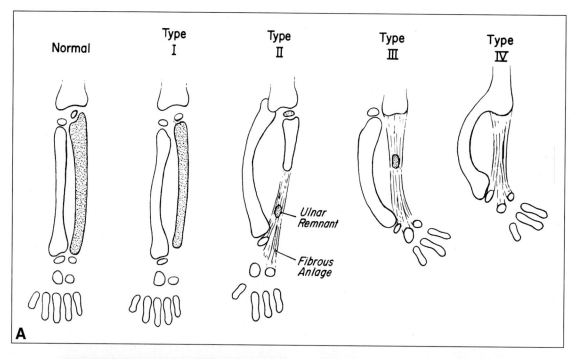

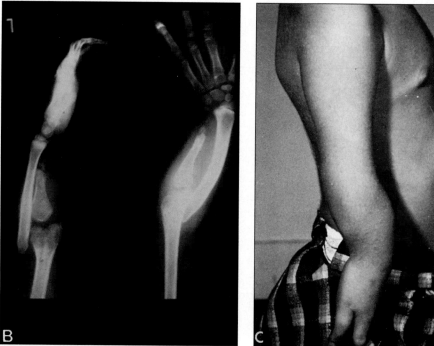

FIGURE 44-11

Ulnar deficiency. **A,** Classification types I through IV. **B,** Type II partial aplasia of ulna (absence of the distal or middle third of ulna). Note associated anomalies in the hand. Treatment is creation of one-bone forearm. **C,** Clinical appearance of ulna with hypoplasia of forearm and congenital deficiency of the hand. (*A and F, From Upton J:* Congenital anomalies of the hand and forearm. *In May JW Jr, Littler JW, editors:* Plastic surgery, *vol 8, The hand, part 2, Philadelphia, 1990, WB Saunders, pp 5213-5398. By permission of the publisher.*)

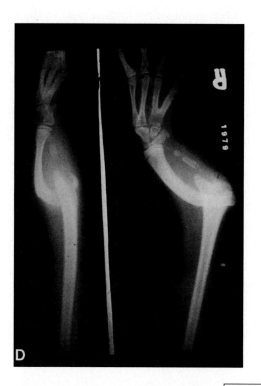

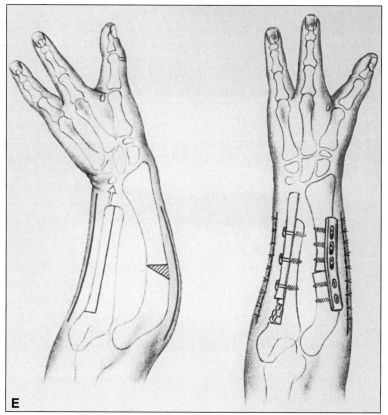

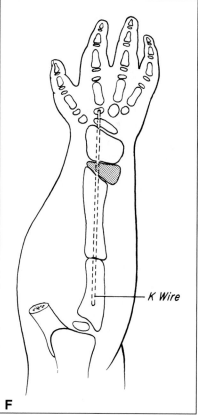

FIGURE 44-11, CONT'D.

D, Type III aplasia of ulna (complete absence of the ulna). Treatment consisted of corrective radial osteotomy with resection of ulnar anlage. **E,** Treatment of type I ulnar deficiency by closing wedge osteotomy; radius and ulna lengthening. *(E, From Blauth W, Schneider-Sickert F: Congenital deformities of the hand: an atlas of their surgical treatment [Translated by UH Weil], Berlin, 1981, Springer-Verlag. By permission of the publisher.)* **F,** Type III ulnar deficiency. Creation of a one-bone forearm using a portion of the radius as an opening wedge bone graft and alignment of the distal and proximal radius with excision of ulnar anlage.

the ulnar side of the wrist. Hand-wrist alignment improves after anlage excision. Others suggest that anlage excision should be more individualized (i.e., will try cast or splints to correct the angulation; is the condition static or progressive? is there wrist or elbow instability?).[14,38,97]

For type III and IV deformities, anlage excision and radial bowing should be treated to relieve tethering and correct alignment (Fig. 44-11, D). Rotational osteotomy of the radius may also be needed when there is an internal rotation deformity of the forearm. Treatment of the radial head dislocation is generally not necessary in type III (complete absence of the ulna) but should be considered in the type II deformity if it is restricting elbow motion.

Type II deformities are the most common and we recommend one-bone forearms in the majority of cases. This operation provides a stable elbow (proximal ulna) with a stable wrist (radius). Ulna anlage excision combined with radius-ulna fusion (fixation) is performed in one stage with care taken to identify ulnar neurovascular structures. Once the anlage is excised, the interosseous membrane can be dissected up to the level of radial osteotomy. Joining proximal ulna and distal radius is performed usually end-to-end with intramedullary K wires or Steinmann pin fixation. Bayne recommends late excision of the radial head if a one-bone-forearm procedure is performed with identification of posterior interosseous nerve.[5] Excision of radial head alone without the one-bone-forearm procedure leads to forearm instability and is contraindicated.

In summary, for the young infant with ulnar deficiency, splinting and casting are recommended, with excision of the ulnar anlage if the deformity is progressive. A preservation of forearm rotation is desirable. For later presentations (ages 1 to 3 years), the treatment depends on the classification. For type II, anlage excision is recommended alone or with creation of a one-bone forearm. The radial head dislocation is left alone unless it limits elbow motion. If there is good forearm stability (i.e., a relatively long ulna without forearm bowing), then excision of the anlage alone may be best.

In the older patient (older than age 3 years), problems include radial angulation, radial head protrusion, and ulnar deviation of the hand. Each condition can be treated individually based on the degree of deformity and effect on limb function. Appropriate corrective osteotomies at one or more levels can be considered, and the radial head can be excised if the forearm is stable.

THE DEFORMED DISTAL ULNA

Deformity of the distal ulna (styloid, head, neck, metaphysis) is fairly common in children, but so far little effect on function has been noted unless the deformity is the residue of trauma.[14] Considerable attention has been paid to the relative lengths of the ulna and radius at the wrist.[28,47,57,82] Ulna neutral, minus, and plus variances are commonly recorded as part of clinical and radiologic examinations. The ideal is thought to be the neutral variance ulna, because ulna plus and ulna minus variances have been associated with an increased incidence of clinical problems. For ulna minus variance, the problems have included Kienböck's disease and scapholunate dissociation. For ulna plus variance, there is a clear association with ulnocarpal impingement, lunotriquetral dissociation, tears of the triangular fibrocartilage complex, and proximal carpal row flexion instability (carpal instability nondissociative-volar intercalated segment instability [CIND-VISI]). Either ulna plus or minus variance may produce asymmetry or incongruence of the distal radioulnar joint. Treatment of these various lesions is discussed in other chapters.

THE CARPUS

CARPAL ANOMALIES

The proximal carpal row is an example of an intercalated segment, i.e., a structural unit in a joint linkage system, that is not directly controlled by motor units.[9,45,67,102] Because the proximal carpal row is also a highly mobile unit, responding to the indirect control of the musculotendinous units that originate proximal and insert distal to it, many factors have been selected as contributing to or detracting from the stability of the proximal carpal row, including the ligament system and the carpal bones (presence, shape, absence of other anomalies).

LIGAMENT LAXITY

The main ligament anomaly to be discussed here is hyperlaxity.[37,55,58,74,111] There are systemic criteria for this condition, which can manifest in syndromes such as Ehlers-Danlos and Marfan syndrome. Hyperlaxity of the wrist may be part of a systemic condition or may occur only at the wrist. There is no consensus on the characteristics of a hyperlax wrist, but these are suggested: Clinical—1) total range of passive wrist motion (extension, flexion, radial deviation, and ulnar deviation) of 280° or more and 2) creation of an obvious carpal deformity with or without a click, catch, thud, or snap during an active provocative maneuver or during an assisted or passive provocative maneuver; and Radiologic—1) radiographic demonstration of a static collapse deformity of either the carpal instability dissociative (CID) type or the CIND type without history of findings suggestive of injury and particularly if both wrists show similar findings and 2) hyperlaxity. Research into the variation in ligament anatomy about the wrist continues,[9,10] but the pattern of developmental deficiencies is not yet cataloged nor a consensus obtained, except for the common deficiency of ligament substance at the space of Poirier.[31,32,102]

SKELETAL ABNORMALITIES OF THE CARPUS

These conditions extend through the spectrum of total to partial absence, coalitions and accessory bones, alterations in shape, and overgrowth. For most of these alterations there is no clear-cut relationship to clinical problems or the clinical problem of the associated hand deformity takes precedence, as in the radial, central, and ulnar deficiencies. Among those congenital or developmental conditions, in which the wrist is the major problem, our experience is as follows.

1) Multiple ossification centers are among the most frequent conditions and are seen in the scaphoid and in the lunate. Not many years ago, it was taught that all scaphoids with evidence of incomplete consolidation at some level of the scaphoid body were congenital bipartite scaphoids.[56] They are of consequence only when misinterpreted as fractures. In fact, most of these are fracture residua* and should not be misinterpreted as congenital or developmental problems.

2) Hypoplasia of the scaphoid or other carpal bones may look like a multipartite bone at certain stages of deterioration under stress loading, but again this is mostly a stress fracture phenomenon,[32,67] usually with associated vascular deficiency. The condition often appears at presentation as Preiser's disease in the scaphoid and Kienböck's disease in the lunate.[35,67,97] Alterations of shape, trabeculation, or articular formation may be factors in more wrist skeletal problems than we know, but they have been discussed in only a few instances to date. One of these, the shape and internal trabecular pattern of the lunate and its predisposition to Kienböck's disease,[3] is discussed in the chapter on Kienböck's disease (see Chapter 18). Another involves the presence or absence of a hamate facet for articulation with the lunate[16,106] and the relationship of that finding with midcarpal arthritis.

3) Accessory bones and coalitions† in or near the carpus are of concern in the differential diagnosis of trauma residua, but they may affect carpal kinematics even if they are congenital. For instance, the common presentation of the proximal carpal row with coalition of the lunate and the triquetrum usually as a VISI deformity is to be expected because the triquetrum is unable to fully extend on the hamate facet. Because this probably increases the stress on the extrinsic ligaments supporting the proximal carpal row and the intrinsic ligaments

between the scaphoid and lunate, one might expect the incidence of both CIND-VISI and scapholunate dissociation (CID-dorsal intercalated segment instability [DISI]) to be somewhat increased, a supposition we believe to be true. Similar speculations can be made about the kinematic influence of scaphotrapezial coalitions, triquetrohamate coalitions, and others. Among the known accessories of the area, the "os styloideum" is probably best known in its common manifestation as a hard mass at the junction of the distal carpal row and third metacarpal base. Treatment will be discussed under Injuries to the Immature Wrist. We have seen several extensive accessories, usually overlying the radial carpus or the ulnar carpus, with a principal manifestation of limited motion and sometimes a fixed position of deviation and flexion. Standardized treatment for these anomalies is not established, but corrective osteotomies for realignment have been used successfully.

4) Associations with hand anomalies* only occasionally require treatment. Radial hemimelia problems are usually those of radial carpus hypoplasia and carpal dislocation, treated as discussed under radial deficiency. Central hemimelia and ulnar hemimelia problems of the carpus are usually absences, hypoplasias, or coalitions and do not usually require specific treatment. The incidence of specific wrist abnormality requiring treatment in the other categories of congenital hand anomalies is low, although there are conditions, mostly syndromes as discussed earlier, in which carpal coalitions are common.

CARPAL DEFORMITIES AND DEVELOPMENTAL CONDITIONS

Most of the significant carpal deformities are associated with bone or joint deficiency or abnormality,† as already reported, but some are secondary to congenital or developmental soft-tissue abnormalities such as arthrogryposis. Skeletal shortening, soft-tissue release, or transfer or combinations of these procedures have been the usual surgical approach for these problems. Supportive splinting preoperatively and postoperatively is a critical part of treatment. A good example of success of these measures for treatment of difficult problems has been reported by Mennen,[76] who has taken the previously reported measures of proximal row carpectomy plus release and transfer of the wrist flexors to obtain satisfactory results for treatment of the arthrogrypotic wrist. In arthrogryposis, the principal difference in application is the use of the procedures when the patient is very young. Treatment early in life is becoming the norm for most congenital and developmental

* References 32,35,52,56,57,61,69,80,97,99,104.
† References 4,8,18,22,23,26,30,34,41,48,52,56–58,61,73,85,97,98,113.

* References 14,35,58,75,85,88,97,98,111.
† References 2,6,21,36,62,96.

problems and for the most part seems to permit easier correction and easier maintenance of correction, provided both static deformities and dynamic imbalances are fully corrected. For the wrist that is both deformed and unstable, wrist shortening may need to be combined with wrist fusion. These measures are particularly applicable to the wrist that is damaged and arthritic from arthropathies.

Arthrogryposis multiplex congenita is a poorly understood congenital syndrome that primarily affects the wrist.[40,44,76,109,112] It is characterized by stiffness and contracture of multiple joints. It can be primarily neurologic or muscle band, and the joint and skeletal changes appear to be secondary. In the upper extremity the characteristic findings are flexion deformity of the wrist, stiff finger joints in moderate flexion, and nearly fixed or fixed extension deformity of the elbow.[76] The musculature surrounding the involved joints is hypoplastic.[109] Skin creases are often diminished or absent, reflecting poor joint function. The condition is commonly bilateral.

Variations on these positions, however, are not uncommon, and associated congenital anomalies such as syndactyly and web space contracture can accompany the joint stiffness. We have found that the primary deficit is usually radial nerve related (i.e., poor triceps function, wrist extension, and finger extension). Triceps muscle contraction causes the lack of elbow flexion while weak wrist extensors lead to wrist flexion and finger flexion posture. Wenner and Saperia[109] found 60% of these patients had a wrist flexion deformity.

The treatment principles involve release of capsular ligaments or bone resection to improve functional position of hand and wrist, with appropriate tendon transfers (Fig. 44-12). The wrist extension and occasional flexion deformity are serious problems limiting hand functional use. Surgical correction of wrist deformity is appropriate if static or dynamic splinting is ineffective.

Combined dorsal and palmar approaches may be necessary to treat arthrogryposis of the wrist. We begin palmarly through an extended carpal tunnel incision. The wrist and finger flexor tendons are examined and they are released if tight. Depending on the degree of tightness, one can elect to lengthen them alone or along with a release of the palmar wrist capsule. We prefer this approach (palmar capsular release and tendon lengthening) in the child younger than age 18 months who presents with arthrogryposis. The wrist flexors are lengthened with a Z-plasty transfer if there is evidence of active wrist extension, or they are transferred dorsally to assist in wrist or finger extension. The finger flexor tendons are also lengthened either by Z-plasty or by profundus-to-sublimis transfer if they are extremely tight. Palmar capsule release is performed to gain 15° to 20° of wrist extension. The wrist is pinned in extension with K wires, with cast immobilization for 4 to 6 weeks. For wrist extension

contracture, lengthening of common wrist extensors is required. This can be combined with release of thumb web space (adduction contracture) and metacarpophalangeal joint intrinsic muscle contractures (Fig. 44-12).

For older children (more than 2 years with arthrogryposis), proximal row carpectomy is a better choice because it 1) readily improves wrist extension by carpal bone excision and 2) indirectly lengthens all of the wrist and finger flexor tendons. We perform proximal row carpectomy (see Chapter 25) through a dorsal curvilinear incision (more transverse than longitudinal). It is important to examine the functional excursion of the wrist extensor tendons because they may be deficient or hypoplastic. Transfer of wrist flexors to finger extensors (or a finger superficialis to a wrist extensor) should be considered when extensor tendons appear deficient. For proximal row carpectomy we excise the entire row, including the entire scaphoid, usually by first dividing the scaphoid with an osteotome and then fragment excision with a scalpel or rongeurs. Capsular flaps, T shaped, are made during the exposure. These can be overlapped at the time of closure to maintain the wrist in extension. K-wire placement, retrograde through the capitate and then back through the radius, is performed to hold the wrist in extension at 25° to 30° (if possible). K wires are removed at 6 weeks and long-term wrist extension splinting is used until active wrist extension can be demonstrated.

Mennen[76] believed that surgery should be performed early at 3 to 6 months when carpal bones are cartilage and easier to excise. This may be too early, however, to routinely recommend proximal row carpectomy, although it does allow for considerable remodeling. We emphasize a later staging and stress the need for tendon transfers.

Wenner and Saperia[109] had five patients who had good results after proximal row excision, but three had recurrences. The patients were older (8 to 12 years) and only one had tendon transfer, which may account for the recurrences that led eventually to wrist arthrodesis. Friedlander, Westin, and Wood[40] reported on 50 wrist deformities, 6 treated by tendon transfer and capsulotomy and 4 by carpectomy, with good results. Osteotomies of the distal radius and ulna have been suggested by other authors,[44] with the potential of increased arc of wrist motion but without addressing tendon-muscle imbalance and need for transfers.

INJURIES TO THE IMMATURE WRIST

THE DISTAL RADIUS

Fracture of the distal radius[32,35,97] is as common in the child as in the adult, but such fractures are made more complicated by the presence of a physis, which is often involved because it is an area of diminished

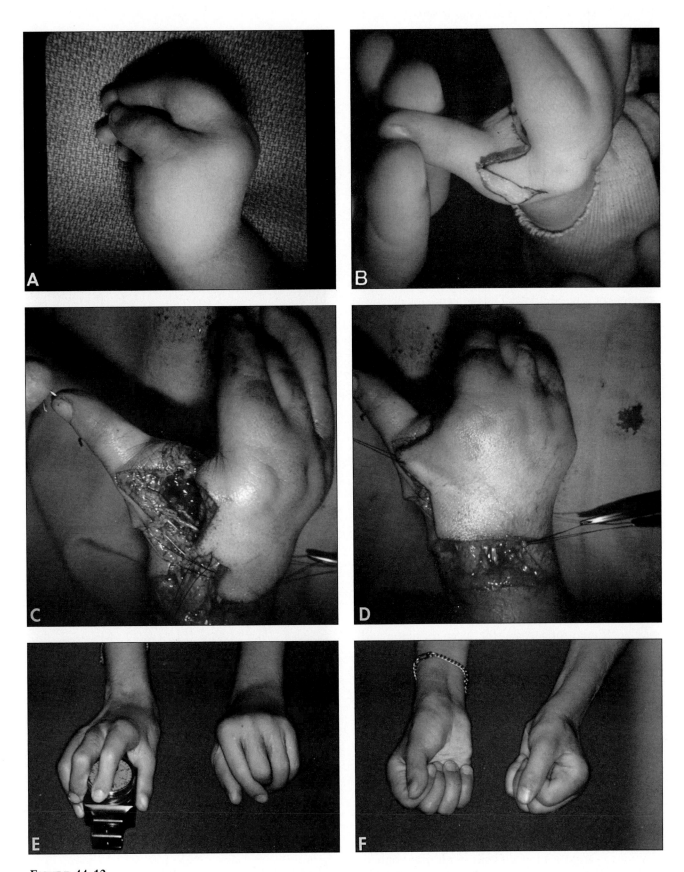

FIGURE 44-12

Arthrogryposis multiplex congenita. **A,** Early deformity of hand and wrist shows thumb adduction contracture, fixed extension of wrist, and flexion of the fingers. **B,** Z-plasty skin release, adductor pollicis lengthening, and first dorsal interosseous release. **C,** Web space deepening and release; Kirschner-wire fixation. **D,** Release of wrist extension contracture. Lengthening wrist extensor tendons. Skin Z-plasty lengthening and flap to cover thumb web space. **E,** Hand function appearance after bilateral wrist, thumb web space, and intrinsic muscle release. Mild flexion contracture of hand and wrist extension contracture. **F,** Bilateral hand grasp. Improved thumb abduction and extension.

resistance compared with bone (Fig. 44-13). These injuries and their treatment, both early and late, are discussed among physeal injuries in children (see Chapter 42). Repetitive stress on these same areas of high risk also produces damage and secondary deformity, particularly when they are related to athletic injuries (see Chapter 45). Carpal deformity can occur with these injuries or secondary to them. The secondary carpal deformities are usually best managed by proper treatment of the distal radius problem. Other than physis injury problems, the distal radius fracture, which is most likely to cause late problems at the distal radioulnar joint or the radiocarpal joint or both, is the fracture with an incompletely reduced rotatory component (Fig. 44-13, C). The problems, usually limited forearm motion or distal radioulnar joint pain, may be sufficient to warrant corrective osteotomy of the radius.

THE DISTAL ULNA

Direct injury to the distal ulna occurs, but it is more often injured in tandem with the distal radius and with the ligament systems that connect the two bones and the adjacent carpus.[7,14,32] The distal ulna also has a physis, and injury to it is similar to that of the distal radius.[66,82] Because the ulna is the smaller of the two forearm bones at the wrist, the problems of dislocation, instability, and malpositioning with lack of joint congruence are usually blamed on the ulna, even though the radius is usually the displaced bone.[47] Severe displacements of the distal ulna may attract early and appropriate attention even to the point of surgical reduction and repair. However, less dramatic injuries are often overlooked unless late problems develop. If joint surfaces are still intact, reduction and stability are often still possible by corrective osteotomy of either the radius or the ulna and repair or reconstruction of the damaged ligament apparatus. The perception of the ulna as an inferior and disposable support at the wrist has not been completely eradicated, and the prominent distal end of the ulna produced by an overly long ulna or overly short radius is a fairly well-known problem even in the child, but the effect of an unstable distal ulna on carpal posture is virtually ignored. The impingement problem can usually be managed adequately by adjusting the lengths of the two forearm bones to an ulna neutral length and an ulna stable configuration. The problem of the malpositioned carpus is more difficult, but it may respond to the same treatment or may require additional stabilizing procedures to the carpus itself.

Ulna lengthening and shortening procedures are now more commonly considered for radial physeal injuries, Madelung's deformity, osteochondromata, and other conditions.[39,42,83] The techniques of ulna shortening and lengthening are best performed independently of

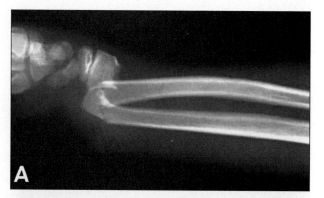
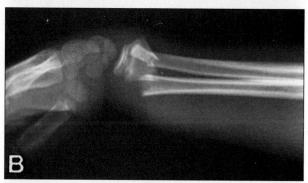
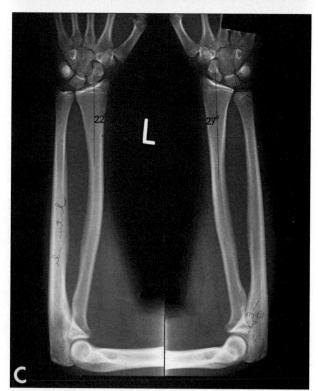

FIGURE 44-13

Distal radius and ulna fracture in the immature wrist. **A,** Oblique view of displaced radius and angulated distal ulna fractures. **B,** Lateral view shows dorsal displaced radius and ulna fractures. **C,** After closed reduction and cast immobilization, forearm alignment is restored. Axial malalignment of the right distal forearm, however, limited forearm supination (because the limb was immobilized in a long arm cast), forearm pronation, and wrist flexion.

any treatment of the radius (see Chapter 33). Ulna shortening is a straightforward procedure that is performed through a longitudinal mid-ulnar approach. A step-cut osteotomy with internal fixation with two to three screws is recommended in children. Control of rotation is also important during the osteotomy. Ulna shortening with internal plate fixation may be considered in older children (adolescents and young adults) with secondary plate removal. Care should be taken to avoid overshortening through the sigmoid fossa of the distal radius. Ulna shortening may be indicated in Madelung's deformity in combination with corrective osteotomy of the radius.

Ulna lengthening may be needed after physeal injuries, osteochondromatosis, growth disturbances related to tumor, or diseases[39] (see Chapter 33). The ulna lengthening can be performed by external fixation techniques such as the Wagner or Orthofix systems or by a one-stage lengthening using dynamic compression plates (and bone grafts), lamina spreaders to gain length, or combinations of external fixation plus plates. We have experience with Ilizarov systems for radial deformity (radial aplasia) but it may be overtreatment for ulna lengthening.

MADELUNG'S DEFORMITY

Madelung's deformity* (see Chapter 41) is a congenital disorder that becomes evident in late childhood and early adolescence as a curving deformity of the wrist. The most common deformity involves abnormal growth of the radial physis, combined with ulna prominence (ulna plus variance). Lesion of the ulnar one-half of the radial physis is the critical lesion that leads to increased radial angulation of the distal radius, secondary ulnar translation of the carpus, and ulnar angulation of the wrist.[105] Associated findings include loss of forearm rotation, subluxation of the wrist, and instability of the distal ulna. The most common radial problems involve 1) palmar subluxation of the carpus, 2) ulnar deviation of the wrist, 3) a dorsal-ulnar curve of the radius, 4) deformity of the physis with closure of the ulnar one-half of the radial physis, and 5) ulnar and palmar angulation of the distal radius articular surface. Ulnar problems include 1) dorsal subluxation, 2) deformity and enlargement of the ulnar head, and 3) decreased ulnar length. Secondary carpal changes that have developed over time involve smaller wedge-shaped scaphoid and lunate of the proximal row and ulnar translation changes, including an arched curvature continuous with the dorsal bar of the radial epiphysis.

Treatment of Madelung's deformity (see Chapter 41) may involve a combined approach on the radius and the ulna. We believe that excision of tethering tissues and

interposition of fat (preferred), methacrylate, or silicone to restore normal physeal growth is best.[66,87,105] Vickers[105] and Peterson[87] suggested that results of such interposition materials can be quite gratifying. We recommend these types of procedures in the patient younger than age 12 years. In the older patient with established deformity, we recommend corrective osteotomy and ulna shortening. Ulna resection alone should not be recommended in the young growing patient. The role of selected epiphysiodesis of radius or ulna is also an important consideration in selected patients. For younger patients, radial and ulnar osteotomy should be delayed in favor of procedures directed at the physeal bar. If the deformity is well established and the child is 12 years or older, lengthening of the ulnar one-half of the radius and shortening of the ulna can be considered. We prefer physiolysis (freeing the distal radius physis of all bone or soft-tissue tether) or the use of external fixator distractor lengthening devices to correct the multiplane and multifactor deformity when possible.

CARPAL INJURY

Instabilities, less than a complete dislocation, occur in the same patterns as in the adult but are rarely diagnosed and even less often reported.* Information is so sparse that nothing definitive can be said, but we have noted these trends: 1) the overall incidence of wrist instability, including dislocations and fracture dislocations, appears to be less than in the adult; 2) the most common instability problem in the child or adolescent appears to be the "instability patterns of the proximal carpal row" rather than scapholunate dissociation; and 3) when diagnosed early, closed positioning and wrist support give a better healing possibility than in the adult; when diagnosed late and symptomatic or malpositioned enough to have surgical treatment considered, soft-tissue repairs or reconstructions are favored.

Carpal dislocations and fracture dislocations are also uncommon in the child or adolescent, but they have been seen and occasionally reported.† Closed reduction is usually adequate, but it should be supplemented by open reduction and appropriate repairs if near-perfect reduction and alignment are not attained and maintained. Both bone and joint remodeling are possible for the child and to a limited extent for the adolescent, but loss of motion and sometimes pain can result from the residual deformities of a poor reduction. Salvage procedures, such as carpal bone excision or carpal fusion, are seldom necessary except in untreated and significantly deformed wrists, and these should be avoided if possible in favor of soft-tissue repair.

Carpal fracture injuries are also infrequently reported,* but enough experience has been obtained to draw these conclusions: 1) scaphoid fracture is the most common carpal fracture, as in the adult, but unlike in the adult, it is usually in the distal third; 2) bone healing usually occurs eventually if there is bone contact, but it can be very slow if reduction is not ideal; 3) even fractures complicated by ischemic changes (mostly Preiser's and Kienböck's) often heal in the child or adolescent age group, if protected from stress for a prolonged time; and 4) diagnosis is complicated by the injury history, which can be confusing or nonexistent, and by the general misperception of pediatric medical managers that congenital, infectious, arthropathy, or even tumor diagnoses are more common in the juvenile than trauma damage. For a long time this perception, even among orthopedists, led to the assumption that the common cause of the "bipartite scaphoid" was congenital and not injury.[69]

The treatment of carpal fractures in this age group occasionally extends to the same open reduction and internal fixation of the bones and repairs of the damaged ligaments that are often required for similar adult fractures. However, healing is quite good in this age group if the fracture position is acceptable and treatment is started early. The critical management feature is early and appropriate diagnosis. Preventive measures are not sufficiently emphasized. Even the normal wrist of the individual with an open physis in the distal radius or ulna should not be expected to accept the forces applied during gymnastics and similar activity without splint positioning and protection and without limiting the high-risk stress intervals, both from the standpoint of time and total involvement as well as the total time of peak increase. There are also special situations that increase risk such as the ulna minus configuration, the degree of lunate coverage by the radius (60% lunate coverage is normal), alterations of radial articular slope, and hypoplasia of carpal bones, particularly the scaphoid and lunate, which are the two primary stress transmitters in the carpus. Special precautions are also indicated for these wrists for both single episode trauma and repetitive stress trauma. Available reports suggest that fracture of the capitate is the next most frequent (after the scaphoid and lunate), but fracture of each of the carpals has been seen in the immature carpus.

SCAPHOID FRACTURES IN CHILDREN

Scaphoid fractures in children are uncommon because physeal separation occurs before the carpal bones fracture.† Nonetheless, scaphoid fractures do occur and must be suspected when wrist pain occurs in older children and young adults (Fig. 44-14). Statistics

suggest that 0.5% of children's upper limb fractures may involve the scaphoid (5/1,000). Our experience suggested that distal one-half to distal one-third fractures are more common whereas proximal one-third fractures are quite rare. We have seen scaphoid fractures either alone or in combination with fracture dislocations of the wrist.[86] Cross-country motocross racers in particular have an increasing incidence of scaphoid fractures and fracture dislocations.

Occasional differential diagnosis between scaphoid fractures and Preiser's avascular ischemia of scaphoid is difficult. In some cases, the relatively cartilaginous scaphoid cannot be imaged well to determine if there has been a fracture. Wrist arthroscopy can be helpful to distinguish between the scaphoid fracture and these other conditions.

Treatment of scaphoid fractures alone is preferably nonoperative. Unless clear displacement occurs or a delay in diagnosis has resulted in a true pseudarthrosis, cast immobilization should be sufficient. If there is displacement, a fracture dislocation of the wrist, or nonunion of the scaphoid (Fig. 44-15, B), operative intervention should be performed. We prefer a dorsal approach for most of these injuries so that both scaphoid fracture and any ligament injuries can be identified and treated. K-wire immobilization is needed in some but there has been no need to date for any type of compression screw, which we would try to avoid.

PREISER'S DISEASE

Preiser's disease is recognized as ischemic changes within the immature and mature scaphoid that give the appearance of scaphoid fracture.

DIFFERENTIAL DIAGNOSIS OF PROBLEMS OF THE IMMATURE WRIST

The managing physician may be lucky enough to see a juvenile with a known injury and obvious consequences or a juvenile with a known congenital or developmental abnormality with an obvious problem at the wrist. However, the more likely introduction will be the story of a gradual development of wrist pain with no pertinent or a confusing history. It is important to remember that: 1) the longitudinal bone growth in the area is endochondral bone formation from the physes, but there is also intramembranous bone formation occurring; 2) there is a high rate of skeletal turnover at all bone remodeling surfaces in the child (trabecular, endosteal, haversian, periosteal) with resulting rapid morphologic changes; and 3) much of the skeletal tissue is still cartilaginous and may not show on radiographs but will affect those nearby areas already ossified. The most likely possibilities for a wrist complaint are described below.

---

* References 25,31,32,69,70,86,97,100,104.
† References 17,35,67,80,86,100,104.

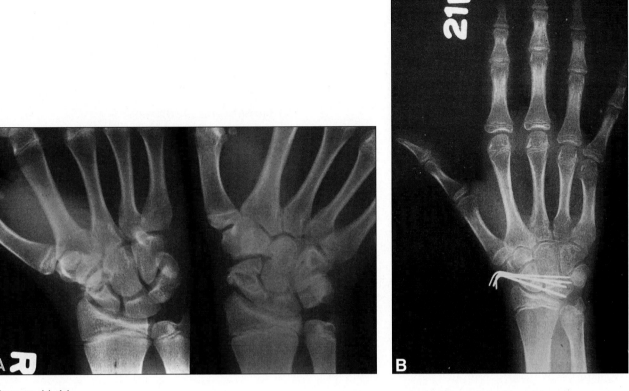

FIGURE 44-14

Scaphoid fracture in immature wrist. **A,** Radial and ulnar deviation views show a stable distal third fracture of the scaphoid. **B,** Treatment involved open reduction bone graft (Rüsse cancellous graft) and internal fixation with Kirschner wires.

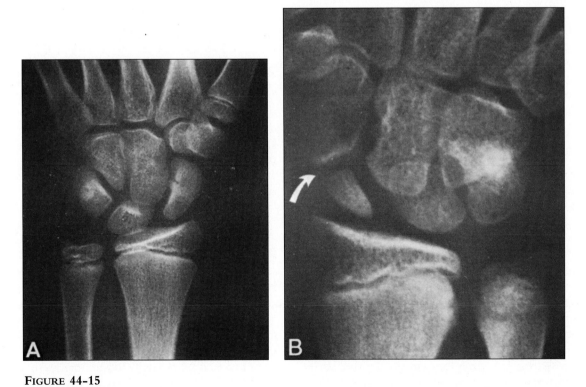

FIGURE 44-15

Scaphoid fracture in immature wrist. **A,** Delayed union (fibrous union) in a mid-third left scaphoid fracture. **B,** Scaphoid nonunion (*arrow*) secondary to ischemic necrosis and original fracture displacement. *(B, From Larson B, Light TR, Ogden JA: Fracture and ischemic necrosis of the immature scaphoid,* J Hand Surg [Am] *12:122-127, 1987. Copyright, American Society for Surgery of the Hand, by permission of Churchill Livingstone.)*

1) TRAUMA

Either single episode or repetitive injury is a possibility and there is also a considerable possibility of occult or hidden trauma from battering,[59] from convulsive episodes, or from fragility of the osseous structures. Specialized imaging may be necessary to differentiate trauma from developmental conditions of the wrist.[*]

2) CONGENITAL OR DEVELOPMENTAL

This diagnostic group includes accessories, coalitions, hypoplasias or absences, or the various deformities associated with the categories of hand anomaly [i.e., 1) failure of formation, 2) failure of differentiation, 3) duplication, 4) overgrowth, 5) undergrowth, 6) congenital constriction bands, and 7) generalized skeletal abnormalities].

3) ARTHROPATHY

Arthropathy may be from infection or disease. This is a particularly difficult category, because the associated swelling, tenderness, and stiffness can closely simulate trauma residua. It is vital that an infectious process be diagnosed early and treated appropriately. It is also important that more chronic conditions, such as juvenile rheumatoid arthritis, be confirmed or at least that the possibility of trauma residua be eliminated. Although the collagen diseases are the most common ones to be considered, such conditions as hemochromatosis, calcium pyrophosphate deposition disease, hypertrophic osteoarthropathy, and sickle disease are potential causes of wrist problems.[†]

4) SKELETAL DYSPLASIA

The many conditions in this category have already been listed in the section on congenital or developmental abnormalities. It is important in detecting this group that a general evaluation be done by an examining physician, because short stature is a common finding.[55,58,74,75,111] Short stature may be within the spectrum of normal, even when individuals are excessively short, or it may be abnormal short stature. If the abnormal short stature is proportionate, endocrine disorders are more likely. If the short stature is disproportionate, some type of osteochondrodysplasia is more likely: short-trunk dysplasia or short-limb dysplasia. The subdivisions of this last group are rhizomelic dysplasia, mesomelic dysplasia, and acromelic dysplasia. In addition to the clinical examination, radiographs of the spine and all the extremities are needed. Consideration of such a diagnosis by a wrist specialist results in referral to a pediatric specialist for appropriate work-up and management.

5) NUTRITIONAL DISORDERS

In much of the world nutritional disorders are becoming a significant part of the differential diagnosis.[35,55,98,99] Even minor degrees of nutritional deficit may result in changes in the rates of skeletal maturation and in accessory ossification centers. More severe deprivation may result in rickets. Chronic total parenteral nutrition may result in copper depletion with generalized demineralization, including lack of ossification of the carpals. These changes and others are similar to another nutritional deprivation disease, scurvy. Excesses are also seen, such as hypervitaminosis A, usually from overdosage of vitamin A as a treatment attempt for acne. These changes, usually hyperostosis of the ulna as far as the wrist area is concerned, are similar to those seen with idiopathic cortical hyperostosis (Caffey's disease).

6) TUMORS

Although almost any neoplasia of either skeletal or soft parts can involve the wrist, the most likely are the various fibromatoses of infancy and childhood, usually benign, and tumors of the blood-forming organs, usually malignant (leukemia).

7) NEUROMUSCULAR DEFICITS

Deformities of the wrist and other skeletal structures due to lack of function, abnormal function, or simply asymmetrical function of the neuromuscular system are a common problem, usually congenital or developmental in origin. Some of these problems, such as arthrogryposis, are included in prior categories; some, such as cerebral palsy, are not.

A DIAGNOSTIC METHODOLOGY FOR PROBLEMS OF THE IMMATURE WRIST

HISTORY

From the standpoint of a wrist management specialist, the initial history naturally is concerned with the wrist problem. Details of its onset and characteristics, clues to its etiology, if any, and management efforts to date should be ascertained, whether sparse or extensive. Even a wrist expert should then proceed to inquire about familial, skeletal, or other system involvement and about the results of pediatric or other consultations.

---

[*] References 11,12,29,35,36,45,46,54,79,81,97,113.
[†] References 1,2,21,36,47,96.

PHYSICAL EXAMINATION

Evaluation of relationships, intelligence, and physical-physiologic-psychologic development proceeds continually as the introductions and examination proceed. Early observation should include observations of stature (short or deformed), limb length (short or deformed), and whether these two features are associated. The status of both wrists and hands and of the upper limbs generally should be ascertained by observation, palpation, and range of motion for anomalies, deformities, malfunction, and signs. The usual signs are swelling or masses and other topographic alterations, crease patterns and other skin alterations, color alterations, temperature alterations, and motion alterations.[*]

PROVOCATIVE MANEUVERS

As with any joint, an important part of a physical examination is reproduction of the symptoms, usually those of pain or abnormal movements or positions. Simple motions or commonplace or special activities may be sufficient to provoke symptoms; if so, they should be performed, described, and analyzed. As in the adult, the next provocative maneuver in the sequence is usually the ascertainment, localization, and prioritization of specific tender areas, particularly those that reprise some element or all of the familiar symptoms. This is done by progressing from light to heavy pressure over various anatomic points within the perceived zone of symptoms. Pressure may be applied with an object such as a pencil eraser, but it is usually best applied with digit tips, because there is stereognostic feedback from this examining tool. In this fashion the amount of pressure is easily titrated from light to heavy with one fingertip, then to reinforced pressure at that fingertip all the way to double thumb maximum pressure, which is sufficient to make even normal structures uncomfortable. This is an extremely valuable provocative maneuver, but it is probably best deferred in the child until last or perhaps not done at all on the first examination, because the amount of pain produced and the degree of cooperation permitted are inversely proportional. Other active provocative maneuvers may be known to the patient or may be easily demonstrated by circumduction, simple grip, range of motion, forearm rotation, digit motions, or various combinations of these.

The most common active maneuver to produce the often symptomatic scapholunate dissociation or the "catch-up clunk" of proximal carpal row instability (CIND-VISI or midcarpal instability in some terminology) consists of wrist motion with slight grip compression and neutral positioning between radial deviation

and ulnar deviation (see Chapter 12). Symptoms are often better demonstrated by passive provocative maneuvers (such as scaphoid stress tests of Watson et al.,[107] lunotriquetral stress test of Reagan et al.,[93] and Kleinman[60]) or simple tests of both joint laxity and symptomatic instabilities: 1) passive range of motion; 2) translational range of motion at all three joints (radioulnocarpal, midcarpal, distal radioulnar) and in four directions (dorsal, palmar, radial, and ulnar); 3) addition of compression to 1 and 2; 4) combinations of pressure and force over bone surfaces, either pushing in the same direction (dorsal pressure on the palmar prominences of the scaphoid tuberosity and the pisiform to translate the proximal carpal row, which may move as a unit or in separate dissociated units) or pushing in opposite directions (dorsal pressure at the palmar pisiform combined with palmar-directed pressure over the dorsal head of the ulna to realign the ulna, triangular fibrocartilage complex, and ulnar carpus; pushing in opposite directions over the dorsal capitate and the palmar forearm to realign the carpal rows); and 5) translocating one or more carpal bones on other articular surfaces, e.g., pisiform on triquetrum, lunate on triquetrum, scaphoid on lunate, proximal carpal row on radius or triangular fibrocartilage.

Some of these maneuvers demonstrate wrist laxity without any particular pathology, although it is known that joint laxity contributes to certain types of wrist injury. The most common wrist area demonstrations of laxity are excessive dorsopalmar range of the distal ulna; collapse of the proximal carpal row into a CIND-VISI (silver fork deformity, clinically) pattern with palmar translation of the hand and distal carpal row on the stabilized forearm, usually more dramatic in ulnar deviation but present also in the midposition with moderate laxity and even in radial deviation with severe laxity; and prominence (near dislocation) of the capitate and distal carpal row with dorsal translation of the hand and distal carpal row on the fixed forearm. A full listing of wrist area provocative maneuvers is beyond the scope of this chapter, but they are important parts of the clinical examination for wrist problems (see Chapter 12).

IMAGING

The current generation of wrist managers are quite uneasy if they cannot confirm clinical suspicions by some type of imaging[*]; as imaging techniques improve, they almost justify such faith. Certainly, no problem possibly pertaining to the wrist articulations should be evaluated without standard, comparison views (posteroanterior and lateral) of both hands and wrists. If a congenital or developmental syndrome or systemic problems are likely, the entire upper limb and appropriate other areas should also be visualized on radiographs, although some of this may be left to the discretion of consultants, if additional consultation is to be requested. Comparison of the wrist radiographs to each other and to age-equated norms can be informative and further imaging may not be required.

However, there are many excellent, additional studies, if needed: 1) radioactive scans to identify reflex

sympathetic dystrophy, vascular alterations, infection, arthropathy, certain tumors; 2) arthrography for communications between joints, joints and spaces, joints and tendon sheaths; 3) tomography for better visualization of ossified structures and their relationships (position of the ulnar head in relation to the sigmoid fossa is best defined in this way); 4) magnetic resonance imaging for better visualization of unossified bones, ligaments, tumors, vascular alterations; 5) ultrasonography

Table 44-4. A Quick Reference for Treatment of Problems of the Immature Wrist*

Problem of the Immature Wrist	Usual Treatment
1. Carpal accessories	Symptoms: treat as fractures or nonunions
2. Carpal coalitions Minnaar 1 and 2	Symptoms: treat as fractures or nonunions
3. Carpal coalitions Minnaar 3 and 4; symptoms from positional stress	Diminish stress loading
4. Carpal coalitions Fixed malposition Limited motion	Restore alignment with osteotomy
5. Carpal dislocation with radial hemimelia	Open reduction with soft-tissue decompression and balancing
6. Carpal deformity with ulnar hemimelia	Excision of ulnar cartilaginous and fibrous tethers and rebalancing of musculotendinous units, if ulnar deviation cannot be reduced to < 20°
7. Arthrogryposis & similar conditions	Proximal row carpectomy and release or transfer of wrist flexors
8. Cerebral palsy & similar diseases	Same as above (7)
9. Fracture of distal forearm	Closed reduction and support (check rotation, physis alignment carefully)
10. Physis-related deformity Growth correction still possible	Physiolysis and block of recurrent scar or bone tether
11. Physis-related deformity No growth correction	Corrective osteotomy with forearm leveling (usually with bone graft)
12. Dislocation or subluxation of distal ulna	Closed reduction (open, if needed) & long arm support
13. Carpal dislocation or subluxation	Closed or open reduction and support
14. Other carpal instability(proximal carpal row instability > scapholunate dissociation > lunotriquetral dissociation)	Closed or open reduction and support
15. Destroyed distal radioulnar joint	Interposition arthroplasty; retain distal ulna physis
16. Destroyed radiocarpal joint	Proximal row carpectomy > radiocarpal fusion
17. Destroyed metacarpal joint	Fusion or arthroplasty (fat)
18. Hypoplastic scaphoid	Diminish loading stress
19. Preiser's disease	Long arm support with or without electric stimulation
20. Preiser's disease (advanced)	Excise scaphoid and interpose fat with or without four-corner fusion
21. Bipartite scaphoid	Treat as fracture, usually with external support
22. Hypoplastic lunate	Diminish loading stress
23. Kienböck's disease	External support with or without electrical stimulation
24. Carpal fractures	Adequate reduction, closed or open, and support
25. Wrist bone or joint infection	Adequate drainage and proper antibiotics
26. Wrist arthropathy	Treat cause; consider synovectomy
27. Wrist tumor	Biopsy or excise or both

* References 7,14,27,31,32,35,39,42,43,51,55,58,64-68,76,80,82,83,86,87,97,100-106,110.

for ganglia, vascular alterations, tumors; 6) special views to demonstrate instability patterns such as stress views, motion studies via passive positions at the extremes via video motion studies (video should include any active provocative maneuvers and possibly include arthrography followed by a repeat of the motion sequences); and 7) three-dimensional reconstructions for carpal relationships and deformities. The development of new and better imaging techniques is competitive with the development of new and better endoscopic techniques. Better visualization of structures, both the normal and the abnormal, buried beneath the enveloping skin surface of the body results from these techniques alone or in combinations. Wrist management benefits from both!

INVASIVE METHODS

Endoscopic methods are used for diagnosis and treatment at the various joints of the wrist and for treatment only in the carpal tunnel area. It is our belief that such methods will be used, eventually, for diagnosis and for treatment even more extensively in the joint systems of the wrist as well as multiple soft-tissue compartments around the wrist. For practical purposes, the immediate current extent of diagnostic assistance from endoscopy relates entirely to arthroscopy of the various wrist joints; even so, much can be learned as follows: 1) visualization and palpation, not perfect but often diagnostic, of joint space, joint cartilage, synovium, many ligaments, and loose bodies as well as bone characteristics such as density, deformity, fracture; 2) stability of the carpal structures under mild stresses; 3) culture of any suspect areas; and 4) biopsy of one or several areas or structures. Such examinations may be aided by cleansing and irrigation and certain treatments may be elected at the same time or at some subsequent time.

Surgery is not often thought of as a diagnostic method, but it is one of the best, because direct inspection at rest and under test is maximum by this technique, although varied by virtue of the direction of and the amount of the exposure. Surgery may, in fact, be done primarily for diagnostic purposes, as for limited visualization of a specific area or structure or specifically for culture or biopsy. Even surgery done specifically for treatment purposes may be instructive with regard to abnormal and pathologic findings; one of the tragedies of this common technique (open surgery) is that both actual observations and the recording of findings are often given short shrift. A lesson, slowly learned, is that extensive exposure, e.g., both dorsal and palmar for wrist dislocations, often pays large dividends in diagnosis and adequate treatment.

SUMMARY

The problems of the immature wrist, whether due to anomalies, injuries, or other causes, are somewhat mysterious because final form and function have not been achieved; metabolic, healing, and reactive responses are so swift; and complaints are different or disguised and growth centers are still open (Table 44-4). There is also a protective instinct operative, which disinclines parents to relinquish responsibility to physicians and one group of physicians to relinquish responsibility to another group. Add to these factors the "hidden iceberg" nature of a large part of the skeleton, which is not yet ossified, and it is not remarkable that skeletal diagnoses are often not made or made only in retrospect. This is further complicated by the fact that healing in the child is so swift after transient episodes of injury, infection, or even disease that medical investigators are often presented with nature's "fait accompli" by the time we are secure with a diagnosis. Rationalize as we may, we can and must do a better job of diagnosing the problems of the immature wrist. With that in mind, this chapter has been constructed, but it will make little difference until all medical managers realize that if a child's wrist is sore, swollen, or stiff, a diagnosis must be made! Whether or what treatment is then required is another matter, but to judge treatment or prognosis with any value we must know what is wrong!

REFERENCES

1. Adamson TC III, Resnik CS, Guerra J Jr, et al.: Hand and wrist arthropathies of hemochromatosis and calcium pyrophosphate deposition disease: distinct radiographic features, *Radiology* 147:377-381, 1983.
2. Ansell BM, Kent PA: Radiological changes in juvenile chronic polyarthritis, *Skeletal Radiol* 1:129-144, 1977.
3. Antuna-Zapico JM: *Morfologia radiologica de los huesos del carpo.* In Antuna-Zapico JM, editor: *Malcia del Semilunar,* Caracas, Venezuela, 1966, Valladolid Secretariado de Publicaciones de la Universidad de Valladolid.
4. Bassöe E, Bassöe HH: The styloid bone and carpe bossu disease, *Am J Roentgenol* 74:886-888, 1955.
5. Bayne LG: *Radial clubhand (radial deficiencies).* In Green DP, editor: *Operative hand surgery,* ed 2, vol 1, New York, 1988, Churchill Livingstone.
6. Beals RK, Bird CB: Carpal and tarsal osteolysis. A case report and review of the literature, *J Bone Joint Surg Am* 57:681-686, 1975.
7. Beals RK, Lovrien EW: Dyschondrosteosis and Madelung's deformity. Report of three kindreds and review of the literature, *Clin Orthop* 116:24-28, 1976.
8. Beatty E: Upper limb tissue differentiation in the human embryo, *Hand Clin* 1:391-403, 1985.
9. Berger RA, Kauer JM, Landsmeer JM: Radioscapholunate ligament: a gross anatomic and histologic study of fetal and adult wrists, *J Hand Surg [Am]* 16:350-355, 1991.
10. Berger RA, Landsmeer JM: The palmar radiocarpal ligaments: a study of adult and fetal human wrist joints, *J Hand Surg [Am]* 15:847-854, 1990.
11. Binkovitz LA, Ehman RL, Cahill DR, et al.: Magnetic resonance imaging of the wrist: normal cross sectional imaging and selected abnormal cases, *Radiographics* 8:1171-1202, 1988.
12. Bond JR, Berquist TH: Radiologic evaluation of hand and wrist motion, *Hand Clin* 7:113-123, 1991.
13. Bora FW Jr, Osterman AL, Kaneda RR, et al.: Radial club-hand deformity. Long-term follow-up, *J Bone Joint Surg Am* 63:741-745, 1981.
14. Broudy AS, Smith RJ: Deformities of the hand and wrist with ulnar deficiency, *J Hand Surg [Am]* 4:304-315, 1979.
15. Buck-Gramcko D: Radialization as a new treatment for radial club hand, *J Hand Surg [Am]* 10:964-968, 1985.
16. Burgess RC: Anatomic variations of the midcarpal joint, *J Hand Surg [Am]* 15:129-131, 1990.
17. Caputo AE, Watson HK, Nissen C: Scaphoid nonunion in a child: a case report, *J Hand Surg [Am]* 20:243-245, 1995.
18. Carlson DH: Coalition of the carpal bones, *Skeletal Radiol* 7:125-127, 1981.
19. Carroll RE, Bowers WH: Congenital deficiency of the ulna, *J Hand Surg [Am]* 2:169-174, 1977.
20. Catagni MA, Szabo RM, Cattaneo R: Preliminary experience with Ilizarov method in late reconstruction of radial hemimelia, *J Hand Surg [Am]* 18:316-321, 1993.
21. Cavanaugh JJA, Holman GH: Hypertrophic osteoarthropathy in childhood, *J Pediatr* 66:27, 1965.
22. Cockshott WP: Carpal fusions, *Am J Roentgenol* 89:1260-1271, 1963.
23. Conway WF, Destouet JM, Gilula LA, et al.: The carpal boss: an overview of radiographic evaluation, *Radiology* 156:29-31, 1985.
24. Cooney WP, Dobyns JH: Radial aplasia results with staged distraction and centralization. Presented at the 48th Annual Meeting of the American Association for Surgery of the Hand, Kansas City, 1993.
25. Cooney WP III, Linscheid RL, Dobyns JH: *Fractures and dislocations of the wrist.* In Rockwood CA Jr, Green DP, Bucholz RW, et al., editors: *Fractures in adults,* ed 4, vol 1, Philadelphia, 1996, Lippincott-Raven, pp 745-867.
26. Cope JR: Carpal coalition, *Clin Radiol* 25:261-266, 1974.
27. Cuono CB, Watson HK: The carpal boss: surgical treatment and etiological considerations, *Plast Reconstr Surg* 63:88-93, 1979.
28. Czitrom AA, Dobyns JH, Linscheid RL: Ulnar variance in carpal instability, *J Hand Surg [Am]* 12:205-208, 1987.
29. Dalinka MK, Meyer S, Kricun ME, et al.: Magnetic resonance imaging of the wrist, *Hand Clin* 7:87-98, 1991.
30. deVilliers Minnaar AB: Congenital fusion of the lunate and triquetral bones in the South African Bantu, *J Bone Joint Surg Br* 34:45-48, 1952.
31. Dobyns JH, Berger RA: *Dislocations of the carpus.* In Chapman MM, Madison M, editors: *Operative orthopaedics,* ed 2, Philadelphia, 1993, JB Lippincott.
32. Dobyns JH, Linscheid RL: *Fractures and dislocations of the wrist.* In Rockwood CA, Green DP, editors: *Fractures in adults,* ed 2, vol 1, Philadelphia, 1984, JB Lippincott.
33. Dobyns JH, Wood VE, Bayne LG, et al.: *Congenital hand deformities.* In Green DP, editor: *Operative hand surgery,* vol 1, New York, 1982, Churchill Livingstone.
34. Ebni B, et al.: Contribucion al estudio de los huesos accesorios de la mano, *Rev Mano* 24:65-76, 1982.
35. Esposito PW, Crawford AH: *Wrist disorders in children.* In Lichtman DM, editor: *The wrist and its disorders,* Philadelphia, 1988, WB Saunders.
36. Feinstein KA, Poznanski AK: *Evaluation of joint disease in the pediatric hand.* In Bora FW Jr, editor: *The pediatric upper extremity: diagnosis and management,* Philadelphia, 1986, WB Saunders.
37. Finsterbush A, Pogrund H: The hypermobility syndrome. Musculoskeletal complaints in 100 consecutive cases of generalized joint hypermobility, *Clin Orthop* 168:124-127, 1982.
38. Flatt AE: *The care of congenital hand anomalies,* ed 2, St. Louis, 1994, Quality Medical Publishing.
39. Fogel GR, McElfresh EC, Peterson HA, et al.: Management of deformities of the forearm in multiple hereditary osteochondromas, *J Bone Joint Surg Am* 66:670-680, 1984.
40. Friedlander HL, Westin GW, Wood WL Jr: Arthrogryposis multiplex congenita. A review of forty-five cases, *J Bone Joint Surg Am* 50:89-112, 1968.
41. Garn SM, Rohmann CG, Davis AA: Genetics of hand-wrist ossification, *Am J Phys Anthrop* 21:33-40, 1963.

42. Gelberman RH, Bauman T: Madelung's deformity and dyschondrosteosis, *J Hand Surg [Am]* 5:338-340, 1980.

43. Gerard FM: Post-traumatic carpal instability in a young child. A case report, *J Bone Joint Surg Am* 62:131-133, 1980.

44. Gibson DA, Urs ND: Arthrogryposis multiplex congenita, *J Bone Joint Surg Br* 52:483-493, 1970.

45. Gilula LA, Destouet JM, Weeks PM, et al.: Roentgenographic diagnosis of the painful wrist, *Clin Orthop* 187:52-64, 1984.

46. Greenan T, Zlatkin MB: Magnetic resonance imaging of the wrist, *Semin Ultrasound CT MRI* 11:267-287, 1990.

47. Hafner R, Poznanski AK, Donovan JM: Ulnar variance in children—standard measurements for evaluation of ulnar shortening in juvenile rheumatoid arthritis, hereditary multiple exostosis and other bone or joint disorders in childhood, *Skeletal Radiol* 18:513-516, 1989.

48. Harle TS, Stevenson JR: Hereditary symphalangism associated with carpal and tarsal fusions, *Radiology* 89:91-94, 1967.

49. Harper HAS, Poznanski AK, Garn SM: The carpal angle in American populations, *Invest Radiol* 9:217-221, 1974.

50. Herrmann J, Zugibe FT, Gilbert EF, et al.: Arthro-dento-osteo dysplasia (Hajdu-Cheney syndrome). Review of a genetic "acro-osteolysis" syndrome, *Z Kinderheilkd* 114:93-110, 1973.

51. Holder LE, Mackinnon SE: Reflex sympathetic dystrophy in the hands: clinical and scintigraphic criteria, *Radiology* 152:517-522, 1984.

52. Hughes PCR, Tanner JM: The development of carpal bone fusion as seen in serial radiographs, *Br J Radiol* 39:943-949, 1966.

53. Johnson J, Omer GE Jr: Congenital ulnar deficiency. Natural history and therapeutic implications, *Hand Clin* 1:499-510, 1985.

54. Jonsson K, Eiken O: Development of carpal bone cysts as revealed by radiography, *Acta Radiol Diagn (Stockh)* 24:231-233, 1983.

55. Kaplan F: *Heritable and endocrine disorders of connective tissue metabolism.* In Bora FW Jr, editor: *The pediatric upper extremity: diagnosis and management,* Philadelphia, 1986, WB Saunders.

56. Keats TE: *An atlas of normal roentgen variants that may simulate disease,* ed 4, Chicago, 1988, Year Book Medical Publishers.

57. Keats TE: Normal variants of the hand and wrist, *Hand Clin* 7:153-166, 1991.

58. Kelikian H: *Congenital deformities of the hand and forearm,* Philadelphia, 1974, WB Saunders.

59. Kleinman PK: *Diagnostic imaging of child abuse,* Baltimore, 1987, Williams & Wilkins.

60. Kleinman W: Lunotriquetral stress examination, *American Society for Surgery of the Hand Correspondence Newsletters,* 1992.

61. Kohler A, Zimmer EA: *Borderlands of the normal and early pathologic in skeletal roentgenology,* ed 3, New York, 1968, Grune & Stratton.

62. Kohler E, Babbitt D, Huizenga B, et al.: Hereditary osteolysis. A clinical, radiological and chemical study, *Radiology* 108:99-105, 1973.

63. Lamb DW: Radial clubhand. A continuing study of sixty-eight patients with one hundred and seventeen club hands, *J Bone Joint Surg Am* 59:1-13, 1977.

64. Lamesch AJ: Dysplasia epiphysealis hemimelica of the carpal bones. Report of a case and review of the literature, *J Bone Joint Surg Am* 65:398-400, 1983.

65. Landsmeer JMF: *Atlas of anatomy of the hand,* New York, 1976, Churchill Livingstone.

66. Langenskiold A, Osterman K: Surgical treatment of partial closure of the epiphysial plate, *Reconstr Surg Traumatol* 17:48-64, 1979.

67. Light TR: Injury to the immature carpus, *Hand Clin* 4:415-424, 1988.

68. Linscheid RL, Dobyns JH, Beabout JW, et al.: Traumatic instability of the wrist. Diagnosis, classification, and pathomechanics, *J Bone Joint Surg Am* 54:1612-1632, 1972.

69. Louis DS, Calhoun TP, Garn SM, et al.: Congenital bipartite scaphoid—fact or fiction? *J Bone Joint Surg Am* 58:1108-1112, 1976.

70. Magid D, Thompson JS, Fishman EK: Computed tomography of the hand and wrist, *Hand Clin* 7:219-233, 1991.

71. Manske PR, McCarroll HR Jr, Swanson K: Centralization of the radial club hand: an ulnar surgical approach, *J Hand Surg [Am]* 6:423-433, 1981.

72. Maurer AH: Nuclear medicine in evaluation of the hand and wrist. *Hand Clin* 7:183-200, 1991.

73. McCredie J: Congenital fusion of bones: radiology, embryology and pathogenesis, *Clin Radiol* 26:47-51, 1975.

74. McKusick VA: *Heritable disorders of connective tissue,* ed 4, St. Louis, 1972, CV Mosby.

75. McKusick VA: *Mendelian inheritance in man: catalogs of autosomal dominant, autosomal recessive, and x-linked phenotypes,* ed 6, Baltimore, 1983, Johns Hopkins University Press.

76. Mennen U: Early corrective surgery of the wrist and elbow in arthrogryposis multiplex congenita, *J Hand Surg [Br]* 18:304-307, 1993.

77. Mesgarzadeh M, Schneck CD, Bonakdarpour A: Carpal tunnel: MR imaging. Part I. Normal anatomy, *Radiology* 171:743-748, 1989.

78. Mesgarzadeh M, Schneck CD, Bonakdarpour A, et al.: Carpal tunnel: MR imaging. Part II. Carpal tunnel syndrome, *Radiology* 171:749-754, 1989.

79. Mrose HE, Rosenthal DI: Arthrography of the hand and wrist, *Hand Clin* 7:201-217, 1991.

80. Mussbichler H: Injuries of the carpal scaphoid in children, *Acta Radiol* 56:361-368, 1961.

81. Nakamura R, Horii E, Tanaka Y, et al.: Three-dimensional CT imaging for wrist disorders, *J Hand Surg [Br]* 14:53-58, 1989.

82. Nelson OA, Buchanan JR, Harrison CS: Distal ulnar growth arrest, *J Hand Surg [Am]* 9:164-170, 1984

83. Nielsen JB: Madelung's deformity. A follow-up study of 26 cases and a review of the literature, *Acta Orthop Scand* 48:379-384, 1977.

84. Ogden JA, Watson HK, Bohne W: Ulnar dysmelia, *J Bone Joint Surg Am* 58:467-475, 1976.

85. O'Rahilly R: A survey of carpal and tarsal anomalies, *J Bone Joint Surg Am* 35:626-642, 1953.

86. Peiro A, Martos F, Mut T, et al.: Trans-scaphoid perilunate dislocation in a child. A case report, *Acta Orthop Scand* 52:31-34, 1981.

87. Peterson HA: *Scanning the bridge.* In Uhthoff HK, Wiley JJ, editors: *Behavior of the growth plate,* New York, 1988, Raven Press.

88. Poznanski AK: *The hand in radiologic diagnosis: with gamuts and pattern profiles,* ed 2, Philadelphia, 1984, WB Saunders.

89. Poznanski AK: Useful measurements in the evaluation of hand radiographs, *Hand Clin* 7:21-36, 1991.

90. Poznanski AK, Hernandez RJ, Guire KE, et al.: Carpal length in children—a useful measurement in the diagnosis of rheumatoid arthritis and some congenital malformation syndromes, *Radiology* 129:661-668, 1978.

91. Pritchett JW: Growth and predictions of growth in the upper extremity, *J Bone Joint Surg Am* 70:520-525, 1988.

92. Ranawat CS, DeFiore J, Straub LR: Madelung's deformity. An end-result study of surgical treatment, *J Bone Joint Surg Am* 57:772-775, 1975.

93. Reagan DS, Linscheid RL, Dobyns JH: Lunotriquetral sprains, *J Hand Surg [Am]* 9:502-514, 1984.

94. Riordan DC: Congenital absence of the radius. A 15-year follow-up (abstract), *J Bone Joint Surg Am* 45:1783, 1963.

95. Riordan DC, Mills EH, Alldredge RH: Congenital absence of the ulna (abstract), *J Bone Joint Surg Am* 43:614, 1961.

96. Schaller JG: Arthritis in children, *Pediatr Clin North Am* 33:1565-1580, 1986.

97. Simmons BP: *Injuries to and developmental deformities of the wrist and carpus.* In Bora FW Jr, editor: *The pediatric upper extremity: diagnosis and management,* Philadelphia, 1986, WB Saunders.

98. Smith DW: *Recognizable patterns of human malformation: genetic, embryologic, and clinical aspects,* ed 2, Philadelphia, 1976, WB Saunders.

99. Snodgrass RM, Dreizen S, Currie C, et al.: The association between anomalous ossification centers in the hand skeleton, nutritional status and rate of skeletal maturation in children five to fourteen years of age, *Am J Roentgenol* 74:1037-1048, 1955.

100. Southcott R, Rosman MA: Non-union of carpal scaphoid fractures in children, *J Bone Joint Surg Br* 59:20-23, 1977.

101. Swanson AB, Tada K, Yonenobu K: Ulnar ray deficiency: its various manifestations, *J Hand Surg [Am]* 9:658-664, 1984.

102. Taleisnik J: *The wrist,* New York, 1985, Churchill Livingstone.

103. Tehranzadeh J, Labosky DA, Gabriele OF: Ganglion cysts and tear of triangular fibrocartilages of both wrists in a cheerleader, *Am J Sports Med* 11:357-359, 1983.

104. Vahvanen V, Westerlund M: Fracture of the carpal scaphoid in children. A clinical and roentgenological study of 108 cases, *Acta Orthop Scand* 51:909-913, 1980.

105. Vickers DW: Langenskiold's operation (physiolysis) for congenital malformation of bone producing Madelung's deformity and clinodactyly (abstract), *J Bone Joint Surg Br* 66:778, 1984.

106. Viegas SF, Wagner K, Patterson R, et al.: Medial (hamate) facet of the lunate, *J Hand Surg [Am]* 15:564-571, 1990.

107. Watson HK, Ashmead D IV, Makhlouf MV: Examination of the scaphoid, *J Hand Surg [Am]* 13:657-660, 1988.

108. Watson HK, Bohne WH: The role of the fibrous hand in ulnar deficient extremities (abstract), *J Bone Joint Surg Am* 53:816, 1971.

109. Wenner SM, Saperia BS: Proximal row carpectomy in arthrogrypotic wrist deformity, *J Hand Surg [Am]* 12:523-525, 1987.

110. Wood VE, Sauser D, Mudge D: The treatment of hereditary multiple exostosis of the upper extremity, *J Hand Surg [Am]* 10:505-513, 1985.

111. Wynn-Davies R: *Heritable disorders in orthopedic practice,* Oxford, 1973, Blackwell Scientific Publications.

112. Wynne-Davies R, Williams PF, O'Connor JC: The 1960s epidemic of arthrogryposis multiplex congenita: a survey from the United Kingdom, Australia and the United States of America, *J Bone Joint Surg Br* 63:76-82, 1981.

113. Zerin JM, Hernandez RJ: Approach to skeletal maturation, *Hand Clin* 7:53-62, 1991.

114. Zinberg EM, Palmer AK, Coren AB, et al.: The triple-injection wrist arthrogram, *J Hand Surg [Am]* 13:803-809, 1988.

45

ATHLETIC INJURIES OF THE WRIST

Steven M. Topper, M.D.
Michael B. Wood, M.D.
William P. Cooney, M.D.

EPIDEMIOLOGY
TENDON-RELATED DISORDERS
  TENDINITIS
  INTERSECTION SYNDROME
  DE QUERVAIN'S TENOSYNOVITIS
  EXTENSOR INSERTIONAL TENOSYNOVITIS
  STENOSING TENOSYNOVITIS OF THE EXTENSOR
    CARPI ULNARIS
  RECURRENT SUBLUXATION OF THE EXTENSOR
    CARPI ULNARIS TENDON
SURGICAL TREATMENT
NERVE DISORDERS
  ETIOLOGY
  CYCLIST'S PALSY (ULNAR NERVE GUYON'S
    CANAL)
  GYMNAST'S PALSY (POSTERIOR INTEROSSEOUS
    NERVE NEUROPATHY)
  WARTENBERG'S SYNDROME (DORSAL SENSORY
    BRANCH RADIAL NERVE)
  CARPAL TUNNEL SYNDROME
VASCULAR DISORDERS
  HYPOTHENAR HAMMER SYNDROME (ULNAR
    ARTERY THROMBOSIS)
BONY INJURIES AND DISORDERS
  SCAPHOID FRACTURES
    CLASSIFICATION

    NONOPERATIVE TREATMENT
    OPERATIVE TREATMENT
    RETURN TO COMPETITION
  CAPITATE FRACTURES
  HOOK OF THE HAMATE FRACTURES
    NONUNION OF THE HAMATE HOOK
    OPERATIVE PROCEDURE
  TRIQUETRUM IMPACTION FRACTURES
  CARPOMETACARPAL FRACTURES AND FRACTURE
    DISLOCATIONS
  GYMNAST'S WRIST
    CHRONIC OSSEOUS INJURIES WITH PHYSEAL
      STRESS REACTION
    DIAGNOSIS AND TREATMENT
  ULNOCARPAL IMPACTION SYNDROME
  DISTAL RADIUS AND ULNA PHYSEAL INJURY
    FROM DISTRACTION
  SCAPHOID IMPACTION SYNDROME
  TRIQUETROLUNATE IMPACTION SYNDROME
ARTHROSCOPY IN TREATMENT OF SPORTS INJURIES
  OF THE WRIST
  INDICATIONS
  LIGAMENT INJURIES
  TRIANGULAR FIBROCARTILAGE COMPLEX
    TREATMENT (PALMER CLASSIFICATION)
SUMMARY

The wrist is exposed to injury in athletics as it serves to position the hand in space and to transmit forces between the hand and forearm. Many sports require repetitive activity of the wrist, making it also vulnerable to overuse disorders. The multiple stresses that cause injury in the athlete are usually one of these two basic types: a one-time excessive uncontrolled force or a persistent, controlled cumulative force. Treatment of the athlete with these conditions differs from that of the nonathlete because of the emphasis on return to a functional level that allows resumption of competition as soon as possible. Focusing on activities of daily living is not adequate for these patients. They require prompt diagnosis and reasonable and adequate intervention in a timely fashion to maximize results. Indeed, returning these patients to a high level of activity is quite challenging to the clinician.

Although wrist injuries are common in sports, they are frequently overlooked or minimized because other injuries receive more attention in the media. Frequently, athletes are able to continue competition with the aid of taping or splints despite a serious ligament injury or fracture. Consequently, wrist injuries are often considered a nuisance rather than a disability. Players, coaches, and fans have a hard time conceptualizing that something as simple as a wrist sprain could be a disabling injury in the long term. Sometimes, it is up to the clinician to thwart the pressure for the athlete to continue competition when it is not in the athlete's best interest. On the other hand, we also must be sensitive to their special needs and help them balance their desire to return to competition with avoidance of adverse long-term sequelae. We often serve them best by being educators as well as clinicians.

Most of the conditions described in this chapter are not peculiar to athletes. Their treatment is often discussed in other chapters in this book. What we have attempted to do is focus on the special needs and extraordinary conditions particular to athletes. In so doing, we highlight management variation and call to the clinician's attention conditions affecting the wrist that are frequently seen in patients who engage in athletic competition.

EPIDEMIOLOGY

Hand and wrist injuries account for roughly 25% of general athletic injuries.[86,163] Few epidemiologic studies have been done that focus on sports injuries to the wrist, but data can be extrapolated from broader studies of upper extremity injuries. In a study by Bergfeld and colleagues,[10] 113 hand and wrist injuries were examined. The most common wrist injuries were fractures of the distal radius ($n = 12$), followed by scaphoid fractures ($n = 11$).

Ellsasser and Stein[51] reported on hand injuries of a professional football team during a 15-year period. There were 46 major hand and wrist injuries involving 21 offensive and 25 defensive players. Although the vast majority of these injuries involved the fingers, there were nine wrist injuries noted. There were five fractures, two fracture dislocations, one dislocation, and one sprain. They also noted that wrist injuries in football are most often caused by tackling and tend to occur in defensive linemen.

Strauss and Lanese[159] studied wrestling tournaments with a total of 1,049 participants. Actual injury sites were not specified, but they noted that there was a fairly equal distribution of injuries across the body, with 21% in the upper extremity. They noted two serious wrist injuries, one of which was a distal radius fracture. Risk of injury did not vary with weight class. There was a high percentage of aggravation of old injuries. This suggested the need for adequate rehabilitation before return to competition.

In a 1-year survey of all hand injuries, Methodist Sports Medicine Center saw 213 injuries in 207 athletes.[135] There was a relatively high frequency of wrist injuries in golf, gymnastics (Table 45-1), and tennis. As would be expected, a higher percentage of injuries occurred during competition (41.1%) than in practice (28.2%) or recreation (15.8%).

During an 8-year period, the Olympic Training Center in Colorado Springs, Colorado, recorded 8,311 athletic injuries. Of these, 204 involved the wrist, representing 2.5% of the total. Sports that had a relatively high percentage of wrist injuries included gymnastics, judo, weight lifting, wrestling, ice hockey, and bicycling.

Although the wrist is exposed to injury in almost every sport, these studies demonstrate a certain clustering in specific types of sports. What they all seem to have in common is high-speed use of the hand or the potential for falls or weightbearing on the upper extremity. One-third of the injuries sustained by gymnasts and bicyclists were to the wrist. Although the total number of injuries in golf and tennis is low, most are to the wrist. Wrestling and judo also involve a high percentage of wrist injuries, which is probably from the twisting and high-impact loading involved in controlling the opponent.

According to Linscheid and Dobyns,[99] 90% of athletic injuries to the wrist occur with the wrist in the dorsiflexed position. Most often this is associated with a compressive load (gymnastics, weight lifting, football). Unfortunately, these injuries are usually unavoidable, because of the nature of hand and wrist involvement dictated by the rules or environment of the sport. An awareness of the risk helps the physician to diagnose and to prevent injury by appropriate training or protective splinting recommendations.

TENDON-RELATED DISORDERS

TENDINITIS

Virtually any tendon that crosses the wrist can become inflamed with stresses related to sports activity.[119,156,179] The mechanism involves sudden initiation of an unaccustomed motion or activity or chronic overloading. The symptoms are usually a vague pain that

Table 45-1. Mechanisms of Loading End Joint Positions in Gymnastic Events

Event	Load	Position
Pommel horse	Compression, rotation	Dorsiflexion, pronation Radial-ulnar deviation
Vault	Compression ± rotation	Dorsiflexion
Beam	Compression	Dorsiflexion
Uneven parallel bars	Compression, traction (especially with dowel grip)	Dorsiflexion, neutral
Floor exercise	Compression	Dorsiflexion
Parallel bars	Compression	Dorsiflexion, neutral
Rings	Compression	Neutral

From Dobyns JH, Gabel GT.[46] By permission of WB Saunders.

radiates along the course of the tendon and is provoked by resisted activation of the involved musculotendinous group. Occasionally, tendinitis causes symptoms referred to the joints over which the tendon passes. Treatment always starts with nonoperative means such as splinting, ice, and nonsteroidal anti-inflammatory medications. Aggravating activities should be avoided during acute inflammation. A flexibility, strength, and endurance program should be initiated after acute inflammation has subsided and before return to vigorous activity. The treating surgeon should also be aware of potential modifications of the athlete's technique or equipment that could prevent reinjury. For example, the stroke of a racquet sport player should be analyzed as well as the size of the grip on the racquet to ensure that it is appropriate. It is difficult for a physician to be conversant with the details of every sport; therefore, help should be sought from trainers or therapists.

INTERSECTION SYNDROME

The term "intersection syndrome" refers to a specific condition characterized by pain, crepitus, tenderness, and swelling where the thumb outriggers cross the radial wrist extensors 6 to 8 cm proximal to Lister's tubercle.[32] This condition has been called peritendinitis crepitans,[83] abductor pollicis longus (APL) bursitis,[180] and oarsman's wrist.[177] It is frequently seen in sports that require repetitive wrist flexion and extension against resistance such as competitive rowing, weight lifting, or gymnastics.[179,180]

Various entities have been implicated as the etiology of this condition. Peritendinous inflammation,[83] myositis,[156] adventitial bursitis,[180] localized compartment syndrome,[177] and second dorsal compartment stenosing tenosynovitis[74] have all been reported. Frequently, patients are able to identify an overuse event temporally related to the onset of their symptoms.

Nonoperative treatment is usually successful.[179] Initial measures include avoidance of aggravating activities, splint immobilization in a thumb spica splint with the thumb interphalangeal joint free and the wrist extended 15°, and nonsteroidal anti-inflammatory medication.

If an initial trial of nonoperative management fails, steroid injection directed to the APL bursa is indicated. The injection is usually done in combination with a local anesthetic such as lidocaine. Usually, a 2- to 3-mL mixture of lidocaine and betamethasone is recommended. Splinting is continued for 2 weeks after the injection. Avoidance of aggravating activities is pursued until the patient is pain free and normal motion and strength have been recovered.

In recalcitrant cases, surgical exploration through a dorsoradial longitudinal incision from the APL muscle belly to the distal edge of the extensor retinaculum is recommended. Some authors[61,74] have suggested that a decompression of the second dorsal compartment is a key component of this procedure. Others have suggested that the pathologic inflamed tissue is found in the area between the thumb outriggers and the second dorsal compartment tendons.[180] Because the true etiology remains in question and bowstringing of the tendons can occur with release of the extensor retinaculum, we do not recommend this as a routine part of the exploration after operation. We advocate careful débridement of all inflamed tissue between the thumb outriggers and the second dorsal compartment tendons. Prolonged protection from aggravating stresses (approximately 3 months) is suggested.[119] We recommend that initial postoperative care consist of a thumb spica splint for the first 2 weeks until the stitches are removed, followed by an early motion program with periodic splinting in an Orthoplast thumb spica splint for an additional 2 to 4 weeks. When motion has returned to near normal, a strengthening program is started and the athlete is allowed to return to competition when grip strength is 80% to 90% of that on the contralateral side.

DE QUERVAIN'S TENOSYNOVITIS

de Quervain's is the most common form of stenosing tenosynovitis reported in athletes. It is most frequently seen in racquet sports.[119] This entity is an inflammation of the first dorsal compartment tendons as they pass through a tight fibro-osseous tunnel at the level of the radial styloid (Fig. 45-1). As a result of repetitive stress, tendons become inflamed by grasping activities associated with repetitive ulnar deviation.

Clinically, the patient presents with pain over the first dorsal compartment, but the pain can radiate along the APL and extensor pollicis brevis tendons (Fig. 45-1, *B*). They often state that the symptoms are related to activity, particularly to thumb use. They complain of stiffness and weakness of oppositional pinch.

Physical examination demonstrates pain and swelling along the course of the tendons on the dorsoradial aspect of the wrist. The diagnosis is confirmed by a positive finding on Finkelstein's test, with pain reproduced by ulnar deviation while the patient holds the thumb tucked in the palm. Occasionally, crepitus can be detected as the tendons slide through the fibro-osseous tunnel with active thumb abduction.

Eighty percent of patients with this condition respond to nonoperative management.[119] We recommend a combination injection of lidocaine and betamethasone given directly into the first dorsal compartment. It is important not to injure the superficial sensory branch of the radial nerve. This can be avoided in most athletes because they are lean and the nerve can be palpated. To avoid an intratendinous injection, the needle is inserted down to bone and the fluid is introduced deep to the tendons. If the fluid does not flow freely, it should not be forced. Often a brisement effect is noted as increased fluid pressure expands the first dorsal compartment. We tend to place our patients in a thumb spica splint for 2 weeks after injection. They return to activity in a graduated fashion. If it is possible, they should avoid the aggravating activity for

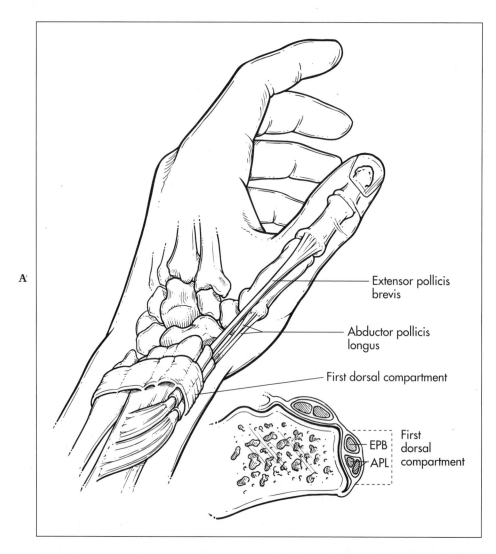

A

Extensor pollicis brevis

Abductor pollicis longus

First dorsal compartment

EPB
APL

First dorsal compartment

FIGURE 45-1

Tenosynovitis of the first extensor compartment. **A,** Anatomy of lateral distal forearm. Note location of superficial branch of radial nerve, extensor retinaculum, radial artery, abductor pollicis longus (*APL*), and extensor pollicis brevis (*EPB*) tendons.

4 to 6 weeks. If not, then a soft silicone thumb spica splint should be worn for support during competition.

In recalcitrant cases, surgical decompression is recommended (Fig. 45-1, *C*). The procedure can be performed quite reliably with local anesthesia. We favor a longitudinal incision to identify and avoid injury to the superficial sensory branch of the radial nerve that can end an athlete's season or career. It is important to visualize the nerve and protect it before release of the retinaculum. The retinacular incision should be made in such a way as to preserve a large palmar-radial flap that will prevent postoperative subluxation of the tendons. This sheath is commonly divided into two separate compartments. Incomplete release can be avoided if the tendons (extensor pollicis longus [EPL] and APL) are identified by observing their function as they are gently tensioned with a smooth retractor. The common mistake is to confuse a slip of the APL with the extensor pollicis brevis. We usually have the patients demonstrate adequate decompression by asking them to move their thumb metacarpal phalangeal and carpometacarpal (CMC) joints after the release is complete. The postoperative dressing limits but does not restrict thumb motion. Sutures are removed at 10 to 14 days, and this is followed by unrestricted motion. The athlete may return to competition as soon as comfort allows.

EXTENSOR INSERTIONAL TENOSYNOVITIS

Insertional tendinitis can occur in any of the extensor tendons that cross the wrist. As with any tendinitis, the patient complains of pain along the course of the tendon. Symptoms are provoked by resisted excursion of the involved tendon. Often, they are locally tender near the insertion and this is occasionally accompanied by demonstrable swelling.

The most common *dorsal extensor tendinitis* in an athlete involves the second compartment tendons—the extensor carpi radialis longus and brevis. This is occasionally associated with a bony thickening at the tendon insertion known as carpal bossing.[99,110,126] This lesion can be mistaken for a dorsal carpal ganglion, but careful examination demonstrates a nonfluctuant consistency, it will not transilluminate, and the location of the mass is distal to the usual ganglion presentation.[47] Routine radiographs confirm the bony nature of the lesion, although the mass is best visualized with the "carpal boss view" (35° supination and 25° ulnar deviation).[132]

B

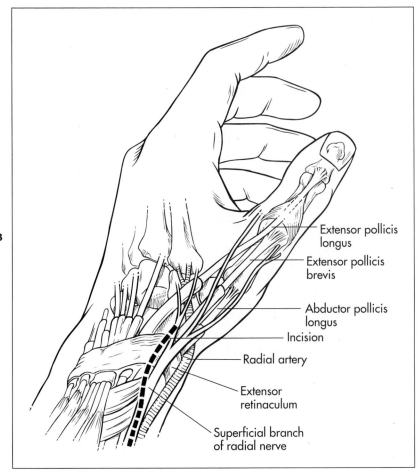

Extensor pollicis longus

Extensor pollicis brevis

Abductor pollicis longus

Incision

Radial artery

Extensor retinaculum

Superficial branch of radial nerve

FIGURE 45-1, CONT'D.

B, Longitudinal curvilinear incision adjacent to the radial nerve between the first and second extensor compartments.

Continued.

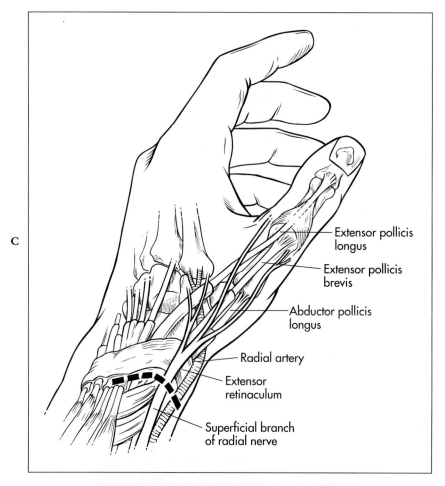

C

Extensor pollicis
longus

Extensor pollicis
brevis

Abductor pollicis
longus

Radial artery

Extensor
retinaculum

Superficial branch
of radial nerve

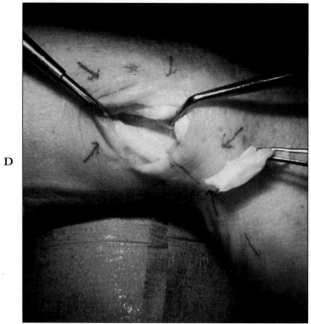

D

FIGURE 45-1, CONT'D.

C, Transverse surgical incision. Distal dorsal transverse incision for release of the first extensor compartment. A more proximal transverse incision can be used for release of intersection syndrome. **D,** Surgical excision of retinacular ganglion cyst on the first extensor compartment in a rowing athlete.

Carpal bossing can be symptomatic.[41] It frequently responds to nonoperative management such as splinting, ice, and anti-inflammatory medication. It is also important to avoid aggravating stresses until the inflammation has subsided and motion and strength have been restored. Although there is little motion in the second and third CMC joints, the bony osteophyte can become quite prominent and irritating to the skin because it is frequently bumped.

Tenosynovitis of the *extensor pollicis longus* and subsequent rupture of the tendon were first reported in Prussian drummers.[90] Hence, the term "drummer's wrist" has been coined for this condition. The EPL is at risk as it courses around Lister's tubercle.[20] Dawson[42] reported rupture in two athletes: a tennis player and a diver. The condition has also been seen in squash players. It is most frequently seen after Colles' fracture.

The patient presents with a history of pain over the radiodorsal aspect of the wrist during activity that requires repetitive extension of the thumb. Examination demonstrates focal tenderness and swelling in the area of Lister's tubercle. Pain can be provoked by resisted thumb extension, and crepitus can often be palpated as the tendon glides around the tubercle.

Nonoperative management includes a wrist or thumb spica splint and anti-inflammatory medication. If the condition is refractory to this approach, an injection of a lidocaine and betamethasone mixture (1.5 mL, ½ lidocaine, ½ betamethasone) about the tendon can be therapeutic and used to confirm the diagnosis. If the patient responds to the injection but later symptoms return, a transposition of the EPL radial to Lister's tubercle can be considered. This procedure is performed through a dorsal transverse incision placed in Langer's lines and carefully deepened to the extensor retinaculum. Care is taken to preserve dorsal cutaneous nerves. The extensor retinaculum is incised over the EPL, and the tendon is translocated out of the third dorsal compartment. It is essential to complete the release proximally so that the tendon or its musculotendinous junction is not kinked. The tendon is allowed to reside superficial to the extensor retinaculum, and the previous incision in the retinaculum is repaired with multiple absorbable simple sutures with the knots buried.

Postoperatively, mobilization is begun at 2 weeks in a thumb spica splint, followed by a gradual strengthening program. Athletic activity is not resumed until motion and strength gains have been maximized.

The *extensor indicis proprius* syndrome was first described in two athletes by Ritter and Inglis.[136] Both of these patients had a lengthy history of vigorous use of the wrist and had activity-related pain and swelling over the fourth dorsal compartment. They received temporary symptomatic relief with immobilization and corticosteroid injections. Eventually, they both had exploratory surgery and were found to have intrusion of the musculotendinous junction into the fourth dorsal compartment. Spinner and Olshansky[152] noted that pain is reproducible by full passive wrist flexion with resisted active index finger extension. It is postulated that the increased volume in the tight compartment causes the inflammation and synovitis associated with this condition. Failing a trial of nonoperative management, good results can be expected reliably with division of the retinaculum and synovectomy.[156] Cauldwell et al.,[24] in a cadaver study, noted that the musculotendinous junction of the extensor indicis proprius passes into the fourth dorsal compartment in 75% of patients and in 4% it passes beyond it.

STENOSING TENOSYNOVITIS OF THE EXTENSOR CARPI ULNARIS

This is an uncommon condition seen in athletes who engage in racquet sports.[76,119] The extensor carpi ulnaris (ECU) is distinct compared with the other extensor tendons that cross the wrist because it has a separate subsheath, described by Spinner and Kaplan.[151] The ECU subsheath is closely related to fibers of the dorsal radioulnar ligament and ulnotriquetral ligament and dorsal cutaneous sensory branches of the ulnar nerve (Fig. 45-2). It is believed to contribute to stability of the distal radioulnar joint. When a patient is evaluated for this condition, underlying ulnar-sided instability of the wrist must be considered and one must be certain that the pain is not neurogenic in origin (e.g., from a crush injury to the dorsal ulnar aspect of the wrist).[81] These patients present with dorsoulnar wrist pain. Swelling of a chronic nature can occur.

Examination demonstrates tenderness over the ECU in the area of the fibro-osseous tunnel.[20,32,46,156] Symptoms may be provoked with ulnar deviation of the wrist and resisted dorsiflexion with the forearm supinated.[76]

Local steroid injection is combined with immobilization for 2 weeks in a long arm splint with the forearm in pronation. Adding lidocaine to the injection can assist in confirming the diagnosis and separating subcutaneous pain from ECU sheath and distal radioulnar joint injuries.[100]

If splint immobilization, rest, and nonsteroidal anti-inflammatory medication fail, surgical release of the subsheath should be considered (Fig. 45-3).[76] It is important to release the subsheath on the radial side so as not to induce an unstable subluxating ECU. This is further reinforced by a meticulous repair of the overlying extensor retinaculum. Postoperatively, the patient is immobilized in a short arm cast with the wrist in 20° extension for 3 weeks. Then, a graduated range of motion and strengthening program is instituted. The athlete should not return to intense training or competition until motion and strength gains are approximately 80% of the uninvolved side.

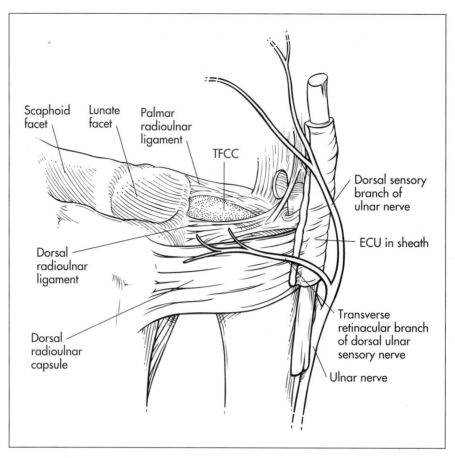

FIGURE 45-2

Transverse retinacular branch of the dorsal sensory branch of the ulnar nerve originates from the dorsal cutaneous branch of the ulnar nerve; retinacular branch crosses on the dorsal ulnar aspect of the extensor retinaculum triangular fibrocartilage complex (*TFCC*). *ECU*, extensor carpi ulnaris.

RECURRENT SUBLUXATION OF THE EXTENSOR CARPI ULNARIS TENDON

A discrete traumatic event is associated with most reported cases of subluxation of the extensor carpi ulnaris.[19,49,130,138] The pathologic lesion is a disruption of the ulnar wall of the fibro-osseous sheath of the sixth dorsal compartment.[179] This occurs secondary to a sudden supination, ulnar deviation, and palmar flexion force. This condition has been reported in tennis, golf, weight lifting, and rodeo.[19,130,138]

The patient complains of a painful ulnar clicking with forearm rotation. Clinical examination demonstrates painful subluxation of the tendon with supination and ulnar deviation of the wrist. A profound and sometimes audible snap can be seen and heard. In some patients this subluxation is not easily demonstrated. In these cases, it is useful to ask the patient to make a tight fist with the wrist in ulnar deviation. The patient then rolls the forearm from a position of pronation to supination, as if using a screwdriver. Reversing this maneuver reduces the tendon. If this condition is detected acutely (within the first 6 weeks), immobilization in pronation and radial deviation should be successful in the acute injury. A long arm cast is recommended to ensure compliance. In a responsible patient, a Munster-type Orthoplast splint is sufficient. In more chronic cases, immobilization may not be effective and the chance of resolution of symptoms while maintaining the same activity level is unlikely.

In chronic cases, several procedures have been described to stabilize the ECU (Fig. 45-3). The majority of these procedures create some type of sling to hold the ECU in the reduced position.[19,49,130,138] We favor a proximal, radially based sling of extensor retinaculum with a meticulous repair or reefing of the subsheath, as described by Burkhart et al.[19]

SURGICAL TREATMENT

The incision is placed dorsoulnarly and curves gently around the head of the ulna. Next, the sensory branch of the ulnar nerve is identified by subcutaneous

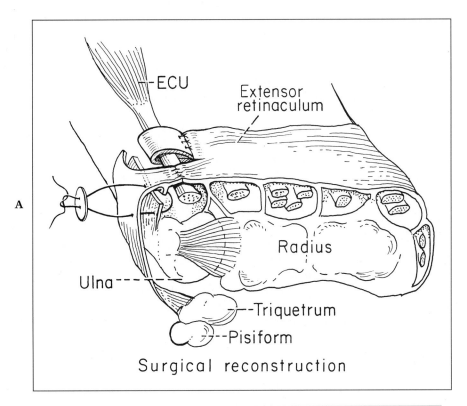

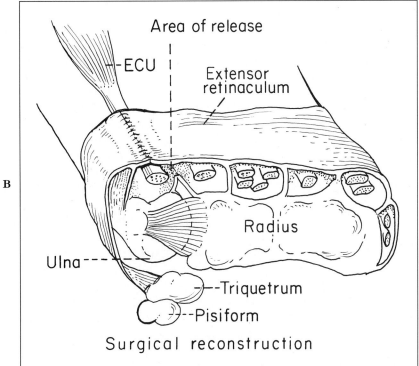

FIGURE 45-3

A, Extensor carpi ulnaris (*ECU*) sheath reconstruction. A radial-based flap from the extensor retinaculum is placed around the ECU tendon to prevent ulnar subluxation. The ulnar wall of the ECU is oversewn to the ulnar extensor retinaculum. *(From Burkhart SS et al.[19] Copyright, American Society for Surgery of the Hand, by permission of Churchill Livingstone.)* **B,** ECU sheath release for constrictive ECU tendinitis.

dissection on the ulnar side of the wound. It is most easily found where it winds around the neck of the ulna to come up to the dorsal side of the hand (Fig. 45-2). Once isolated, it is protected throughout the remainder of the operative procedure. A common mistake is to injure the transverse joint articular branch, which can lead to postoperative neuroma (Fig. 45-2). Once identified, the extensor retinaculum is exposed both proximally and distally. The sling is radially based, incorporating the proximal one-third of the retinaculum. The ulnarmost portion of the sling is detached from the medial border of the ulna to ensure adequate length. The sling is first designed and then incised. The remainder of the retinaculum is taken down in the standard fashion with a longitudinal incision proceeding proximal to distal over the sixth dorsal compartment. The subsheath is then inspected. If it is disrupted, it is simply repaired. If it is attenuated, then it is released longitudinally on the radial side and reefed in a pants-over-vest fashion. The retinacular sling is routed palmar to the ECU tendon and wrapped back over the tendon and sewn to itself (Fig. 45-3).

Once this is completed, it is important to ensure that the ECU tendon glides freely, because stenosis of this compartment has also been reported.[76] We also put the forearm through a gentle range of motion to observe the positions of the forearm in which the tendon is best reduced. Typically, this is forearm pronation or midrotation with radial deviation of the wrist. Postoperatively, the patient is placed in a sugar tongs splint, with positioning in the splint based on intraoperative observation of the reduction of the tendon. A Munster cast is used for 6 weeks postoperatively. Motion is regained by a monitored therapy program focusing on pronation and supination of the forearm. Once motion is restored, a graduated strengthening program is started. Aggressive training or competition can be resumed once motion and strength have returned.

NERVE DISORDERS

Neurologic disorders of the wrist occur relatively infrequently in the athlete.[6,43,47,60] Hirasawa and Sakakida[81] reported a 19% incidence of ulnar, median, and digital nerve involvement in 66 athletic peripheral nerve injuries. However, there are certain athletic endeavors in which the incidence is relatively more frequent, such as bicycling, baseball, karate, rugby, and handball.[60,84] Nerve entrapment syndromes in the wrists of athletes include carpal tunnel syndrome (median nerve),[12,55,127,160] cyclist's palsy (Guyon's canal syndrome),* gymnast's palsy (posterior interosseous nerve compression),[44] and Wartenberg's

---
* References 30,84,87,91,94,115,146,148.

disease (superficial sensory branch of the radial nerve compression).[134,167]

ETIOLOGY

Entrapment neuropathies develop when a mechanical compression from local tissue edema, blunt trauma, adjacent joint synovitis, or equipment constraints causes compression and vascular compromise of the involved nerve, with symmetric segmented vessels carried in the mesoneurium (Fig. 45-4).[12] It is likely that mechanical compression causes venous obstruction and subsequent vascular congestion and circulatory embarrassment. Anoxia of the involved nerve segment results in cell damage and edema, which can exacerbate the effect of the original compression. As this process continues, eventually the healing response causes a fibroblastic proliferation that can constrict the nerve and compromise axoplasmic flow and hence nerve cell body nutrition and function permanently.[160]

CYCLIST'S PALSY (ULNAR NERVE GUYON'S CANAL)

Long-distance cyclists frequently develop numbness and paresthesias in the digits innervated by the ulnar nerve secondary to compression of the ulnar nerve in and distal to Guyon's canal. This is also seen in other sports that involve repetitive contusion of the ulnar palm or aspect of the palm such as racquet sports and handball. Occasionally, findings are restricted to the deep motor branch associated with ulnar intrinsic weakness and paralysis with absence of sensory symptoms.[30,84,91,140,179]

The ulnar nerve at the wrist is vulnerable in the area of Guyon's canal. Here the nerve is tethered by the borders of the canal. Shea and McClain[146] have divided compression of the ulnar nerve at the wrist into three types that can be distinguished on clinical examination. Type 1 involves both the motor and sensory branches and occurs proximal to the canal to just within it. Type 2 involves the middle third of the canal to the area of the hook of the hamate. There is selective involvement of the motor branch. In type 3 the lesion involves just the sensory branch and occurs in the distal third of the canal.

These patients present with symptoms of paresthesias in the fingers innervated by the ulnar nerve. They have tenderness over Guyon's canal and a positive Tinel sign in this area, with radiation to the small finger and ulnar half of the ring finger. In advanced cases, they complain of weakness of grasp: 40% of grip strength is related to the muscles in the hand innervated by the ulnar nerve.[134] Loss of motor strength can be demonstrated by weakness of the first dorsal interosseous muscle, weakness of the thumb adductor muscle (positive Froment's sign), or weakness of the third palmar interosseous muscle, which leads to unopposed activity of the extensor digiti minimi (positive Wartenberg's sign). In

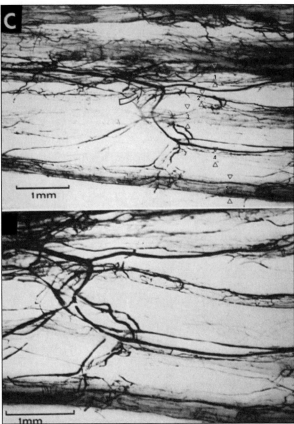

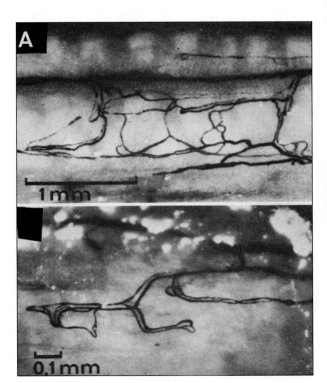

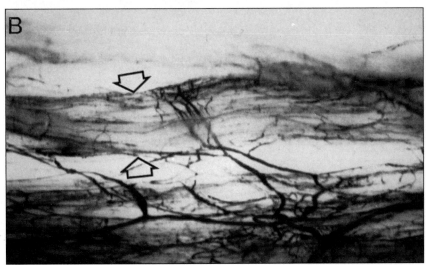

FIGURE 45-4

A, *Top:* The surface microvascular pattern on the perineurial epithelium of the ulnar nerve motor branch in Guyon's canal (India ink perfusion). *Bottom:* Details of perineurial microvascular plexus show well-defined capillary loops. **B,** Microangiogram illustrates the intrinsic vascularization of the human median nerve from the carpal tunnel region. Arrows indicate outline of one fascicle. **C,** *Top:* Median nerve in the carpal tunnel. India ink perfused and clarified. Curved arrow shows location of epineurial vascular cord supplied by numbers 1 through 5. *Bottom:* Higher magnification of site identified by arrow. *(From Lundborg G: The intrinsic vascularization of human peripheral nerves: structural and functional aspects, J Hand Surg 4:34-41, 1979. Copyright, British Society for Surgery of the Hand, by permission of Churchill Livingstone.)*

advanced cases, there is a deficit in two-point discrimination. It is essential that Allen's test be performed in these patients so that ulnar artery thrombosis,* which can compress the ulnar nerve due to mass effect, is not missed. The examiner should also be aware of other etiologies of nerve compression in this area, such as a fracture of the hook of the hamate, ganglion, and anomalous muscles.[52,91,134] These etiologies should be eliminated as possibilities because of their relatively high incidence in athletes.

Factors that have been shown to contribute to the frequent development of this condition in cyclists include worn-out gloves, unpadded handlebars, vibration from rough roads, riding a poorly fitted bicycle, and prolonged grasping of dropped handlebars.[30,84,94,115] Jackson[87] studied 20 cyclists who rode more than 100 miles per week. He found that 9 of the 20 complained of paresthesias while riding that resolved on completion of the ride. Three had symptoms in the ulnar nerve distribution. None had motor weakness, and all 20 had normal electromyograms. The cyclists attributed this

condition to failing to change hand position frequently enough. The author was unable to recommend the ideal hand position but did advocate frequent changing of position. Other authors[84,110] have emphasized frequent changes in hand position as well as proper bicycle fit, padded handlebars, and proper cycling gloves. In regard to bicycle fit, it is generally believed that body weight is best distributed when the distance from the nose of the saddle to the point where the handlebars attach to the stem is equal to the distance from the cyclist's elbow to the tip of the outstretched fingers (Fig. 45-5). New glove designs with a gel pad or sorbothane pads seem to be particularly effective. This condition merits the name "handlebar palsy."[60,148]

Treatment includes cessation of direct pressure over the hypothenar eminence until symptoms have resolved. A splint, anti-inflammatory medication, and cryotherapy can be useful. If these measures are ineffective, then decompression of Guyon's canal may be required. When nonoperative management has failed and surgical intervention is being considered, we have found electromyography helpful to confirm the diagnosis, judge the severity of compression, and localize

---

* References 6,29,70,72,82,96,105,108,112,128,184.

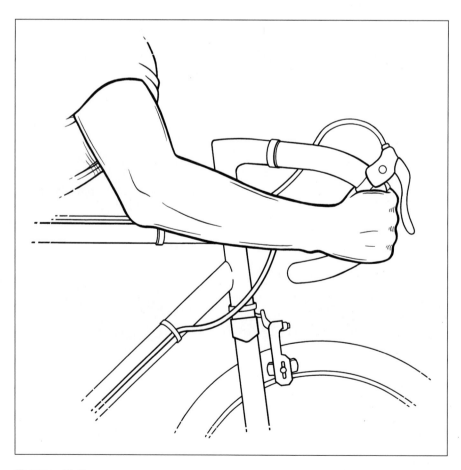

FIGURE 45-5

Hand and forearm position to relax stress on the wrist during bicycle riding.

the level of compression. If there is a sustained measurable loss of sensation or demonstrable motor loss, surgical intervention is advisable and should not be delayed.

Return to sports should be avoided until symptoms are resolved or can be ameliorated by padded gloves or appropriate equipment and technique modification. After surgical treatment, return to competitive cycling should be delayed a minimum of 6 weeks to allow for reinnervation and to prevent adverse fibrous tissue scar response.

GYMNAST'S PALSY (POSTERIOR INTEROSSEOUS NERVE NEUROPATHY)

Posterior interosseous nerve palsy is caused by direct compression or injury to the nerve or from repeated hyperextension of the wrist.[6,44,47] Pain can be localized at the wrist extension crease and can be reproduced by direct compression over this area. Nonoperative treatment is recommended. This includes avoidance of hyperextension and use of a soft wrist splint in the competitive environment.

If nonoperative management fails, a posterior interosseous neurectomy may be required.[179] This procedure is performed through a small transverse incision in the wrist extension crease just over the fourth dorsal compartment tendons. Care is taken not to injure longitudinal subcutaneous sensory branches. A longitudinal incision is made in the extensor retinaculum, and the fourth compartment tendons are retracted (Fig. 45-6). The nerve is easily identified and separated from the posterior interosseous artery by careful longitudinal spreading in the floor of the compartment. Once found, the nerve is exposed over a 1.5- to 2-cm segment, and this portion is sharply resected. A meticulous repair of the extensor retinaculum is performed when closing the wrist.

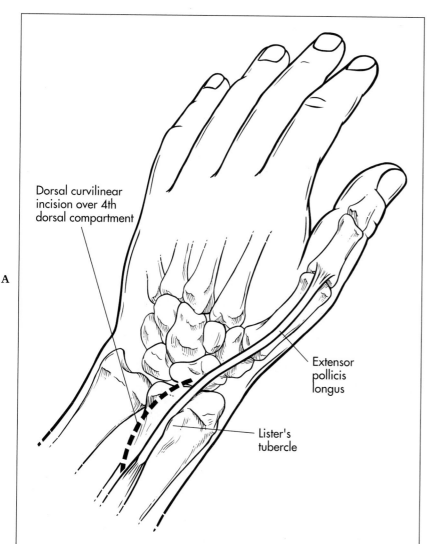

Dorsal curvilinear incision over 4th dorsal compartment

Extensor pollicis longus

Lister's tubercle

A

FIGURE 45-6

Posterior interosseous neurectomy (PIN).
A, A curvilinear incision over the fourth dorsal compartment.

Continued.

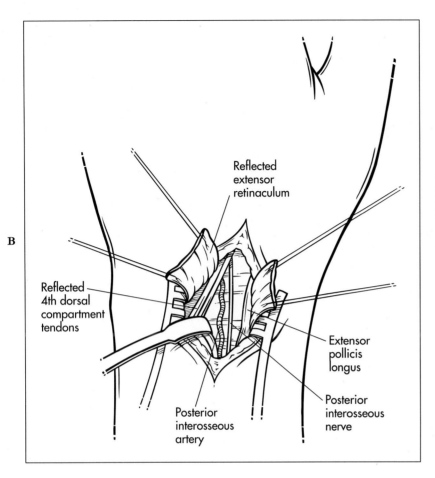

B

Reflected
extensor
retinaculum

Reflected
4th dorsal
compartment
tendons

Posterior
interosseous
artery

Extensor
pollicis
longus

Posterior
interosseous
nerve

FIGURE 45-6, CONT'D.

B, With retraction of the extensor pollicis longus tendon, the posterior interosseous nerve and artery are observed overlying the interosseous membrane. After PIN, the anterior interosseous nerve (sensory compartment) can also be divided by creating a window in the interosseous membrane and locating the nerve adjacent to the distal radius.

WARTENBERG'S SYNDROME (DORSAL SENSORY BRANCH RADIAL NERVE)

Athletes involved in sports that require repetitive forearm rotation along with ulnar deviation of the wrist can develop a traction neuropathy of the superficial sensory branch of the radial nerve that was originally described in nonathletes by Wartenberg.[167] This condition is also seen in athletes who wear equipment that encompasses the wrist, such as wrist straps in weight lifters or doweled grips in gymnasts.[6] Anatomically, the radial sensory nerve is located in a subcutaneous position between the extensor carpi radialis longus and the brachioradialis at the junction of the mid and distal thirds of the forearm. The fascia at this point of transition sends fibers from the musculotendinous area of the brachioradialis to the extensor carpi radialis longus. This creates a relatively unyielding bridge under the nerve and is the most common location of entrapment.

The patient presents with pain and numbness over the dorsoradial aspect of the hand and thumb. Pertinent physical findings include Tinel's sign over the nerve and exacerbation of symptoms with wrist flexion and ulnar deviation.

Dellon and Mackinnon[43] reported on 58 cases of compression of the superficial sensory branch of the radial nerve. They recommended nonoperative management in early cases (6-12 months) with splinting in supination. The best results were noted when the neuropathy developed from brief periods of increased physical activity or from one-time contusions of the nerve. Nonoperative management of these lesions in the athlete should include rest from the aggravating activity until symptoms abate, ice, and splinting in a palmar cock-up-type Orthoplast splint for 2 to 3 weeks. If an adequate trial of nonoperative measures fails, then surgical decompression of the nerve is warranted. Dellon and Mackinnon were able to achieve 86% good to excellent results, with 43% return to preinjury activity level after external neurolysis of the radial nerve.

We approach the nerve through a 3- to 4-cm longitudinal incision over the dorsoradial aspect of the forearm (Fig. 45-1). This incision should be centered over the point of maximal Tinel's sign, which should approximate the area where the nerve changes from a deep to a superficial location. The incision is deepened to the level of the brachial fascia, taking care not to injure the lateral antebrachial cutaneous nerve. The brachioradialis is identified and retracted radially. Careful longitudinal spreading allows the nerve to be identified. With the nerve in view, the fascia that connects the brachioradialis to the extensor carpi radialis is divided.

considered less than 3 weeks, delayed from 4 to 6 months, and established nonunions when there is no healing at greater than 6 months. The location of the fracture in the bone is important because of the tenuous blood supply of the scaphoid.[68,162] Fractures through the proximal third take an average of 6 to 11 weeks longer to heal than fractures of the waist and are associated with avascular necrosis rates from 14% to 39%.

Russe[142] emphasized the fact that the configuration of the fracture has prognostic significance. He suggested that the vertical oblique fractures, although the least common (5%), are the most unstable and therefore require longer immobilization (10-12 weeks) (Fig. 45-9). McLaughlin and Parkes[111] proposed a system to help predict which nondisplaced fractures were more likely to displace with closed treatment. Type three fractures with any displacement at all are inherently unstable. They recommended operative fixation of selected type two and all type three fractures. A Mayo Clinic series reported on 45 patients in whom the union rate for displaced fractures was 54% compared with a union rate of 94% for nondisplaced fractures.[34] Included in the seven unions were three malunions. Significant displacement was defined as 1) displacement greater than 1 mm, 2) scapholunate angle greater than 45°, and 3) capitolunate angle greater than 15°. Subsequently, the criterion for significant scapholunate angulation has

been relaxed to greater than 60° as a better understanding of normal variation in angulation has been gained.

The poor outcome occurs when displaced fractures of the scaphoid are treated closed as emphasized by Szabo and Manske.[161] In their series, fractures that were displaced greater than 1 mm were associated with a nonunion rate of 55% and a 50% incidence of avascular necrosis. The criteria of significant displacement give the clinician hard data on which to base treatment decisions. If the fracture configuration is outside of these limits, the expected results decrease dramatically from excellent to poor.

The most comprehensive classification system of scaphoid fractures and nonunions has been proposed by Herbert.[78,79] This system recommends operative internal fixation for all but the most stable incomplete fractures (Type A). This obviously shows a bias toward internal fixation, no doubt based on the excellent results that have been reported by Herbert and Fisher.[79] In the athlete, there is increased justification for internal fixation with a compression screw. Others* are more inclined to treat all nondisplaced fractures closed, with reported rates of union in the 90% to 95% range. The challenge put forward by

---

* References 3,13,34,36,38,39,69,93,99,116,142,149,157,161,166,170, 183.

TYPES OF FRACTURE AND RECOMMENDED TIME OF IMMOBILIZATION		
TYPE IN RELATION TO LONG AXIS OF NAVICULAR		**IMMOBILIZATION**
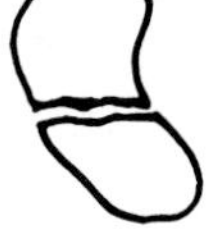	HORIZONTAL OBLIQUE 35 %	DISTAL THIRD 6 WEEKS MIDDLE THIRD 6 WEEKS PROXIMAL THIRD 10-12 WEEKS
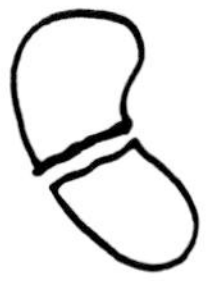	TRANSVERSE 60 %	6 WEEKS (+ 4 TO 6 WEEKS)
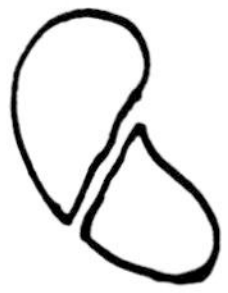	VERTICAL OBLIQUE 5 %	10 - 12 WEEKS

FIGURE 45-9

Russe classification. Fracture immobilization time. *(From Russe O.[142] By permission of the journal.)*

Herbert's classification system echoes back to points made by Russe[142] and McLaughlin and Parkes[111] that all nondisplaced fractures are not the same. Perhaps, nondisplaced fractures with a vertical oblique orientation that are complete should be primarily internally fixed. If a trial of nonoperative management is selected in these cases, they at least should be followed very closely.

Nonoperative Treatment. If an acute scaphoid fracture is not displaced in the athlete, the preferred treatment is a long arm thumb spica cast for the first 6 weeks and then a short arm thumb spica cast until the fracture is clinically and radiographically healed. The study by Gellman and associates[69] confirmed faster (and better) scaphoid healing as well as decreased rates of nonunion in the group treated in this fashion. In regard to position, Weber and Chao[170] have demonstrated that the displacement forces are minimized with the wrist in slight flexion and radial deviation. In fact, by utilizing this positioning, Weber[169] reported a union rate of 100% in 19 patients.

Fractures of the scaphoid should be followed for early displacement. If there is any question of subsequent displacement, appropriate imaging is obtained to answer the question before treatment proceeds. When patients are switched to a short arm cast, we recommend seeing them every third week until the fracture is healed. We recommend tomograms to confirm union if there is any question regarding fracture healing.

Operative Treatment. There is continued controversy about selecting operative management for displaced scaphoid fractures.[34,36,78,161] Most authorities believe that the configuration of these fractures represents a type of interfragmentary instability[149] that requires reduction and stable fixation. The consequences of scaphoid malunion[4] and nonunion[104,141] are well known and can herald the end of an athlete's career. The type of fixation selected by the surgeon to hold an operatively reduced scaphoid fracture is based on the fracture appearance, degree of comminution and displacement, and the surgeon's preference. Smooth Kirschner (K) wires, cancellous bone screws, and

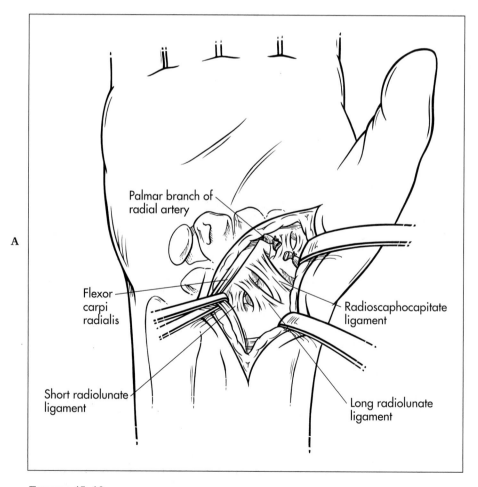

FIGURE 45-10

A, Palmar approach to the scaphoid (after Herbert). A radial-palmar skin incision is made; division of the palmar branch of the radial artery; flexor carpi radialis tendon retracted ulnarly and radial artery radially.

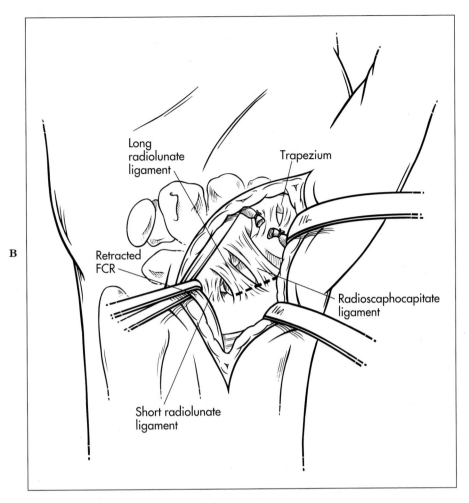

B

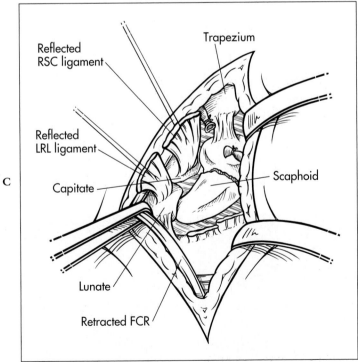

C

FIGURE 45-10, CONT'D.

B, Palmar approach with division of the palmar radioscaphocapitate and long radiolunate ligaments parallel to the articular surface of the distal radius (radial styloid). **C,** Reflection of the radioscaphocapitate (*RSC*) ligament and long radiolunate (*LRL*) ligament exposes the scaphoid and radial side of the lunate, preserved short radiolunate ligament, and retracted flexor carpi radialis (*FCR*).

various scaphoid screws have all been used successfully. The advantage of K wires is the ease of insertion. The disadvantages are that they produce no compressive forces and can migrate and the pin sites must be meticulously cared for to avoid infection. Cancellous bone screws offer the most compression (17-kg force),[145] but the head is prominent and a second operation is often required to treat or prevent hardware impingement problems. This type of screw fixation, however, is an option and has been used successfully.[59,98]

The Herbert screw introduced in 1984 offers several advantages as a result of its unique and original design. It is countersunk below the articular cartilage, obviating the need for subsequent removal. It achieves compression by a unique differential thread pitch design (4.4-kg force).[78,145] It uses the Huene jig that assists with operative reduction and compression before screw insertion.[78,85] It can be difficult to use. As Barton[8] so aptly stated regarding its difficulty, "but so are other advanced surgical techniques and that is no excuse for not learning to do them properly." Herbert and Fisher[79] reported a 100% union rate using this implant for fresh acute fractures, and we have noted similar success.

A new compression screw has been introduced by Whipple. The screw is cannulated and has self-tapping threads. These design modifications allow for less manipulation of the bone once reduction has been accomplished and provide for arthroscopic-assisted reduction and implantation of the screw.[175] We generally recommend the Herbert or Herbert-Whipple screw for acute unstable fractures. The palmar approach is favored for fractures of the distal two-thirds (Fig. 45-10). A dorsal approach is recommended for the proximal one-third, with antegrade insertion of the screw. The pitfall of the palmar approach is alteration of the tension on the palmar radiocarpal ligaments, which can lead to a postoperative instability pattern. Garcia-Elias and associates[66] have reported a significant increase in scapholunate and lunocapitate

angulation with the palmar approach when these ligaments are not repaired. The pitfall of the dorsal approach is the need for freehand insertion of the Herbert or Whipple screw.

For the preferred operative procedure (Herbert screw insertion) for acute fractures, regional or general anesthesia is used. When a structural bone graft may be needed, we favor the iliac crest. An anterior Russe-type incision is normally used for fractures of the distal two-thirds of the bone. The incision is centered over the tubercle of the scaphoid. The distal limb of the incision is gently curved radially. The proximal limb of the incision extends approximately 3 cm along the radial border of the flexor carpi radialis. The incision is deepened and the radial artery is identified and secured with a vessel loop and retracted radially. It is often necessary to ligate the superficial palmar branch of the radial artery, which crosses the wound at the base of the thenar muscle origin (Fig. 45-10). The sheath of the flexor carpi radialis is opened and the tendon is retracted ulnarly, exposing the palmar radiocarpal ligaments. The radioscaphocapitate ligament and long radiolunate ligament are identified coursing from their origin on the radial styloid. These two ligaments are the only radiocarpal ligaments that need to be disturbed with this approach. They can be sharply detached near their origin and retracted distally and ulnarly (Figs. 45-10, B and C). After scaphoid bone grafting, they must be repaired directly back to their origin by preserving a cuff of tissue on the styloid or by using a bone anchor device, in which case preserving a cuff of tissue is not necessary.

The scaphotrapezial joint is identified and the capsule is divided transversely to gain access to the distal pole of the scaphoid. A trial reduction is done to assess the character of the fracture to decide if a temporary K-wire fixation or a bone graft will be needed. The blade of the Huene jig is set for the appropriate wrist (right or left) and then carefully hooked around the proximal pole of the scaphoid (Figs. 45-11 and 45-12).

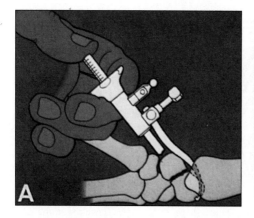 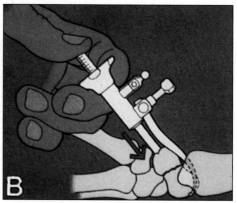

FIGURE 45-11

A and **B**, Placement of the Huene jig for compression of the two components of the scaphoid fracture (palmar approach). *(From Herbert TJ.[78] By permission of the publisher.)*

Distraction and ulnar deviation are helpful when applying the Huene jig. We often use a Lorenz elevator placed in the radioscaphoid joint to facilitate distraction of the radioscaphoid articulation. Once the hook of the Huene jig has been seated on the proximal scaphoid, distraction is relaxed and the wrist is gently dorsiflexed, bringing the distal pole of the scaphoid into view. The end of the guide is then engaged on the tubercle of the scaphoid and the fracture is compressed (Fig. 45-12).

It is sometimes necessary to cut a trough out of the lateral aspect of the trapezium to make room for the application of the end of the guide. While the compression maneuver is being applied to the scaphoid, a special Herbert elevator is used to raise the proximal pole into place. It is usually necessary to use a temporary K wire to prevent rotational malalignment of the scaphoid. At this point, either fluoroscopic or hard film images are obtained to confirm adequate reduction of the scaphoid, correct placement of the K wire, and length of the K wire.

Next, the length of the screw is measured off the jig (Fig. 45-12, *B*). Instrumentation then proceeds, inserting first the starting drill and then the main drill to their full depth. The appropriate size Herbert screw is then inserted in the barrel of the jig and set firmly across the fracture site, applying additional compression (Fig. 45-13). The K wires and jig are removed. Depending on the rotational stability of the construct, a parallel K wire can be left behind. Intraoperative images are then obtained to confirm adequate reduction and placement of the screw. The tourniquet is released, hemostasis is obtained, the area is irrigated, and closure is accomplished. It is vital that the radioscaphocapitate and long radiolunate ligaments are repaired anatomically by one of the options previously

mentioned. We use a bulky hand dressing with a thumb spica splint for initial postoperative care.

Fractures of the proximal one-third are best managed through a dorsal approach[45] (see Chapter 17). We use a transverse incision placed in the wrist extension crease or a dorsoradial curvilinear incision. The extensor retinaculum is divided longitudinally over the third dorsal compartment. The EPL is translocated radially and the radial wrist extensors are retracted in the same direction. To increase the exposure, the fourth dorsal compartment can be subperiosteally dissected off the radius and retracted ulnarly. The dorsal capsule is divided in line with the fibers of the dorsal radiocarpal and intercarpal ligaments, and the capsule is then reflected radially. This type of capsular approach involves little dissection in the area of the dorsal scaphoid and thereby avoids injury to the dorsal blood supply. The scaphoid is then reduced and fixed with a K wire. The screw is inserted freehand (Fig. 45-13, *F*), as the jig was not designed for this approach. It is advisable to leave a parallel K wire behind for rotational stability. An anatomic repair of the dorsal capsule is facilitated by preserving a rim of tissue on the triquetrum when it is taken down.

When the internal fixation is stable, short arm cast immobilization is sufficient. Initially, a well-padded thumb spica splint is used for the first 10 days until the sutures are removed. A short arm cast is applied until 6 weeks postoperatively. This may need to be extended if bone graft was necessary or if the fixation was tenuous. After that period, an Orthoplast thumb spica splint is used. The patients are then generally reviewed at 6-week intervals until union is documented.

Return to Competition. There are no clear guidelines available regarding when it is safe to return an athlete

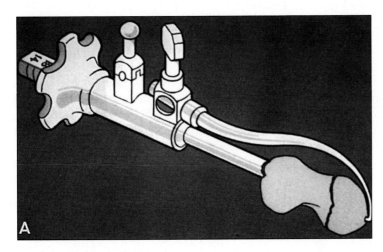

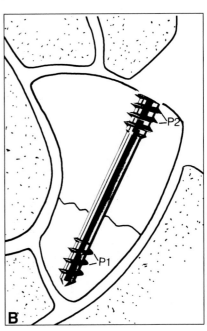

FIGURE 45-12

A, Compression of the scaphoid results from ratcheting down the Huene jig. **B,** Differential pitch P2 and P1 provide added compression, locking the proximal and distal halves of the scaphoid. Note that the smooth barrel alone crosses the fracture site. *(From Herbert TJ.[78] By permission of the publisher.)*

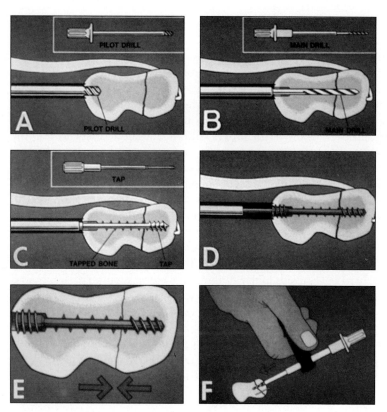

FIGURE 45-13

Technique of insertion of Herbert bone screw. **A,** Pilot drill, overdrilling the distal component. **B,** Main drill, inserted across the pilot drill hole, across the fracture site and into the proximal component. **C,** Bone tapped across the drill hole. **D,** Insertion of the Herbert screw; note lag effect across the fracture site. **E,** Final compression of the scaphoid fracture site. **F,** Freehand placement of the Herbert screw in proximal scaphoid. *(From Herbert TJ.[78] By permission of the publisher.)*

with a scaphoid fracture to competition. There are two points that most would agree on. The first is that it is reasonably safe to return after the fracture has healed, and the second is that a malunion or nonunion of the scaphoid can be a career-ending event for an athlete. Some authors advocate return to competitive athletics in a silicone cast as soon as pain permits in a stable fracture not requiring operative intervention.[39,110] Unfortunately, there are no large series available to support the hypothesis that this is safe. In fact, Culver and Anderson[39] mentioned that they have seen many athletes who were told that their fractures had healed, and on resumption of impact loading, the fracture either displaces or is refractured with minimal trauma. Unofficially, some surgeons have advocated operative intervention for stable nondisplaced fractures in the athlete with the hope of return to competition sooner. This obviously represents a willingness on the part of the surgeon and the athlete to accept the inherent risks of surgical intervention to treat a fracture that has a 95% chance of healing closed.[116]

Huene[85] reported allowing patients to return to contact sports 6 to 8 weeks after internal fixation of scaphoid fractures. He had four athletes in the series and, although no long-term data are presented, it appears that all four of them healed. He used a standard AO partially threaded cancellous screw and took it out after union. Herbert[78] has recommended that contact sports should be avoided for at least 3 months after operative fixation with his implant. Individual patient concerns should be considered. Are there financial issues at stake (scholarship and professional athletes), what position or sport do they play (what type of stresses are they likely to encounter), how vital are they to the team (is peer pressure involved), what time in the season is it (is early return to activity really that important), what are their plans for after their athletic career, and how much risk are they willing to take? Many patients seem to have an expectation that there is a cookbook answer to the question "When can I play again?" We have generally found that, if time is taken and the appropriate questions are asked and the risks explained, a mutually agreeable consensus can be reached. In view of the devastating long-term consequences of post-traumatic arthritis associated with a scaphoid nonunion, we encourage the player to avoid impact loading until the fracture has healed and then continue to protect it in a silicone cast or splint worn during competition for an additional 3 months. We do not think that the Herbert bone screw represents rigid enough fixation to justify early impact loading. Therefore, we do not recommend operative fixation of nondisplaced fractures.

CAPITATE FRACTURES

Injury to the capitate occurs from direct blunt trauma or by extreme dorsiflexion of the wrist. This particular fracture is not associated with any specific sport in regard to frequency, but rather is seen as a result of accident in high-impact high-velocity sports.

The mechanism of injury has been elucidated by Stein and Siegel.[155] They demonstrated that, with the wrist in extreme dorsiflexion, the energy of sudden impact is dissipated through the greater arc of the wrist. First, the scaphoid fails in tension. This allows the capitate to come into contact with the dorsal rim of the radius, which creates force concentration which in turn causes a fracture. As the hyperextension is relaxed, the proximal pole of the capitate can rotate up to 180° in the plane of the palm. The proximal capitate is devoid of soft-tissue attachments, so it often undergoes osteonecrosis leading to the scaphocapitate syndrome, which has been described as a result of this injury.[18]

The patients present with a typical history of dorsiflexion or direct blunt trauma.[58] The swelling is diffuse, and isolating pain to the capitate is difficult because the scaphoid is often involved. The key to diagnosis is an awareness of the injury.

Radiographs are hard to interpret because of superimposition of other carpal bones. If clinical suspicion is high and routine radiographs with oblique views fail to clearly show the neck of the capitate, tomograms will be required.[58,101]

Owing to the frequency of nonunions, avascular necrosis, and functional limitations with this injury, primary excision of the head fragment has been suggested.[33,57,99] We agree with authors who favor anatomic reduction and internal fixation. If avascular necrosis develops, this is managed later with either bone grafting or midcarpal fusion. Large fragments and all displaced fragments do better with open reduction and pin fixation through a dorsal approach. A Herbert screw also can be used. If there is a coexistent scaphoid fracture, this can be managed through either the same dorsal approach or an additional palmar approach, depending on the location of the fracture in the scaphoid. Stable fixation of the scaphoid is recommended. Casting is continued until there is evidence of fracture healing or it is obvious that further treatment is necessary.

HOOK OF THE HAMATE FRACTURES

Fracture of the hook of the hamate in the athlete is an infrequent but important injury, accounting for about 2.5% of all carpal fractures.[75] It results from a direct contact or racquet sport–type injury.[*] The hamate hook projects into the palm in the area of the hypothenar eminence and serves as an attachment point for the transverse carpal ligament and the pisohamate ligament. The flexor digiti minimi and the palmaris brevis originate from the hook of the hamate. The deep branch of the ulnar nerve traverses the base of the hook, where it is in direct contact with bone. The superficial branch of the ulnar nerve lies in proximity to the tip of the hook. The ulnar contents of the

carpal tunnel are also in proximity to the hamate hook. These structures are at risk of injury with a fracture of the hook of the hamate.

Direct blunt trauma is the usual cause for hamate hook fracture, but indirect forces transmitted through ligamentous attachments can and do cause fracture as well. In athletics, these fractures most commonly occur while swinging an instrument such as a tennis racquet, baseball bat, or golf club. When a racquet, bat, or club is gripped in the palm, the end of the handle is over the hypothenar region (Fig. 45-14). If centrifugal forces overcome grip with a powerful swing or a dubbed shot, the handle can strike and fracture the hook of the hamate. Most frequently the hook is fractured near the base, but it can fracture anywhere along its surface. Stark et al.[153] reported in a review of 62 hamate hook fractures that 11% were through the palmar one-third, 13% were through the mid one-third, and 76% were through the dorsal one-third or the base (Fig. 45-15). Stark et al.[154] also suggested that in baseball the fracture occurs at the end of a checked swing, not when the ball is hit. In racquet sports, it results when the player loses control of the racquet. In golf it tends to occur with dubbed shots affecting the lead wrist (left wrist in a right-handed golfer).

The most common sports in which this injury is seen are golf, tennis, and baseball, but any sport that uses equipment that has a handle puts the hamate hook at risk. A 7-year review of these injuries at the Mayo Clinic isolated 21 cases, 12 of which were caused by sports, and the distribution of the type of sport that caused injury is shown in Figure 45-16.[11]

Clinically, the most common symptom is pain in the palm aggravated by grasp. Patients can often point directly to the area of tenderness that they experience with gripping activities. Loss of grip strength and dorsal wrist pain are also common complaints. Symptoms of ulnar nerve paresthesias and weakness or problems with the contents of the carpal canal, including tenosynovitis, tendon fraying, or mild carpal tunnel syndrome, are present in about 25% of cases.[*]

Examination demonstrates tenderness over the hook of the hamate, which can be difficult to palpate secondary to overlying fibrofatty tissue. The hook can be identified along a line from the pisiform to the flexion crease of the index finger.[27] Ulnar nerve paresthesias or palsy, tendinitis, or rupture of the flexor profundus tendon to the small finger is not infrequently seen.

The diagnosis of hook fracture is confirmed radiographically. Routine radiographs may not show the fracture.[110] Norman et al.[114] reported that there are clues readily seen on routine posteroanterior views: absence of the hook of the hamate, sclerosis of the hook, and lack of cortical density (i.e., a barely visible outline of the hamulus). A common mistake is to

* References 3,11,75,99,110,124,154,172.

* References 11,22,75,124,153,154.

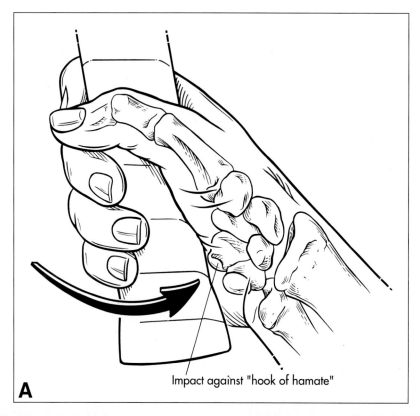

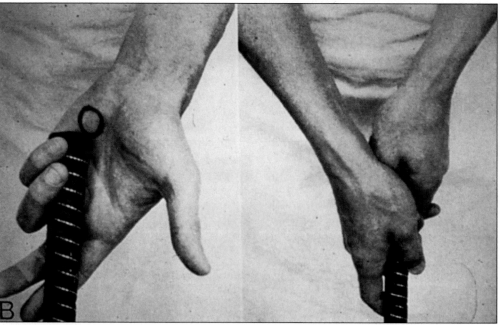

FIGURE 45-14

Mechanism of hook of hamate fracture. **A,** Racquet sports: impaction against the base of the racquet handle can cause a hamate fracture. **B,** *Left:* Golf-related hamate fracture with butt end of the club on the left (or dominant) palm against the hook of the hamate. *Right:* Full golf grip.

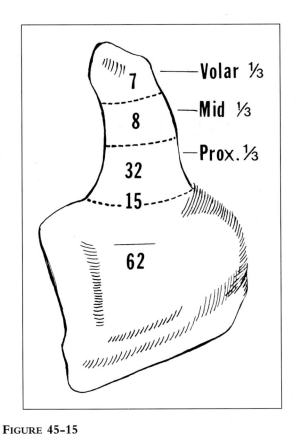

FIGURE 45-15

Common locations of hook of hamate fractures in series. *(From Stark HH et al.[153] By permission of the journal.)*

interpret a congenitally absent or hypoplastic hook as a fracture.[114,132] This is often bilateral and usually can be eliminated as a possibility with views of the opposite side. Bishop and Beckenbaugh[11] reported a 53% sensitivity with the carpal tunnel view in the Mayo Clinic series (Fig. 45-17). They commented that the inconsistent variable was technician positioning of the patient. As with other plain radiographic examinations of the carpus, the problem is caused by superimposition of other carpal bones. A two-dimensional view of a three-dimensional structure can easily be misinterpreted in the carpus. We think that when clinical suspicion is high it is unsafe to eliminate fracture as a possibility based on plain radiographs. We agree with those who recommend biplanar imaging (computed tomography) (Fig. 45-17, *B*) to visualize fractures of the hamate hook.[11,22,50,114,124]

Nonunion of the Hamate Hook. The incidence of nonunion in hamate fractures is significant. Displacement is secondary to the pull of muscular attachments and the relatively poor blood supply of the hook, which leads to delayed healing.[110] One case of osteonecrosis has been reported.[53] Although good results can be reliably achieved with excision of the fracture fragment,* several surgeons have reported

---

* References 11,22,75,93,124,153,154.

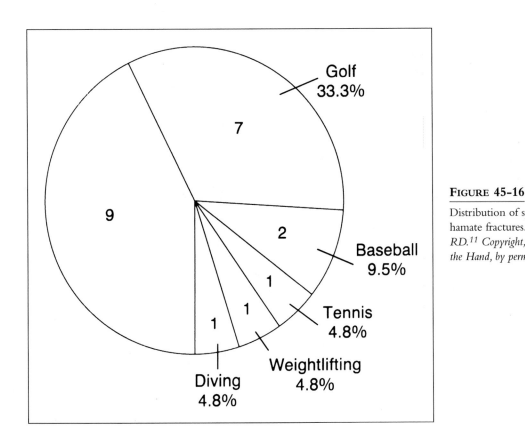

FIGURE 45-16

Distribution of sports that caused hook of hamate fractures. *(From Bishop AT, Beckenbaugh RD.[11] Copyright, American Society for Surgery of the Hand, by permission of Churchill Livingstone.)*

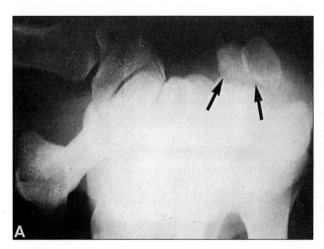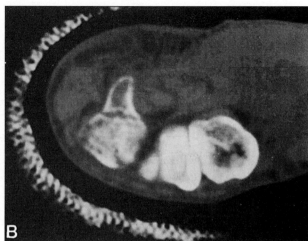

FIGURE 45-17

Diagnosis of hook of hamate fractures. **A,** Carpal tunnel view shows fracture (*arrows*) adjacent to the pisiform. **B,** Computed tomography (axial) shows a fracture through the base of the hamate.

success with cast treatment of acute fractures.[114,144,173] Whalen et al.[173] reported on a series of eight patients from the Mayo Clinic who were treated with a short arm gauntlet-type cast. They divided the group into acute (< 7 days from injury) and subacute (> 7 days from injury). All fractures were nondisplaced. Seven of the eight fractures healed. In one patient in the subacute group who was noncompliant with treatment, a nonunion developed. They concluded that a poor prognosis was associated with diagnostic delays and the failure to institute appropriate immobilization. This study suggests that, if caught early, immobilization may be effective and avoids a surgical intervention. Allowing the athletes to return to competition only after the fracture is healed is recommended and protection in a silicone gauntlet cast should be considered.[110]

Leading surgeons recommend excision for nonunion of hook of the hamate. Uniformly good results have been reported after primary excision of the fracture fragment.* In general, a brief 2- to 3-week period of immobilization postoperatively followed by early return to full activity once scar tenderness has subsided is recommended.[93] There does not appear to be any long-term sequela in regard to function when the hook is excised.

Surgical open reduction and internal fixation can be considered in those acute or delayed diagnosed fractures if they are displaced. Currently, we recommend a trial of cast treatment for acute nondisplaced fractures (< 2 weeks from injury). They have a potential to heal, and surgical complications, such as infection or iatrogenic damage to neurovascular structures, can be avoided. However, if the fracture is displaced or diagnosed late (> 2 weeks from injury) or has associated

findings such as tendon ruptures or ulnar neurapraxia, surgical open reduction and either excision of the fracture fragment or internal fixation is recommended. Although open reduction and internal fixation is feasible, it does not appear to offer any advantage over primary excision.[11]

Operative Procedure. The operation is performed during regional or general anesthesia with tourniquet control. A curvilinear palmar incision is placed over the hook of the hamate, which has been previously marked by the technique described above.[27] Care is taken to identify and protect the ulnar nerve and artery. Sharp subperiosteal dissection is used to isolate the fracture fragment. Often the fracture fragment is surprisingly stable from periosteal attachments or fibrous nonunion. Once the periosteum is released, it is usually easy to isolate the fracture plane. We try to preserve a flap of periosteum to cover the raw cancellous surface once the fragment is removed. It is important to spend time smoothing out the bed from which the fragment is removed to eliminate sharp edges that could cause tendon fraying. The periosteal flap is then closed with an absorbable suture. We use a compressive hand dressing with an ulnar gutter splint postoperatively. This is removed at 10 to 14 days, and the sutures are removed. Return to competition is deferred until scar tenderness has abated, usually by 4 to 6 weeks postoperatively.

TRIQUETRUM IMPACTION FRACTURES

Fractures of the triquetrum are the second[9] or third[18] most common fractures of the carpus. This injury is not uncommonly seen in the athlete, and it can be associated with perilunate and axial pattern fracture dislocations.[33,63-65] This injury has no consistent

---

* References 11,22,75,93,124,153,154.

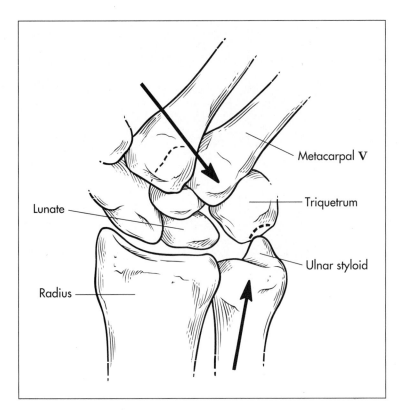

FIGURE 45-18

Mechanism of triquetral impaction fractures. The ulnar styloid strikes against the ulnar proximal aspect of the triquetrum.

association with any particular sport. It tends to happen as a result of a fall or blunt trauma to the dorsum of the hand. The mechanism of this injury is not fully understood. Because of the strong dorsal attachments of the radiotriquetral ligament and the intercarpal ligament, it has long been thought to represent an avulsion fracture.[73,107] The fact that most of these injuries occur with the wrist in dorsiflexion and ulnar deviation[54] has led some to question this mechanism.

Levy et al.[97] first suggested that the fracture occurs by impaction of the dorsal triquetrum against the ulnar styloid. They demonstrated that this was mechanically possible by means of cadaver dissections and radiographic analysis. Garcia-Elias[63] compared 76 patients with dorsal triquetrum fractures to 100 uninjured patients. There was a statistically significant incidence of long ulnar styloid processes in the population with sustained dorsal triquetrum fractures. It is generally thought, based on these studies, that most of these fractures do occur by impaction (Fig. 45-18). However, most of those with associated carpal instability or that occur from an extreme palmar flexion injury probably do represent avulsion fractures.

The patients present with dorsoulnar wrist pain and a history of injury. They are usually focally tender over the triquetrum. Placing the wrist in a position of dorsiflexion and ulnar deviation reproduces their pain. It is important to consider associated carpal instability and perform the routine provocative tests to eliminate this possibility. Other causes of ulnar-sided wrist pain

are also included in the differential diagnosis, such as triangular fibrocartilage complex (TFCC) tears, injury to the dorsal radioulnar joint, sprains of the lunatotriquetral interval, and impaction injuries of the triquetral hamate joint.*

The diagnosis is confirmed radiographically. These fractures are often missed on standard posteroanterior and lateral views. The best plain radiographic view is a 45° pronated oblique. Planar imaging studies are also helpful but rarely necessary.

Immobilization is all that is needed. We use a short arm gauntlet-type cast in neutral position. After 4 weeks, pain subsides and athletes can generally return to competition.[183] Poor results occur when associated injuries are overlooked.

CARPOMETACARPAL FRACTURES AND FRACTURE DISLOCATIONS

Injuries to the CMC joints are relatively rare. The concavoconvex articulations and stout ligamentous restraints provide for significant intrinsic stability.[77] Excluding the thumb ray, the most frequently injured CMC joints are the hamate metacarpal articulations of the ring and small fingers.[21,64,102] The mechanism of injury is not clearly defined. It has been postulated that it occurs by one or in a combination of three ways: a palmar applied force to a dorsiflexed hand, a

---

* References 16,21,37,48,64,71,102,106,182.

dorsal applied force to a palmar flexed hand, or an axially applied force such as when a clenched fist strikes an unyielding object. The largest series of hamatometacarpal fracture dislocations was reported by Cain et al.[21] They reported on a young military population in which the predominant mechanism of injury was an axial load applied to a clenched fist. They commented that these injuries are frequently missed on standard posteroanterior and lateral views and that a 45° pronated oblique view was essential to visualize the fracture (Fig. 45-19).

Garcia-Elias et al.[64] reported on the Mayo Clinic experience with these injuries. They suggested that the most effective way to diagnose these fractures is with axial or lateral polytomography. Not only is the fracture clearly defined but the morphology, articular congruency, and displacement can be assessed with accuracy. When diagnosed early and treated with open reduction and stabilization, patients experienced uniformly excellent results. Five patients in that series presented late, and even with bone grafting and stabilization until fracture consolidation, the results were not as good.

The key to dealing with this injury successfully is making the diagnosis early. If it is suspected, as part of the initial radiographic survey a 45° pronated oblique view should be obtained.[21] If there are further questions about the morphology of the fracture or the degree of articular involvement, polytomography provides adequate visualization.

Garcia-Elias modified Cain's original classification system to include the radial two CMC joints and associated injury at the midcarpal level. The classification is as follows: type I, CMC dislocations with no carpal fracture (Ia) or small dorsal chip fractures of the distal carpal bones (Ib); type II, CMC dislocation with a major fracture affecting only the dorsal aspect of the carpal bone; type III, coronal carpal fracture involving both the CMC and midcarpal joint; and type IV, dorsal subluxation or dislocation of the midcarpal joint without (IVa) or with (IVb) fracture of the palmar aspect of the carpal bone representing ligamentous avulsion (Fig. 45-20).

Because reduction is often easy to obtain but difficult to hold, we believe that this fracture should be managed in a setting where stable fixation can be added. We favor an attempt at closed reduction during regional or general anesthesia by applying longitudinal traction to the involved rays. Occasionally, direct manual pressure is also helpful in obtaining a reduction. This is then stabilized by percutaneous pin fixation to an adjacent stable metacarpal ray and proximally from the involved metacarpal to an adjacent carpal bone much like the typical stabilization of Bennett's fracture.

If reduction is unobtainable by closed means or there is significant comminution that requires bone grafting, the fracture should be opened.[64,65] This is done through a dorsal curvilinear incision. Cutaneous nerves are protected and the extensor tendons are retracted. The

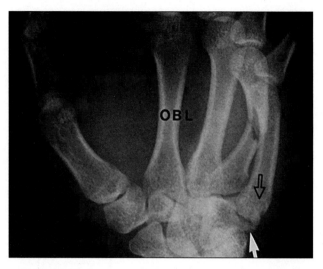

FIGURE 45-19

Hamatometacarpal fracture dislocation best seen in a 45° pronation oblique (*OBL*) view: note proximal migration of the fifth metacarpal shaft (*open arrow*) and comminuted dorsal hamate fracture (*solid arrow*) along with fourth metacarpal shaft fracture. *(From Cain JE et al.[21] Copyright, American Society for Surgery of the Hand, by permission of Churchill Livingstone.)*

fracture is exposed subperiosteally, and the joint is exposed with a transverse incision through adjacent ligaments and the joint capsule. This should be done carefully so that these important ligamentous restraints can be repaired. Bone grafting is helpful in maintaining reduction of depressed fracture fragments that require open manipulation. During the process of manipulative reduction, longitudinal traction should be used.

Type IVa and IVb injuries do not create midcarpal or CMC joint incongruity, but they are associated with significant ligamentous damage at the midcarpal joint level which should be repaired. Once the joint surfaces and ligamentous relationships have been restored and adequately stabilized, the wound is closed in layers. Postoperatively, the patients are placed in a cast that includes the metacarpophalangeal joints of the involved metacarpals. Metacarpophalangeal joint motion is allowed after the third week. K wires are removed after 4 to 6 weeks and casting is continued until the fracture has consolidated, which is usually 6 to 8 weeks. After removal of the cast, motion is followed by strengthening therapy. Athletic competition is avoided until range of motion has been restored. If this is not acceptable, a padded splint should be used during practice and competition.

GYMNAST'S WRIST

Over the past two decades, the popularity of gymnastics has exploded. This is probably the result of increased media coverage of Olympic athletes and an

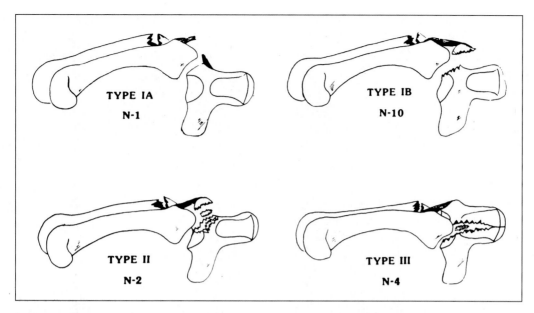

FIGURE 45-20

Classification of carpometacarpal fracture dislocations. Type IA: Subluxation or dislocation of the fifth metacarpal base accompanied by dorsal carpometacarpal ligament disruption. No hamate injury is apparent. Type IB: Demonstrates a dorsal hamate fracture. Type II: Dorsal hamate comminution. Type III: Coronal splitting of the hamate. Frequency of the injury represented by the letter "N." Type IV: Dorsal subluxation or dislocation of the midcarpal joint without (IVA) or with (IVB) fracture of the palmar aspect of a carpal bone (not illustrated). *(From Cain JE et al.[21] Copyright, American Society for Surgery of the Hand, by permission of Churchill Livingstone.)*

overall increase in physical fitness awareness. Many schools incorporate gymnastics as part of their physical fitness curriculum. It is estimated that 600,000 students are involved in gymnastics on an annual basis.[46] In addition, there has been an increasing number of gymnastics studios opening in cities across the country, making training and club competition available. Entry level involvement generally begins around age 7 to 8 years. Peak involvement and performance usually occur around age 13 to 16 years. Men's events include the pommel horse, rings, parallel bars, floor exercises, vault, and horizontal bar. Women's events include floor exercises, balance beam, vault, and uneven parallel bars. Each of these events places high levels of stress on the wrist joint, with high-level loading and extremes of joint positioning. The type of load and joint position during loading for each event are listed in Table 45-1.[46] The principal load type is compression, with dorsiflexion being the most frequent position. The degree, direction, and frequency of forces transmitted across the gymnast's wrist during training and competition are such that the wrist becomes a weightbearing joint. This, superimposed on skeletal immaturity, leads to various problems. Wrist problems in gymnasts are so common that Aronen[5] stated that wrist pain is perceived as a direct result of the sport.

The overall relative incidence of chronic injuries in gymnastics ranges from 17%[126] to 43%.[171] Of these, 80% to 90% represent chronic overuse at the level of the wrist.[46] The injury rate in a nationally ranked women's collegiate gymnastics program has been reported as 0.95 per participant per season. Several authors have reported that injury rates increase as the level of competition increases.[67,103,109,126]

Chronic Osseous Injuries With Physeal Stress Reaction. Chronic repetitive compressive stress on the distal radius can have an adverse effect on enchondral ossification. Repeated microtrauma can disrupt the integrity of the metaphyseal vascular network that is required for proper ossification of the primary spongiosa. The result is that chondrogenesis continues in the germinal zone; however, the transformation of cartilage to bone is impeded. This causes a widened irregular growth plate (especially on the metaphyseal side) (Fig. 45-21). Fortunately, as is seen in fractures, once circulation is reestablished the calcified cartilage is rapidly ossified and there usually are no long-term sequelae.[131]

Patients typically present with a prolonged history of dorsal wrist pain and swelling that is exacerbated by activities. Typical findings include local swelling over the dorsal distal radius, exacerbated by axial loading and dorsiflexion.[131,139]

Radiographic findings characteristically show 1) widening of the distal radial physis, 2) cystic changes and irregularity of the metaphyseal margin of the plate, 3) palmar and radial beaking adjacent to the physis, and 4) haziness of the physis (Fig. 45-21).[139]

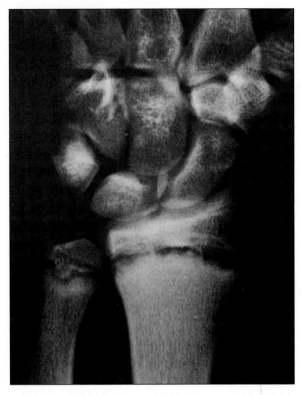

FIGURE 45-21

Distal radius stress fracture. Note widening of distal radius and ulnar physes. *(From Carter SR et al.[23] By permission of the British Institute of Radiology.)*

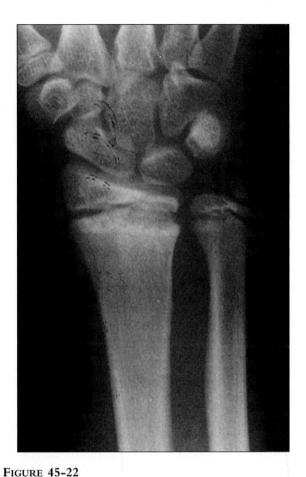

FIGURE 45-22

Premature closure of the physis of the distal radius, ulnar half, with associated ulnar styloid fracture in a young gymnast. *(From Weiker GG.[172] By permission of WB Saunders.)*

Bone scintigraphy may show increased uptake, often in both wrists.

The etiology of this process appears to be extreme dorsiflexion associated with axial compression and torsion on a chronic repetitive basis. The name "dorsiflexion jam syndrome" has been coined for this condition.[172]

Diagnosis and Treatment. The cornerstone of treatment is early diagnosis and cessation of aggravating activities. Those patients with radiographic findings take longer to recover than those who are identified early. Weightbearing on the affected extremity should not be resumed until the wrist is asymptomatic, full motion has been regained, and the wrist is nontender to provocative maneuvers such as axial loading with forced dorsiflexion or a handstand. Whether or not full activity can be resumed before complete radiographic healing has taken place is unknown.[46] Usually, radiographic healing requires a minimum of 3 months.[23]

Several authors have reported no permanent growth alterations of the limb; however, follow-up to skeletal maturity was rarely performed.[23,117,139] Permanent alterations such as Madelung's deformity[165] and

premature physeal closure (Fig. 45-22) leading to the ulna plus variant have been noted.[2,139,172]

Mandelbaum et al.[106] reported ulna variance that was related to duration of participation in 29 male collegiate gymnasts. The first group averaged 10 years of participation (11) and a positive variance of 2.82 mm. The second averaged 8 years of experience (18) and a variance of 1.28 mm. This is striking compared with an age-matched control group with ulna variance of -0.62 mm. As would be expected with the relatively high incidence of positive ulna variance in the gymnast, ulnocarpal impaction syndrome is common. These same authors reported that 87.5% of the collegiate gymnasts in their series had ulnar-sided wrist pain. In 68% of these, it was exacerbated with ulnar deviation. af Ekenstam et al.[1] found that ulnar deviation (25°) and pronation (75°) increased ulnar-sided load from 15% to 24% and 37%, respectively. The position of pronation and ulnar deviation is common on the vault (Fig. 45-23), and this position of the wrist may be responsible for the high incidence of ulnocarpal impaction in gymnasts.

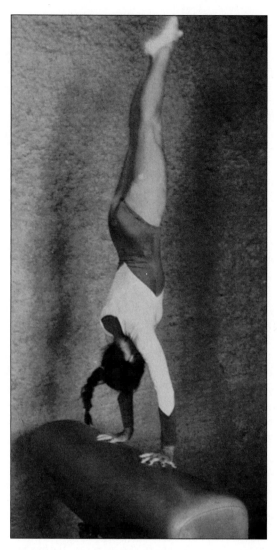

FIGURE 45-23

Hyperextension of the wrist in the vault may induce compression loads across the distal radius physes and potential physeal closure. *(From Weiker GG.172 By permission of WB Saunders.)*

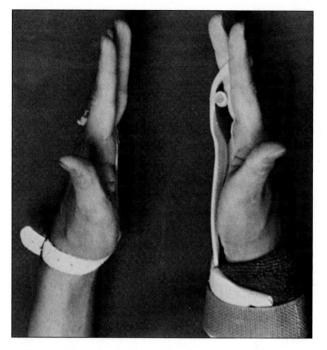

FIGURE 45-24

Dowel grips for use in gymnastics; *left,* traditional grips fitted for female athlete; *right,* dowelled grip fitted for female athlete. *(From Weiker GG.172 By permission of WB Saunders.)*

Ulnocarpal Impaction Syndrome

Patients with ulnocarpal impaction present with ulnar-sided wrist pain aggravated by activity (see Chapter 33).* Typical findings include tenderness over the proximal lunate and triquetrum. Pain is aggravated by forced ulnar deviation, especially when the ulnar head is translated anterior-posterior.

Radiographs frequently show ulna positive variance and can also demonstrate rarefaction of the triquetrum and lunate in the areas of impingement. Arthrography or arthroscopy can often be helpful in determining the integrity of the TFCC and triquetrolunate interosseous membrane.[31,35,137] If less invasive means have

been exhausted, arthroscopy can add valuable information in establishing the diagnosis and planning further treatment.[14,175,176]

Nonoperative management involves the avoidance of aggravating activities and anti-inflammatory medication. Initially, simple cessation of training or training modifications should be tried. If this fails to resolve the symptoms, then the extremity should be immobilized for 4 to 6 weeks. Persistent pain may require operative intervention. Arthroscopic débridement of TFCC tears[118,120] has been infrequently reported in gymnasts.[106] Distal ulna shortening or an arthroscopic wafer resection should be considered in cases with ulna plus variance.[15,40,46,56,178]

Distal Radius and Ulna Physeal Injury from Distraction

Most maneuvers in gymnastics avoid distraction forces across the wrist. Even in events such as the high bar or uneven parallel bar, the distraction forces are borne by the forearm digital flexors. Contraction of these muscle groups actually applies a compression load to the radius and ulna.[46,172] A dowel grip is often used to decrease muscular contraction forces required to maintain grip (Fig. 45-24). This device works by passively transferring distraction forces to the wrist. It effectively suspends the forearm and the body from

---

* References 23,46,99,106,172,182.

the hand and wrist. Yong-Hing and co-workers[182] have reported a traction-induced distal radius physeal stress reaction in a young gymnast. The history differed from the usual compression stress reaction in that the symptoms were aggravated by the rings and high bar rather than the pommel horse. The patient did admit to frequent use of the dowel grips over many years of intense training. Physical examination revealed provocation of symptoms with axial distraction. Radiographic evidence of healing was complete at 4 months from initiation of treatment, which was simply cessation of the aggravating activity. The authors commented that dowel grips should be avoided in the skeletally immature.

SCAPHOID IMPACTION SYNDROME

Repeated hyperextension of the wrist can result in impingement between the dorsal rim of the radius and the proximal carpal row. This injury is frequently seen in gymnastic events such as the pommel horse or floor exercises, but it can also be seen in weight lifters or push-up enthusiasts.[41,99] Biomechanical analysis has demonstrated that when the wrist is in dorsiflexion its range is limited by the dorsal articular surfaces, which are coapted under compression. In radial deviation, the dorsal rims of the radius and scaphoid impact, whereas in ulnar deviation the dorsal aspects of the triquetrum and hamate impact.[170] Linscheid and Dobyns[99] described such stresses resulting in pain and point tenderness over the dorsal rim of the scaphoid reproduced by hyperdorsiflexion. Weiker[172] noted that a frequent finding in gymnasts with wrist pain is a relative lack of finger and wrist flexor strength. He theorized that with fatigue the athlete loses the dynamic cushioning effect on the dorsiflexion moment. At that

point, the limit to wrist dorsiflexion is only the ligaments and the skeleton, which leads to impingement.

Diagnosis is made by careful history and physical examination with findings of pain with hyperextension of the wrist.[46,106,126] Radiographs often reveal ossicles or a hypertrophic dorsal scaphoid or radial rim on lateral views taken in slight flexion.[99] Often if the patient presents with signs and symptoms that are characteristic before radiographic changes have occurred, a local steroid injection can help ameliorate synovitis. Symptoms usually resolve with 2 weeks' rest, temporary splinting, and avoidance of hyperdorsiflexion stresses.

Nonoperative treatment should include not only rest but also a strengthening program for the wrist and finger flexors. During this period of restrengthening, an orthosis that limits maximum dorsiflexion is helpful (Fig. 45-25).

Surgical exploration is rarely necessary but occasionally required for recalcitrant symptoms.[172] Exploration can reveal chondromalacia, synovitis, capsular stripping, or osteophytosis. Good results can be obtained with cheilotomy of either or both opposing surfaces.[46] This is followed by a 2-week period in a short arm cast. After the cast is off and sutures are out, a graduated range of motion program is started. The athlete should not return to competitive level participation until full motion has returned and strength is comparable to that on the uninvolved side.

TRIQUETROLUNATE IMPACTION SYNDROME

Similar to the scaphoid impaction syndrome, the triquetrum or the lunate (or both) can be affected when ulnar deviation is added to dorsiflexion. Floor exercises and pommel horse, which require extremes of dorsiflexion, are associated causal factors. An acute injury

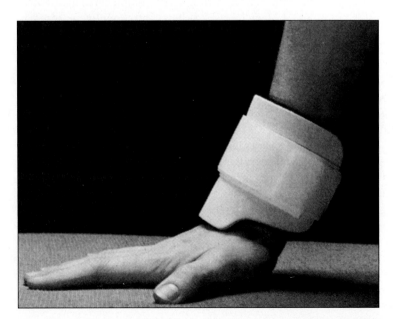

FIGURE 45-25

Dorsal wrist block splint (support) to limit wrist dorsiflexion (extension) and prevent hyperextension injury in gymnast. *(From Weiker GG.[172] By permission of WB Saunders.)*

to functional activity. Generally, 2 mm of bone is removed. Knowing the diameter of the bur assists in judging the depth of resection. Pronation and supination assist in exposing the entire ulnar head. An intraoperative hard copy film is taken to confirm adequate recession of the ulnar head.

Postoperatively, the patients are placed in a sugar tongs splint until wound stability has been achieved and sutures are removed. A range of motion program is instituted focusing on forearm pronation and supination. Once adequate motion has been restored, a strengthening program is instituted. Resumption of competition is allowed when grip strength is 80% of the uninvolved side.

Arthroscopy represents a new technique in the wrist with great therapeutic usefulness. Investigators

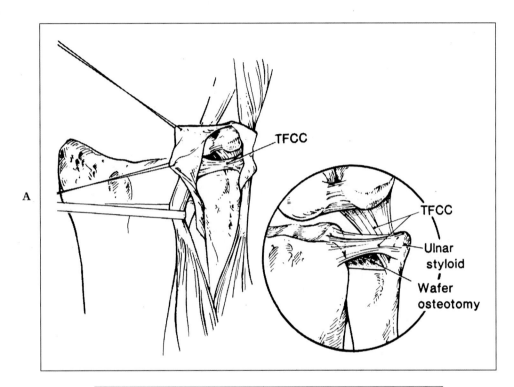

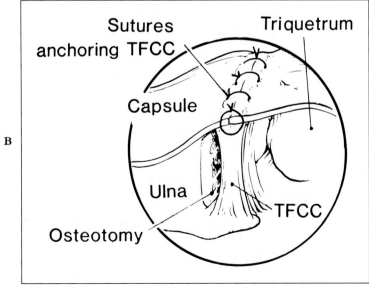

FIGURE 45-27

A, Wafer excision of the distal ulna. *Left:* exposure through a capsule of the distal radioulnar joint shows triangular fibrocartilage complex (*TFCC*) and distal articular surface of the ulna. *Right:* wafer osteotomy of the distal ulna, preserving the ulnar styloid and the TFCC. **B,** Capsular repair to the dorsal edge of the TFCC after excision of the distal ulna. (*From Feldon P et al.*[56] *Copyright, American Society for Surgery of the Hand, by permission of Churchill Livingstone.*)

who deal with athletes have seen the promise of this minimally invasive procedure and have pioneered new techniques. As time and experience have increased, arthroscopy has become a vital tool of the hand surgeon. It allows for a close-up accurate view of the anatomy and pathologic features, which in many cases can be attended to through a few small incisions.

SUMMARY

Athletic injuries of the wrist require special attention. We have discussed this unique group of patients in a separate chapter to provide a more comprehensive approach to management of the athlete. Details of many of the techniques used for injury treatment of the athlete are found elsewhere in this book. Special conditions such as gymnast's wrist, scaphoid impaction syndrome, and compressive neuropathies are found primarily in the athlete and are given greater attention.

Rehabilitation is emphasized as an important element of returning the athlete to competition. It is an essential element of patient athlete management to include full rehabilitation of motion and strength before returning the athlete to competition. Newer procedures such as wrist arthroscopy may lessen the time requirement for rehabilitation in certain athletic wrist problems.

REFERENCES

1. af Ekenstam FW, Palmer AK, Glisson RR: The load on the radius and ulna in different positions of the wrist and forearm. A cadaver study, *Acta Orthop Scand* 55:363-365, 1984.
2. Albanese SA, Palmer AK, Kerr DR, et al.: Wrist pain and distal growth plate closure of the radius in gymnasts, *J Pediatr Orthop* 9:23-28, 1989.
3. Amadio PC: Epidemiology of hand and wrist injuries in sports, *Hand Clin* 6:379-381, 1990.
4. Amadio PC, Berquist TH, Smith DK, et al.: Scaphoid malunion, *J Hand Surg [Am]* 14:679-687, 1989.
5. Aronen JG: Problems of the upper extremity in gymnasts, *Clin Sports Med* 4:61-71, 1985.
6. Aulicino PL: Neurovascular injuries in the hands of athletes, *Hand Clin* 6:455-466, 1990.
7. Barker NW, Hines EA Jr: Arterial occlusion in the hands and fingers associated with repeated occupational trauma, *Proc Staff Meet Mayo Clin* 19:345-349, 1944.
8. Barton NJ: Twenty questions about scaphoid fractures, *J Hand Surg [Br]* 17:289-310, 1992.
9. Bartone NF, Grieco RV: Fractures of the triquetrum, *J Bone Joint Surg Am* 38:353-356, 1956.
10. Bergfeld JA, Weiker GG, Andrish JT, et al.: Soft playing splint for protection of significant hand and wrist injuries in sports, *Am J Sports Med* 10:293-296, 1982.
11. Bishop AT, Beckenbaugh RD: Fracture of the hamate hook, *J Hand Surg [Am]* 13:135-139, 1988.
12. Blunt MJ: The vascular anatomy of the median nerve in the forearm and hand, *J Anat* 93:15-22, 1959.
13. Borgeskov S, Christiansen B, Kjaer A, et al.: Fractures of the carpal bones, *Acta Orthop Scand* 37:276-287, 1966
14. Botte MJ, Cooney WP, Linscheid RL: Arthroscopy of the wrist: anatomy and technique, *J Hand Surg [Am]* 14:313-316, 1989.
15. Boulas HJ, Milek MA: Ulnar shortening for tears of the triangular fibrocartilaginous complex, *J Hand Surg [Am]* 15:415-420, 1990.
16. Bowers WH: *Distal radioulnar joint.* In Green DP, editor: *Operative hand surgery,* New York, 1975, Churchill Livingstone, pp 743-769.
17. Bowers WH: Instability of the distal radioulnar articulation, *Hand Clin* 7:311-327, 1991.
18. Bryan RS, Dobyns JH: Fractures of the carpal bones other than lunate and navicular, *Clin Orthop* 149:107-111, 1980.
19. Burkhart SS, Wood MB, Linscheid RL: Posttraumatic recurrent subluxation of the extensor carpi ulnaris tendon, *J Hand Surg [Am]* 7:1-3, 1982.
20. Burman M: Stenosing tendovaginitis of the dorsal and volar compartments of the wrist, *Arch Surg* 65:752-762, 1952.
21. Cain JE Jr, Shepler TR, Wilson MR: Hematometacarpal fracture-dislocation: classification and treatment, *J Hand Surg [Am]* 12:762-767, 1987.
22. Carter PR, Eaton RG, Littler JW: Ununited fracture of the hook of the hamate, *J Bone Joint Surg Am* 59:583-588, 1977.
23. Carter SR, Aldridge MJ, Fitzgerald R, et al.: Stress changes of the wrist in adolescent gymnasts, *Br J Radiol* 61:109-112, 1988.
24. Cauldwell EW, Anson BJ, Wright RR: Extensor indicis proprius muscle: study of 263 consecutive specimens, *Quart Bull Northwestern Univ Med School* 17:267-279, 1943.
25. Chen SC: The scaphoid compression test, *J Hand Surg [Br]* 14:323-325, 1989.
26. Chidgey LK: Histologic anatomy of the triangular fibrocartilage, *Hand Clin* 7:249-262, 1991.
27. Cobb TK, Cooney WP, An KN: Clinical location of hook of hamate: a technical note for endoscopic carpal tunnel release, *J Hand Surg [Am]* 19:516-518, 1994.

28. Coleman SS, Anson BJ: Arterial patterns in the hand based upon a study of 650 specimens, *Surg Gynecol Obstet* 113:408-424, 1961.

29. Conn J Jr, Bergan JJ, Bell JL: Hypothenar hammer syndrome: posttraumatic digital ischemia, *Surgery* 68:1122-1128, 1970.

30. Converse TA: Cyclist's palsy (letter to the editor), *N Engl J Med* 301:1397-1398, 1979.

31. Cooney WP: Evaluation of chronic wrist pain by arthrography, arthroscopy, and arthrotomy, *J Hand Surg [Am]* 18:815-822, 1993.

32. Cooney WP III: Sports injuries to the upper extremity: how to recognize and deal with some common problems, *Postgrad Med* 76(4):45-50, 1984.

33. Cooney WP, Bussey R, Dobyns JH, et al.: Difficult wrist fractures. Perilunate fracture-dislocations of the wrist, *Clin Orthop* 214:136-147, 1987.

34. Cooney WP, Dobyns JH, Linscheid RL: Fractures of the scaphoid: a rational approach to management, *Clin Orthop* 149:90-97, 1980.

35. Cooney WP, Dobyns JH, Linscheid RL: Arthroscopy of the wrist: anatomy and classification of carpal instability, *Arthroscopy* 6:133-140, 1990.

36. Cooney WP, Linscheid RL, Dobyns JH: Scaphoid fractures. Problems associated with nonunion and avascular necrosis, *Orthop Clin North Am* 15:381-391, 1984.

37. Cooney WP, Linscheid RL, Dobyns JH: Triangular fibrocartilage tears, *J Hand Surg [Am]* 19:143-154, 1994.

38. Cooney WP, Linscheid RL, Dobyns JH, et al.: Scaphoid nonunion: role of anterior interpositional bone grafts, *J Hand Surg [Am]* 13:635-650, 1988.

39. Culver JE, Anderson TE: Fractures of the hand and wrist in the athlete, *Clin Sports Med* 11:101-128, 1992.

40. Darrow JC Jr, Linscheid RL, Dobyns JH, et al.: Distal ulnar recession for disorders of the distal radioulnar joint, *J Hand Surg [Am]* 10:482-491, 1985.

41. Dauphine RT, Linscheid RL: Unrecognized sprain patterns of the wrist (abstract), *J Bone Joint Surg Am* 57:727, 1975.

42. Dawson WJ: Sports-induced spontaneous rupture of the extensor pollicis longus tendon, *J Hand Surg [Am]* 17:457-458, 1992.

43. Dellon AL, Mackinnon SE: Radial sensory nerve entrapment in the forearm, *J Hand Surg [Am]* 11:199-205, 1986.

44. Dellon AL, Seif SS: Anatomic dissections relating the posterior interosseous nerve to the carpus, and the etiology of dorsal wrist ganglion pain, *J Hand Surg [Am]* 3:326-332, 1978.

45. DeMaagd RL, Engber WD: Retrograde Herbert screw fixation for treatment of proximal pole scaphoid nonunions, *J Hand Surg [Am]* 14:996-1003, 1989.

46. Dobyns JH, Gabel GT: Gymnast's wrist, *Hand Clin* 6:493-505, 1990.

47. Dobyns JH, Sim FH, Linscheid RL: Sports stress syndromes of the hand and wrist, *Am J Sports Med* 6:236-254, 1978.

48. Drewniany JJ, Palmer AK: Injuries to the distal radioulnar joint, *Orthop Clin North Am* 17:451-459, 1986.

49. Eckhardt WA, Palmer AK: Recurrent dislocation of extensor carpi ulnaris tendon, *J Hand Surg [Am]* 6:629-631, 1981.

50. Egawa M, Asai T: Fracture of the hook of the hamate: report of six cases and the suitability of computerized tomography, *J Hand Surg [Am]* 8:393-398, 1983.

51. Ellsasser JC, Stein AH: Management of hand injuries in a professional football team. Review of 15 years of experience with one team, *Am J Sports Med* 7:178-182, 1979.

52. Fahrer M, Millroy PJ: Ulnar compression neuropathy due to an anomalous abductor digiti minimi—clinical and anatomic study, *J Hand Surg [Am]* 6:266-268, 1981.

53. Failla JM: Osteonecrosis associated with nonunion of the hook of the hamate, *Orthopedics* 16:217-218, 1993.

54. Fairbank TJ: Chip fractures of os triquetrum (carpal cuneiform), *Br Med J* 2:310-311, 1942.

55. Feinstein PA: Endoscopic carpal tunnel release in a community-based series, *J Hand Surg [Am]* 18:451-454, 1993.

56. Feldon P, Terrono AL, Belsky MR: Wafer distal ulna resection for triangular fibrocartilage tears and/or ulna impaction syndrome, *J Hand Surg [Am]* 17:731-737, 1992.

57. Fenton RL: The naviculo-capitate fracture syndrome, *J Bone Joint Surg Am* 38:681-684, 1956.

58. Fenton RL, Rosen H: Fracture of capitate bone—report of 2 cases, *Bull Hosp Joint Dis* 11:134-139, 1950.

59. Fernandez DL: Anterior bone grafting and conventional lag screw fixation to treat scaphoid nonunions, *J Hand Surg [Am]* 15:140-147, 1990.

60. Finelli PF: Handlebar palsy (letter to the editor), *N Engl J Med* 292:702, 1975.

61. Froimson AI: *Tenosynovitis and tennis elbow.* In Green DP, editor: *Operative hand surgery,* ed 3, New York, 1993, Churchill Livingstone, pp 1989-2006.

62. Ganel A, Engel J, Oster Z, et al.: Bone scanning in the assessment of fractures of the scaphoid, *J Hand Surg [Am]* 4:540-543, 1979.

63. Garcia-Elias M: Dorsal fractures of the triquetrum—avulsion or compression fractures? *J Hand Surg [Am]* 12:266-268, 1987.

64. Garcia-Elias M, Bishop AT, Dobyns JH, et al.: Transcarpal carpometacarpal dislocations, excluding the thumb, *J Hand Surg [Am]* 15:531-540, 1990.

65. Garcia-Elias M, Dobyns JH, Cooney WP III, et al.: Traumatic axial dislocations of the carpus, *J Hand Surg [Am]* 14:446-457, 1989.

66. Garcia-Elias M, Vall A, Salo JM, et al.: Carpal alignment after different surgical approaches to the scaphoid: a comparative study, *J Hand Surg [Am]* 13:604-612, 1988.

67. Garrick JG, Requa RK: Epidemiology of women's gymnastics injuries, *Am J Sports Med* 8:261-264, 1980.

68. Gelberman RH, Menon J: The vascularity of the scaphoid bone, *J Hand Surg [Am]* 5:508-513, 1980.

69. Gellman H, Caputo RJ, Carter V, et al.: Comparison of short and long thumb-spica casts for non-displaced fractures of the carpal scaphoid, *J Bone Joint Surg Am* 71:354-357, 1989.

70. Given KS, Puckett CL, Kleinert HE: Ulnar artery thrombosis, *Plast Reconstr Surg* 61:405-411, 1978

71. Golimbu CN, Firooznia H, Melone CP Jr, et al.: Tears of the triangular fibrocartilage of the wrist: MR imaging, *Radiology* 173:731-733, 1989.

72. Goren ML: Palmar intramural thrombosis of the ulnar artery, *Calif Med* 89:424-425, 1958.

73. Greening WP: Isolated fracture of carpal cuneiform, *Br Med J* 1:221-222, 1942.

74. Grundberg AB, Reagan DS: Pathologic anatomy of the forearm: intersection syndrome, *J Hand Surg [Am]* 10:299-302, 1985.

75. Gupta A, Risitano G, Crawford R, et al.: Fractures of the hook of the hamate, *Injury* 20:284-286, 1989.

76. Hajj AA, Wood MB: Stenosing tenosynovitis of the extensor carpi ulnaris, *J Hand Surg [Am]* 11:519-520, 1986.

77. Hankin FM, Peel SM: Sport-related fractures and dislocations in the hand, *Hand Clin* 6:429-453, 1990.

78. Herbert TJ: *The fractured scaphoid,* St. Louis, 1990, Quality Medical Publishing.

79. Herbert TJ, Fisher WE: Management of the fractured scaphoid using a new bone screw, *J Bone Joint Surg Br* 66:114-123, 1984.

80. Hermansdorfer JD, Kleinman WB: Management of chronic peripheral tears of the triangular fibrocartilage complex, *J Hand Surg [Am]* 16:340-346, 1991.

81. Hirasawa Y, Sakakida K: Sports and peripheral nerve injury, *Am J Sports Med* 11:420-426, 1983.

82. Ho PK, Dellon AL, Wilgis EF: True aneurysms of the hand resulting from athletic injury. Report of two cases, *Am J Sports Med* 13:136-138, 1985.

83. Howard NJ: Peritendinitis crepitans: a muscle-effort syndrome, *J Bone Joint Surg Am* 19:447-459, 1937.

84. Hoyt CS: Ulnar neuropathy in bicycle riders (letter to the editor), *Arch Neurol* 33:372, 1976.

85. Huene DR: Primary internal fixation of carpal navicular fractures in the athlete, *Am J Sports Med* 7:175-177, 1979.

86. Hursh LM: Numbers and types of sports injuries (letter to the editor), *JAMA* 199:507, 1967.

87. Jackson DL: Electrodiagnostic studies of median and ulnar nerves in cyclists, *Phys Sports Med* 17:137-148, Sept 1989.

88. Jantea CL, Baltzer A, Ruther W: Arthroscopic repair of radial-sided lesions of the triangular fibrocartilage complex, *Hand Clin* 11:31-36, 1995.

89. Jorgensen TM, Andresen JH, Thommesen P, et al.: Scanning and radiology of the carpal scaphoid bone, *Acta Orthop Scand* 50:663-665, 1979.

90. Kiefhaber TR, Stern PJ: Upper extremity tendinitis and overuse syndromes in the athlete, *Clin Sports Med* 11:39-55, 1992.

91. Kleinert HE, Hayes JE: The ulnar tunnel syndrome, *Plast Reconstr Surg* 47:21-24, 1971.

92. Kleinert HE, Volianitis GJ: Thrombosis of the palmar arterial arch and its tributaries: etiology and newer concepts in treatment, *J Trauma* 5:447-457, 1965.

93. Koman LA, Mooney JF III, Poehling GC: Fractures and ligamentous injuries of the wrist, *Hand Clin* 6:477-491, 1990.

94. Kulund DN, Brubaker CE: Injuries in the Bikecentennial tour, *Phys Sports Med* 6:74-78, June 1978.

95. Langhoff O, Andersen JL: Consequences of late immobilization of scaphoid fractures, *J Hand Surg [Br]* 13:77-79, 1988.

96. Lawrence RR, Wilson JN: Ulnar artery thrombosis in the palm. Case reports, *Plast Reconstr Surg* 36:604-608, 1965.

97. Levy M, Fischel RE, Stern GM, et al.: Chip fractures of the os triquetrum: the mechanism of injury, *J Bone Joint Surg Br* 61:355-357, 1979.

98. Leyshon A, Ireland J, Trickey EL: The treatment of delayed union and non-union of the carpal scaphoid by screw fixation, *J Bone Joint Surg Br* 66:124-127, 1984.

99. Linscheid RL, Dobyns JH: Athletic injuries of the wrist, *Clin Orthop* 198:141-151, 1985.

100. Linscheid RL, Dobyns JH: *Wrist sprains.* In Tubiana R, editor: *The hand,* Philadelphia, 1985, WB Saunders, pp 970-985.

101. Linscheid RL, Dobyns JH, Younge DK: Trispiral tomography in the evaluation of wrist injury, *Bull Hosp Jt Dis Orthop Inst* 44:297-308, 1984.

102. Loth TS, McMillan MD: Coronal dorsal hamate fractures, *J Hand Surg [Am]* 13:616-618, 1988.

103. Lowry CB, Leveau BF: A retrospective study of gymnastics injuries to competitors and noncompetitors in private clubs, *Am J Sports Med* 10:237-239, 1982.

104. Mack GR, Bosse MJ, Gelberman RH, et al.: The natural history of scaphoid non-union, *J Bone Joint Surg Am* 66:504-509, 1984.

105. Malloch JD: Palmar-arch thrombosis, *Br Med J* 2:28, 1962.

106. Mandelbaum BR, Bartolozzi AR, Davis CA, et al.: Wrist pain syndrome in the gymnast. Pathogenetic, diagnostic, and therapeutic considerations, *Am J Sports Med* 17:305-317, 1989.

107. Mark LK: Fractures of the triquetrum, *Am J Roentgenol* 83:676-799, 1960.

108. Martin AF: Ulnar artery thrombosis in the palm. A case report, *Clin Orthop* 17:373-376, 1960.

109. McAuley E, Hudash G, Shields K, et al.: Injuries in women's gymnastics. The state of the art, *Am J Sports Med* 16 Suppl 1:S124-S131, 1988.

110. McCue FC III, Baugher WH, Kulund DN, et al.: Hand and wrist injuries in the athlete, *Am J Sports Med* 7:275-286, 1979.

111. McLaughlin HL, Parkes JC II: Fracture of the carpal navicular (scaphoid) bone: gradations in therapy based upon pathology, *J Trauma* 9:311-319, 1969.

112. Mehlhoff TL, Wood MB: Ulnar artery thrombosis and the role of interposition vein grafting: patency with microsurgical technique, *J Hand Surg [Am]* 16:274-278, 1991.

113. Nakamura R, Imaeda T, Horii E, et al.: Analysis of scaphoid fracture displacement by three-dimensional computed tomography, *J Hand Surg [Am]* 16:485-492, 1991.

114. Norman A, Nelson J, Green S: Fractures of the hook of the hamate: radiographic signs, *Radiology* 154:49-53, 1985.

115. Noth J, Dietz V, Mauritz KH: Cyclist's palsy: neurological and EMG study in 4 cases with distal ulnar lesions, *J Neurol Sci* 47:111-116, 1980.

116. O'Brien ET: Acute fractures and dislocations of the carpus, *Orthop Clin North Am* 15:237-258, 1984.

117. Ogden JA: *The uniqueness of growing bone.* In Rockwood CA Jr, Wilkins KE, King RE, editors: *Fractures in children,* ed 3, New York, 1991, JB Lippincott, pp 42-43.

118. Osterman AL: Arthroscopic debridement of triangular fibrocartilage complex tears, *Arthroscopy* 6:120-124, 1990.

119. Osterman AL, Moskow L, Low DW: Soft-tissue injuries of the hand and wrist in racquet sports, *Clin Sports Med* 7:329-348, 1988.

120. Osterman AL, Terrill RG: Arthroscopic treatment of TFCC lesions, *Hand Clin* 7:277-281, 1991.

121. Palmer AK: Triangular fibrocartilage complex lesions: a classification, *J Hand Surg [Am]* 14:594-606, 1989.

122. Palmer AK: Triangular fibrocartilage disorders: injury patterns and treatment, *Arthroscopy* 6:125-132, 1990.

123. Palmer AK, Werner FW: The triangular fibrocartilage complex of the wrist—anatomy and function, *J Hand Surg [Am]* 6:153-162, 1981.

124. Parker RD, Berkowitz MS, Brahms MA, et al.: Hook of the hamate fractures in athletes, *Am J Sports Med* 14:517-523, 1986.

125. Perlik PC, Guilford WB: Magnetic resonance imaging to assess vascularity of scaphoid nonunions, *J Hand Surg [Am]* 16:479-484, 1991.

126. Pettrone FA, Ricciardelli E: Gymnastic injuries: the Virginia experience 1982-1983, *Am J Sports Med* 15:59-62, 1987.

127. Phalen GS: The carpal-tunnel syndrome: seventeen years' experience in diagnosis and treatment of six hundred fifty-four hands, *J Bone Joint Surg Am* 48:211-228, 1966.

128. Porubsky GL, Brown SI, Urbaniak JR: Ulnar artery thrombosis: a sports-related injury, *Am J Sports Med* 14:170-175, 1986.

129. Powell JM, Lloyd GJ, Rintoul RF: New clinical test for fracture of the scaphoid, *Can J Surg* 31:237-238, 1988.

130. Rayan GM: Recurrent dislocation of the extensor carpi ulnaris in athletes, *Am J Sports Med* 11:183-184, 1983.

131. Read MT: Stress fractures of the distal radius in adolescent gymnasts, *Br J Sports Med* 15:272-276, 1981.

132. Recht MP, Burk DL Jr, Dalinka MK: Radiology of wrist and hand injuries in athletes, *Clin Sports Med* 6:811-828, 1987.

133. Redler I: Meniscoid of the wrist, *Clin Orthop* 88:138-141, 1972.

134. Rettig AC: Neurovascular injuries in the wrists and hands of athletes, *Clin Sports Med* 9:389-417, 1990.

135. Rettig AC, Ryan RO, Stone JA: *Epidemiology of hand injuries in sports.* In Strickland JW, Rettig AC, editors: *Hand injuries in athletes,* Philadelphia, 1992, WB Saunders, pp 37-48.

136. Ritter MA, Inglis AE: The extensor indicis proprius syndrome, *J Bone Joint Surg Am* 51:1645-1648, 1969.

137. Roth JH, Haddad RG: Radiocarpal arthroscopy and arthrography in the diagnosis of ulnar wrist pain, *Arthroscopy* 2:234-243, 1986.

138. Rowland SA: Acute traumatic subluxation of the extensor carpi ulnaris tendon at the wrist, *J Hand Surg [Am]* 11:809-811, 1986.

139. Roy S, Caine D, Singer KM: Stress changes of the distal radial epiphysis in young gymnasts. A report of twenty-one cases and a review of the literature, *Am J Sports Med* 13:301-308, 1985.

140. Ruby LK: Common hand injuries in the athlete, *Orthop Clin North Am* 11:819-839, 1980.

141. Ruby LK, Stinson J, Belsky MR: The natural history of scaphoid non-union. A review of fifty-five cases, *J Bone Joint Surg Am* 67:428-432, 1985.

142. Russe O: Fracture of the carpal navicular: diagnosis, non-operative treatment, and operative treatment, *J Bone Joint Surg Am* 42:759-768, 1960.

143. Sanders WE: Evaluation of the humpback scaphoid by computed tomography in the longitudinal axial plane of the scaphoid, *J Hand Surg [Am]* 13:182-187, 1988.

144. Schlosser H, Murray JF: Fracture of the hook of the hamate, *Can J Surg* 27:587-589, 1984.

145. Shaw JA: A biomechanical comparison of scaphoid screws, *J Hand Surg [Am]* 12:347-353, 1987.

146. Shea JD, McClain EJ: Ulnar-nerve compression syndromes at and below the wrist, *J Bone Joint Surg Am* 51:1095-1103, 1969.

147. Short W: Repair of radial triangular fibrocartilage tear, *J Hand Surg* (in press).

148. Smail DF: Handlebar palsy (letter to the editor), *N Engl J Med* 292:322, 1975.

149. Smith DK, An KN, Cooney WP III, et al.: Effects of a scaphoid waist osteotomy on carpal kinematics, *J Orthop Res* 7:590-598, 1989.

150. Smith DK, Linscheid RL, Amadio PC, et al.: Scaphoid anatomy: evaluation with complex motion tomography, *Radiology* 173:177-180, 1989.

151. Spinner M, Kaplan EB: Extensor carpi ulnaris: its relationship to the stability of the distal radio-ulnar joint, *Clin Orthop* 68:124-129, 1970.

152. Spinner M, Olshansky K: The *extensor indicis proprius* syndrome: a clinical test, *Plast Reconstr Surg* 51:134-138, 1973.

153. Stark HH, Chao EK, Zemel NP, et al.: Fracture of the hook of the hamate, *J Bone Joint Surg Am* 71:1202-1207, 1989.

154. Stark HH, Jobe FW, Boyes JH, et al.: Fracture of the hook of the hamate in athletes, *J Bone Joint Surg Am* 59:575-582, 1977

155. Stein F, Siegel MW: Naviculocapitate fracture syndrome: a case report: new thoughts on the mechanism of injury, *J Bone Joint Surg Am* 51:391-395, 1969.

156. Stern PJ: Tendinitis, overuse syndromes, and tendon injuries, *Hand Clin* 6:467-476, 1990.

157. Stewart MJ: Fractures of the carpal navicular (scaphoid): a report of 436 cases, *J Bone Joint Surg [Am]* 36:998-1006, 1954.

158. Stordahl A, Schjoth A, Woxholt G, et al.: Bone scanning of fractures of the scaphoid, *J Hand Surg [Br]* 9:189-190, 1984.

159. Strauss RH, Lanese RR: Injuries among wrestlers in school and college tournaments, *JAMA* 248:2016-2019, 1982.

160. Sunderland S: The nerve lesion in the carpal tunnel syndrome, *J Neurol Neurosurg Psychiatry* 39:615-626, 1976.

161. Szabo RM, Manske D: Displaced fractures of the scaphoid, *Clin Orthop* 230:30-38, 1988.

162. Taleisnik J, Kelly PJ: The extraosseous and intraosseous blood supply of the scaphoid bone, *J Bone Joint Surg Am* 48:1125-1137, 1966.

163. Thiebault J: Le risque sportif: etude de 43093 dossiers concernant 57 disciplines (sport amateur), *Rev Franc Dom Corp* 6:319, 1980.

164. Thiru-Pathi RG, Ferlic DC, Clayton ML, et al.: Arterial anatomy of the triangular fibrocartilage of the wrist and its surgical significance, *J Hand Surg [Am]* 11:258-263, 1986.

165. Vender MI, Watson HK: Acquired Madelung-like deformity in a gymnast, *J Hand Surg [Am]* 13:19-21, 1988.

166. Verdan C: Fractures of the scaphoid, *Surg Clin North Am* 40:461-464, 1960.

167. Wartenberg R: Cheiralgia paraesthetica (Isolierte Neuritis des Ramus superficialis nervi radialis). *Ztschr Ges Neurol Psychiat* 141:145-155, 1932.

168. Watson HK, Ashmead D IV, Makhlouf MV: Examination of the scaphoid, *J Hand Surg [Am]* 13:657-660, 1988.

169. Weber ER: Biomechanical implications of scaphoid waist fractures, *Clin Orthop* 149:83-89, 1980.

170. Weber ER, Chao EY: An experimental approach to the mechanism of scaphoid waist fractures, *J Hand Surg [Am]* 3:142-148, 1978.

171. Weiker GG: Club gymnastics, *Clin Sports Med* 4:39-43, 1985.

172. Weiker GG: Hand and wrist problems in the gymnast, *Clin Sports Med* 11:189-202, 1992.

173. Whalen JL, Bishop AT, Linscheid RL: Nonoperative treatment of acute hamate hook fractures, *J Hand Surg [Am]* 17:507-511, 1992.

174. Whipple TL: *Arthroscopic surgery—the wrist,* Philadelphia, 1992, JB Lippincott.

175. Whipple TL: The role of arthroscopy in the treatment of wrist injuries in the athlete, *Clin Sports Med* 11:227-238, 1992.

176. Whipple TL, Marotta JJ, Powell JH III: Techniques of wrist arthroscopy, *Arthroscopy* 2:244-252, 1986.

177. Williams JG: Surgical management of traumatic non-infective tenosynovitis of the wrist extensors, *J Bone Joint Surg Br* 59:408-410, 1977.

178. Wnorowski DC, Palmer AK, Werner FW, et al.: Anatomic and biomechanical analysis of the arthroscopic waver procedure, *Arthroscopy* 8:204-212, 1992.

179. Wood MB, Dobyns JH: Sports-related extraarticular wrist syndromes, *Clin Orthop* 202:93-102, 1986.

180. Wood MB, Linscheid RL: Abductor pollicis longus bursitis, *Clin Orthop* 93:293-296, 1973.

181. Wood MR: Hydrocortisone injections for carpal tunnel syndrome, *Hand* 12:62-64, 1980.

182. Yong-Hing K, Wedge JH, Bowen CV: Chronic injury to the distal ulnar and radial growth plates in an adolescent gymnast. A case report, *J Bone Joint Surg Am* 70:1087-1089, 1988.

183. Zemel NP, Stark HH: Fractures and dislocations of the carpal bones, *Clin Sports Med* 5:709-724, 1986.

184. Zweig J, Lie KK, Posch JL, et al.: Thrombosis of the ulnar artery following blunt trauma to the hand, *J Bone Joint Surg Am* 51:1191-1198, 1969.

XII

COMPLICATIONS OF WRIST INJURIES AND TREATMENT

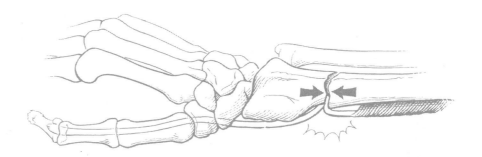

46

COMPLICATIONS OF INJURIES OF THE WRIST (AND CHRONIC PAIN MANAGEMENT)

William P. Cooney, M.D.
Owen J. Moy, M.D.
Michael B. Wood, M.D.

SOFT-TISSUE INJURIES
  SKIN
  TENDONS
  NERVE
    MEDIAN NEUROPATHY (CARPAL TUNNEL
      SYNDROME)
    ULNAR NEUROPATHY
    CUTANEOUS NEUROPATHY
    TREATMENT
BONE AND JOINT

FRACTURE REDUCTIONS
NONUNION
MALUNION
CARPAL INSTABILITY
PAIN SYNDROMES
  SYMPATHETIC DYSTROPHY
  SOMATIC NERVE PAIN
  PREFERRED TREATMENT PLAN
  TREATMENT ALTERNATIVES FOR SOMATIC PAIN
    VERSUS SYMPATHETIC PAIN

Complications related to injury or surgery on the wrist are being recognized and reported with increasing frequency. To make a decision or judgment regarding various types of treatment (either operative or nonoperative), knowledge of the risks of complication(s) is important for the patient as well as the treating physician. Complications can result from the initial injury, be related to the disease process, or result from treatment programs. It is our desire to maximize the treatment benefits while minimizing and eliminating any and all complications. The treatment outcome will be judged by the patient, insurance carrier or other provider, and physician based on the ultimate outcome. An awareness of potential complications not only helps in preparation for operative and nonoperative treatment but should allow for early intervention to minimize or prevent permanent damage. In this chapter, we review the more common complications associated with injuries to the wrist and their operative treatment.

SOFT-TISSUE INJURIES

SKIN

Most complications of the skin are the result of the original injury that produces swelling and soft-tissue injury. The problem is exacerbated by the incorrect timing or application of a cast, dressing, or fixation supports (Fig. 46-1). Constricting bandages or casts do not allow for swelling, and as a result skin-pressure necrosis and even compartment syndromes can result.[67-69,73] Most casts should be applied only after time to allow the swelling to subside (Fig. 46-2). We recommend either dorsal or palmar splints or use of a sugar tongs splint for the initial immobilization of wrist injuries. Excessive hematoma injection should also be avoided (Fig. 46-3).

Cast application after fractures of the distal radius or other carpal injuries is best 24 to 48 hours after the injury.[19,44,63] Reestablishment of soft tissue and bone length may be needed, and we recommend application of the cast while the limb is under traction. The cast should be well padded, particularly around bone prominences such as the radial styloid, ulnar styloid, and medial and lateral epicondyles. Careful molding of the cast will not only assist with maintaining fracture reduction but also prevent pressure areas. Around pins or wires, we suggest sponge padding that will give if the cast loosens or shifts. A window over the pins or wires is a second option to avoid pressure or motion on the pin site. The choice of cast material can also influence sites of pressure, with plaster cast providing better molding and few rough or sharp edges compared with the currently popular plastic materials.[52]

Generally, soft-tissue injury to the wrist is overlooked. The tendency of most surgeons is to examine the underlying bone or joint injury.[12] Skin avulsions, crush, or abrasions can result from the initial injury,

making treatment of the bone or joint injury more difficult. Planning for soft-tissue coverage becomes essential when the skin loss extends beyond or deep to the superficial fascia, with direct contact on the extensor or flexor tendons (Fig. 46-4).[37] Local rotation flaps of skin or more commonly island pedicle vascularized flaps, such as the radial forearm flap or posterior interosseous artery retrograde flap, are commonly needed.[41] A distal pedicle flap such as the groin flap may also need to be considered for soft-tissue coverage. Free-tissue transfers are a third consideration. For the dorsal aspect of the hand and wrist, the lateral arm flap, fascia lata flap, or dorsalis pedis-based free-tissue transfers provide excellent skin and soft-tissue coverage. Free flaps also provide the opportunity for composite tissue transfer, such as the lateral arm flap's ability to include bone and nerve tissue. Distant, local, or free-flap transfers are rarely primary procedures; rather, they are deferred until after wrist bone stabilization and wound débridement. As swelling subsides, the soft-tissue defect may not require major flap coverage but delayed primary closure. Prevention of soft-tissue loss but adherence to principles of tensionless wound closure and clean wounds often minimizes the need for soft-tissue flaps about the wrist.

TENDONS

Tendon injuries can result from crush, laceration, or compression within closed spaces. With many fractures of the carpus or distal radius, abrasion injury to flexor and extensor tendons has occurred.[6,11,20,39] The most common extensor tendon injury is to the extensor pollicis longus after a distal radius fracture (Fig. 46-5).[24,34,39] It may be difficult to prevent because it is most common with undisplaced fractures. Finger flexor tendon injuries are associated with scaphoid and hamate fractures that go unrecognized

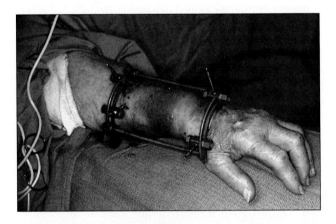

FIGURE 46-1

Skin abrasions, swelling, and ecchymosis related to a severely displaced fracture of the distal radius. Release of the skin around the pin sites was required.

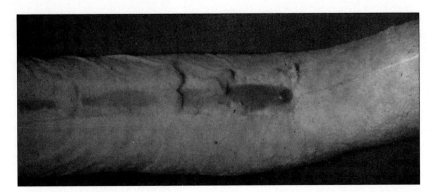

FIGURE 46-2

Swelling about a cast that was applied immediately after a fracture dislocation of the wrist. Note the extended amount of swelling despite splitting the cast over the distal forearm. Complete release of the cast and all cast padding and stockinette is required to prevent a compartment syndrome.

and occasionally become entrapped within the fracture site (Fig. 46-6).[6,20,77] Compression forces within a closed compartment are frequent after fracture, and synovitis may occur in several areas. The carpal tunnel, first dorsal compartment, and fourth dorsal compartment are the most common sites of increased compressive forces that lead to tendon rupture.[24,28,39] Recognition of synovitis early can assist in maintaining a full range of finger motion and prevent finger and wrist joint stiffness.

For tendon injuries from fracture or direct crush or laceration within the extensor retinaculum or flexor compartments, treatment by primary tendon graft or tendon transfer is required (Fig. 46-7).[20,34] For tendon lacerations outside of flexor or extensor compartments, tendon repair may be possible. With the attrition tear, tendon repair is rarely possible. For the extensor pollicis longus, which is the most common tendon rupture, we prefer the extensor indicis proprius transfer (Fig. 46-7) from the index finger to the extensor pollicis longus at a level just proximal to the metacarpophalangeal joint of the thumb.[22,41] A tendon graft (palmaris or plantaris) is performed in selected cases by bypassing the injured tendon as it is passed beneath the extensor retinaculum. Extensor pollicis longus tendon rupture can occur either early or late, with the interval ranging from a day to years. Accurate fracture reduction in general helps to decrease the risk of late rupture.

For adhesions or synovitis,[47] the first level of treatment is local injections of cortisone, physiotherapy, and active motion. Peritendinous adhesions that significantly restrict tendon gliding may require surgical intervention followed by early active motion. Adhesion release is best performed during local anesthesia, if possible, so that full motion can be confirmed and demonstrated to the patient. Stenosing tenosynovitis of the

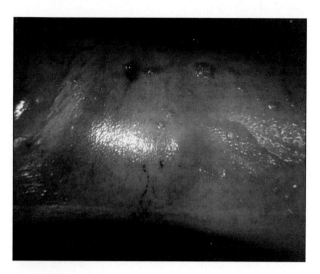

FIGURE 46-3

Excessive hematoma formation associated with a lidocaine block before assisted closed reduction of a distal radius fracture. The amount of fracture displacement suggested that a proximal axillary block or Bier block would have been a better choice for anesthesia of the upper limb for fracture reduction.

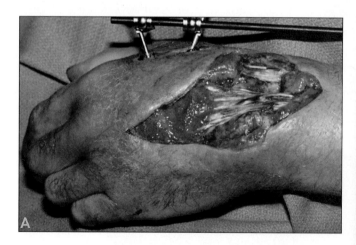

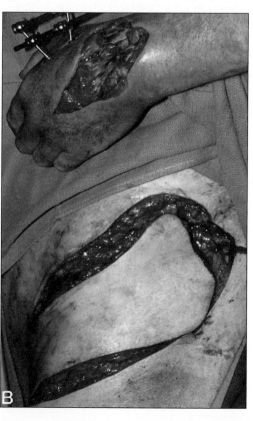

FIGURE 46-4

Groin flap coverage for an infected open fracture of the distal radius in a diabetic patient. **A,** Open wound with exposed extensor tendons. **B,** Prepositioning of hand wound and groin before insetting.

first extensor compartment (de Quervain's) on the other hand is treated effectively by cortisone injection, supportive splint, and assisted motion, and only with persistent, unresponsive cases is release of the first dorsal extensor compartment required. Local anesthesia is again recommended to be sure that all compartments (abductor pollicis longus and extensor pollicis brevis compartments) are released.

Entrapment of flexor and extensor tendons (or muscle) can occur but is rare.[11,25,71] Failure to reduce a distal radius fracture may suggest interposition of muscle (pronator quadratus) or tendon (Fig. 46-8). Tendon dysfunction may be a clue to entrapment

within the fracture site (Fig. 46-6). Not only will the fracture not reduce, but with careful clinical examination tendon excursion will be decreased or eliminated and the tenodesing effect that should be present with wrist motion will not be present. Early recognition is essential so that open extraction of the tendon or muscle can be performed along with reduction of the fracture (or wrist dislocation) as the case requires.

Entrapment of extensor tendons can occur with fractures of the distal radius within the fracture site or within the distal radioulnar joint (Fig. 46-9).[11,77] The affected tendon can be the extensor carpi ulnaris, extensor digiti minimi (distal radioulnar joint), or

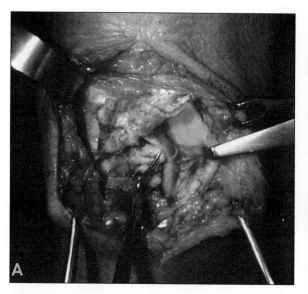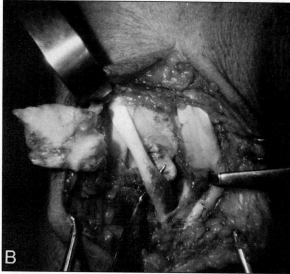

FIGURE 46-5

A, Extensor pollicis longus fraying around Lister's tubercle associated with a fracture of the distal radius. **B,** Release of the extensor pollicis longus tendon sheath along with the extensor retinaculum.

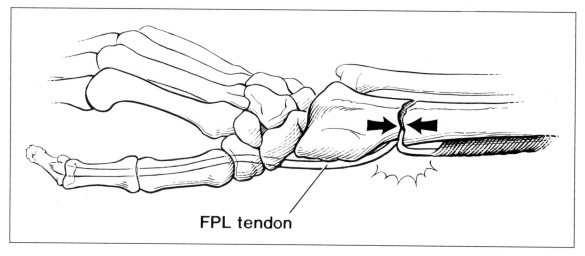

FPL tendon

FIGURE 46-6

Entrapment of the flexor pollicis longus tendon (*FPL*) within a proximal radius fracture site (*arrows*). (*From Kozin SH, Wood MB.[41] By permission of Mayo Foundation.*)

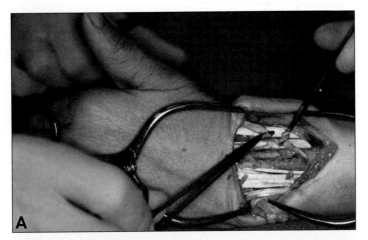

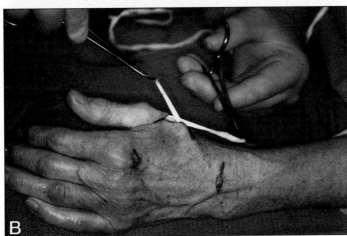

FIGURE 46-7

Transfer of the extensor indicis proprius in the treatment of a rupture of the extensor pollicis longus tendon after treatment of a distal radius fracture. **A,** Rupture of the extensor pollicis longus tendon. **B,** Incisions at the index metacarpophalangeal joint, distal radius, and just proximal to the thumb metacarpophalangeal joint for extensor indicis proprius transfer to restore thumb extension. *(From Kozin SH, Wood MB.⁴¹ By permission of the journal.)*

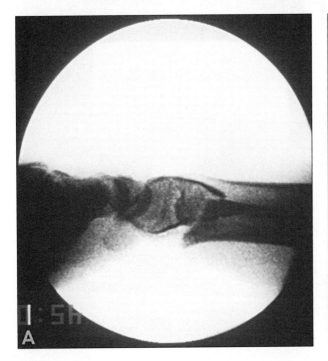

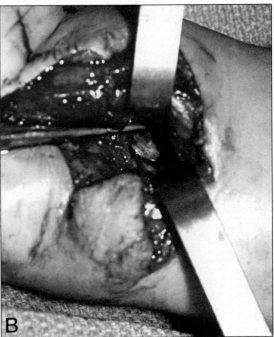

FIGURE 46-8

A, Pronator quadratus interposition blocking reduction an extra-articular fracture of the distal radius. Note failure to align the palmar cortices of the distal radius. **B,** Extended carpal tunnel approach, including release of the pronator quadratus (between the retractors), with a problem elevating the fracture to allow for reduction.

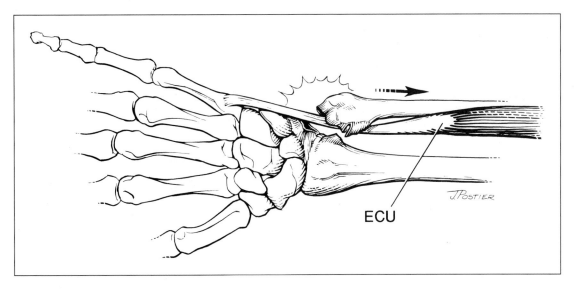

FIGURE 46-9

Entrapment of the extensor carpi ulnaris (*ECU*) tendon within the distal radioulnar joint. *(From Kozin SH, Wood MB.*[41] *By permission of Mayo Foundation.)*

extensor pollicis longus (distal radius fracture site). Failure to reduce the fracture or inability to reduce the distal radioulnar joint should increase suspicion of tendon interposition. Look for a widened distal radioulnar joint and vacant extensor carpi ulnaris sulcus (empty sulcus sign) in diagnosis of tendon entrapment within the dorsal radioulnar joint.

For treatment, open reduction of the distal radioulnar joint, extraction of the tendon, and repair of the extensor carpi ulnaris fibro-osseous sheath is recommended. For the entrapment of extensor tendons within the fracture site, after extraction, the fracture should be anatomically reduced and part (distal half) of the extensor retinaculum should be placed deep to the tendon to prevent further attrition injury or vascular compromise.

NERVE

Trauma related to laceration, compression, or contusion to peripheral nerves is not uncommon in injuries around the wrist.* There is little soft-tissue protection for the subcutaneous nerves and nerve-related paresthesias are frequent (Fig. 46-10). The surgeon needs to remember that not only the median, ulnar, and sensory branches of the radial nerve cross the wrist but also other cutaneous branches such as the lateral antebrachial cutaneous nerve and the dorsal cutaneous branch of the ulnar nerve can be injured and produce dysesthesias.† It is particularly important to determine serious nerve-related injuries (such as

compression of the median nerve within the carpal tunnel or within the fracture site) (Figs. 46-10, *A* and *B*).* The radial sensory and dorsal ulnar sensory nerves are also at risk for serious direct injury (Fig. 46-11).† The ulnar nerve within Guyon's space is less commonly involved because it lies in more of a "space" than a closed compartment.[36,42,78] Fractures of the distal radius are associated with the highest frequency of nerve damage.[10] These injuries may result in long-term disability exceeding that of the bony injury. Iatrogenic injury to these nerves can also occur during surgical treatment of bone or joint injury. The mechanism of injury can be direct blow or contusion, transection, entrapment, or compressive neuropathy. The frequency of such injuries ranges from 0.2% to 17%.[19,71,73]

Although the neurologic injury secondary to transection and entrapment of the nerve is rare, compression and contusion are well documented. In our previous communication of this subject,[19] median nerve injury was the most common complication associated with fractures of the distal radius. Proximity to the distal radius and its confinement within the carpal tunnel make the median nerve quite prone to compression and contusion (Table 46-1). According to anatomic studies performed by Vance and Gelberman,[74] the distance between the median nerve and the radius at the midforearm level is 10 mm, whereas at the wrist the distance is only 3 mm. In a simulated fracture of the distal radius with dorsal displacement of the distal radius, the distance between the median nerve and the

---

* References 1,9,14,15,21,27,42,44,50,53,59,60.
† References 2,13,15,23,36,44,51.

* References 9,14,19,27,50,54.
† References 13,23,44,51,66,70,72,74.

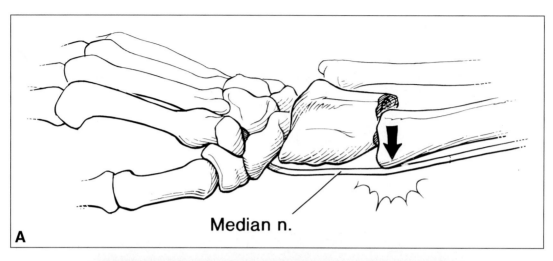

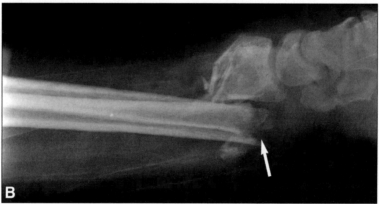

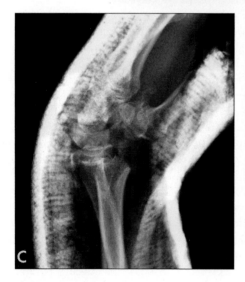

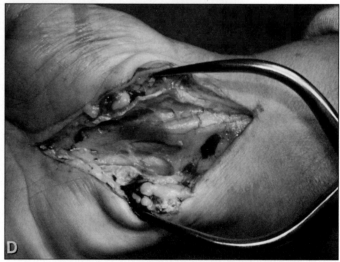

FIGURE 46–10

A, Direct contusion of the median nerve (*n.*) by a displaced proximal fragment of a fracture of the distal radius (*arrow*). *(From Kozin SH, Wood MB.[41] By permission of Mayo Foundation.)* **B,** Clinical example of severe direct compression with partial impaling of the median nerve by a displaced fracture of the distal radius (*arrow*). **C,** Dorsal Barton's fracture dislocation of the wrist left unreduced and treated in a cast resulted in an acute median neuropathy. **D,** Extended carpal tunnel incision for release of the median nerve associated with a displaced distal radius fracture. The incision crosses the wrist crease and must extend at least 3 cm proximally on the forearm.

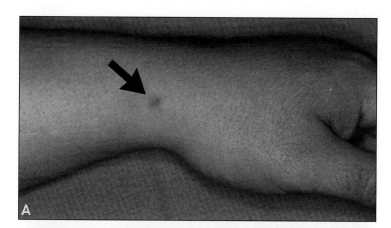

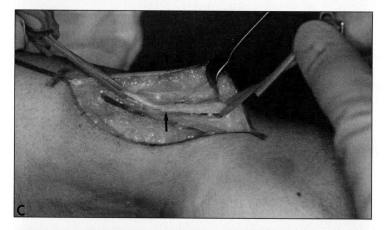

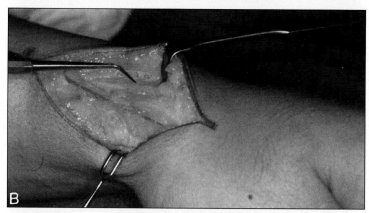

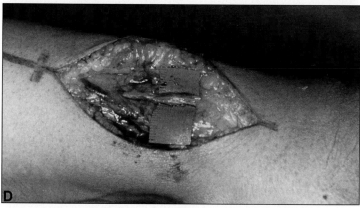

FIGURE 46-11

Injury of the radial sensory nerve. **A,** Puncture site (*arrow*) over the radial aspect of the distal forearm. **B,** Site of injury noted at the distal end of the pointer (nerve probe). **C,** Area of injury (*arrow*) demonstrated on the superficial main branch of the radial nerve between the two nerve-vessel loops. **D,** After neurolysis of the radial sensory nerve.

Table 46-1. Distance of Nerves to the Radius and Ulna in the Forearms of Cadavers

| | Distance (mm) | | | |
| | Radius | | Ulna | |
Nerve	Initial	Post-Osteotomy	Initial	Post-Osteotomy
Median				
At midforearm	10	10	>10	>10
At pronator quadratus	5	5	>10	>10
At wrist	3	< 2	>10	>10
Ulnar				
At midforearm	>10	10	10	10
At pronator quadratus	>10	5	5	5
At wrist	3	< 2	3	Tethered

From Vance RM, Gelberman R.H.[74] By permission of the journal.

radius was less than 2 mm. Such close approximation makes this nerve prone not only to compression and contusion by fracture fragments but also to transection or entrapment within the fracture site.

Median Neuropathy (Carpal Tunnel Syndrome).

Median neuropathy can occur immediately at the time of the fracture (Fig. 46-10, A), secondary to the fracture reduction technique, late associated with the position of fracture immobilization (cotton-loader position), or as a chronic complication related to malunion of the fracture and compromise of the carpal tunnel (Fig. 46-10, B).* Early in the presentation of a distal radius fracture, fracture fragments can impale the median nerve, producing partial or complete laceration or even occasionally entrapment of the nerve in an open fracture within the fracture site itself. Presentation several weeks after the injury usually relates to tightness or compartment compression syndromes from cast immobilization, the wrist flexion position, or hematoma formation.[28,53] Measurement of carpal tunnel pressures has been suggested in this subacute presentation. Electromyography is still the most valuable technique to determine the extent of nerve compression or injury. Patient complaints combined with increased carpal tunnel pressure measurements or conduction delays of the median nerve indicate the need for early surgical intervention.

Late presentation of carpal tunnel syndrome can occur months or years after the original fracture as a result of narrowing of the carpal tunnel or repetitive traction along the median nerve due to the excessive fracture callous or persistent palmar displacement of the fracture. Malunion of the distal radius and chronic

perilunate dislocation (Fig. 46-12), for example, have been associated with chronic median neuropathy and have required not only carpal tunnel release but also proximal row carpectomy or corrective osteotomy of the distal radius.[19,73,77]

Ulnar Neuropathy.

The ulnar nerve, which lies parallel to the median nerve, is also in close proximity to the distal end of the radius and ulna (Table 46-1).[42,74] In simulated fractures of the distal radius and ulna, the nerve has come to within 3 mm of the proximal fracture fragments. In the presence of dorsal displacement, the nerve can be tethered over the proximal fragment or entrapped at the fracture site. Despite these possibilities of ulnar nerve injury, it is quite uncommonly associated with injuries of the wrist because it is less tightly confined to a closed compartment.[64] In a series of 38 fracture dislocations of the wrist, there were 26 associated soft-tissue injuries. Of these, 10 involved the median nerve and 2 involved the ulnar nerve.[18] Compared with the carpal canal, Guyon's canal is shorter and more distal to the radiocarpal joint, allowing for greater excursion of the ulnar nerve. After fractures of carpal bones, in fact, the motor branch of the ulnar nerve is more susceptible to injury than sensory nerve components. Although most often occurring as isolated injuries, combined median and ulnar nerve injuries[42,60,66] can occur and are most often associated with fractures of both the radius and ulna.

Cutaneous Neuropathy.

The superficial branch of the radial nerve (RSN) and the intimately associated terminal branches of the lateral antebrachial cutaneous nerve can also be injured during bony trauma (Fig. 46-11).[44,51] The RSN assumes a subcutaneous position approximately 9 cm proximal to the radial styloid.[2] It

---

* References 1,8,14,15,50,54,59,60,76.

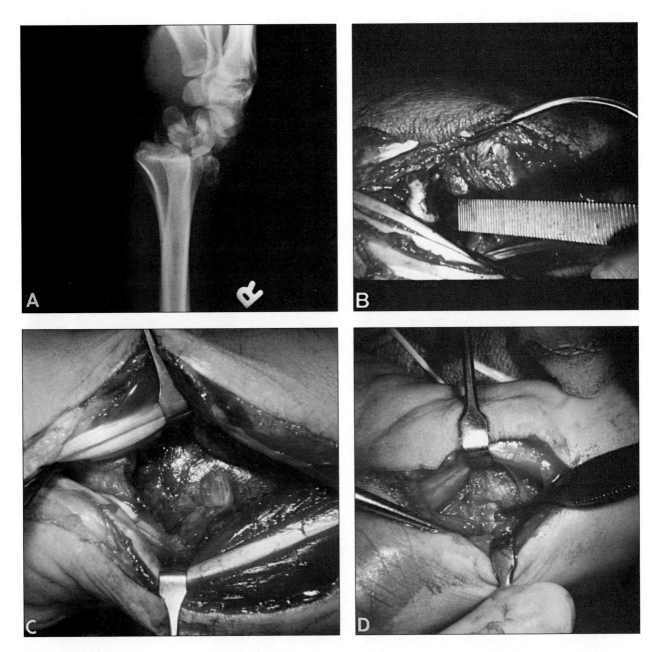

FIGURE 46-12

Perilunate dislocation of the wrist causes complications of the wrist. **A,** Dorsal dislocation of the wrist associated with compressive neuropathy of median and ulnar nerves requires open release (carpal tunnel and Guyon's canal release). **B,** Lunate dislocation into the carpal tunnel shown beneath the Carroll elevator. With release of the space of Poirier, the lunate is reduced back into alignment with the lunate fossa of the distal radius. **C,** Reduced perilunate dislocation shows the floor of the carpal tunnel and radial and central edge of the space of Poirier. Repair of the palmar carpal ligaments is recommended, closing the space of Poirier. **D,** Forceps point to the site of repair of the palmar carpal ligament. The median nerve is gently retracted radially.

divides into its respective branches approximately 5 cm proximal to the radial styloid and supplies the dorsum of the thumb, the first web space, and the index and middle fingers. The RSN in 75% of cases overlaps the terminal branches of the lateral antebrachial cutaneous nerve in the area of the thumb, the first web space, and the index and middle fingers.[51]

The RSN and the lateral antebrachial cutaneous nerves are subject to contusion during initial trauma or close manipulation or from a cast or splint applied to immobilize the bony injury.[53] These nerves, as well as the dorsal sensory branch of the ulnar nerve and the palmar cutaneous branches of both median and ulnar nerves,[13,21,23,36,72] are also prone to injury during surgical treatment. This includes injury from percutaneous Kirschner (K) wires as well as from larger-sized pins used to apply external fixation devices (Fig. 46-13).[31,33,61-63] Of more recent concern

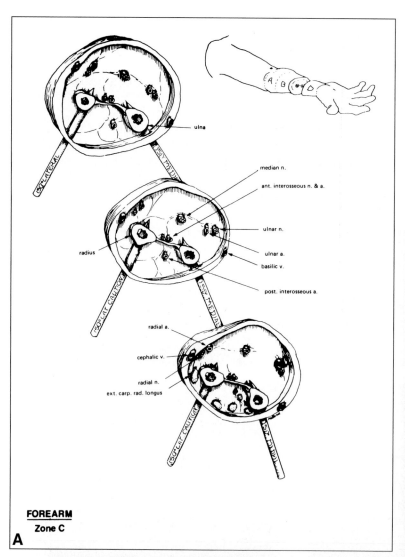

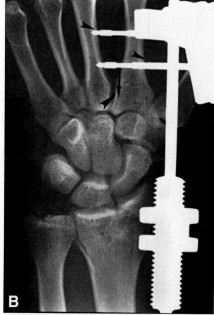

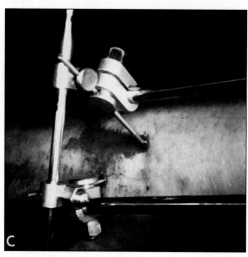

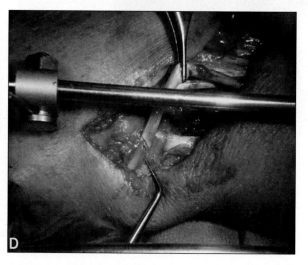

FIGURE 46-13

External fixation of the distal radius can be associated with complications related to pin placement. **A,** Preferred sites of placement of percutaneous (or preferably open) pins within the distal radius and ulna. *a.,* artery; *ant.,* anterior; *carp.,* carpi; *ext.,* extensor; *LAT,* lateral; *n.,* nerve; *post.,* posterior; *rad.,* radialis; *v.,* vein. *(From Green SA: Complications of external skeletal fixation: causes, prevention, and treatment, Springfield, Illinois, 1981, Charles C Thomas. By permission of the author.)* **B,** External fixation of a distal radius fracture with interrupted threaded pins placed through the base of the index metacarpal. Pins are placed to far distal and extend through the cortices *(arrowheads)*; a more proximal placement *(arrow)* is recommended along with continuously threaded pins. Pin loosening resulted. **C,** Percutaneous nonthreaded pins placed dorsally into the distal radius with Roger Anderson frame. Injury to the extensor tendons of the fingers and thumb can result from this method of pin placement. Open placement of pins from a lateral (radial) direction into the distal radius is preferred, with care taken to identify and protect the radial sensory nerve. **D,** Partial laceration of the extensor pollicis longus (at the end of the dental probe) associated with percutaneous placement of transfixation pins into the distal radius.

is the possible injury to cutaneous nerves from arthroscopic portals used during wrist arthroscopy to evaluate chronic ligamentous injuries of the wrist, fracture reduction of the distal radius, and associated injuries to the triangular fibrocartilage complex.

In the diagnosis of nerve injuries associated with wrist trauma, careful history and physical examination are fundamental to the evaluation. Motor and sensory function are evaluated for each nerve distribution, particularly in the patient who is unable to respond. Two-point discrimination is a critical part of the sensory examination and should be performed without exception. Although difficult to perform in an emergency room, Gelberman and associates[28] have shown that von Frey and vibratory testing may be more accurate than two-point discrimination in identifying early changes in nerve function. Radiographs reveal the degree of fracture displacement and angulation that can result in stretching and tethering of the surrounding neurovascular structures (Figs. 46-10, B and C). Radiographs also reveal the presence of a palmarly displaced fracture component or carpal bone, which may produce direct compression to a nerve and contribute to increased pressures within the carpal tunnel or Guyon's canal (Fig. 46-12, B). After either closed or open manipulation of the fracture, a repeat physical examination is of fundamental importance.

It is not unusual for patients with fractures of the distal radius to report paresthesias in the median nerve distribution. In most cases, if two-point discrimination is normal, further treatment is not required.[9,27] In the event of abnormal results of a neurologic examination, which have remained unchanged from premanipulation or have deteriorated after treatment of the fracture, additional evaluation is mandatory. Carpal tunnel and forearm compartment pressure measurements may be warranted. The utility of measuring carpal tunnel pressure may be of special benefit in evaluating the comatose patient who has suffered significant trauma to the wrist area. Evaluation of late neurologic changes and deficits can be facilitated with electrodiagnostic studies, including nerve conduction velocity and electromyography, as mentioned earlier.

Treatment. Specific treatment of nerve injuries, as previously noted, depends on the history of the injury and changes brought on by treatment. Cutaneous nerves, which are injured secondary to contusion either from the initial trauma or therapy, are treated nonsurgically by observation and desensitization with modalities such as transcutaneous electrical nerve stimulation (TENS), ice massage, desensitization fabrics, and massage. If symptoms are nonresponsive and become chronic, exploration and neurolysis or neurectomy may be necessary. If the injury is the result of excessive pressure from an overlying cast or splint, early recognition is essential and reapplication of a better-fitting splint or

cast is recommended. Protective padding (such as silicone or elastomer padding) and relief of pressure from a splint (remolded splint) may be needed. Direct penetrating injuries resulting from the initial trauma or from an iatrogenic injury such as a surgical incision, percutaneous K-wire insertion, or application of an external fixator pin should be treated with wire and pin removal and observation. Primary nerve exploration and nerve resection and repair may occasionally be required. If such an injury is recognized later after primary repair is no longer feasible, depending on the location of injury and symptoms, treatment may involve therapy consisting of a trial of desensitization (TENS), local nerve blocks, and protective splinting. If symptoms remain unresolved, surgical exploration with excision of neuromata and nerve grafting may be required.

Treatment of injuries to the median or the ulnar nerve is determined by the presence and progression of findings such as loss of sensory or motor function after reduction. Decisions on treatment are based in large part on clinical judgment (Fig. 46-14). Although many patients complain of symptoms consistent with paresthesias in the median or ulnar nerve distributions (or both), most report improvement on observation after reduction. Exploration and decompression of the median or ulnar nerve should be considered for patients who have objective neurologic abnormalities, such as increased two-point discrimination, loss of sweating, and loss of motor function, both prereduction and postreduction.

Treatment of compressive neuropathies and other traumatic conditions resistant to conservative treatment generally requires operative intervention.[9,16,36,41,54] For the median nerve compression at the wrist, release of the carpal tunnel (transverse carpal ligament) along with division of the fascia of the distal third of the forearm is recommended (see Chapter 51). For malunited distal radius fractures, a corrective osteotomy alone or combined with carpal tunnel release should be considered (see Chapter 16). Prevention of compressive neuropathy can be achieved by minimizing the need for repeated closed reduction of fractures, avoiding excessive palmar flexion in immobilization of the distal radius fracture, and carefully avoiding any form of constricting cast or dressings.

With other wrist injuries such as fracture dislocations of the wrist,[18] either contusion or stretch injury of the median nerve may have occurred. For severe carpal dislocations or fracture dislocations, a palmar approach to repair the ligaments is usually indicated. Open release and inspection of the median nerve can be performed as part of this procedure (Fig. 46-12) (see Chapters 26 and 27). Careful retraction of the median nerve is necessary to avoid added injury to the likely contused median nerve.

For the remaining potential nerve complications that can complicate wrist injuries, treatment is generally conservative. Most of the lesions are stretch injuries that improve with time, but the crush or contusions can produce long-lasting distress and permanent neuroma that are particularly difficult to treat.

Iatrogenic causes of peripheral neuropathy need to be prevented. A cast or braces must avoid producing pressure on the bony prominence about the wrist. With the insertion of pins or a K wire in the treatment of distal radius fractures or carpal injuries, open insertion should be considered when the path of the pin or wire is potentially in the anatomic area of the cutaneous nerve, particularly if a threaded pin or K wire is used. Patient complaints of nerve dysesthetic pain should be attended to promptly by removal of the offending cast or dressing or the removal of the pin (or both).

For persistent cases of peripheral neuritis after wrist injuries, physical therapy for desensitization about the cutaneous nerve combined with TENS and peripheral nerve blocks can be helpful. We have had success with both continuous and repetitive blocks of the radial, ulnar, and median nerves as well as dorsal and palmar cutaneous nerves in providing lasting pain relief. Blocks are performed by either repeated injections over 2- to 3-day intervals or by placing a plastic angiocatheter subcutaneously adjacent to the involved nerve and injecting bupivacaine (0.5%) every 4 to 6 hours.

The patient can be involved in the treatment program by self-administration of bupivacaine (0.5 to 1 mL) every 4 to 6 hours through the angiocatheter attached to a heparin lock. As a last resort, surgical treatment by neurolysis, placement of silicone sheeting between the nerve and scar tissue, or proximal transection of the nerve may be necessary. We do not believe that it is necessary to bury the nerve in bone or muscle. Resecting the involved nerve proximal enough so that there is sufficient soft tissue around the nerve to provide protection is sufficient. A new neuroma will always form, and hopefully it will not be painful.

In summary, neurologic lesions commonly accompany injuries about the wrist. Patients who have an abnormal neurologic examination prereduction and postreduction require no further initial treatment other than prudent observation. On the other hand, if results of the physical examination are abnormal after reduction of fractures or dislocations, one should look for palmar displaced fracture fragments or carpal bones, immobilization positions of excessive wrist flexion, or a constrictive splint or cast as the underlying cause. If a fracture reduction cannot be maintained without placing the wrist in an extreme position of flexion, then alternative means of maintaining reduction by external fixation or open reduction and

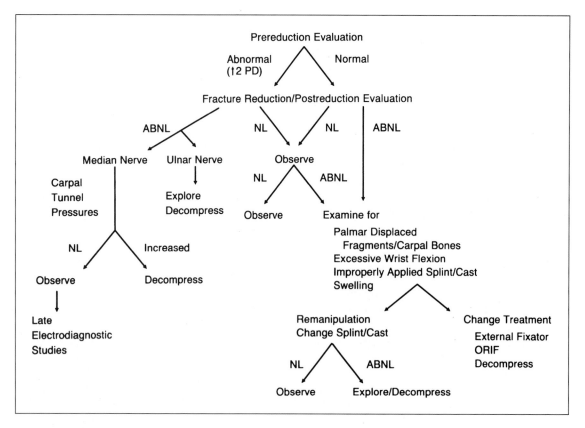

FIGURE 46-14

Treatment plan for median- and ulnar-nerve related compression neuropathy. *ABNL*, abnormal; *NL*, normal; *ORIF*, open reduction and internal fixation; *PD*, two-point discrimination.

internal fixation (or both) need to be considered. In the presence of a persistent, palmarly displaced bone spike or carpal bone, surgical intervention is indicated to decompress the involved area (see Chapter 51).

Late neurologic compromise is defined as conditions that persist following primary healing of the bony or ligamentous injury. If neurologic symptoms are secondary to a correctable bony lesion such as a malunited fracture, decompression and correction of bony alignment are recommended. If no offending bony lesion can be identified, these symptoms can be approached like any primary compressive neuropathy at the wrist. In the evaluation of nerve complications about the wrist, prevention of nerve injury by awareness of anatomy during pin placement and surgical intervention by prompt treatment of compressive or direct trauma to the nerve should help to decrease the incidence of this complication.

BONE AND JOINT

FRACTURE REDUCTIONS

Loss of reduction after closed treatment of distal radius fractures and recurrence of instability after conservative (nonoperative) treatment of carpal dislocations are among the most frequent complications after injury of the wrist (Fig. 46-15).[16,18,22,26,41] In previous series[8,19] evaluating complications of distal radius fractures, loss of reduction was the most common complication after peripheral (median) neuropathy (Fig. 46-16). With efforts at repeat reduction of distal radius fractures, the incidence of other complications such as

pain dystrophy, median neuropathy, and instability of the distal radioulnar joint was noted.[63] The application of longitudinal traction for the reduction combined with sufficient peripheral nerve block (axillary block or Bier block) has helped avoid this problem. When it is time for cast reapplication, the extremity is again placed in traction with finger traps and countertraction across the arm (elbow at 90°) so that distraction (ligamentataxis) is again beneficial. Use of external fixation, which provides continued ligamentataxis, has provided an excellent method of avoiding loss of reduction, although some reports[61,62] demonstrate mild-moderate loss of reduction despite external fixation. When comminution is extensive, open reduction, bone graft, and fracture stabilization with external or internal fixation should be considered (Fig. 46-17).

Every effort should be made in the treatment of fractures of the distal radius to first obtain and then maintain anatomic reduction of the fracture. It is always preferable to avoid repetitive reductions. Care must be taken to avoid cast, splints, or percutaneous pins if they will not be sufficient to hold and maintain fracture alignment. Failure to follow these principles can have significant effects on the final result when the loss of reduction becomes permanent (Fig. 46-18).

In many patients with Colles' fractures, painful motions and "stiffness" may abate or simply become more tolerable to the patient. We recommend waiting a minimum of 6 months and usually 1 year once union is present before determining the need for any remedial or reconstructive surgical intervention. After a period of "conservative" treatment has passed, options for surgical intervention can then be better discussed and assessed.[55] In Chapters 15 and 16, the specific procedures for

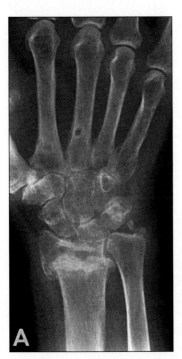

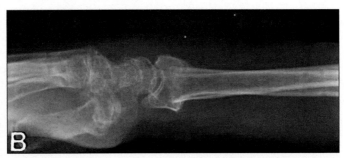

FIGURE 46-15

A and **B**, Loss of reduction of fractures of the distal radius has consequences demonstrated in these posteroanterior and lateral radiographs of radial shortening, loss of radial tilt, radioulnar displacement, and dorsal angulation of the distal radius, producing consequences of ulnar carpal abutment, incongruity of the distal radioulnar joint, and radiocarpal instability.

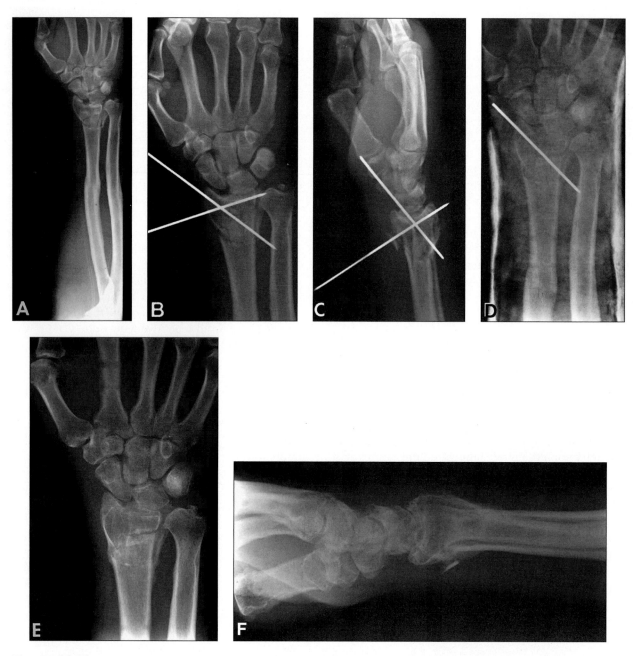

FIGURE 46-16

Incomplete reduction and improper immobilization of a comminuted fracture of the distal radius. **A,** Comminuted fracture of the distal radius involving radioscaphoid and radiolunate joints; prominent distal ulna. **B** and **C,** Posteroanterior and lateral radiographs of a closed reduction and percutaneous pin fixation with 0.045-in. Kirschner wires. **D,** Cast immobilization with one remaining percutaneous pin. (Second pin removed as result of loosening.) **E** and **F,** Posteroanterior and lateral radiographs of the final result show malunion of the intra-articular component of the fracture along with loss of radial length. Post-traumatic arthritis.

treatment of Colles' fracture malunion are presented. In the majority of cases, we recommend open corrective osteotomy for patients who live an active life and want full restoration (as possible) of motion and strength to their wrist. As a result of corrective osteotomy, not only do radiocarpal and midcarpal joint motion (kinematics) change and improve but the distal radioulnar joint alignment is restored. Forearm pronation and supination dramatically improve after this procedure.

Darrach resections and other forms of distal ulna resection with or without soft-tissue interposition are suggested in elderly patients who would be expected to put fewer functional demands on their wrists (see Chapter 34). The type of procedure is adjusted to patient needs and expectations. Ulna resection rather than radius lengthening may also be considered if ulnocarpal abutment is the major concern. In patients younger than age 60 years with active lives, ulna

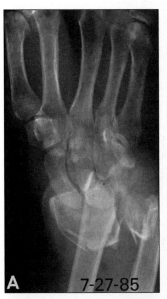

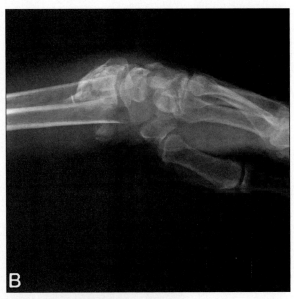

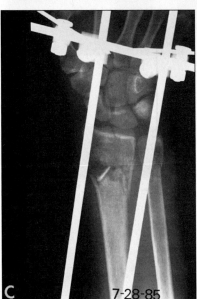

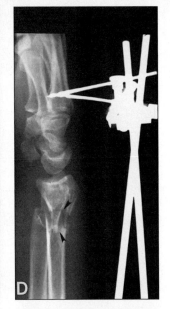

FIGURE 46–17

Delayed fracture union. Displaced comminuted fracture of the distal radius in an elderly woman. **A** and **B,** Postero-anterior and lateral radiographs demonstrate significant dorsal and proximal displacement of both the radial and ulnar fracture components. **C** and **D,** Treatment with distraction reduction and external fixation. Note the bone deficit on both the posteroanterior and lateral (*arrowheads*) radiographs of the distal radius. **E,** Bone graft from the iliac crest was inserted through a limited dorsal incision. The graft was tightly packed into the deficit created by the distal radius fracture. **F,** Early union of the fracture 3 months later with further consolidation expected. Full maintenance of radial and ulnar length.

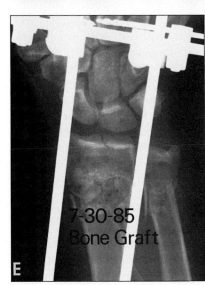

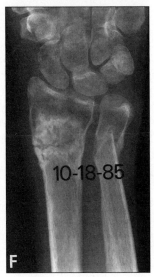

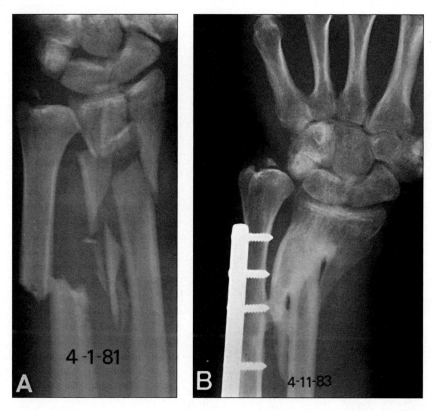

FIGURE 46-18

Comminuted fracture of the distal radius metaphysis and diaphysis with a midshaft fracture of the ulna. **A,** Posteroanterior radiograph shows the fracture extension into the radiocarpal joint along with both spiral butterfly fragments and proximal displacement of the radius. Medial offset fracture of the ulna. **B,** Plate fixation of the ulna was performed combined with external fixation of the distal radius. Open reduction and internal fixation with bone graft was not considered for the radius because the fracture was open (inside out). Unfortunate late result of a healed but badly shortened distal radius. Salvage by excision of distal ulna. Delayed bone grafting and internal fixation of the radius may have been preferred.

shortening is preferred to ulna resection, assuming that other forms of carpal malalignment are not a serious component of the malunion when corrective osteotomy of the radius would be preferred.

NONUNION

Nonunion is rare after fractures of the distal radius.[19] There are few reports in the literature describing this complication. Harper and Jones[35] described two cases in which nonunion occurred after closed reduction and plaster cast immobilization. Nonunion has also followed incomplete fracture reduction (Figs. 46-19, *A* through *D*). Others[69,77] reported nonunion in cases of severe high-energy trauma (Fig. 46-20). Our own experience involves cases in which adequate length of immobilization was not used (less than 6 weeks) and cases with external fixation in which distraction was excessive. We have not observed nonunion when appropriate open reduction, bone grafting, and internal fracture fixation were elected.

Treatment of nonunion almost always requires open reduction and internal fixation with distal radius plates and screws, bone grafting, and appropriate cast support. External fixation may be needed to supplement the internal fixation, and bone graft with supplemental internal fixation (K wires) is needed in the very unstable nonunions. Nonunion should be preventable, but patients with bone loss from the original trauma or from osteoporosis may simply not have adequate bone stock to provide the foundation for fracture healing (Fig. 46-20). Today, such circumstances are recognized more frequently, and bone grafting of distal radius fractures is not infrequently reported as a usual or even customary treatment modality.

MALUNION

With failure to either obtain or maintain fracture alignment, loss of reduction can lead to malunion (Fig. 46-21) (see Chapter 16). The malunion is a significant complication when the extent of dorsal angulation

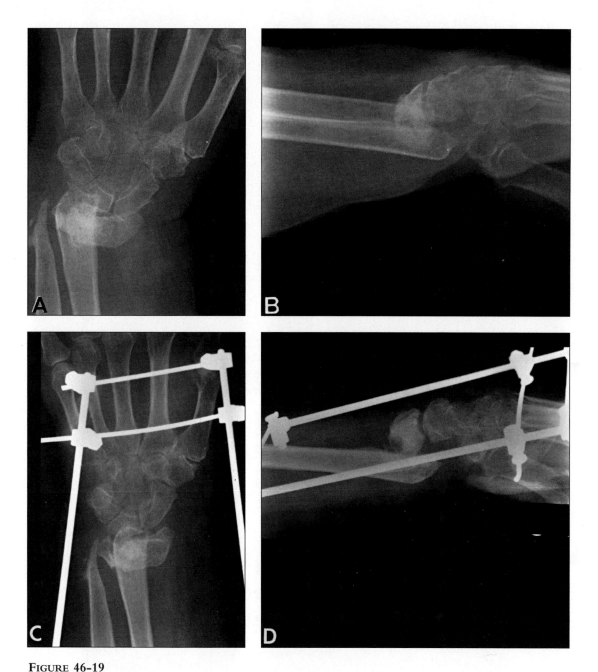

FIGURE 46-19

Nonunion of the distal radius. **A** and **B**, Posteroanterior and lateral views of a severely displaced fracture of the distal radius. **C** and **D**, Immobilization with external fixation, yet failure to reduce the fracture. Nonunion resulted.

exceeds 20° (total of 30° from the normal palmar tilt of the distal radius), loss of radial length exceeds 5 mm, or radial angulation is 10° or less, which represents a loss of 10° to 15° from normal 22° of radial angulation.[5,19,55] These factors of malunion have primary consequences of ulnar carpal abutment, incongruity, or distal radioulnar joint and radiocarpal joint instability (Fig. 46-15).[17,22] Secondarily, carpal malalignment occurs at the midcarpal joint.[10,21] The result of malunion thereby affects not just the radiocarpal joint but the wrist midcarpal joint. These factors can lead to painful or reduced motion (flexion-extension as well as

pronation and supination), carpal instability, and reduced or fatigued strength.[8,19,21]

Treatment of malunion (Fig. 46-22) is determined by many factors, not the least of which are patient age, level of activity, and work or home activity demands.

CARPAL INSTABILITY

Carpal instability associated with fractures of the distal radius can be primary as a result of the original injury as well as secondary, as noted above with fracture malunion. We more commonly recognize carpal

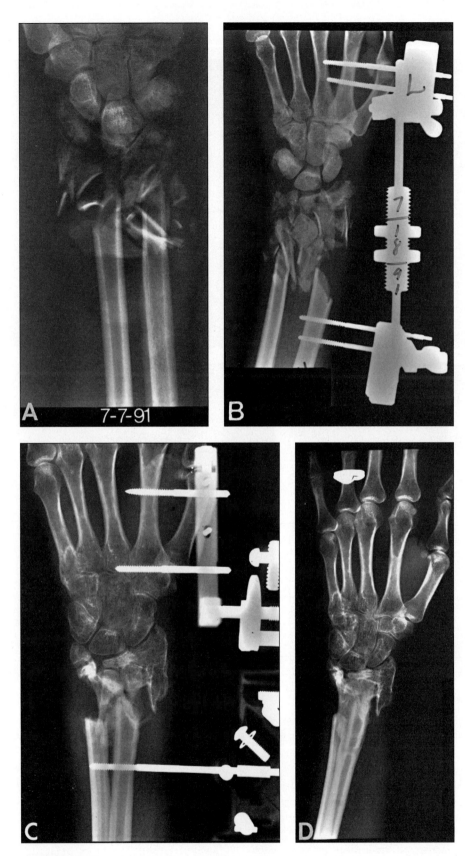

FIGURE 46–20

A, Explosive comminuted fracture of the distal radius. **B,** Stabilization with a C-series Hoffmann external fixator to maintain length. **C,** Agee-WristJack *(Hand Biomechanics Lab, Inc., Sacramento, California)* applied to allow for fracture reduction combined with bone grafting from the iliac crest. Excision of the distal ulna. **D,** Union of the distal radius but with a cross union to the ulna, resulting in loss of forearm rotation.

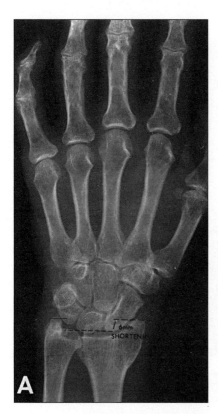

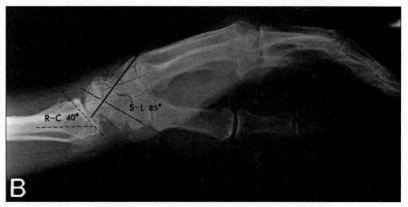

Figure 46-21

Malunion of the distal radius. **A** and **B,** Radial shortening of 6 mm noted on the posteroanterior film along with 40° of dorsal radiocarpal (*R-C*) angulation and 85° of secondary scapholunate (*S-L*) carpal instability.

instability today than we did in the past, but it is still not uncommon to not recognize the combination of fracture and intracarpal ligament injury.

One should be alerted to the potential for ligament injuries within the wrist when there are fractures of the radial styloid and scaphoid fossa of the distal radius. These fractures can have an extension through the scapholunate interval leading to scapholunate dissociation. With fractures extending into the distal radioulnar joint, tears of the triangular fibrocartilage and instability (subluxation or dislocation) of the distal radioulnar joint may be present. For both conditions, it is important to test stability of the distal radioulnar joint after reduction and fixation of the distal radius fracture.

Combined carpal instability may occur in which the carpal instability is the result of both malunion of the distal radius and an intracarpal ligament injury. Some of the carpal instabilities (Fig. 46-23) can be quite subtle and only recognized on careful clinical examination combined with wrist arthrography or arthroscopy. In general, adequate treatment of the distal radius fracture also provides the proper support for ligament healing. However, inadequate reduction of the fracture combined with inappropriate cast support or the application of external fixation systems may lead to secondary displacement and carpal instability. One should be alert for abnormal patterns of carpal instability on routine posteroanterior and lateral radiographs when treating fractures of the distal radius or other injuries of the wrist.

PAIN SYNDROMES

Chronic persistent peripheral nerve pain is one of the most difficult ailments and often the most difficult complaint that an individual has to endure after an injury or complication from surgical treatment of the wrist. We have observed patients completely disabled from peripheral nerve pain after minor injuries or "simple" surgical procedures on the wrist. Pain not only makes work impossible but often disturbs even light daily tasks and makes sleep difficult or impossible, culminating in increasing psychologic stress.[3] These conditions have many names. Based on recent studies, they are now generically referred to as "complex regional pain syndromes (CRPS)," the term we prefer[57] and will use in this section (Table 46-2).

Before determining how to best treat the patient with peripheral nerve pain, we have found that the physician and surgeon need to first distinguish sympathetic-related peripheral nerve pain from somatic-related peripheral nerve pain because the conditions are quite different.

Sympathetic Dystrophy

Sympathetic dystrophy and sympathetic-mediated pain dysfunction are the most serious of the complications that can occur after injuries about the wrist.*

---

* References 4,7,29,32,38,41,43,75.

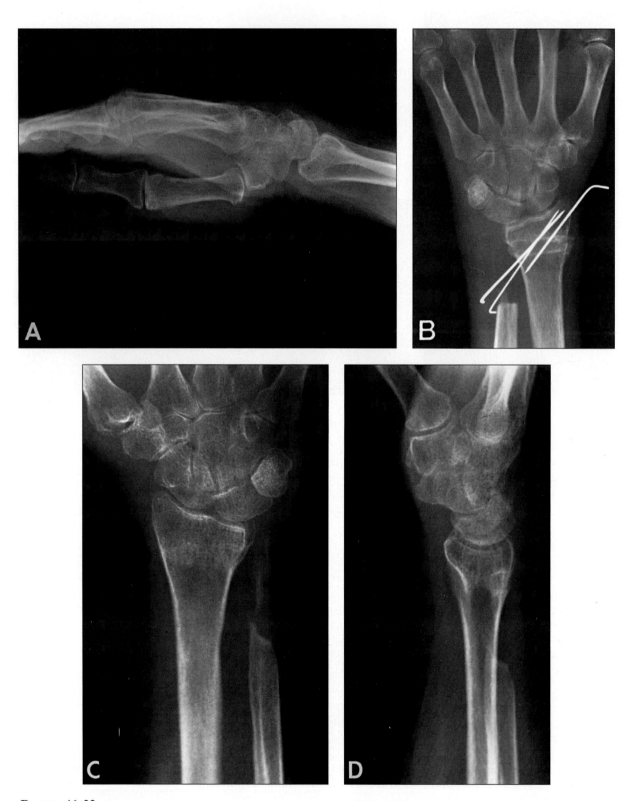

FIGURE 46-22

Malunion of the distal radius and adaptive carpal instability treated by corrective osteotomy. **A,** Lateral view of the wrist shows dorsal angulation of the distal radius of 25° combined with secondary carpal instability. Note palmar tilt of the lunate and dorsal shift of the capitate with increased scapholunate angle. **B,** Corrective osteotomy was performed combined with excision of the distal ulna. An iliac crest graft was used to regain radial length and restore lost dorsal-palmar angulation. Internal fixation with three Kirschner wires. Note mild scapholunate gap. Dorsal plate fixation might have been used today. **C** and **D,** Excellent result with full healing of the distal radius; a stable distal ulna after excision; only mild carpal instability with palmar tilt of the lunate.

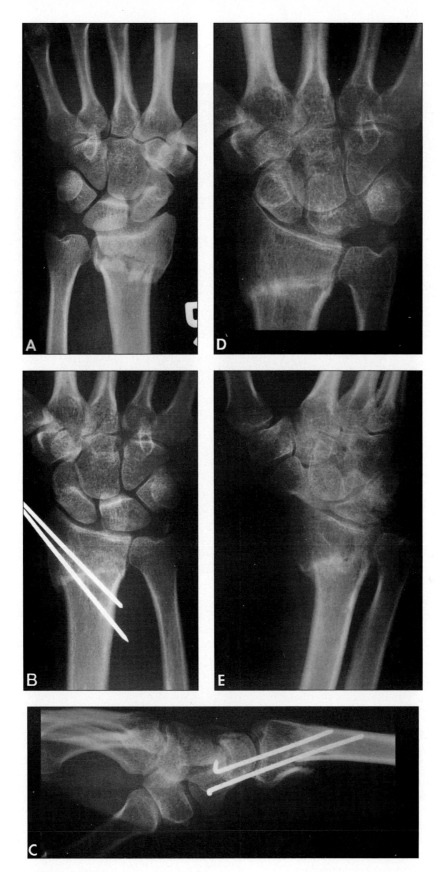

FIGURE 46-23

Secondary carpal instability associated with a distal radius fracture. **A,** Anteroposterior radiograph of the distal radius shows a mildly displaced extra-articular fracture with displaced ulnar styloid. **B** and **C,** Posteroanterior and lateral radiographs of the wrist. Treatment by closed reduction and percutaneous pin (Kirschner wire) fixation. **D** and **E,** Posteroanterior and oblique radiographs. Late result demonstrates a healed fracture of the radius but associated with carpal instability. Palmar flexion of both the scaphoid and lunate.   *Continued.*

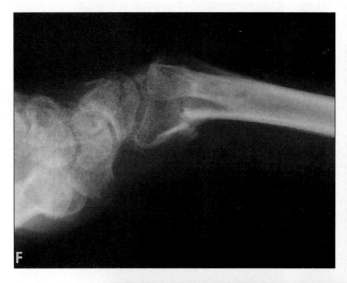
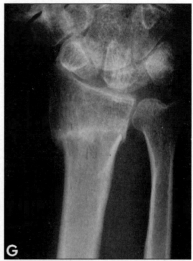
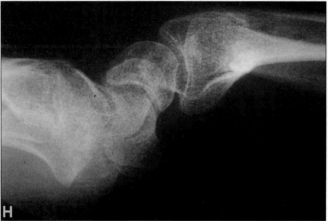

FIGURE 46-23, CONT'D.

F, Lateral view of the wrist confirms palmar flexion of the lunate and scaphoid despite relatively normal appearance of the distal radius angulation. **G** and **H,** Final appearance demonstrates further progression of primary carpal instability associated with this seemingly benign extra-articular fracture of the distal radius. Note severe palmar angulation (tilt) of the proximal carpal row.

Table 46-2. Classification of Pain Dysfunction

Complex Regional Pain: Type I

Reflex sympathetic dystrophy: A syndrome that develops after an initiating noxious event, not limited to the distribution of a single nerve, and pain not proportional to the initiating event; it is characterized by abnormal sudomotor activity, allodynia, and hyperalgesia

Complex Regional Pain: Type II

Causalgia: A syndrome that develops after acute trauma to a peripheral nerve; it is characterized by burning pain and hyperpathia usually isolated to one major nerve or its branches; partial nerve injury is a common initiating event

Sympathetic pain is a diffuse, disabling hypersensitivity in one or more peripheral nerve autonomous zones that starts with burning pain, cold sensitivity, hyperhidrosis, and often painful motion.[57] It presents an exaggerated response of the extremity to injury, producing intense and prolonged pain, vasomotor disturbance, and associated trophic changes. It crosses several dermatome distributions. Protection and guarding of the extremity by the patient, often holding or carrying the hand and wrist, or limiting use of the limb in pinch, grasp, and daily activities are characteristic. The patient will protect the limb from physician or therapist, not allowing palpation or percussion or even light touch around the affected nerve(s) (stage I) (Table 46-3).[40] If the condition is not recognized and treated early, the limb suffers further with loss of use (Fig. 46-24). Stiffness of soft tissues, loss of joint motion, and contracture develop. The skin atrophies, the previous

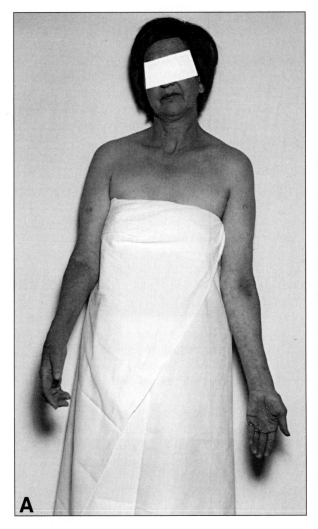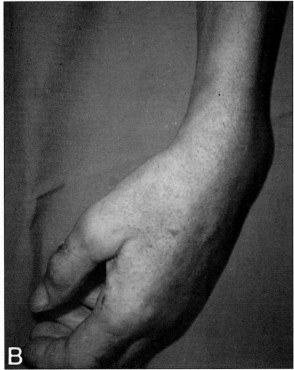

FIGURE 46-24

Sympathetic dysfunction, typically with limb disuse, can be observed on inspection of the patient as a whole or the hand and wrist in particular. **A,** Sympathetic dysfunction of the left upper extremity. Patient presents with shoulder stiffness, forearm and hand muscle atrophy, pain, weakness, and joint stiffness of the fingers and thumb. **B,** Dysfunction of the hand and wrist with swelling, palmar erythema, joint stiffness, and contracture ("wounded paw" appearance). Trophic changes with vasomotor disturbance are noted.

Table 46-3. Clinical Stages of Reflex Sympathetic Dystrophy

Factor	Stage I	Stage II	Stage III
Time since onset	Early	3 months	6 to 9 months
Appearance	Erythema	Cyanotic	Pale, cool
	Heat	Loss of creases	Glossy, tight skin
		Tight, shiny skin	
		Palmar nodules	
		Finger tapering	
Swelling	Soft, puffy	Brawny fusiform	Minimal
Sensation	Hyperesthesia	Hyperesthesia	Increase or decrease
Hidrosis	Increased	Increased or neutral	Dry
Osteoporosis	Spotty or polar	More diffuse	Homogeneous
			Thinned cortices
Contractures	No	Variable	Yes

From Inhofe PD, Garcia-Moral CA.[38] By permission of Excerpta Medica.

warmth of hypervascularity turns to coldness, and strength and function diminish further (stage II). The late stage of sympathetic dystrophy sets in with shiny, dry skin, degeneration of muscle tone, further joint stiffness, and both joint and muscle contracture (stage III).

Diagnosis initially is by clinical symptoms and signs of painful disuse of the hand and wrist, a high degree of awareness, and supportive laboratory testing.[43] Positive bone scans (Fig. 46-25), hypervascularity (thermography), positive sweat test with autonomic dysfunction (quantitative sudomotor axon reflex test [QSART]), and later osteoporosis can help confirm the diagnosis.* Sympathetic nerve blocks, which can be effective in treating this condition, can help confirm the diagnosis.[4,12,32,45] The sympathetic dystrophy scale (Wilson)[75] has recently been effective in confirming and rating the severity of this sympathetic-mediated CRPS (Table 46-4).

Treatment of sympathetic-mediated dystrophy can be difficult and prolonged. The most important principle is that control of pain is essential before initiating any form of muscle, joint, or nerve-related physical therapy. Local nerve blocks may help, but more commonly sympathetic nerve blocks are performed on several consecutive days with physical therapy after each of the blocks. For more difficult cases, a continuous sympathetic nerve block with a catheter in the supraclavicular area and performed by an anesthesiologist is recommended.[3,30,45] With pain under control, the physical therapist can then work toward improvement in motion and gradual active use of the extremity. Splints may be needed to provide assisted correction of deformity or to hold resting functional positions. The splints or passive motion provided by splints, however, must not be painful.

Surgical treatment is to be avoided in cases of sympathetic dystrophy, unless a specific compressive neuropathy such as median neuropathy in the carpal tunnel can be identified. If a series of sympathetic blocks is helpful, then sympathectomy may be considered in the recalcitrant, long-standing cases. The treatment program can often be extended over many months. It requires significant physician-patient interaction, in particular, patient encouragement and reinforcement that pain control (by sympathetic, axillary, or local nerve blocks) and physical therapy will be successful. The patient must play an active role in the program. Once pain is under control, active motion of the affected extremity by the

---

Table 46-4. Putative Diagnostic Criteria for Reflex Sympathetic Dystrophy

Clinical Symptoms and Signs
1. Burning pain
2. Hyperpathia or allodynia
3. Temperature or color changes
4. Edema
5. Hair or nail growth changes

Laboratory Results
6. Thermometry or thermography
7. Bone radiograph
8. 3-Phase bone scan
9. Quantitative sweat test
10. Response to sympathetic block

Interpretation: If Total of Positive Findings Is
> 6	Probable RSD
3-5	Possible RSD
< 3	Unlikely RSD

RSD, reflex sympathetic dystrophy.

---

* References 4,12,32,38,48,49,65.

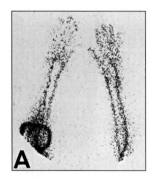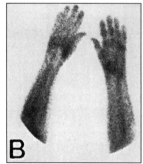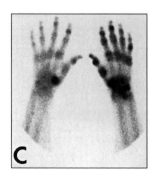

FIGURE 46-25

Triphasic bone scan in sympathetic dystrophy. **A,** Injection phase outlines the vascular pattern of the forearm, wrist, and hand. **B,** Early phase demonstrates relative symmetry between the two extremities. **C,** Late phase suggests a degenerative process of the left thumb carpometacarpal joint and diffuse uptake on the right compatible with a clinical diagnosis of sympathetic dystrophy involving the wrist and all of the finger joints.

patient is essential. If the condition presents late, fixed contracture may have developed. Release of joints and pinning in a better position for function, followed by active motion, may be required.

SOMATIC NERVE PAIN

Somatic peripheral nerve pain is different from sympathetic pain, although they may occasionally coexist in the same injured extremity (Table 46-5).[12,57,70] It involves characteristically only *one* peripheral nerve in the area of pain distribution. The pain is sharp, lancinating along a single cutaneous or deep peripheral nerve. Nerve response tests such as Tinel's sign or passive nerve stretch signs provoke the patient's complaints. Direct compression or contusion to a peripheral nerve results in a nerve injury that often produces sensory loss but without a significant sympathetic or motor component. The median nerve, for example, may present the picture of an acute injury after dislocations of the wrist or with a severely displaced distal radius fracture. The dorsal and palmar cutaneous nerves can be injured during surgical approaches to the wrist.

The radial nerve, which is quite superficial over the distal forearm, may sustain a direct blow or other injury. These direct nerve injuries produce a clinical picture different from that of sympathetic dystrophy. They are *somatic-mediated* with pain and weakness and do not have overt sympathetic-related findings. There is pain, but it is once again localized to a single autonomous zone. The pain is shooting or lancinating, producing paresthesia in the affected peripheral nerve distribution. Once again, sensory nerve loss may be present but not severe, and motor involvement is rare. Sympathetic components of pain, if they are present, are minor and localized to a single nerve rather than general distribution. QSART, bone scan, and other tests of sympathetic dysfunction usually have normal results. Sympathetic nerve blocks are not helpful. Rather, the first approach is a specific isolated block of the affected nerve that usually confirms the diagnosis and repeated, isolated nerve blocks often benefit the patient greatly.

A second approach is surgical neurolysis combined with soft-tissue coverage. For the median nerve within the carpal tunnel, vascular hypothenar muscle or fascia flaps can be effective, but improvement can be difficult to predict. Other options include a vascular omental or radial forearm flap, wrapping the affected nerve with vein graft, or using direct nerve stimulation proximal to the level of nerve injury. We have experienced success with several of these treatment modalities in properly selected patients. They are generally considered when the more conservative methods of nerve blocks and therapy have failed or when the patient presents late with established pain patterns or fibrosis and scarring about the injured peripheral nerve. Our experience suggests that vascular soft-tissue flaps in particular can

increase nerve gliding and decrease pain provided the primary problem is fibrosis external to the involved nerve. When internal fibrosis is present, there may be no successful form of treatment other than nerve ablation.

Our last resort as a treatment alternative for failed conservative treatment has been direct peripheral nerve stimulation.[58,70] We have had reasonable success (about 75% improvement in pain) in selected patients with such a program. When we can demonstrate that nerve pain is relieved by two or more consecutive nerve blocks of a single peripheral nerve and that the pain is in one specific dermatome distribution only (Fig. 46-26), we proceed with implantation of a direct electrical nerve stimulation system. The purpose of direct electrical nerve stimulation is to control somatic nerve pain by the alternating low-intensity pulses of electrical stimulation. These patients often have pain for many months or even years.[58,70] We strongly recommend and use psychologic testing on all of these patients. In our experience, pain is often relieved (70% to 80%) but not eliminated. Sleep improves and the need for narcotic pain medication is decreased or eliminated. Such

---

Table 46-5. Differential Diagnosis and Treatment of Somatic and Sympathetic Pain

Somatic	Sympathetic
Diagnosis	
Isolated nerve	Diffuse nerve
Dermatomal distribution	General distribution
Dysesthesias + paresthesias	Dystrophic changes (↑ color, sweat, cold response)
Shooting, lancinating pain	Burning, dystrophic pain
	Thermography +
Sweat test −	Sweat test +
Bone scan − (unless a fracture)	Bone scan −
Treatment	
1. Nerve block (isolated)	1. Warmth
2. TENS	2. Glove or garment
3. Continuous catheter	3. Sympathetic blocks
4. Nerve ablation	4. Sympathectomy
5. Protection (splint or padding)	5. Physical therapy— active use of extremity
6. Physical therapy— active use	6. Psychologic support
7. Psychologic support	

TENS, transcutaneous electrical nerve stimulation.

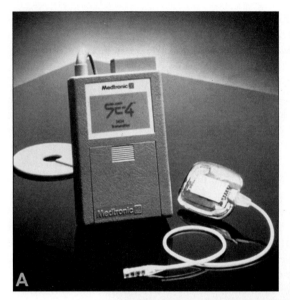
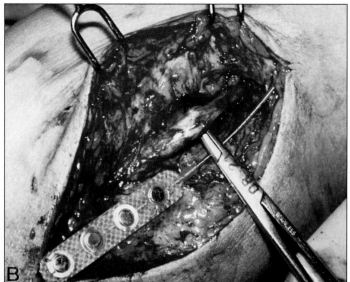
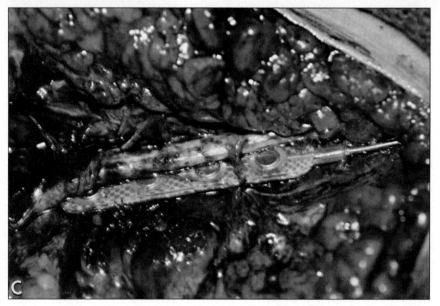

FIGURE 46-26

Direct electrical stimulation of painful peripheral nerves. **A,** The components of the system include a nerve electrode pad, a connecting lead, and a pulse generator similar to a pacemaker. **B** and **C,** The electrode is placed directly adjacent to the involved peripheral nerve.

treatment is again beneficial primarily for somatic nerve pain. Psychologic support is also required during this time because patients are typically depressed and fatigued as a consequence of the chronic pain, lack of sleep, low self-esteem, and anxiety over failure to get well. These programs, as one might expect, will not be successful in patients with secondary gain, hostility, or extended work compensation claims.

By way of definition, we prefer not to use the terminology of reflex sympathetic dystrophy unless the criteria for this diagnosis are clearly met.[3,29,57,75] A reflex sympathetic dystrophy score, as mentioned earlier, is quite helpful in this regard (Table 46-4).[75]

Chronic upper limb pain should be distinguished as either causalgia (somatic or isolated peripheral nerve pain) or as sympathetic pain (that associated with increased sympathetic-mediated pain response). In the classification of chronic pain syndromes, the taxonomy prepared by Mersky and Bogduk[57] is again helpful in distinguishing CRPS. These authors stressed this association of sympathetically maintained pain with reflex sympathetic dystrophy but note that it may not necessarily always be predominant. In contrast, causalgia (somatic) pain has a direct nerve injury component whereas the sympathetic component is minor or absent (Table 46-5).

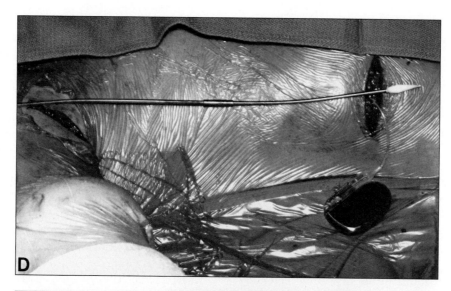

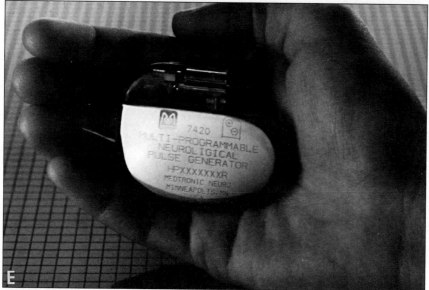

Figure 46-26, cont'd.

D, The connecting leads are placed subcutaneously from the electrode to a pulse generator placed in the flank. The amplitude and rate of stimulation can be adjusted to match the needs of the patient for pain control. **E,** Programmable pulse generator (Itrel) that is placed in the flank and attached to the connecting lead.

PREFERRED TREATMENT PLAN

The most difficult question facing upper limb surgeons is what to do with these serious incapacitating complaints of pain in the patient with a previous wrist injury. The general treatment plans for sympathetic and somatic pain have been discussed. For the specifics, one needs first to separate the somatic pain from the sympathetic-mediated pain. For both evaluation and treatment of somatic pain, we start with isolated peripheral nerve blocks. Ice massage or contrasting ice and heat massage in between the series of peripheral nerve blocks is recommended. TENS is also helpful in selected patients to control pain between the peripheral nerve blocks. A protective splint or pad over the affected nerve helps to prevent further injury. If the pain persists, an indwelling catheter (angiocatheter) placed adjacent to the affected nerve for continuous nerve block is effective in many patients. We have the patient inject bupivacaine (0.5%) every 4 to 6 hours for pain relief. This is followed by physical therapy. When a specific diagnosis of nerve entrapment can be made (e.g., median nerve compression at the wrist), surgical intervention may be indicated. Supportive evidence of such a compression neuropathy by electromyography and nerve conduction studies should be obtained. Ill-advised surgical intervention only makes the pain dysfunction worse if there is not a compressive neuropathy to treat.

TREATMENT ALTERNATIVES FOR SOMATIC PAIN VERSUS SYMPATHETIC PAIN

Once the diagnosis of somatic-mediated pain is made, then treatment of somatic pain can begin immediately. Controlling the pain focus or trigger area should be performed by one of several methods. Repeated local injections with a long-acting analgesic (bupivacaine 0.5%) or the placement of a catheter (e.g., within the carpal tunnel or distal forearm adjacent to the median nerve or proximal to the first dorsal extensor compartment for isolated radial sensory neuropathy) can be effective in controlling and often eliminating chronic nerve pain.

Once pain is controlled, continued use of TENS for several weeks helps prevent recurrence. Surgical intervention may occasionally be needed if these pain-alleviating measures are unsuccessful. Cases needing surgical treatment include a neuroma of a cutaneous nerve best approached by nerve ablation proximal to the area of injury or by soft-tissue transfer into muscle or fascia about the injured nerve in an effort to provide increased vascularity and a scar-free bed.

Treatment of these conditions using peripheral nerve blocks, TENS, and direct electrical stimulation is based on the hypothesis of Livingston[46] that a cycle of chronic nerve irritation increases afferent input, usually in an increased internuncial pool, with continuous stimulation of sympathetic and motor afferent fibers. Blocking this afferent signal is proposed by the "gate control theory" of Melzack and Wall,[12,56] who suggested that activation of blocking afferent signals "closes the gate" and controls the internuncial pool of overactivity.

In general, treatment should also be separated into early and late treatment alternatives.* For the patient with early presentation of pain dysfunction, the isolated nerve problems need to be identified and corrected. If a K wire or pin is adjacent to a peripheral or cutaneous nerve, the pin must be removed. If the patient has progressing signs of carpal tunnel syndrome, the median nerve needs to be decompressed. If the external fixation system is causing psychologic problems related to pins penetrating the skin and results in failure of the patient to use the hand, then it must be removed and another method of fracture immobilization selected. It is a poor choice to simply observe or delay evaluation of the patient with persistent pain associated with fracture or other injury about the wrist. Continued use of narcotic pain medication in such patients must be

strongly discouraged. Injured limbs should be relatively painless after 48 to 72 hours of treatment for fracture or soft-tissue injury. Narcotics should not be given for chronic pain. If patients have persisting pain, then the cause of the pain must be sought.

Early in the treatment of pain dysfunction, physical therapy is quite useful, but it must be as pain free as possible. "No pain no gain" does not apply to the treatment of the patient with a painful wrist. Local or regional nerve blocks should be used to minimize the pain and maximize the outcome from physical therapy. A coordinated program of pain management helps greatly in this regard. Early treatment of suspected pain dysfunction (causalgia or sympathetic) is extremely important to prevent the late sequelae and improve overall treatment results.

Late presentation of sympathetic pain dysfunction, which is more commonly seen, may be in either the second or third stages and treatment here may vary.[43] For the patient with the full-blown sympathetic dystrophy, the use of stellate ganglion or interscalene blocks is essential.[30,32] When the patient has a positive reflex sympathetic dystrophy score, studies demonstrate improved response to therapy and pain with proximal nerve blocks as part of the management program. We recommend a series of blocks extending over a period of 2 to 3 weeks (not just a single block). The procedures are best performed by a qualified anesthesiologist experienced in pain management. After the pain decreases, the patients can be effective contributors to their own treatment program. Patients must be educated that the improvement depends in part on their own active involvement in exercises and pain control.

Patients without sympathetic pain dystrophy will also benefit from proximal nerve blocks such as axillary or interscalene blocks or axillary nerve blocks. The level of anesthesia can be titrated such that it controls pain but does not eliminate active motion. Local and regional blocks in our experience allow the patient to tolerate physical therapy much better.

The surgeon's direct role in the treatment of chronic pain is limited. However, the surgeon must always assist in the overall direction of patient management and can be involved in placement of percutaneous catheters for continuous anesthesia of isolated peripheral nerve injuries and trials of individual peripheral blocks. Single nerve injections may benefit the patient and help to distinguish sympathetic from causalgia pain. Surgery is limited to compressive neuropathies, electromyographically proven, and to treatment of stiff joints by manipulation and pinning in the very late stages of the problem. A supportive role and encouragement by the surgeon are most helpful and appreciated by the patient. It is essential for the surgeon to stay involved with the care of his or her patients because they need direction, support, and guidance.

* References 30,38,40,43,45,58.

REFERENCES

1. Abbott LC, Saunders JBCM: Injuries of the median nerve in fractures of the lower end of the radius, *Surg Gynecol Obstet* 57:507-516, 1933.
2. Abrams RA, Brown RA, Botte MJ: The superficial branch of the radial nerve: an anatomic study with surgical implications, *J Hand Surg [Am]* 17:1037-1041, 1992.
3. Amadio PC: Pain dysfunction syndromes, *J Bone Joint Surg Am* 70:944-949, 1988.
4. Amadio PC, Mackinnon SE, Merritt WH, et al.: Reflex sympathetic dystrophy syndrome: consensus report of an ad hoc committee of the American Association for Hand Surgery on the definition of reflex sympathetic dystrophy syndrome, *Plast Reconstr Surg* 87:371-375, 1991.
5. Aro HT, Koivunen T: Minor axial shortening of the radius affects outcome of Colles' fracture treatment, *J Hand Surg [Am]* 16:392-398, 1991.
6. Ashall G: Flexor pollicis longus rupture after fracture of the distal radius, *Injury* 22:153-155, 1991.
7. Atkins RM, Duckworth T, Kanis JA: Features of algodystrophy after Colles' fracture, *J Bone Joint Surg Br* 72:105-110, 1990.
8. Bacorn RW, Kurtzke JF: Colles' fracture. A study of two thousand cases from New York State Workmen's Compensation Board, *J Bone Joint Surg [Am]* 35:643-658, 1953.
9. Bauman TD, Gelberman RH, Mubarak SJ, et al.: The acute carpal tunnel syndrome, *Clin Orthop* 156:151-156, 1981.
10. Bickerstaff DR, Bell MJ: Carpal malalignment in Colles' fractures, *J Hand Surg [Br]* 14:155-160, 1989.
11. Biyani A, Bhan S: Dual extensor tendon entrapment in Galeazzi fracture-dislocation: a case report, *J Trauma* 29:1295-1297, 1989.
12. Bonica JJ: Causalgia and other reflex sympathetic dystrophies, *Adv Pain Res Ther* 3:141-166, 1979.
13. Botte MJ, Cohen MS, Lavernia CJ, et al.: The dorsal branch of the ulnar nerve: an anatomic study, *J Hand Surg [Am]* 15:603-607, 1990.
14. Bourrel P, Ferro RM: Nerve complications in closed fractures of the lower end of the radius, *Ann Chir Main* 1:119-126, 1982.
15. Brain WR, Wright AD, Wilkinson M: Spontaneous compression of both median nerves in the carpal tunnel. Six cases treated surgically, *Lancet* 1:277-282, 1947.
16. Bryan RS, Dobyns JH: Fractures of the carpal bones other than lunate and navicular, *Clin Orthop* 149:107-111, 1980.
17. Cassebaum WH: Colles' fracture. A study of end results, *JAMA* 143:963-965, 1950.
18. Cooney WP, Bussey R, Dobyns JH, et al.: Difficult wrist fractures. Perilunate fracture-dislocations of the wrist, *Clin Orthop* 214:136-147, 1987.
19. Cooney WP III, Dobyns JH, Linscheid RL: Complications of Colles' fractures, *J Bone Joint Surg Am* 62:613-619, 1980.
20. Diamond JP, Newman JH: Multiple flexor tendon ruptures following Colles' fractures: a case report, *J Hand Surg [Br]* 12:112-114, 1987.
21. Dias JJ, McMohan A: Effect of Colles' fracture malunion on carpal alignment, *J R Coll Surg Edinb* 33:303-305, 1988.
22. Dobyns JH, Linscheid RL: *Complications of treatment of fractures and dislocations of the wrist.* In Epps CH Jr, editor: *Complications in orthopaedic surgery,* ed 2, vol 1, Philadelphia, 1986, JB Lippincott, pp 339-417.
23. Engber WD, Gmeiner JG: Palmar cutaneous branch of the ulnar nerve, *J Hand Surg [Am]* 5:26-29, 1980.
24. Engkvist O, Lundborg G: Rupture of the extensor pollicis longus tendon after fracture of the lower end of the radius—a clinical and microangiographic study, *Hand* 11:76-86, 1979.
25. Fernandez DL: Irreducible radiocarpal fracture-dislocation and radioulnar dissociation with entrapment of the ulnar nerve, artery and flexor profundus II-V-case report, *J Hand Surg [Am]* 6:456-461, 1981.
26. Gartland JJ Jr, Werley CW: Evaluation of healed Colles' fractures, *J Bone Joint Surg Am* 33:895-907, 1951.
27. Gelberman RH: *Acute carpal tunnel syndrome.* In Gelberman RH, editor: *Operative nerve repair and reconstruction,* vol 2, Philadelphia, 1991, JB Lippincott, pp 939-948.
28. Gelberman RH, Szabo RM, Mortensen WW: Carpal tunnel pressures and wrist position in patients with Colles' fractures, *J Trauma* 24:747-749, 1984.
29. Gibbons JJ, Wilson PR: RSD score: criteria for the diagnosis of reflex sympathetic dystrophy and causalgia, *Clin J Pain* 8:260-263, 1992.
30. Gibbons JJ, Wilson PR, Lamer TS, et al.: Interscalene blocks for chronic upper extremity pain, *Reg Anesth* 13:50-56, 1988.
31. Goldie BS, Powell JM: Bony transfixion of the median nerve following Colles' fracture. A case report, *Clin Orthop* 273:275-277, 1991.
32. Goldner JL: Causes and prevention of reflex sympathetic dystrophy (letter to the editor), *J Hand Surg [Am]* 5:295-296, 1980.
33. Green DP: Pins and plaster treatment of comminuted fractures of the distal end of the radius, *J Bone Joint Surg Am* 57:304-310, 1975.
34. Hamlin C, Littler JW: Restoration of the extensor pollicis longus tendon by an intercalated graft, *J Bone Joint Surg Am* 59:412-414, 1977.
35. Harper WM, Jones JM: Non-union of Colles' fracture: report of two cases, *J Hand Surg [Br]* 15:121-123, 1990.
36. Howard FM: Ulnar-nerve palsy in wrist fractures, *J Bone Joint Surg Am* 43:1197-1201, 1961.
37. Hueston JT: Dupuytren's contracture and specific injury, *Med J Aust* 1:1084-1085, 1968.
38. Inhofe PD, Garcia-Moral CA: Reflex sympathetic dystrophy. A review of the literature and a long-term outcome study, *Orthop Rev* 23:655-661, 1994.
39. Jenkins NH, Mackie IG: Late rupture of the extensor pollicis longus tendon: the case against attrition, *J Hand Surg [Br]* 13:448-449, 1988.

40. Kleinert HE, Cole NM, Wayne L, et al.: Post-traumatic sympathetic dystrophy, *Orthop Clin North Am* 4:917-927, 1973.

41. Kozin SH, Wood MB: Early soft-tissue complications after fractures of the distal part of the radius, *J Bone Joint Surg Am* 75:144-153, 1993.

42. Kumar A: Median and ulnar nerve injury secondary to a comminuted Colles fracture, *J Trauma* 30:118-119, 1990.

43. Lankford LL, Thompson JE: Reflex sympathetic dystrophy, upper and lower extremity. Diagnosis and management, *Instruct Course Lect* 26:163-178, 1977.

44. Linscheid RL: Injuries to radial nerve at wrist, *Arch Surg* 91:942-946, 1965.

45. Linson MA, Leffert R, Todd DP: The treatment of upper extremity reflex sympathetic dystrophy with prolonged continuous stellate ganglion blockade, *J Hand Surg [Am]* 8:153-159, 1983.

46. Livingston WK: *Pain mechanisms: a physiologic interpretation of causalgia and its related states,* New York, 1943, Macmillan.

47. Lombardi RM, Wood MB, Linscheid RL: Symptomatic restrictive thumb-index flexor tenosynovitis: incidence of musculotendinous anomalies and results of treatment, *J Hand Surg [Am]* 13:325-328, 1988.

48. Low PA, Amadio PC, Wilson PR, et al.: Laboratory findings in reflex sympathetic dystrophy: a preliminary report, *Clin J Pain* 10:235-239, 1994.

49. Low PA, Caskey PE, Tuck RR, et al.: Quantitative sudomotor axon reflex test in normal and neuropathic subjects, *Ann Neurol* 14:573-580, 1983.

50. Lynch AC, Lipscomb PR: The carpal tunnel syndrome and Colles' fractures, *JAMA* 185:363-366, 1963.

51. Mackinnon SE, Dellon AL: The overlap pattern of the lateral antebrachial cutaneous nerve and the superficial branch of the radial nerve, *J Hand Surg [Am]* 10:522-526, 1985.

52. Marson BM, Keenan MA: Skin surface pressures under short leg casts, *J Orthop Trauma* 7:275-278, 1993.

53. McCarroll HR Jr: Nerve injuries associated with wrist trauma, *Orthop Clin North Am* 15:279-287, 1984.

54. McClain EJ, Wissinger HA: The acute carpal tunnel syndrome: nine case reports, *J Trauma* 16:75-78, 1976.

55. McQueen M, Caspers J: Colles fracture: does the anatomical result affect the final function? *J Bone Joint Surg Br* 70:649-651, 1988.

56. Melzack R, Wall PD: Pain mechanisms. A new theory, *Science* 150:971-979, 1965.

57. Mersky H, Bogduk N: *Classification of chronic pain,* ed 2, Seattle, 1990, IASP Press.

58. Nashold BS Jr, Goldner JL, Mullen JB, et al.: Long-term pain control by direct peripheral-nerve stimulation, *J Bone Joint Surg Am* 64:1-10, 1982.

59. Paley D, McMurtry RY: Median nerve compression by volarly displaced fragments of the distal radius, *Clin Orthop* 215:139-147, 1987.

60. Rychak JS, Kalenak A: Injury to the median and ulnar nerves secondary to fracture of the radius. A case report, *J Bone Joint Surg Am* 59:414-415, 1977.

61. Sanders RA, Keppel FL, Waldrop JI: External fixation of distal radial fractures: results and complications, *J Hand Surg [Am]* 16:385-391, 1991.

62. Schuind F, Donkerwolcke M, Burny F: External fixation of wrist fractures, *Orthopedics* 7:841-844, 1984.

63. Seitz WH Jr: Complications and problems in the management of distal radius fractures, *Hand Clin* 10:117-123, 1994.

64. Shea JD, McClain EJ: Ulnar-nerve compression syndromes at and below the wrist, *J Bone Joint Surg Am* 51:1095-1103, 1969.

65. Sherman RA, Barja RH, Bruno GM: Thermographic correlates of chronic pain: analysis of 125 patients incorporating evaluations by a blind panel, *Arch Phys Med Rehabil* 68:273-279, 1987.

66. Siegel RS, Weiden I: Combined median and ulnar nerve lesions complicating fractures of the distal radius and ulna. Two case reports, *J Trauma* 8:1114-1118, 1968.

67. Smith RJ: *Intrinsic contracture.* In Green DP, editor: *Operative hand surgery,* ed 2, vol 1, New York, 1988, Churchill Livingstone, pp 609-631.

68. Spinner M, Aiache A, Silver L, et al.: Impending ischemic contracture of the hand. Early diagnosis and management, *Plast Reconstr Surg* 50:341-349, 1972.

69. Stewart HD, Innes AR, Burke FD: The hand complications of Colles' fractures, *J Hand Surg [Br]* 10:103-106, 1985.

70. Strege DW, Cooney WP, Wood MB, et al.: Chronic peripheral nerve pain treated with direct electrical nerve stimulation, *J Hand Surg [Am]* 19:931-939, 1994.

71. Sumner JM, Khuri SM: Entrapment of the median nerve and flexor pollicis longus tendon in an epiphyseal fracture-dislocation of the distal radioulnar joint: a case report, *J Hand Surg [Am]* 9:711-714, 1984.

72. Taleisnik J: The palmar cutaneous branch of the median nerve and the approach to the carpal tunnel. An anatomical study, *J Bone Joint Surg Am* 55:1212-1217, 1973.

73. Taleisnik J: *Complications of fractures, dislocations, and ligamentous injuries of the wrist.* In Boswick JA Jr, editor: *Complications in hand surgery,* Philadelphia, 1986, WB Saunders, pp 154-196.

74. Vance RM, Gelberman RH: Acute ulnar neuropathy with fractures at the wrist, *J Bone Joint Surg Am* 60:962-965, 1978.

75. Wilson PR: *Sympathetically maintained pain. Diagnosis, measurement, and efficacy of treatment.* In Stanton Hicks M, editor: *Pain and the sympathetic nervous system,* Dordrecht, 1990, Klüwer Academic Publishers, pp 91-124.

76. Younge D: Haematoma block for fractures of the wrist: a cause of compartment syndrome, *J Hand Surg [Br]* 14:194-195, 1989.

77. Zemel NP: The prevention and treatment of complications from fractures of the distal radius and ulna, *Hand Clin* 3:1-11, 1987.

78. Zoega H: Fracture of the lower end of the radius with ulnar nerve palsy, *J Bone Joint Surg Br* 48:514-516, 1966.

47

COMPARTMENT SYNDROMES AND ISCHEMIC CONTRACTURE: HAND, WRIST, AND FOREARM

Joseph M. Failla, M.D.

ANATOMY
BIOMECHANICS
HISTORY
ETIOLOGY
CLINICAL DIAGNOSIS OF ACUTE COMPARTMENT
  SYNDROME
COMPARTMENT PRESSURE MEASUREMENTS
COMPARTMENT PRESSURE MEASUREMENT
  TECHNIQUES

SURGICAL TREATMENT OF ACUTE COMPARTMENT
  SYNDROME
  SURGICAL TECHNIQUE: HAND AND WRIST
  SURGICAL TECHNIQUE: FOREARM
SURGICAL TREATMENT OF ESTABLISHED
  VOLKMANN'S CONTRACTURE
PREFERRED SURGICAL APPROACH

Compartment syndrome is a condition that can result when a rigid treatment philosophy leads to unintended patient morbidity. On the other hand, performing a fasciotomy when a compartment pressure measurement is above an arbitrary normal value, without regard to the patient's clinical symptoms, can result in unsightly scars and potentially damaged neurovascular structures. Reliance on an equivocal clinical examination in an unconscious patient without measurement of compartment pressure can be far more dangerous, leading to a late or omitted fasciotomy. This chapter presents a general view of the history, physiology, and diagnosis and a surgical treatment philosophy of compartment syndrome affecting the forearm, wrist, and hand. New concepts related to diagnosis and treatment of this condition are presented to increase understanding of the clinical behavior of compartment syndrome, making treatment more rational and providing a basis for prevention.

ANATOMY

It is not possible to write about compartment syndrome affecting the wrist alone other than in carpal tunnel syndrome (see Chapter 51). The wrist is, however, affected in Volkmann's contracture secondary to pathologic events in the forearm, just as wrist motion normally is indirectly brought about by the tendons that cross over and around it rather than inserting directly on carpal bones. The wrist in compartment syndrome is thus relegated to being an "intercalated segment" between the forearm and the hand, much as the proximal carpal row is between the distal radius and the distal carpal row.[34] The wrist does contain a compartment (i.e., the carpal tunnel); there is now little debate about whether the space is open or closed (Fig. 47-1). The carpal tunnel has been shown to be a functional compartment in which pressure can increase with chronic compression from a normal of zero pressure to pathologic values greater than 30 mm Hg.[19] Carpal tunnel pressures do not appear to reflect changes in forearm compartment syndrome (Fig. 47-1, D), and each condition should be treated independently and separately. However, increased pressure may not be the only force on the median nerve in compartment syndrome, because there is also an element of frictional forces from the swollen lumbrical or profundus lying within swollen tenosynovium directly adjacent to the median nerve.

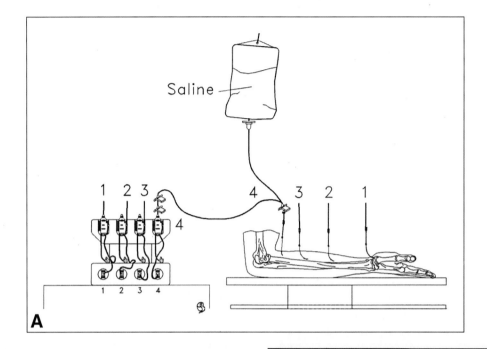

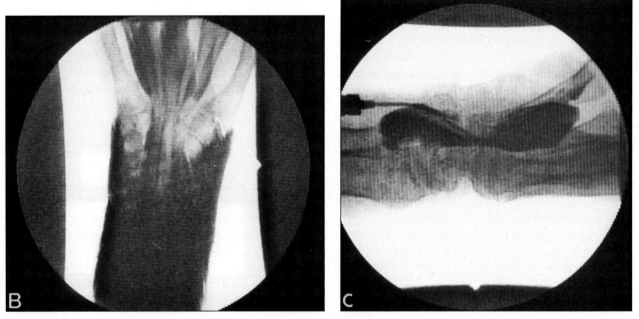

FIGURE 47-1

Compartment pressure measurements: carpal tunnel and forearm. **A,** This line drawing shows position of catheters in the carpal tunnel (*1*) and in various positions in the forearm (*2,3,4*). **B,** Posteroanterior radiographic film of Hypaque infusion into the forearm of a cadaver specimen shows a high concentration in the forearm with only late, incomplete filling of the carpal canal. **C,** Lateral radiographic film of cadaver specimen after infusion of Hypaque solution into the carpal tunnel. Note proximal limitation of the contrast medium at the distal forearm–carpal tunnel junction.

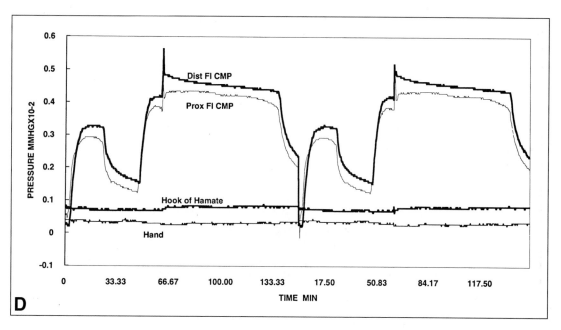

FIGURE 47-1, CONT'D.

D, Infusion pressure measurements show high pressure in the forearm (distal flexor compartment and proximal flexor compartment) compared with the carpal tunnel (hook of hamate or within the hand). *Dist Fl CMP,* distal portion of flexor compartment; *Prox Fl CMP,* proximal portion of flexor compartment. *(From Cobb TK, Cooney WP, An K-N: Pressure dynamics of the carpal tunnel and flexor compartment of the forearm,* J Hand Surg [Am] *20:193-198, 1995. Copyright, American Society for Surgery of the Hand, by permission of Churchill Livingstone.)*

As the wrist is affected by the forearm, the hand is in turn affected by the wrist. Pathologic wrist flexion causes long digital extensor tenodesis with metacarpophalangeal (MCP) joint extension, which is superimposed on shortened long digital flexors, causing interphalangeal clawing and a possible element of median and ulnar intrinsic palsy, worsening the clawing. The interphalangeal joints can remain supple, and in this setting active digital extension is possible only with further wrist flexion. Thenar and hypothenar weakness and fibrosis lead to an adducted thumb, contracted first web, and flattened palmar arch. However, the intrinsic muscle contractures cannot directly affect the wrist because these muscles originate on or distal to the transverse carpal ligament or distal carpal bones and are distal to even the most distal axis of wrist motion (Fig. 47-2). Lumbricals contract not only for digit extension but also have excursion into the carpal tunnel caused by contraction of profundus tendons during finger flexion.

These complex related deformities must be considered when planning stages of surgical release of established Volkmann's contracture. Release of intrinsic hand deformity may not be indicated at the same time as release of forearm contracture because the latter may allow lumbrical excursion sufficient to improve digit contracture. Extensive single-stage surgery may lead to excessive swelling and pain, which would limit motion that is often greatly needed after contracture release. Distal intrinsic release or joint contracture release, however, may improve motion.

BIOMECHANICS

In Volkmann's contracture, the digital flexors and occasionally wrist flexors are involved in ischemic insult that results in extreme positions of finger and wrist flexion. Even if excursion is left in the fibrosed musculotendinous units, a large percentage of this excursion is used for wrist motion, with only the remainder left for digital flexion. Active extension of the digits can occur only with the wrist maintained in extreme flexion so that excursion can be directed toward the fingers. Any active wrist extension results in tight flexion (Fig. 47-3) secondary to the tenodesis effect of contracted finger flexors.

A specific clinical case can illustrate a method of calculating how much excursion needs to be restored to the flexors in the forearm to improve wrist motion and finger motion.

A 45-year-old right-handed female homemaker sustained a radius and ulnar shaft fracture at age 7 years. Volkmann's ischemic contracture resulted (Fig. 47-3, *B*).

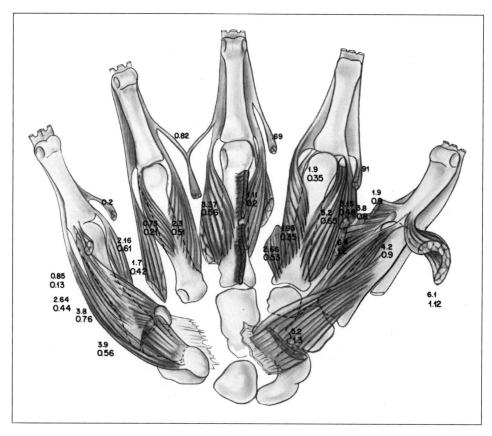

FIGURE 47-2

Intrinsic muscles of the hand. Note that all of the intrinsic muscles have muscle origin and insertion distal to the wrist and that intrinsic muscle tightness or contracture would not affect wrist motion or cause a wrist contracture.

She functioned well despite a deformity of wrist and finger flexion. She presented with a complaint of permanent wrist flexion (30°) and the fingers resting in a clawed posture (MCP extension 0°; the proximal and distal interphalangeal joints flexed to 50°). When she actively flexed the wrist to 60°, digital extension at the interphalangeal joints was much improved but not full. Wrist active extension was possible to a neutral position, but this caused the fingers to be pulled passively into tight flexion, limiting any function. In planning surgical treatment for this patient, it was noted that she could benefit from a change in wrist position and finger position. However, the extent of tendon release on lengthening was not clear. She specifically desired the ability to extend the wrist more without bothersome flexion tenodesis of the fingers.

In planning operative release, one option is to consider the radian method[6] to calculate the amount of digital flexor excursion that would be necessary by surgical release to allow the wrist to extend and the fingers to extend (Fig. 47-4). If the goal is to extend the wrist to neutral without causing the fingers to flex

tightly, then the amount of excursion necessary for this could be calculated by roughly assuming a radius of wrist motion of 2 cm with the axis at the midcarpal joint (head of capitate). A 30° increase in wrist extension to the neutral position would result from 1.4 cm of added flexor profundus excursion. If the wrist moves from 30° flexion to neutral, it would move along the circle of motion a certain portion of a radian. If it moves through one radian, it moves 57.29°. If it moves the width of the radius, which in this case is 2 cm, then a 30° motion can be calculated to equal 1.04 cm. If 1.04 cm of excursion is added to the flexor tendons, the wrist could then move to a neutral position without causing flexor tenodesis of the fingers. If the proximal and distal interphalangeal joints need to move from a position of -50° to 0° extension, this would require additional excursion. If one assumes that the radius of motion at the head of the proximal phalanx and at the middle phalanx is 0.5 cm, the excursion needed at each joint would be 0.43 cm, for a total of 0.86 cm. These calculations are estimates that provide a rough guide to preoperative planning in such patients.

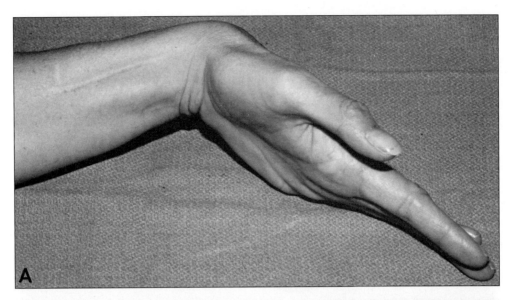

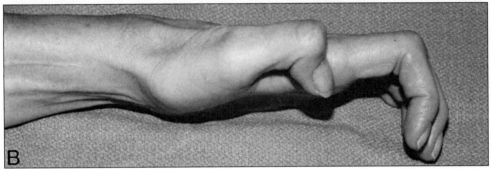

FIGURE 47-3

A, Active digital extension in a 45-year-old patient with untreated palmar forearm Volkmann's contracture since childhood. Full digital extension is only possible with maximal wrist flexion. **B,** Any attempt at wrist extension, in this case to neutral, causes tight flexor tenodesis of the fingers and thumb at all joints, showing involvement of the flexor pollicis longus and flexor profundus in Volkmann's contracture.

HISTORY

It is probable that the concepts that led to early understanding of compartment syndrome of the forearm did not simply suddenly appear in the 19th century. Physicians of antiquity dealt primarily with life-threatening wounds, including those involving the extremities. Egyptian medicine, as recounted in the Edwin Smith papyrus "Book of Wounds," describes linen pads and bark splints used to immobilize forearm fractures[17] (Fig. 47-5).

Hippocratic writings of the 4th century BC, specifically the chapter on "Fractures and Joints," described in a detailed and careful way a method of treatment of forearm fractures by dressings applied in layers, with carefully increasing tension to immobilize fractures. Recommendations were included on position of immobilization for forearm fractures. He also warned that excessive hand swelling and pain are indications of

a dressing placed too tightly and recommended that dressings be replaced daily, until by the seventh day "the fractured bones will be more mobile and ready for adjustment."[29] Although Hippocrates also did not specifically describe compartment syndrome, he evidently was aware of the possibility of dangerous amounts of swelling after forearm fracture.

Galen, in the 2nd century AD in Rome, treated wounds of the gladiators, sutured muscles and tendons with silk, and did animal dissections but essentially did not increase knowledge from the Hippocratic writings.[35] Although the Dark Ages continued along the lines of Hippocratic medicine, there was no shortage of extremity wounds that could result in compartment syndrome during these years and it would not be surprising if some reference to this condition was found in writings of physicians before the 19th century.

The history of the understanding of compartment syndrome can be divided into three phases. The first

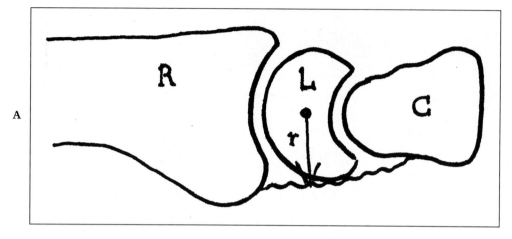

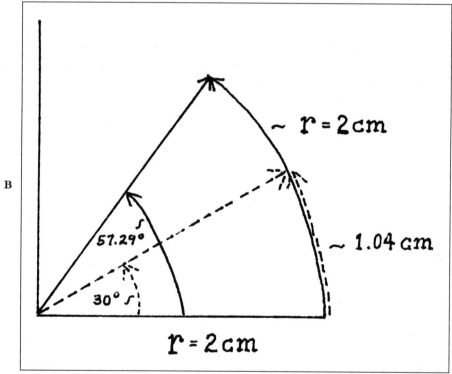

FIGURE 47-4

A, The radian method allows calculation of the amount of tendon excursion necessary to allow a known amount of angular motion to occur at a joint, when the radius of the arc of motion is known. For example, in the wrist joint, a radius of 2 cm can be drawn from the center of the lunate in a palmar direction to the palmar capsule. *C,* capitate; *L,* lunate; *r,* radius of wrist arc of motion; *R,* radius. **B,** If the wrist moves 57.29°, then the linear distance of motion along the motion arc is 1 radian, which is the length of the radius, or 2 cm in this example. If the wrist moved only 30°, for example, from 30° flexion to neutral, this would trace a portion of a radian of 2 cm, which could be calculated to be 1.04 cm. This is the amount of flexor tendon excursion required to allow this wrist extension to occur.

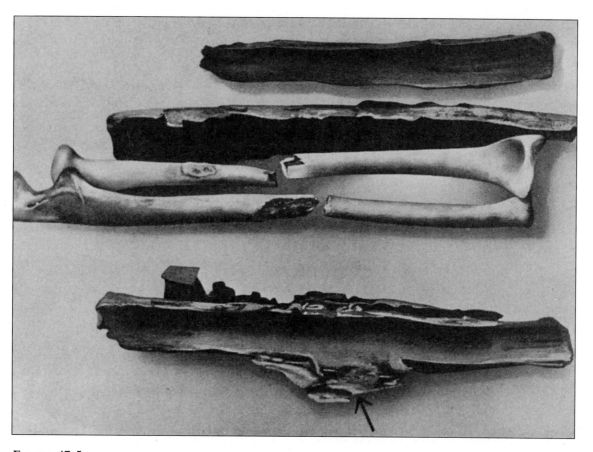

FIGURE 47-5

Radius and ulnar fractures treated with bark splints by Egyptian physicians in the 3rd millennium BC. *(From Majno.[35] By permission of the President and Fellows of Harvard College. Reprinted from Smith GE: The most ancient splints, BMJ 1:732-734, 1908.)*

phase was the last half of the 19th century and the beginning of the 20th century. The second and third blend into each other in the 20th century. The first phase is a descriptive or clinical era containing mostly case reports that cluster at the end of the 19th century and the beginning of the 20th century, with Volkmann's work credited as seminal in 1881.[58] This original work is available in English translation.[59] Volkmann, born in Leipzig (1830), was surgeon general to the Prussian army in 1870 during the Franco-Prussian war. He had considerable experience with fractures, which may have been a factor in his understanding of the pathology of ischemic muscle contracture. He reported treating 31 patients who had open fractures with Lister's aseptic technique. No infections developed, which was a great advance for his time. He recognized that open treatment of fractures was possible and that one could avoid ischemic muscle contracture by opening (surgically) fascial compartments.

In 1926, Jepson,[30] from the Mayo Clinic, reported an experimental study dealing with ischemic muscle contracture and reviewed the literature of his time. He referenced many case reports, particularly emphasizing one by Leser of Germany[33] and crediting him with drawing

attention to the clinical condition of ischemic contracture. Jepson, in fact, referred to this as "Volkmann-Leser contraction" and quoted a report by a German investigator named Hildebrand in 1906[28] of a case described by Hamilton in 1850. Not only did Hamilton warn against damage to forearm muscles after radius fracture and tight bandaging, but he credited Dupuytren with the earliest case reports.[21,22]

Frank Hastings Hamilton was a prolific American bone and joint surgeon who wrote extensively on the treatment of fractures and was a founder of the University of Buffalo School of Medicine in 1843. Hamilton's general orthopedic writings had received no acknowledgment in orthopedic literature until Jepson's mention of the 1850 case report on forearm ischemia after distal radius fracture. Hamilton appears to have predated Volkmann in his ideas about compartment syndrome. However, Hamilton did not precisely understand or describe the nature of the muscle injury in compartment syndrome, as Volkmann did. He simply pointed out the danger of tight dressings on an acutely swollen forearm after fracture.

Dupuytren's writings of 1828 credit him with a detailed description of extreme swelling and pain after tight bandaging of an extremity injury. Dupuytren's description, relayed by Hamilton, may be the first detailed description of a developing compartment syndrome.

> The fracture was reduced... an apparatus was applied, but fast and too tightly; and not withstanding the great swelling and acute pain which the patient endured, it was not removed until the fourth day, when the hand was cold and edematous, and the forearm red, painful, and covered with vessications.... Portions of the flexor muscles subsequently sloughed, and the skin subsequently mortified.

Hamilton concluded by saying, "finally, whatever may be the mode of dressing, let me repeat the injunction to examine the arm frequently. No surgeon can do justice to himself or to his patient, who does not look at the arm at least once in 24 hours during the first 10 or 14 days, and in some cases the patient ought to be seen twice daily."

It is interesting that art imitated nature in this same era, almost to the year, in the writings of Gustave Flaubert, a contemporary of Dupuytren and Hamilton (*Madame Bovary,* from which the following quotation is taken, was published in 1857). In the novel *Madame Bovary,* Flaubert describes the results of an ill-conceived operation for clubfoot by Dr. Charles Bovary.[16] The operation was a percutaneous Achilles tenotomy followed by forced reduction of the equinovarus deformity maintained by splints and straps.

> The interesting patient was writhing in dreadful convulsions, so violent that the contraption in that his foot was locked almost beat down the wall. With many precautions, in order not to disturb the position of the limb, the box was removed, and an awful spectacle came into view. The outlines of the foot disappeared into such a swelling that the entire skin seemed about to burst; moreover, the leg was covered with bruises caused by the famous machine. Hyppolyte (the patient) had abundantly complained, but nobody had paid any attention to him.

It is interesting that a recent passage from an article on Volkmann's contracture complicating Colles' fractures is hauntingly similar in tone. Cooney et al.[11] described patients with this complication, "three of whom had had a constricting cast that was retained despite the patient's complaints of persisting pain. Continued use of analgesics in two patients further masked the symptoms."

The second stage of literature on compartment syndrome was less clinically descriptive and more experimental. Theories on the etiology of compartment syndrome began to appear, and gradually it was realized that the syndrome could occur in the absence of tight bandages. Steindler[53] warned that acute elbow flexion in supracondylar humerus fractures was the main problem rather than tight bandages, saying "it appears doubtful that much blame can be placed upon the circular dressing as such provided a good plaster technique is used." Early theories were summarized by Bunnell[9] in his text. These theories

included 1) blocked venous flow[4,30]; 2) "the vasomotor theory" attributed by Bunnell[9] to Leriche, Griffiths, and Foisie; 3) subfascial hematoma attributed by Benjamin[5] to the French authors Moulonquet and Jorge; and 4) arterial spasm.[20,43] Bunnell[9] had the foresight to summarize all these theories of his time by saying "a closed fascial space under pressure, in addition to partial venous and arterial obstruction furnishes the requirement to result in Volkmann's contracture. The circulation is slowed and congested, not stopped." This era also includes early reports on the histology of muscle death in Volkmann's ischemia.[7] Fasciotomy as a means of preventing ischemic fracture was suggested by Murphy,[42] who described hemorrhage into muscle in 1914. Jepson[30] stated in 1926, "The tension in the subfascial zone in the forearm can be so great as to cause cyanosis of the whole forearm and hand."

These early suggestions on how to prevent the development of ischemic contracture herald the third phase of compartment syndrome literature, which deals more with experimentation and understanding the pathophysiology of the microcirculation,[2,20,26] advances in measurements of compartment pressure as a prelude to fasciotomy,[41,45,60] advances in the details of fasciotomy technique,[1,13] and an extensive catalog of the varied causes of compartment syndrome.[46] This phase of literature is obviously ongoing.

ETIOLOGY

There are several injuries that have historically been emphasized so well that they virtually have become red flags for surgeons treating extremity injuries. With the potential for compartment syndrome, care is taken in the treatment of supracondylar humerus fracture in children immobilized in acute flexion, in the management of forearm fracture associated with severe crushing[47] or vascular injury, and in the reduction and immobilization of distal radius fractures.[12,27,50,54] Despite strong clinical suspicion, compartment syndrome can still develop insidiously in these common settings. Clinical experience has uncovered new causes of compartment syndrome that are not readily associated with it. These include low-velocity gunshot wounds to the forearm,[32] minor forearm crush injury,[1] toxic shock syndrome,[32] leukemic infiltrates,[56] compartment syndrome masked by epidural anesthesia,[55] hemophilic bleed into muscle, and compartment syndrome masked by inability to feel pain as a result of nerve palsy.[61]

The specific anatomic causes of the various compartment syndromes can differ widely.[43] Arterial injury with bleeding into a compartment is obviously different from brachial artery damage in a supracondylar humerus fracture. The pathophysiology of compartment syndrome, however, must explain on a microcirculatory

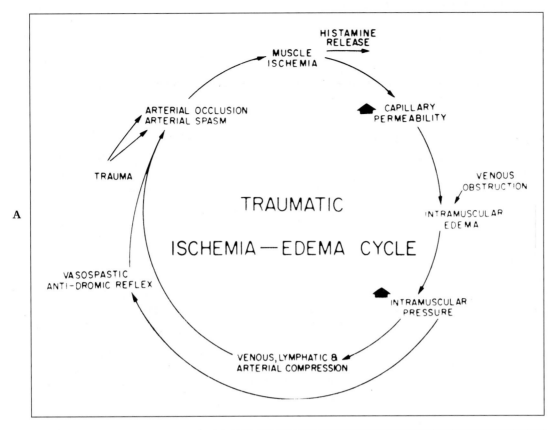

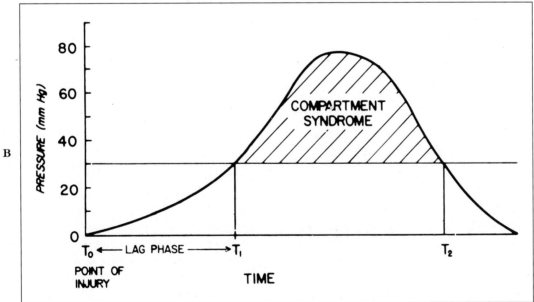

FIGURE 47-6

A, Traumatic ischemia-edema cycle. Initiated by nonspecific trauma, arterial flow into a specific region is decreased by occlusion, compression, or spasm. Such a reduction in perfusion creates a proportionate degree of ischemia in the individual muscles. Within the muscle substance, anoxia develops. Histamine-like substances increase capillary permeability and promote a transudation of plasma into the muscle. The summation of this effect is increasing intramuscular edema. Subsequently, a progressive increase in intramuscular intrinsic pressure is compounded by any unyielding dressings encircling the arm. Occlusive dressings add to the venous compression, causing a further increase in intrinsic tissue pressure. Vasospasm reinforces and perpetuates the initial vascular compromise and a destructive ischemia-edema cycle develops. *(From Eaton and Green.[13] By permission of WB Saunders.)* **B,** The time between injury and the onset of clinical findings in compartment syndrome may range from hours to days (*LAG PHASE T_0-T_1*). The ischemia of muscle and nerves in the compartment does not take place until pressures are greater than 30 mm Hg (*horizontal line*). The time from injury diagnosis and treatment is only a relative indicator of the ischemic period unless tissue pressures are monitored from the time of injury. *(From Gelberman et al.[18] By permission of JB Lippincott.)*

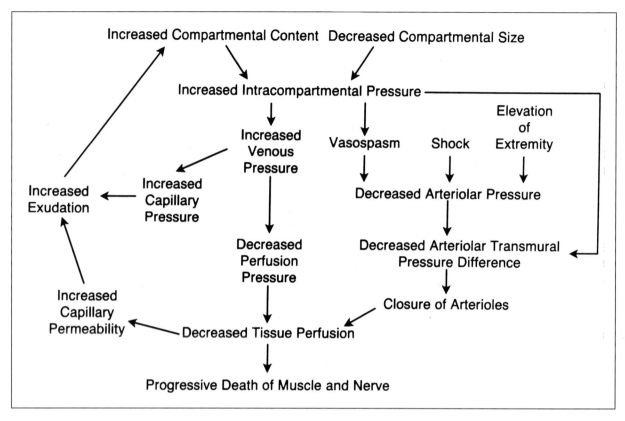

FIGURE 47-7

Some of the pathophysiologic events that may occur in a compartment syndrome.

basis how both these different mechanisms lead to muscle ischemia and ultimately increased compartment pressure (Fig. 47-6). The main theme of all proposed theories is that muscle ischemia produced by different mechanisms leads to increased capillary bed permeability and leaking of a plasma filtrate out of the capillaries; sludging of red blood cells in the capillary, decreasing flow; and muscle edema (Fig. 47-7). Edema then leads to increased compartment pressure, decreased venous return, and eventually arteriovenous shunting and capillary closure by extramural compression as tissue pressures increase (Fig. 47-6, *B*). As tissue pressure exceeds arterial perfusion, more ischemia develops and a sustained vicious cycle results, with muscle necrosis, peripheral nerve ischemia, entrapment, fibrosis, and end-stage Volkmann's contracture.

The hypotheses on the primary etiology of compartment syndrome are, however, still qualitative. The main two include 1) the "critical closing pressure" of arterioles is exceeded and 2) the compression of thin-walled veins prevents venous return as a result of increasing tissue pressure.[2,10] These theories each explain the presence of high tissue pressure but not the actual initiating event. Specifically, the cellular mediator of capillary leaking, which is presumably the main

event, is not known. For example, if histamine release by muscle mast cells in response to ischemia is causing cellular changes that cause capillaries to leak, then perhaps delivery of an antihistamine or an inhibitor of mast cell degranulation to the compartment could prevent these initiating events. There are many chemical mediators that operate on the cellular level to cause capillary leaking and ischemic muscle, and knowledge of these exact mechanisms could help prevent the development of compartment syndrome.

CLINICAL DIAGNOSIS OF ACUTE COMPARTMENT SYNDROME

The clinical history is the first step in making the diagnosis of a compartment syndrome. Knowledge of injuries commonly and uncommonly associated with compartment syndrome is crucial. Also important is knowledge of the amount of time since injury because of its relation to muscle and nerve recovery in established compartment syndrome. With an increased awareness based on history of the injury mechanism and patient complaints of deep aching pain and painful limb movements, the physical examination of the patient with a developing compartment syndrome becomes essential.[9,31,46,53] The history should include severe pain described as "out of proportion to the injury" and severe enough in intensity to be obvious during the initial patient examination and subsequently on reexamination.

Steindler[53] placed cyanosis before pain as an important sign in developing compartment syndrome but said that "the usual signs indicating impending contracture develop in the course of a few days, or a week at the most; sometimes even within a few hours. They are, in sequence: coldness, cyanosis, swelling, paraesthesias, pain, paralysis, contracture of the muscles and the appearance of the claw hand, or 'main en griffe.' " Pain often appears, however, immediately after the application of the cast and can be continuous and unrelenting. It is commonly known that all layers of a dressing, including cast padding, plaster, and stockinette, must be removed not only to prevent compartment syndrome in such a setting but also to do an adequate examination of the extremity. Bunnell[9] prosaically described pain as "sudden and severe, accompanied by much restlessness and the constant intense pain of tightness, of tissues dying from ischemia... the fingers are semiflexed, and any attempt to extend them increases the pain." This is perhaps the first reference to the useful examination maneuver of passive digital extension to check for palmar compartment ischemia.[9]

All of the patients with fasciotomy reported by Gelberman et al.[18] had pain on passive digital extension. Pain is also described as the most consistent symptom, persistent, progressive, and unrelieved by immobilization.[31] Although there is a long time between the injury, elevation of pressures, and clinical findings of compartment syndrome (Fig. 47-6, B), it is often stressed that pulses remain intact despite full-blown compartment syndrome. Paresthesia and hypoesthesia in the hand are stressed as reliable signs,[9,44] and loss of two-point discrimination in many patients was stressed as well.[18] Skin color changes can range from cyanosis to pallor and are not specific enough for early diagnosis of compartment syndrome. Loss of function (e.g., active finger flexion) due to pain is an early sign, but actual muscle paralysis is late and should not be relied on for early diagnosis. Compartment pressures that are high enough to stop microcirculation will produce, over 6 hours, muscle and nerve damage that leads to paralysis. Early signs of muscle damage at the cellular level[26] result in paralysis that can give valuable information in a patient's history of onset of compartment syndrome and may help provide a prognosis for muscle recovery.

The exception to pain as a reliable sign in the diagnosis of compartment syndrome occurs in patients who cannot respond well to questions and to characterizing the pain (e.g., children and unconscious patients). Patients with nerve palsy can have an "occult" compartment syndrome as a result of inability to feel pain. Reported examples include patients with Charcot-Marie-Tooth disease and patients with tibial fracture and peroneal palsy.[61] However, with the exception of these types of difficult patients, excessive unremitting pain should be the cornerstone of clinical diagnosis of compartment syndrome. Ischemic extremity muscle associated with severe extremity injury should produce pain. It is doubtful if a "silent" compartment syndrome such as silent myocardial infarction can occur. However, if high levels of narcotic pain medication have been initiated, the pain may be blocked sufficiently that the patient is asymptomatic. Another reliable sign is a tense compartment on palpation with a gloved finger. Gentle palpation should elicit pain in a compartment affected by compartment syndrome.

A normal extremity compartment should be soft and compressible and should feel softer than a tennis ball, whereas an extremity compartment with full-blown compartment syndrome should feel as firm as a baseball. Gentle passive extension of the fingers with a common muscle belly in the palmar compartment (e.g., the flexor digitorum profundus) causes extreme pain. This pain, however, must be distinguished from local muscle or tendon damage. For example, a palmar forearm low-velocity gunshot wound or knife wound in which isolated single musculotendinous units may be injured can be responsible for the pain. This requires a subtle distinction to make the diagnosis; the patient's ability to actively flex and passively extend adjacent digits without pain does not support the diagnosis of compartment syndrome. If there is doubt after physical examination in any situation in which compartment syndrome is suspected, then compartment pressures should be measured to answer the question. Patients with severe pain, loss of active muscle function, and increased pain on passive motion with local fascial compartment tenseness should be assumed to have a compartment syndrome. When in doubt, a fasciotomy should be done. The risks of fasciotomy are minimal compared with those of a missed compartment syndrome.

COMPARTMENT PRESSURE MEASUREMENTS

Compartment pressures measure the resting interstitial pressures between fascial or bone-fascial areas. Normal compartment pressure in an uninjured extremity should be 0 to 8 mm Hg.[41] Normal capillary pressure ranges from 20 to 25 mm Hg. A pressure greater than 30 mm Hg can theoretically stop the microcirculation and has been suggested as an indication for a fasciotomy.[23] This is consistent with experiments with compression of the forearm by a rigid plastic splint that stopped capillary flow at 30 mm Hg.[2] Despite this information, there is not uniform agreement on a compartment pressure value that is an absolute trigger for a fasciotomy.

Heppenstall et al.[26] related compartment pressure to the driving pressure head set outside the extremity, or the mean arterial pressure. A higher actual pressure can be tolerated better than a lower mean arterial pressure. When the difference between the mean arterial pressure and the compartment pressure was less than 30 mm Hg, fasciotomy was recommended because muscle damage has been detected by magnetic resonance methods.[26] It was pointed out that hypotension lowers the patient's ability to tolerate a given compartment pressure. Whitesides et al.,[60] taking into account the concept of critical closing pressure, suggested relating compartment pressure to diastolic pressure. It was suggested that fasciotomy be done if the difference between the compartment pressure and diastolic pressure was at least 10 to 30 mm Hg. A normotensive patient would require fasciotomy if compartment pressure was 40 to 45 mm Hg. Accordingly, a hypotensive patient could tolerate only lower compartment pressures. Matsen et al.[38] pointed out that clinically there is no absolute value for compartment pressure that would lead to fasciotomy. Thirteen of their patients had compartment pressure greater than 30 mm Hg and negative results of a clinical examination for compartment syndrome. No fasciotomy was done in these patients and none had sequelae such as Volkmann's contracture.

Nerve and muscle cell damage have been shown to increase with time of compartment ischemia. Hargens et al.[24] quantitated nerve damage in an animal model showing conduction block and histologic changes with a pressure greater than 30 mm Hg for 6 to 8 hours. Matsen[36] and Matsen and Rorabeck[37] pointed out that 30 min of ischemia leads to paresthesias, with irreversible damage in 12 to 24 hours. Muscle is damaged after 3 hours, with irreversible changes leading to contracture after 4 to 12 hours. These data reveal the importance of a detailed clinical history to determine the amount of time compartment syndrome has been present and the likelihood of tissue damage before fasciotomy. Clinical evidence has shown that if fasciotomy is performed less than 12 hours after the onset of compartment syndrome there is a much higher incidence of good results than if it is performed more than 12 hours after onset.[51]

When compartment syndrome is obvious by history and physical examination, compartment pressures are often measured to check severity[21] and to document the compartment syndrome for medicolegal purposes. Without the latter consideration and focusing primarily on the medical care of the patient, the clinical diagnosis of compartment syndrome, when obvious, is an absolute indication for a fasciotomy. In the presence of a solid clinical diagnosis of compartment syndrome, even with a low compartment pressure measurement (e.g., 15 mm Hg), my colleagues and I believe that this is an indication for fasciotomy. Fasciotomy should not be delayed in a patient with clinical compartment syndrome simply because of a low pressure measurement. The low pressure in this setting is an early point in time on the graph of a relentlessly developing compartment syndrome, which, if present clinically, will undoubtedly show increasing compartment pressure to damaging levels in time. Early fasciotomy can prevent this from happening. If there is doubt about the clinical diagnosis, then serial examinations and pressure measurements can be performed, but fasciotomy should not be delayed until an arbitrary high compartment pressure is reached.[48]

Pressure measurements automatically done for all injuries potentially associated with compartment syndrome can lead to unnecessary fasciotomy if the patient has no sign of compartment syndrome clinically and if the treating physician has an arbitrary compartment pressure value at which fasciotomy is performed. For example, a patient with no clinical signs of compartment syndrome after an extremity injury with moderate swelling may have a compartment pressure value of 30 mm Hg. The clinical picture determined by careful detailed history and physical examination serially should reveal clearly that muscle and nerve circulation are compromised and should point to the need for compartment pressure measurements and not vice versa.[37] A shotgun approach in which all patients with swollen injured extremities, even in the absence of clinical compartment syndrome, have compartment pressures measured is improper. In contrast, compartment pressure measurement is mandatory in patients in whom the clinical diagnosis cannot be certain, such as the unconscious patient, those with coexisting nerve palsy, children, and those with lack of sensation in the extremity.

In summary, when deciding on the critical level of compartment pressure, because a sustained compartment pressure of 30 mm Hg is enough to stop microcirculation to nerve and muscle, this pressure level should be of great concern when associated with the clinical features of compartment syndrome. This pressure value in the setting of an unsure diagnosis or a difficult patient is a reasonable trigger for a fasciotomy.

COMPARTMENT PRESSURE MEASUREMENT TECHNIQUES

All techniques of compartment pressure measurement involve placing a column of fluid between the fluid inside the extremity compartment at risk and a pressure-monitoring device. Whitesides et al.[60] described the needle manometer technique of

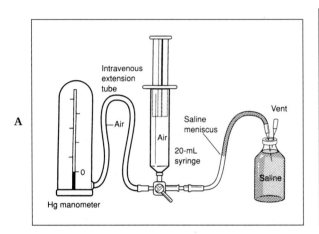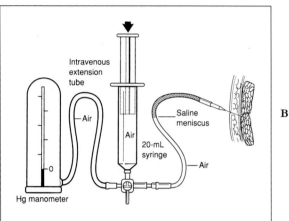

FIGURE 47-8

Whitesides technique. Tissue pressure is measured by determining the amount of pressure within a closed system that is required to overcome the pressure in a closed compartment. **A,** Assembled equipment for the Whitesides infusion technique just before placement of needle into area to be tested. **B,** Configuration of equipment for test. The valve has been turned to an open position, making a "T" of the open tubing. *(From Whitesides TE Jr, Heckman MM: Acute compartment syndrome: update on diagnosis and treatment,* J Am Acad Orthop Surg *4:209-218, 1996. By permission of the American Academy of Orthopaedic Surgeons.)*

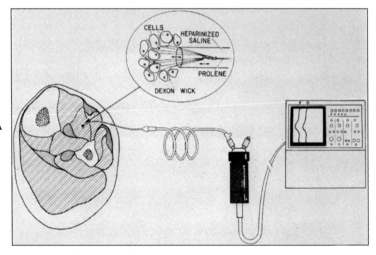

FIGURE 47-9

Wick catheter technique. **A,** Schematic representation of the tip of the wick catheter of multiple Dexon fibers in place within the anterior compartment of the leg. The fibers prevent tissue blockage of the orifice of the catheter and allow free exchange of fluid between the interstitium and the fluid-filled catheter. **B,** Increasing compartment pressure in a patient after tibial osteotomy. Cast splitting causes a marked decrease in pressure and relief of symptoms. *I.M.,* intramuscular. *(From Mubarak et al.[40] By permission of the journal.)*

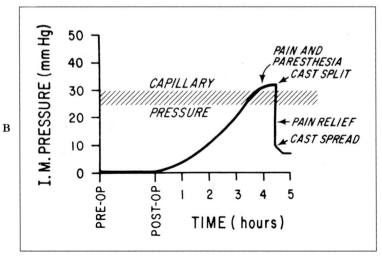

compartment pressure measurement (Fig. 47-8). The equipment for this technique includes an 18-G needle, a three-way stopcock, intravenous extension tubing, and blood pressure manometer, all of which are relatively simple to obtain. The method has been well described and although it is straightforward, practice is required for rapid, reproducible, and accurate use of the device. This method can be quickly and easily used and does not rely on sophisticated electronic equipment, which may not always be available or functioning well. It is essential that this method be mastered by all those dealing with compartment syndrome.

Many modifications of this original needle-manometer technique have been described. They all involve a variation on the simple 18-G needle portion of the technique in an effort to improve accuracy. Mubarak et al.[40] described a "wick" catheter that has the theoretical advantage of low likelihood of clotting at the tip (Fig. 47-9). The wick tip is essentially an unraveled suture, the filaments of which establish small channels of fluid in contact with compartment fluid. The slit catheter is a modification in which five cuts are made in the tip of the catheter, creating six small flaps in contact with the compartment fluid. This catheter was more accurate than the wick or needle manometer technique for continuous monitoring in a dog leg model.[45] A continuous infusion technique through a regular intravenous catheter connected to a pressure transducer has also been described; it has the theoretical advantage of increased patency at the tip of the catheter.[38] A modification of the 18-G needle technique of Whitesides uses a needle with an additional opening of 1.5 mm on a "side port" proximal to the needle tip.[3] A study[39] comparing the side-port needle to the slit catheter showed no statistical difference in compartment pressure measurements in a dog leg model. There was, however, a statistical difference between these two methods and the needle-manometer technique of Whitesides, which gave an average 18 mm Hg higher reading (i.e., tending to overdiagnose compartment pressure elevation).

All these techniques are effective. Whitesides' needle-manometer technique is basic and essential. If all else fails and special catheters and electronic equipment are not available, as is often the case outside the tertiary hospital setting, the needle manometer equipment is easily obtained and used. It should be well understood by all residents in training before the use of more sophisticated techniques. If this technique tends to overstate the compartment pressure, as has been suggested, this is a relatively safe tendency compared with understating the pressure. Because compartment pressure measurements rarely are ever used alone to decide on fasciotomy, the Whitesides method is a useful technique.

Table 47-1. Reported Compartmental Syndromes With Some of Their Associated Physical Signs and Symptoms

Compartment	Sensory Loss	Muscles Weakened	Painful Passive Movement	Location of Tenseness
Forearm				
Dorsal	—	Thumb and finger extensors	Thumb and finger flexion	Dorsal forearm
Palmar	Ulnar and median nerves	Thumb and finger extensors	Thumb and finger extension	Palmar forearm
Hand				
Interosseous	—	Interosseous muscles	Adduction and abduction of metacarpophalangeal joints	Dorsum of hand between metacarpals
Leg				
Anterior	Deep peroneal nerve	Toe extensors and tibialis anterior	Toe flexion	Anterior aspect of leg
Lateral	Superficial and deep peroneal nerves	Peroneal muscles	Foot inversion	Lateral aspect of leg over fibula
Superficial posterior	—	Soleus and gastrocnemius	Foot dorsiflexion	Calf
Deep posterior	Posterior tibial nerve	Toe flexors and tibialis posterior	Toe extension	Distal medial leg between Achilles tendon and tibia

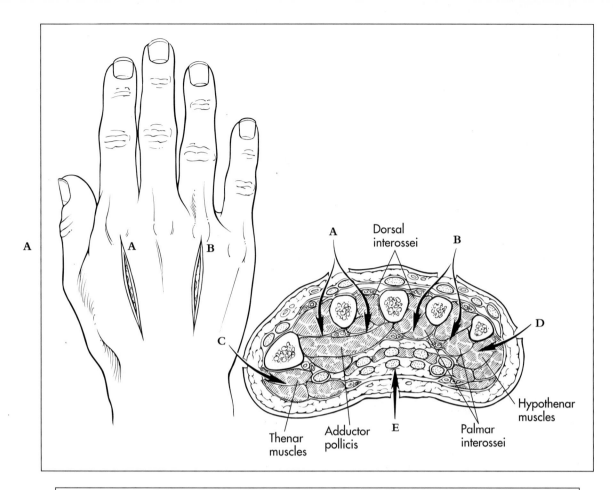

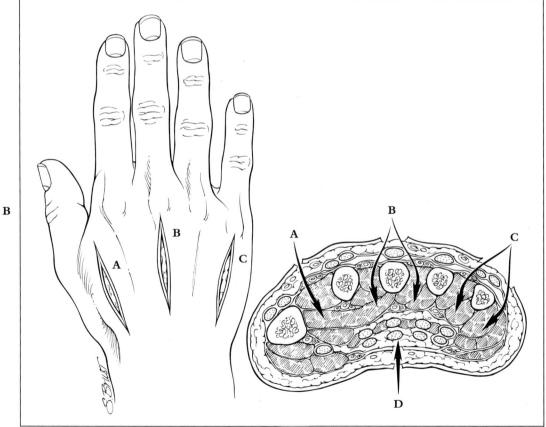

Figure 47-10

Surgical technique: hand. Release of ischemic contracture and intrinsic muscles. **A,** Two dorsal incisions (*A* and *B*) provide access to intrinsic muscles. Separate thumb web and thenar (*C*), hypothenar (*D*), and carpal tunnel (*E*) incisions may also be required. **B,** Four incisions for intrinsic release. *A,* thumb web space; *B,* dorsal third metacarpal; *C,* ulnar between 4th and 5th metacarpal; *D,* carpal tunnel. *(Modified from Rowland.[46] By permission of the publisher.)*

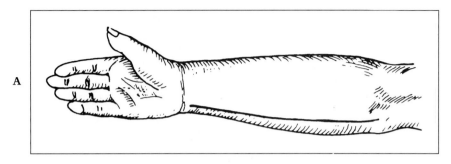

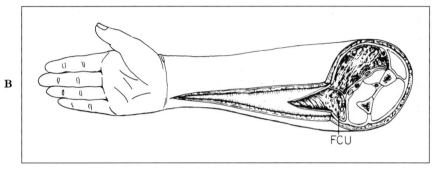

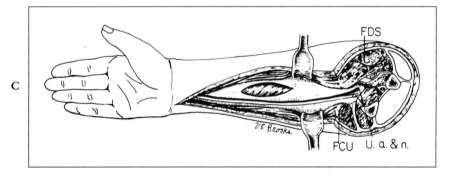

FIGURE 47-11

Surgical technique: forearm. **A,** The incision from the medial epicondyle to the ulnar-most extent of the flexor crease of the wrist. **B,** Lacertus fibrosus and fascia overlying the flexor carpi ulnaris (*FCU*) are opened. **C,** The FCU is retracted ulnarly and the flexor digitorum superficialis (*FDS*) is retracted radially to permit opening of the fascia of the deep palmar compartment. Care is taken to avoid the ulnar artery (*U.a.*) and nerve (*U.n.*). *(From Matsen et al.[38] By permission of the journal.)*

SURGICAL TREATMENT OF ACUTE COMPARTMENT SYNDROME

Detailed knowledge of the compartments of the finger, hand, wrist, and forearm is essential for all surgeons who perform compartment release (Table 47-1). The hand has 10 separate compartments: thenar, hypothenar, four dorsal interosseous compartments, three palmar interosseous compartments, and the adductor compartment (Fig. 47-10). The wrist contains two compartments: carpal tunnel and Guyon's canal. The forearm contains the palmar compartment, divided into superficial and deep, or the superficialis muscle and the profundus and flexor pollicis longus muscles, respectively (Figs. 47-11 and 47-12, *B*). There is also a dorsal compartment and the compartment containing the mobile wad muscles (the brachioradialis and the radial wrist extensors).[46]

In rare situations both the hand and the forearm will be involved—e.g., if both are crushed or severely burned or with vascular injury proximal to the hand with severe upper extremity hand swelling. The hand alone can be involved after injection injury, severe local crush or burn, or multiple, closed hand fractures.

Safe release of the thenar compartment can be accomplished with an incision on the radial border of the thumb metacarpal through the thenar fascia near the bone (Fig. 47-10). This keeps the dissection well away from tendons, vessels, and nerves. A small branch of the radial sensory nerve can be encountered in this area and should be protected. A similar method is used to release the hypothenar compartment, with an incision at the ulnar border of the fifth metacarpal, again keeping dissection away from nerve and vessel (Fig. 47-10). The dorsal ulnar sensory branch of the ulnar nerve can be encountered in this area and should be protected. In both areas this leaves the scar slightly dorsal to the muscle compartment where more extensile dorsal skin can stretch to allow swollen muscle to bulge adequately and keeps scar away from the potentially sensitive palmar surface.

SURGICAL TECHNIQUE: HAND AND WRIST

Release of the interosseous compartments (Fig. 47-10) can be accomplished by two dorsal longitudinal incisions: one is placed over the index and the other over the ring metacarpal.[46] This is the preferred

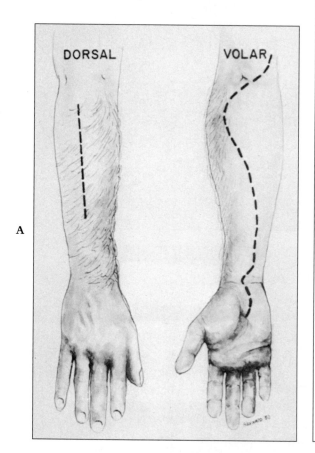

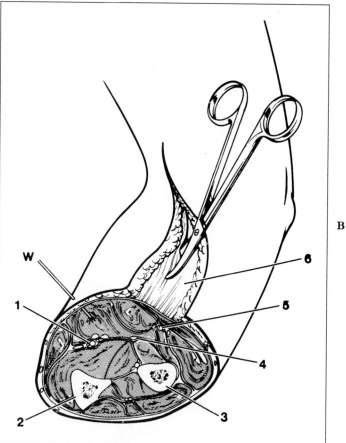

FIGURE 47-12

A, *Left:* The dorsal midline longitudinal incision between the extensor carpi radialis and the extensor digitorum communis muscles is preferred, with care to extend the release down to the deep muscles overlying the interosseous membrane. *Right:* The preferred palmar incision begins proximally in the antecubital fossa and extends distally in a curvilinear fashion to the wrist, where it crosses the carpal tunnel in a zigzag or curvilinear incision. **B,** Diagrammatic cross section of the left midforearm with the Wick catheter (*W*) in place and the surgical scissors releasing the superficial fascia (*6*). *1,* ulnar nerve; *2,* ulna; *3,* radius; *4,* median nerve; *5,* radial nerve. *(From Gelberman et al.[18] By permission of JB Lippincott.)*

technique. An alternative is to use a transverse dorsal incision over the metacarpals[52] or three dorsal incisions. With three incisions, there is the least undermining of skin flaps. In this technique, one incision is placed over the first web longitudinally and allows release of the first dorsal interosseous and abductor pollicis muscles. A second incision is placed in line with the third metacarpal. Just radial to this incision, the fascia of the second dorsal interosseous and first palmar interosseous muscles can be released. Ulnar to this incision, the fascia of the third dorsal interosseous and second palmar interosseous muscles can be released. The third incision is placed between the fourth and fifth metacarpals for release of the fourth dorsal interosseous muscle and third palmar interosseous fascia.

The wrist compartments can both be released by a standard open carpal tunnel release technique. This is performed at the same time as a palmar forearm release and in fact can be the first step in the forearm release. The incision is placed longitudinally between the third and fourth metacarpals, at the ulnar aspect of the carpal tunnel, then curves ulnarward across the wrist flexion crease, in line with the linear portion of the incision ulnar to the palmaris longus tendon for release of the distal forearm fascia (see Chapter 51). Retraction of the ulnar flap in an ulnar direction, everting its edge, reveals the fascia over Guyon's canal, which is easily released with the ulnar nerve and artery under direct vision.

SURGICAL TECHNIQUE: FOREARM

The palmar forearm release incision has been described as curvilinear,[46] zigzag, and straight ulnar.[38] The shape of the incision (Figs. 47-11 and 47-12) is not as important as the principle that the release should be extensile, from above the antecubital fossa to the end of the carpal tunnel. The general principles

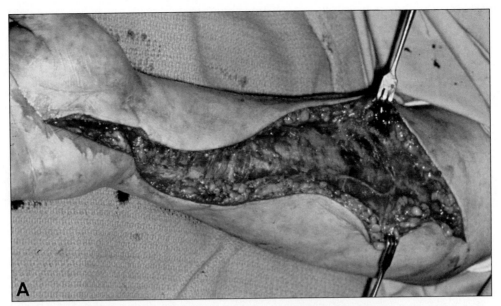

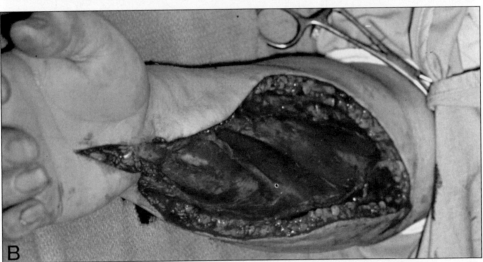

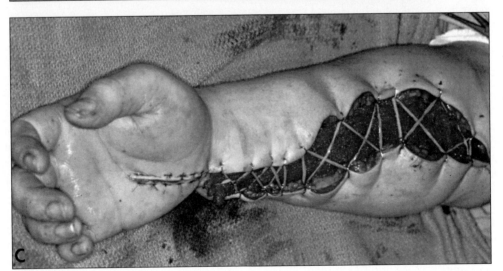

FIGURE 47-13

A, Acute forearm compartment syndrome in a 36-year-old woman with toxic shock syndrome and swollen upper and lower extremities. The incision for release of the forearm begins at the carpal tunnel, crosses the wrist flexion crease obliquely and ulnarly, and curves radially toward the proximal forearm and back ulnarly to include the antecubital fossa. Forearm fascia is clearly identified the length of the incision. Skin release alone does not release muscle compartments or relieve increased pressure. **B,** After incision of the fascia, the swollen muscle is able to bulge freely. **C,** Partial closure of the wound proximally and distally is performed without tension or avascular skin edges.

are that the incision must be oriented primarily in a longitudinal way without transverse elements that would cross skin creases in a straight line. It should create skin flaps that allow access to the forearm fascia in an extensile fashion; that do not place the ulnar nerve and artery, the median nerve, or the radial nerve and artery at risk during the release; and that allow these structures to remain covered despite muscle bulging after release. The interval between the flexor digitorum superficialis and the flexor digitorum profundus with the median nerve lying between them (i.e., the area of greatest potential of muscle and nerve ischemia) must be accessible for individual muscle release. A special consideration would be a need for exploration of either the radial or ulnar artery when vascular damage is suspected; the incision can be centered over the particular area of interest. If brachial artery damage is suspected, the incision can be extended further proximally above the antecubital crease and medial to the biceps tendons.

My colleagues and I prefer a curvilinear incision (Fig. 47-12), beginning with release of the carpal tunnel. The incision curves gently from ulnar to radial at the level of the middle third of the forearm after release of the distal forearm fascia in line with the transverse carpal ligament and ulnar to the palmaris longus tendon. The incision continues to curve radially until the proximal third level of the forearm, where it curves back again in an ulnar direction into the antecubital crease and continues longitudinally ulnar to the biceps tendon. Proximally, the distal fascia of the arm, the lacertus fibrosus, and the proximal forearm fascia are released (Figs. 47-11, B and C). If median paresthesias are a prominent feature of the compartment syndrome, then the median nerve is released between the heads of the pronator muscle and beneath the superficialis arch.[18] The palmar forearm fascia is released the entire remaining length of the forearm (Fig. 47-13). The median nerve is traced from distal at the level of the tendons to proximal, beneath and within the superficialis muscle (Figs. 47-14, A through C). Individual superficialis, profundus, and flexor pollicis longus muscle releases are performed as needed. Individual arteries are inspected, as indicated by the injury.

Sheridan and Matsen[51] alluded to a "closed" fasciotomy technique. The controversial modification of the standard open extensile release for palmar fasciotomy is the partially closed fasciotomy. This technique, which could be considered in early compartment syndrome, endeavors to leave a bridge of skin intact over the distal third of the forearm under which a well-visualized subcutaneous fasciotomy is done. The rationale for this technique is that the distal third of the forearm contains mostly tendons and little or no muscle and that intact skin over a short area could make later wound closure easier. Potential disadvantages of this technique are incomplete fasciotomy

(especially deep fascia and epimysium) or injury to the median nerve or ulnar neurovascular bundle.

Dorsal forearm compartment release is accomplished with a straight incision over the dorsal midline of the middle third of the forearm, through which the mobile wad and dorsal forearm muscles can be approached. This incision may not be necessary, however, because palmar compartment release may lower dorsal forearm compartment pressures, and dorsal compartment pressure measurements after palmar fasciotomy have been recommended to determine the need for dorsal fasciotomy.[18] My colleagues and I prefer, however, to release the dorsal compartment whenever indicated preoperatively by the clinical examination and appropriate pressure measurements. Isolated dorsal compartment syndrome without palmar compartment ischemia can lead to wrist and finger extension contracture. A separate incision to prevent this complication should be addressed by the incision described above.

After fasciotomy, the skin is not closed. Skin edges can be loosely approximated with sutures, leaving ample room for the wound to spread and to allow muscle bulging and for good circulation to remain in the skin flaps (Fig. 47-13, C). Coverage should be with non-adherent dressings and bulky gauze, with the fingers free for motion. Wound coverage can occur in 48 hours by either direct skin closure, if muscle swelling is markedly decreased, or by split-thickness skin graft and partial closure, as necessary. Dressings are similar for release of hand compartments. If swelling is severe, including intrinsic minus posturing that is difficult to overcome passively, then MCP joints can be pinned in flexion to avoid potential collateral ligament fibrotic shortening.

SURGICAL TREATMENT OF ESTABLISHED VOLKMANN'S CONTRACTURE

Volkmann's contracture affecting the hand alone involves severe intrinsic tightness and first web contracture secondary to thumb adductor ischemia (Figs. 47-15, A through C). Details on release of the contracture should center on precisely localizing the site of pathology. Is the primary contracture at the level of the interosseous muscle bellies, the tendons, the collateral ligaments of the MCP joints, or the palmar plate and more distally at the level of the lateral bands? Determining these factors allows one to focus the surgical release and to decide whether the proximal interphalangeal joint is affected alone or with the MCP joint (Fig. 47-14, C). Release can occur at the distal intrinsic level and progress proximally as needed to the level of the interosseous tendons at the base of the proximal phalanx or more proximally at the interosseous muscle insertions on the metacarpals, as described in detail by Smith.[52]

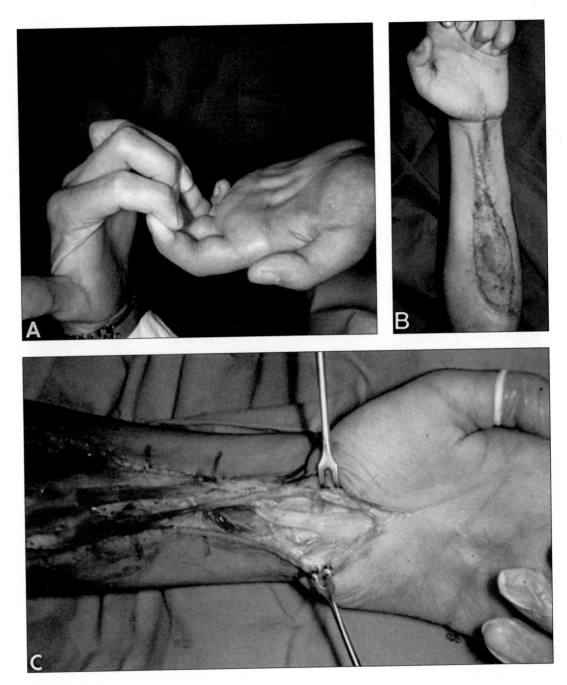

FIGURE 47-14

A and **B,** Passive extension and active flexion in a 26-year-old man after palmar forearm release and split-thickness skin closure for chronic compartment syndrome, resulting from being repeatedly struck in the forearm with a shovel. Despite compartment release, Volkmann's ischemic contracture gradually developed. **C,** The median nerve is identified in the carpal canal and traced proximally into the scar.

Volkmann's contracture affects the wrist most commonly by causing wrist flexion, but wrist extension contracture secondary to isolated dorsal compartment syndrome is also possible. Bunnell[9] described release of the pronator quadratus and pronator teres for wrist pronation contracture. Isolated wrist contracture, however, is rare and is considered an element of forearm ischemic contracture. Historical salvage procedures directed at the wrist, such as carpectomy or wrist fusion, are not performed because release of the forearm contracture by excision of the infarct improves wrist position adequately in the majority of cases. Steindler[53] pointed out that Z lengthening of contracted wrist flexors is useful, and he discouraged the use of bony procedures on the wrist.

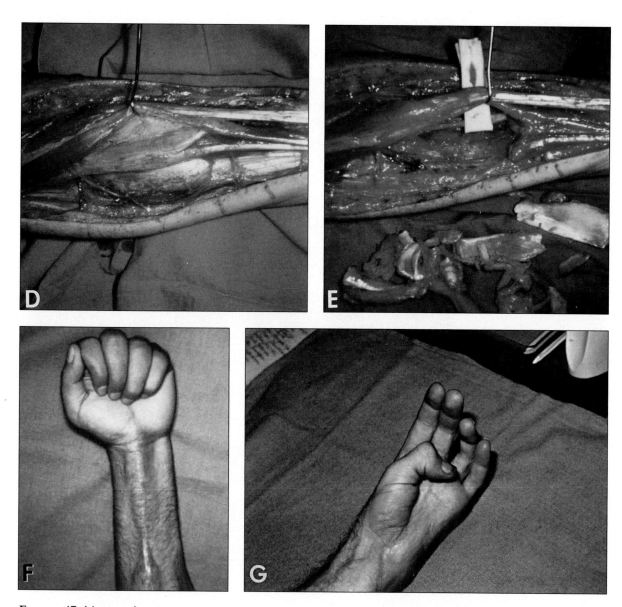

FIGURE 47-14, CONT'D.

D and **E,** Extensile palmar forearm incision for excision of infarcted flexor muscle group. Avascular muscle will appear yellowish gray. The flexor pollicis longus, flexor superficialis, flexor profundus, and the wrist flexors were excised. The Penrose drain protects the median nerve after it is freed from scar. **F,** Active thumb and digital flexion after secondary reconstruction by transfer of the brachioradialis to the flexor pollicis longus and **(G)** the extensor carpi radialis to the flexor digitorum profundus.

Seddon's[49] description of the gross pathology and surgical anatomy in forearm ischemic contracture is accurate and useful. He described an infarct as a three-dimensional ellipse, the center axis of which is the anterior interosseous arch, surrounding the flexor pollicis longus, flexor profundus, and flexor superficialis. The ulnar neurovascular bundle is at the periphery of the infarct and less often involved. He distinguished between muscle fibrosis and necrosis and recommended a waiting period before exploration because of the partial ability of muscle to regenerate. He described a detailed surgical approach, the principle of which was excision of all necrotic tissue (guided by gross appearance of nerve and muscle and response to nerve stimulation), complete neurolysis, and reconstruction by tendon transfer.

Eaton and Green[13,14] reviewed surgical procedures in established Volkmann's contracture and found that proximal flexor pronator muscle release, median and ulnar neurolysis, and tendon transfer could be useful. Buck-Gramcko and Fry[8] described four stages of established forearm contracture based on muscle and nerve changes. The earliest stage did best with muscle slide procedures and the most severe stage was treated with wrist fusion, neurolysis, scar excision, muscle slide procedures, and extensor to flexor transfers.

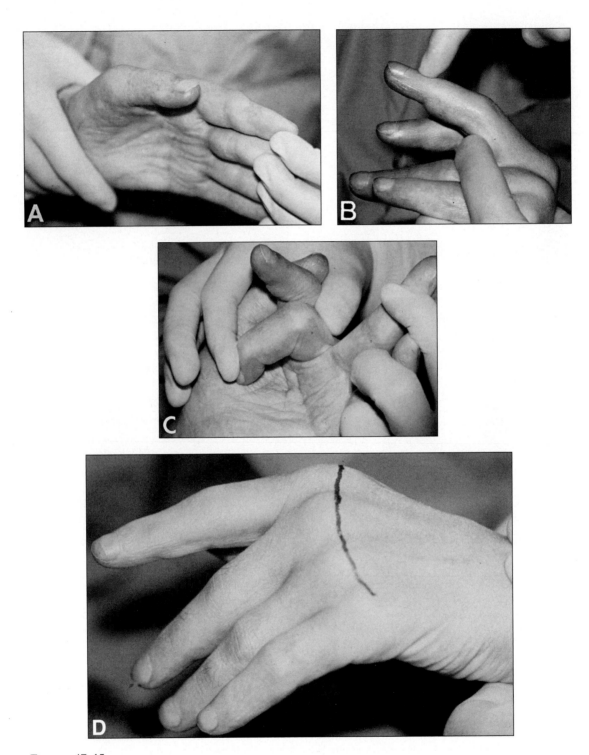

FIGURE 47–15

Intrinsic contracture and Volkmann's contracture of the forearm secondary to axillary artery disruption. Note **(A)** limited passive metacarpophalangeal extension and a positive intrinsic tightness test **(B** and **C)**. **D,** Dorsal transverse incision over the metacarpophalangeal joints for release of metacarpophalangeal joint contracture, lengthening of the interosseous muscle, and distal intrinsic tendon release.

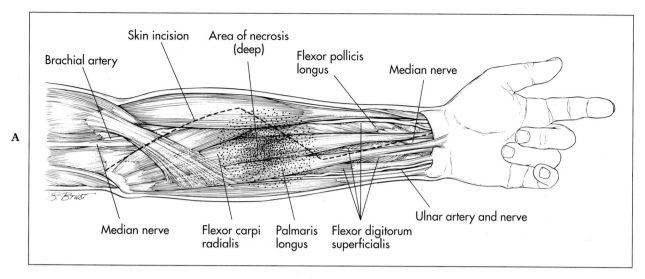

A

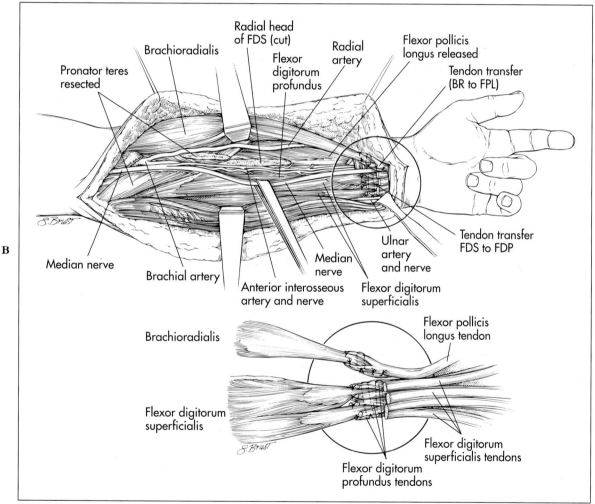

B

FIGURE 47-16

Treatment options for Volkmann's contracture based on the degree of muscle ischemia and necrosis. **A,** The area of necrosis described by Seddon is deep to the palmaris longus and flexor superficialis muscles, involving the flexor digitorum profundus and the flexor pollicis longus (*FPL*). Surgical treatment generally involves an extended forearm incision beginning in the antecubital fossa where the median nerve and brachial artery can be identified. The incision is extended distally in a zigzag fashion to the wrist and the carpal tunnel. **B,** For the mild to moderate cases of Volkmann's contracture, it is necessary to perform a complete neurolysis of the median nerve, to release the anterior interosseous nerve, and to release the flexor digitorum profundus and the flexor pollicis longus. After their release, tendon transfers are performed: flexor digitorum superficialis (*FDS*) to the flexor digitorum profundus (*FDP*) and brachioradialis (*BR*) to the FPL.

Continued.

C

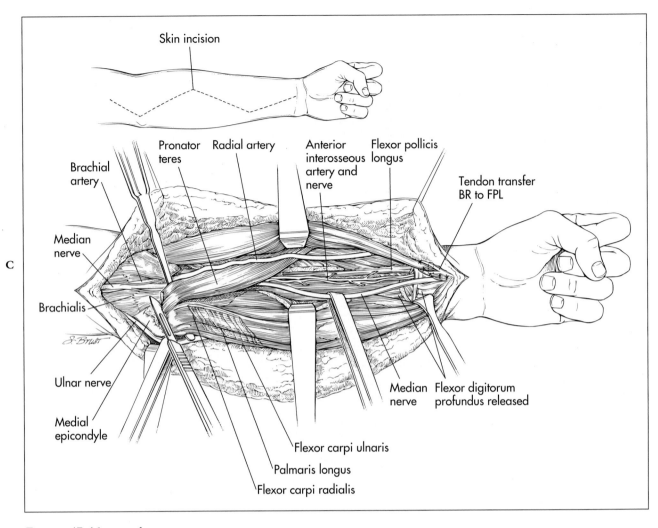

FIGURE 47-16, CONT'D.

C, For the more moderate to severe cases, the flexor pronator slide may be more efficient than tendon transfer. Neurolysis of the median nerve and the anterior interosseous nerve is performed deep to the superficial muscles, beginning proximally at the elbow and distally at the wrist and then moving to the area of compression and scarring. The flexor profundus and flexor pollicis longus (*FPL*) usually need to be released. The brachioradialis (*BR*) can be transferred to the FPL; the flexor pronator origin can then be released from the medial epicondyle, proximal to middle third of the ulna, with care taken to identify and protect the ulnar nerve, brachial artery, and its radial and ulnar branches.

Tsuge,[57] borrowing heavily from Seddon's original description of ischemic contracture pathology, described three stages of contracture: 1) mild, involving isolated flexor profundus units and no fixed joint or intrinsic contracture; 2) moderate, including flexor profundus and flexor pollicis longus contracture, with or without superficialis or wrist flexor involvement; and 3) severe, with all flexors and some extensors involved and severe nerve compression. Extensive muscle slide procedures were recommended, with neurolysis in early stages and muscle excision and reconstruction for the late severe type.

In the planning for surgery of established Volkmann's contracture of the forearm,[17] the first step is to establish realistic functional goals with the patient and family. Often hand function is extremely limited and even a small increase in function is appreciated by the patient. If contracture has been present for a long enough time for the patient to have adapted well to it, surgery should not be done for cosmetic reasons alone. Each case is individualized, requiring more or less release of fascial tissues and extensive dissection, depending on the amount of necrotic muscle and nerve compression (Fig. 47-16).

The essential plan is to excise necrotic muscle and to perform a neurolysis. A flexor-pronator origin release may be appropriate if there is a wrist flexion and pronation contracture, but muscle slide procedures that do not address the necrotic muscle are not as direct an approach to the deformity. Muscle release alone should be reserved for musculotendinous units that retain some contractility. A lengthening done at

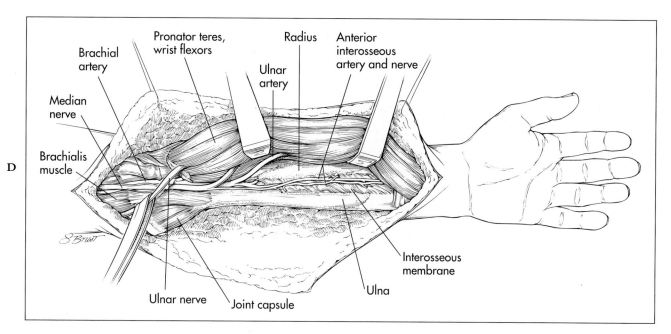

D

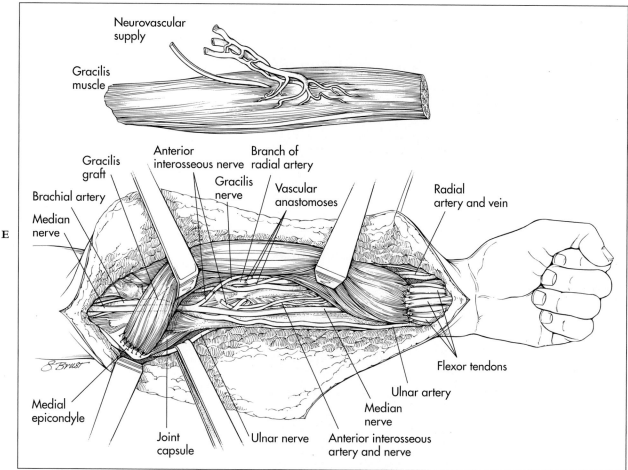

E

FIGURE 47-16, CONT'D.

D, The dissection and release of the flexor pronator origin, which should include the flexor carpi radialis, palmaris longus, and flexor carpi ulnaris, starts proximally at the medial epicondyle and proceeds distally along the ulna and interosseous membrane, with the degree of muscle release related to the flexion contracture of the wrist and fingers. A goal is wrist extension of 20° with near full finger extension. Neurolysis of the median nerve and anterior interosseous nerve should be performed and care should be taken to protect the vascular structures deep in the forearm. The ulnar nerve may need anterior transposition or may be left in its normal position, depending on the degree of release of the flexor carpi ulnaris muscle. **E,** For the severe case in which there is complete muscle degeneration often including the superficial muscles, a free muscle transfer may be indicated. Muscle options include the pectoralis major, latissimus dorsi, or gracilis. The gracilis, after harvest from the medial aspect of the proximal thigh, fits the length needed quite well. It is first reinnervated through a normal part of the anterior interosseous nerve (confirmed by frozen section) and revascularized by the radial or brachial artery. The proximal end of the muscle is then attached to the medial epicondyle, and distally the flexor tendons (flexor profundus and flexor pollicis longus) are interwoven into the muscle or muscle-tendon junction with tension of the fingers judged with the wrist in neutral flexion-extension. If there is a skin and soft-tissue contracture and scarring, a myocutaneous transfer can be considered.

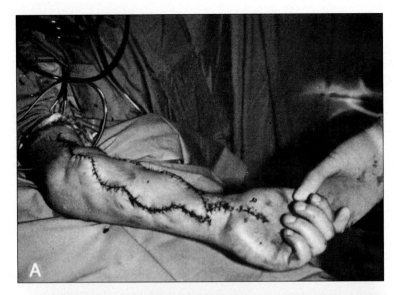

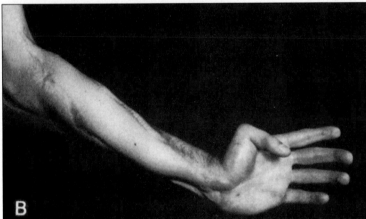

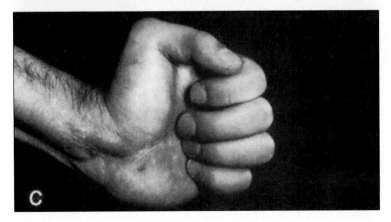

FIGURE 47-17

A, Microvascular treatment of Volkmann's ischemic contracture by transfer of a latissimus dorsi musculo-cutaneous flap in an 11-year-old boy. Immediate post-transfer appearance demonstrates the cutaneous transfer and extended incision for release of the transverse carpal ligament distally and lacertus fibrosus and biceps aponeurosis proximally. Nerve repair was performed by connecting the long thoracic nerve of the latissimus to the anterior interosseous nerve. **B,** At a 7-year follow-up, maximum active wrist and finger extension are demonstrated. There is a residual flexion contracture of the thumb, which was not included in the flexor tendon release and free muscle transfer. **C,** Active flexion of the fingers with extension of the wrist demonstrates complete release of the flexor contracture. *(From Favero KJ, Wood MB, Meland NB: Transfer of innervated latissimus dorsi free musculo-cutaneous flap for the restoration of finger flexion, J Hand Surg [Am] 18:535-540, 1993. Copyright, American Society for Surgery of the Hand, by permission of Churchill Livingstone.)*

the musculotendinous junction in these cases may be preferable to one done more proximally. Tendon transfers such as brachioradialis to the flexor pollicis longus and flexor superficialis to flexor profundus may be selected in mild to moderate cases, and the flexor slide procedures may be used in mild (minimal release 1-2 cm) or severe (complete release of 3-4 cm) cases when muscle-tendon transfer from scar or contracture is not possible. Finally, free muscle transfer (gracilis,

pectoralis major, or latissimus dorsi) can be performed when there is severe contracture without possibility of tendon lengthening or release (Figs. 47-17 and 47-18).

The timing of operation is individualized as well. A waiting period of 3 months is appropriate to allow muscle recovery to occur and the degree of muscle necrosis to stabilize. The quality of nerve recovery is directly related to a thorough neurolysis; thus, there is some urgency to operate on the patient with severe

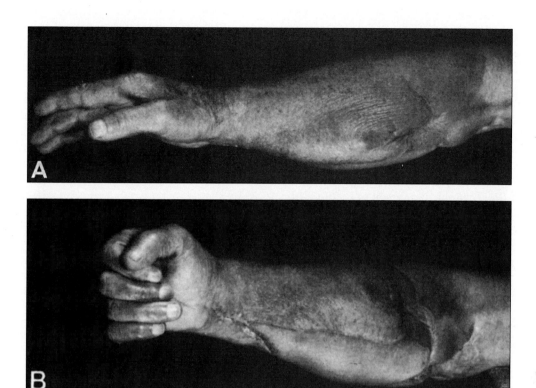

FIGURE 47-18

A 24-year-old man demonstrates finger extension **(A)** and flexion **(B)** after latissimus dorsi free muscu-locutaneous transfer for Volkmann's ischemic contracture. *(From Favero KJ, Wood MB, Meland NB: Transfer of innervated latissimus dorsi free musculocutaneous flap for the restoration of finger flexion,* J Hand Surg [Am] *18:535-540, 1993. Copyright, American Society for Surgery of the Hand, by permission of Churchill Livingstone.)*

nerve involvement. It is assumed that the nerve lesion can recover, if only partially, and nerve excision, as described by Seddon from actual necrosis, should be rare. Neurolysis may need to be supplemented by epineurotomy or group fascicular neurolysis, but rarely is a nerve necrotic enough to require complete excision.

PREFERRED SURGICAL APPROACH

Surgery is performed with tourniquet control to improve identification of viable muscle and because the infarct area is usually obvious. Dead muscle is yellow to gray. It is essentially fibrous tissue partially stained by hemosiderin. The surgical plan is to begin at the carpal tunnel, with complete release, and trace the median nerve in a proximal direction (Fig. 47-14). Carpal tunnel release should be done in almost all cases. It would be an unusual case that would not require carpal tunnel surgery. An example might be a patient with minimal nerve dysfunction and a wrist contracture suggesting that the nerve is caught in scar predominantly in the forearm. Most patients with forearm infarcts and contractures do not also have hand contracture unless there has been crush of both.

In patients with isolated hand contracture, carpal tunnel release and intrinsic muscle release should be included as part of Volkmann's contracture release.

Beginning the approach distally is preferable to beginning proximally, because at the level of the tendons in the distal third of the forearm the damage and scarring are least. The median nerve is essentially caught between superficial and deep infarcts, usually between the flexor superficialis and the flexor profundus tendons. The concept of the median nerve as a "satellite" of the superficialis muscle, as put forth by Henry,[25] is helpful in tracing the median nerve through the scarred superficialis muscle. Surgical intervention primarily involves neurolysis of median and ulnar nerves, carefully separating the nerve from the scarred muscle, with excision of the dead muscle. Proximal to distal dissection of median and ulnar nerves and brachial radial and ulnar arteries is carefully performed with loop magnification. Dissection proceeds in an orderly fashion from superficial to deep and from ulnar to radial. In addition to the ulnar neurovascular bundle, median nerve, radial artery, and radial nerve, the anterior interosseous artery is at risk and should be identified and protected. Scar and fibrosis may be so dense that the dissection needs to proceed proximal to the antecubital fossa, identifying nerve and vessel proximally and then tracing distally to meet the distal nerve and vessel dissection. Identification of the median nerve proximally where it appears to be normal, with dissection progressing distally toward the damaged muscle, helps prevent unwanted nerve and vessel damage.

It is rare that the hand and forearm are both involved. If this is the case, the intrinsic release can work against correction of finger deformity because it will increase proximal interphalangeal joint flexion, which is the primary problem or result of the forearm contracture. Excision of the forearm infarct should result in almost full correction of the wrist and finger flexion deformity. Bony procedures such as wrist fusion or carpectomy are necessary only in late, fixed deformity. The exceptions to correction of finger deformity after infarct incision in the forearm are the MCP joints. Residual flexion contracture at this level may be due to intrinsic contracture, specifically of the interosseous muscles tightly holding the MCP joints in flexion (Fig. 47-15). If this is the case, release of intrinsic muscles from their skeletal origin is then suggested. First web contracture may also be present due to a necrotic adductor muscle that may require partial excision and release.

After incision of the forearm infarct, reconstruction should be done secondarily. Options include tendon transfer (Fig. 47-16, *B*), muscle release (flexor-pronator slide) (Fig. 47-16, *C*), or free muscle transfer (Figs. 47-17 and 47-18). For any of these procedures, the general principles of tendon transfer apply. These include a stable wound free of inflammation and time, which allows for tissue planes to be reestablished along the plane of infarct excision. Scar should be mobile, extensile, and supple. The joints of the hand and wrist should be supple, and there should be no hand or forearm edema.

In tendon transfer, the muscles most likely to be available are the brachioradialis and wrist extensors (i.e., the mobile wad muscles), which are rarely necrotic. The brachioradialis muscle has been particularly useful in providing thumb flexion,[15] and either the healthy flexor superficialis or extensor carpi radialis longus can be used effectively for finger flexors.

Postoperative care is mandatory to prevent recurrence and to maximize the surgical release and transfers. Cast and splint immobilization should be continued a minimum of 3 and upward to 6 months. The goals include wrist extension to 20° (or more) and full finger extension with the wrist in neutral position to 20° extension.

REFERENCES

1. Aerts P, De Boeck HD, Casteleyn PP, et al.: Deep volar compartment syndrome of the forearm following minor crush injury, *J Pediatr Orthop* 9:69-71, 1989.

2. Ashton H: The effect of increased tissue pressure on blood flow, *Clin Orthop* 113:15-26, 1975.

3. Awbrey BJ, Sienkiewicz PS, Mankin HJ: Chronic exercise-induced compartment pressure elevation measured with a miniaturized fluid pressure monitor. A laboratory and clinical study, *Am J Sports Med* 16:610-615, 1988.

4. Bardenheuer H: Die Entstehung und Behandlung der ischämischen Muskelkontraktur und Gangrän, *Dtsch Z Chir Leipz* 108:44-201, 1910-1911.

5. Benjamin A: The relief of traumatic arterial spasm in threatened Volkmann's ischaemic contracture, *J Bone Joint Surg Br* 39:711-713, 1957.

6. Brand PW: *Clinical mechanics of the hand,* St. Louis, CV Mosby, 1985.

7. Brooks B: Pathologic changes in muscle as a result of disturbances of circulation: an experimental study of Volkmann's ischemic paralysis, *Arch Surg* 5:188-216, 1922.

8. Buck-Gramcko D, Fry C: Ischemic contracture of the forearm and hand. Staging and indications for surgical treatment [German]. *Handchir Mikrochir Plast Chir* 23:128-143, 1991.

9. Bunnell S: *Surgery of the hand,* ed 2, Philadelphia, 1948, JB Lippincott, pp 221-231.

10. Burton AC: On physical equilibrium of small blood vessels, *Am J Physiol* 164:319-329, 1951.

11. Cooney WP III, Dobyns JH, Linscheid RL: Complications of Colles' fractures, *J Bone Joint Surg Am* 62:613-619, 1980.

12. Denolf F, Roos J, Feyen J: Compartment syndrome after fracture of the distal radius, *Acta Orthop Belg* 60:339-342, 1994.

13. Eaton RG, Green WT: Epimysiotomy and fasciotomy in the treatment of Volkmann's ischemic contracture, *Orthop Clin North Am* 3:175-186, 1972.

14. Eaton RG, Green WT: Volkmann's ischemia. A volar compartment syndrome of the forearm, *Clin Orthop* 113:58-64, 1975.

15. Failla JM, Peimer CA, Sherwin FS: Brachioradialis transfer for digital palsy, *J Hand Surg [Br]* 15:312-316, 1990.

16. Flaubert G: *Madame Bovary: background and sources, essays in criticism.* In De Man P, editor: New York, 1965, WW Norton, pp 128-129.

17. Geary N: Late surgical decompression for compartment syndrome of the forearm, *J Bone Joint Surg Br* 66:745-748, 1984.

18. Gelberman RH, Garfin SR, Hergenroeder PT, et al.: Compartment syndromes of the forearm: diagnosis and treatment, *Clin Orthop* 161:252-261, 1981.

19. Gelberman RH, Hergenroeder PT, Hargens AR, et al.: The carpal tunnel syndrome. A study of carpal canal pressures, *J Bone Joint Surg Am* 63:380-383, 1981.

20. Griffiths DL: Volkmann's ischaemic contracture, *Br J Surg* 28:239-260, 1940.

21. Hamilton FH: *Deformities after fractures,* Philadelphia, 1856, TK & PG Collins (reproduced from *Tr Am Med Assoc* 8:1855).

22. Hamilton FH: *A practical treatise on fractures and dislocations,* Philadelphia, 1860, Blanchard and Lea, pp 266-325.

23. Hargens AR, Akeson WH, Mubarak SJ, et al.: Fluid balance within the canine anterolateral compartment and its relationship to compartment syndromes, *J Bone Joint Surg Am* 60:499-505, 1978.

24. Hargens AR, Romine JS, Sipe JC, et al.: Peripheral nerve-conduction block by high muscle-compartment pressure, *J Bone Joint Surg Am* 61:192-200, 1979.

25. Henry AK: *Extensile exposure,* ed 2, Edinburgh, 1973, Churchill Livingstone, pp 97-98.

26. Heppenstall RB, Sapega AA, Izant T, et al.: Compartment syndrome: a quantitative study of high-energy phosphorus compounds using ^{31}P-magnetic resonance spectroscopy, *J Trauma* 29:1113-1119, 1989.

27. Hernandez J Jr, Peterson HA: Fracture of the distal radial physis complicated by compartment syndrome and premature physeal closure, *J Pediatr Orthop* 6:627-630, 1986.

28. Hildebrand O: Die Lehre von den ischämischen muskellähmungen und Kontrakturen, *Samml Klin Vortr Leipz n F,* No. 437 (Chir, No. 122), 559-584, 1906.

29. Hippocrates. *Loeb classics,* vol 3. (English translation by ET Whitington Trans.) Cambridge, 1984, Harvard University Press, pp 95-115.

30. Jepson PN: Ischaemic contracture: experimental study, *Ann Surg* 84:785-795, 1926.

31. Jobe MT: *Volkmann's contracture and compartment syndromes.* In Crenshaw AH, editor: *Campbell's operative orthopaedics,* ed 8, vol 5, St. Louis, 1992, Mosby–Year Book, pp 3341-3345.

32. Knezevich S, Torch M: Streptococcal toxic shocklike syndrome leading to bilateral lower extremity compartment syndrome and renal failure. Report of a case, *Clin Orthop* 254:247-250, 1990.

33. Leser E: Untersuchungen über ischämische Muskellähmungen und Muskelcontracturen, *Samml Klin Vortr Leipz* No. 249 (Chir, No. 77), 2087-2114, 2 pl, 1884.

34. Linscheid RL, Dobyns JH, Beabout JW, et al.: Traumatic instability of the wrist. Diagnosis, classification, and pathomechanics, *J Bone Joint Surg Am* 54:1612-1632, 1972.

35. Majno G: *The healing hand: man and wound in the ancient world,* Cambridge, 1975, Harvard University Press, pp 395-427.

36. Matsen FA III: Compartmental syndrome. A unified concept, *Clin Orthop* 113:8-14, 1975.

37. Matsen FA III, Rorabeck CH: Compartment syndromes, *Instr Course Lect* 38:463-472, 1989.

38. Matsen FA III, Winquist RA, Krugmire RB Jr: Diagnosis and management of compartmental syndromes, *J Bone Joint Surg Am* 62:286-291, 1980.

39. Moed BR, Thorderson PK: Measurement of intracompartmental pressure: a comparison of the slit catheter, side-ported needle, and simple needle, *J Bone Joint Surg Am* 75:231-235, 1993.

40. Mubarak SJ, Hargens AR, Owen CA, et al.: The wick catheter technique for measurement of intramuscular pressure. A new research and clinical tool, *J Bone Joint Surg Am* 58:1016-1020, 1976.

41. Mubarak SJ, Owen CA, Hargens AR, et al.: Acute compartment syndromes: diagnosis and treatment with the aid of the wick catheter, *J Bone Joint Surg Am* 60:1091-1095, 1978.

42. Murphy JB: Myositis: ischemic myositis: infiltration myositis: cicatricial muscular or tendon fixation in forearm: internal, external and combined compression myositis, with subsequent musculotendinous shortening, *JAMA* 63:1249-1254, 1914.

43. Naidu SH, Heppenstall RB: Compartment syndrome of the forearm and hand, *Hand Clin* 10:13-27, 1994.

44. Pellegrini VD: *Complications.* In McCollister C, editor: *Fractures and dislocations,* ed 3, Philadelphia, 1991, JB Lippincott, pp 335-396.

45. Rorabeck CH, Castle GS, Hardie R, et al.: Compartmental pressure measurements: an experimental investigation using the slit catheter, *J Trauma* 21:446-449, 1981.

46. Rowland SA: *Fasciotomy: the treatment of compartment syndrome.* In Green DP, editor: *Operative hand surgery,* ed 2, vol 1, New York, 1988, Churchill Livingstone, pp 665-707.

47. Royle SG: Compartment syndrome following forearm fracture in children, *Injury* 21:73-76, 1990.

48. Royle SG: The role of tissue pressure recording in forearm fractures in children, *Injury* 23:549-552, 1992.

49. Seddon HJ: Volkmann's contracture: treatment by excision of the infarct, *J Bone Joint Surg Br* 38:152-174, 1956.

50. Shall J, Cohn BT, Froimson AI: Acute compartment syndrome of the forearm in association with fracture of the distal end of the radius. Report of two cases, *J Bone Joint Surg Am* 68:1451-1454, 1986.

51. Sheridan GW, Matsen FA III: Fasciotomy in the treatment of the acute compartment syndrome, *J Bone Joint Surg Am* 58:112-115, 1976.

52. Smith RJ: *Intrinsic contracture.* In Green DP, editor: *Operative hand surgery,* ed 2, vol 1, New York, 1988, Churchill Livingstone, pp 609-631.

53. Steindler A: *Traumatic deformities and disabilities of the upper extremity,* Springfield, Illinois, 1946, Charles C Thomas, p 279.

54. Stockley I, Harvey IA, Getty CJM: Acute volar compartment syndrome of the forearm secondary to fractures of the distal radius, *Injury* 19:101-104, 1988.

55. Strecker WB, Wood MB, Bieber EJ: Compartment syndrome masked by epidural anesthesia for postoperative pain. Report of a case, *J Bone Joint Surg Am* 68:1447-1448, 1986.

56. Trumble T: Forearm compartment syndrome secondary to leukemic infiltrates, *J Hand Surg [Am]* 12:563-565, 1987.

57. Tsuge K: *Management of established Volkmann's contracture.* In Green DP, editor: *Operative hand surgery,* ed 2, vol 1, New York, 1988, Churchill Livingstone, pp 591-607.

58. Volkmann R: Die ischämische Muskellähmungen und kontrakturen, *Centralbl Chir Leipz* 8:801-803, 1881.

59. Volkmann R: *Classic 27. Ischaemic muscle paralyses and contractures.* In Bick EM, editor: *Classics of orthopaedics,* Philadelphia, 1976, JB Lippincott.

60. Whitesides TE, Haney TC, Morimoto K, et al.: Tissue pressure measurements as a determinant for the need of fasciotomy, *Clin Orthop* 113:43-51, 1975.

61. Wright JG, Bogoch ER, Hastings DE: The "occult" compartment syndrome, *J Trauma* 29:133-134, 1989.

48

SYNOVITIS OF THE WRIST

Peter M. Murray, M.D.
Richard A. Berger, M.D., Ph.D.

RHEUMATOID SYNOVITIS
  PATHOMECHANICS
  WRIST SYNOVITIS
  SYNOVECTOMY
  AUTHORS' PREFERRED METHOD OF TREATMENT
OSTEOARTHRITIS
CRYSTALLINE-INDUCED SYNOVITIS
JUVENILE RHEUMATOID ARTHRITIS
OTHER FORMS OF SYNOVITIS
SILICONE SYNOVITIS
SURGICAL TECHNIQUE: AUTHORS' PREFERENCE

DORSAL WRIST SYNOVECTOMY
  SILICONE SYNOVITIS
  WRIST JOINT CLOSURE AND RETINACULUM
    TRANSFER
PALMAR TENOSYNOVECTOMY IN CARPAL TUNNEL
  RELEASE
ARTHROSCOPIC SYNOVECTOMY
  EQUIPMENT
  PROCEDURE
  POSTOPERATIVE MANAGEMENT

The wrist is a diarthrodial joint containing two rows of carpal bones and is lined by an extensive synovial membrane derived from embryonic mesenchyma. The word "synovia," Greek for "with egg," was applied to the fluid secreted by the synovium, which to the early observers resembled egg albumin. The synovium has villose projections into the joint, with an intima containing two types of cells: A and B. Type A cells predominate and are characterized by surface pila podia and many intracellular organelles. Type B cells are less well developed but are active in the production of synovial fluid protein.

Benjamin C. Brody was the first to recognize the pathologic importance of "synovitis" in patients with rheumatoid arthritis.[85] It was Swett[88] in 1923 who first popularized the technique of synovectomy when he reported on the results of 15 patients so treated. He believed that removal of diseased synovial tissue could slow down or even halt the progression of a disease process by enabling normal synovial tissue to regenerate. Subsequently, this hypothesis has been shared by many others, particularly as it relates to rheumatoid

arthritis.* Other arthritic processes, such as gout, pseudogout, septic arthritis, seronegative spondylopathies, and particulate debris synovitis, can ultimately attribute joint destruction to an active synovial membrane, irrespective of the joint involved.

RHEUMATOID SYNOVITIS

In 1948, O. J. Vaughan-Jackson of London, England, described the rupture of extensor tendons as a result of rheumatoid arthritis involving the distal radioulnar joint (DRUJ).[91] Before this, rheumatoid deformities of the wrist were essentially untreated. The description of these cases[91,92] helped physicians recognize the natural progression of wrist synovitis due to rheumatoid arthritis and perhaps heralded the modern era of rheumatoid hand and wrist surgical reconstruction.[29]

Although intensive research has been devoted to understanding rheumatoid arthritis, the actual etiology

---

* References 1,12,13,27,46,48,52,56,61,63,79,80,89,90.

still eludes investigators. Rheumatoid synovitis is similar to many viral conditions in animals, and the measles virus and parvovirus have been cultured from some patients with seronegative arthritides.[76] Increased numbers of antibodies to Epstein-Barr virus have also been observed in these patients. Early synovial changes in patients with rheumatoid arthritis include cell lining proliferation, edema of subsynovial tissue along with microvascular changes, and polymorphonuclear leukocyte invasion of the synovium.[76] Subsequently, the synovium becomes more edematous, with elongated villi projected into the joint and proliferation of lining cells from the typical three layers to three to four times this number. Vascular changes ultimately occur, with thrombosis and paravascular hemorrhages. Histologically, chronic rheumatoid synovium harbors T-cell lymphocytes as well as immunoglobulin G-producing plasma cells.[76,97]

PATHOMECHANICS

The progression and natural history of rheumatoid disease about the wrist have been debated. Most feel the wrist is affected within the first few years, with destruction of the digits following somewhat later.[14,43] The inciting events about the wrist are the result of changes in the synovium, which expands, stretches, and ultimately destroys the wrist joint capsule as well as the intraosseous ligaments.[92] These initial events later produce carpal collapse, with scaphoid rotatory instability ultimately causing palmar subluxation of the proximal carpal row.[54,80]

Hindley and Stanley[43] suggested that in the first 5 years of rheumatoid disease, radiocarpal involvement predominates. In a retrospective radiographic review of 50 wrists, they identified the lunate fossa as the most severely involved during the initial 5 years of rheumatoid disease, followed by the scaphoid fossa, with the midcarpal joint being relatively spared. After a mean follow-up of 9.56 years, the lunate fossa was still the most severely involved, but there was a "catching up" of the metacarpophalangeal joints with respect to severity of involvement. There was also significant early involvement of the distal radiolunate articulation (50%), but it was radiographically considered moderate.[26,74]

Straub and Ranawat[80] suggested from their observations that rheumatoid disease about the wrist begins in the extensor carpi ulnaris (ECU) tendon sheath, which later leads to involvement of the DRUJ. This causes destruction of the triangular fibrocartilage complex, leading to DRUJ subluxation and ultimately tendon rupture or the "Vaughan-Jackson lesion" (Fig. 48-1). They observed synovial involvement of the radiocarpal joint later in the disease process. Their recommendation was synovectomy early in the course of the disease (Fig. 48-2).

Buckland-Wright and Walker[14] performed a macroradiographic assessment of 40 patients with rheumatoid arthritis of the wrist and hand. They found that, on average, twice as many erosions occurred in the wrist as in the hand, with the largest number of erosions occurring in the scaphoid. Taleisnik[89] suggested that these scaphoid erosions result from "notching" or grooving of the scaphoid due to synovitis involving the radioscaphocapitate ligament. Ultimately, palmar ligamentous incompetence as a result of synovitis leads to ulnar translocation and palmar subluxation of the carpus. Martel and others[55] found ulnar styloid involvement in 46% of radiographs reviewed. Taleisnik[89] suggested that these findings indicate palmar synovitis of the ulnar carpal ligamentous complex insertion, and it is the incompetence of this ligamentous complex that ultimately leads to palmar subluxation of the carpus. It is also this resultant palmar subluxation that creates a relative supination of the carpus, allowing the ulnar head to become prominent dorsally.[89] This tendency is perhaps accentuated by synovial destruction of the triangular fibrocartilage and ECU tendon sheath, creating one of the early subtle physical findings of rheumatoid arthritis.

WRIST SYNOVITIS

Persistent synovitis eventually leads to interosseous ligament destruction, particularly the scapholunate interosseous ligament. Rotatory subluxation of the scaphoid follows.[79] The carpal collapse can be most easily appreciated radiographically by detection of an increasing scapholunate diastasis on the anteroposterior film and an increase in the scapholunate angle beyond 60° on the lateral view. Other less subtle physical findings of synovitis about the wrist include a generalized boggy, sometimes tender swelling over the dorsoradial and dorsoulnar aspects of the wrist. On clinical inspection, there is loss of the concave junction between the base of the thumb and the distal forearm along with an increased convexity occurring along the ulnar border of the wrist and forearm. Range of motion in all planes is diminished, as is grip strength. Easily overlooked is synovitis of the palmar aspect of the wrist. Inspection of the palmar aspect of the wrist in the patient with rheumatoid arthritis may reveal a generalized fullness with loss of observable tendon silhouettes beneath the skin. Local tenderness is present on palpation of the flexor tendons.[20] Patients with rheumatoid arthritis frequently have signs and symptoms of carpal tunnel syndrome that require carpal tunnel release. Barnes and Currey[5] studied history, physical findings, and electrodiagnostic tests in 45 randomly selected patients with seropositive rheumatoid arthritis, comparing them with 25 control patients. They found 69% of rheumatoid arthritis patients had findings consistent with carpal tunnel syndrome compared with only 15% in the control group.

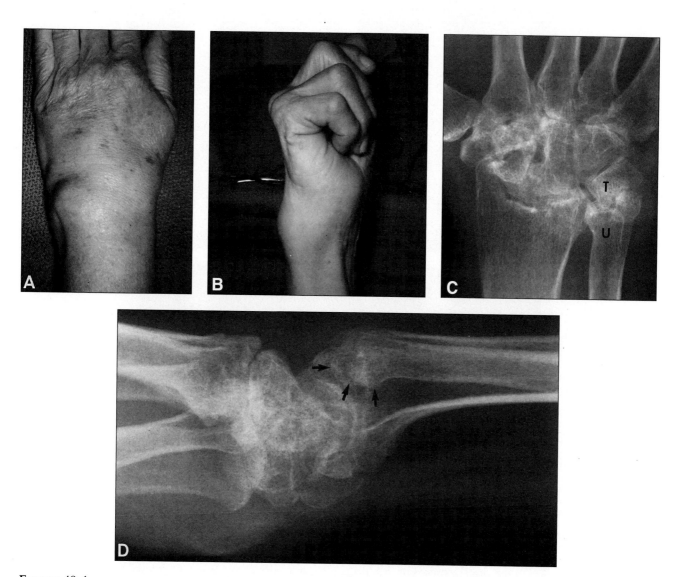

FIGURE 48-1

Instability of the distal radioulnar joint—"Vaughan-Jackson lesion." **A,** Dorsal subluxation of the ulna associated with rheumatoid synovitis. **B,** Ulnar aspect of the wrist shows prominent distal ulna and carpal supination. **C** and **D,** Posteroanterior **(C)** and lateral **(D)** radiographs of the right wrist of a patient with advanced changes associated with rheumatoid arthritis. **C,** Note the loss of carpal height from scapholunate dissociation and radiolunate subluxation. This results in palmar and proximal migration of the triquetrum (*T*), placing the head of the ulna (*U*) dorsal to the carpus. This is particularly evident in **D** (*arrows*). This creates the bony foundation for the "caput ulnae syndrome."

SYNOVECTOMY

Swett[88] was the first to introduce the concept of synovectomy as a means of removal of the etiologic agent in rheumatoid arthritis of the wrist. Although "complete synovectomy" is impossible, evidence suggests that limited synovectomy has at least some short-lived value in the early treatment of rheumatoid arthritis of the wrist.* Before surgical intervention, medical treatment should be maximized for 4 to 6 months.[34,56] Drugs such as prednisone, methotrexate, hydroxychloroquine, and various nonsteroidal anti-inflammatory agents can significantly arrest progression of wrist synovitis in rheumatoid patients. If this conservative approach to the treatment of wrist synovitis is chosen, the patient should also wear nighttime resting splints. Our preference is a forearm-based Orthoplast splint with the wrist in prehensile dorsiflexion of 30° and the digits in the patient's natural "resting position" (Fig. 48-3). Other nonoperative treatments have included chemical synovectomies using osmic acid, gold, rifamycin, phenylbutazone, or sodium salicylate—all having only limited success.[76]

When synovitis cannot be controlled medically, surgical intervention is indicated as long as the radiocarpal articulation has not been significantly involved. The Wrightington classification as described by

---

* References 1,13,46,48,56,58,71,89,90.

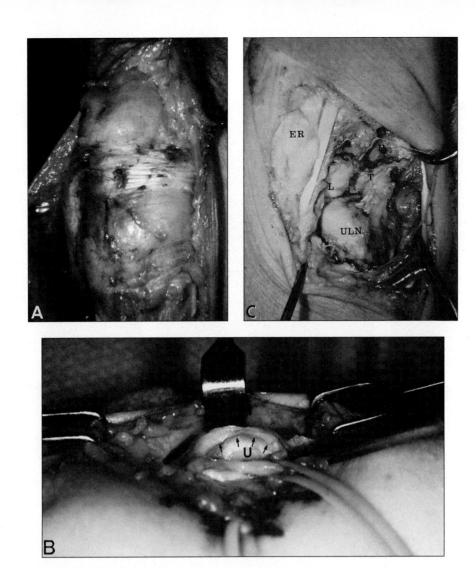

FIGURE 48-2

Synovitis of the wrist and distal radioulnar joint. **A,** Surgical dorsal-ulnar view shows extensive synovitis distal and proximal to the extensor retinaculum. **B,** Intraoperative view of a wrist with the "caput ulnae syndrome" approached through a dorsal incision, from a radial perspective. The head of the ulna (*U*) erupted through the dorsal joint capsule of the distal radioulnar joint (*arrows*). The vessel loop is around a "pseudotendon" remnant of the extensor digiti minimi, which was disrupted as a consequence of the prominent ulna. **C,** Postsynovectomy of midcarpal, radiocarpal, and distal radioulnar joints; extensor retinaculum (*ER*) reflected ulnarly. *H,* hamate; *L,* lunate; *T,* triquetrum; *ULN,* ulna.

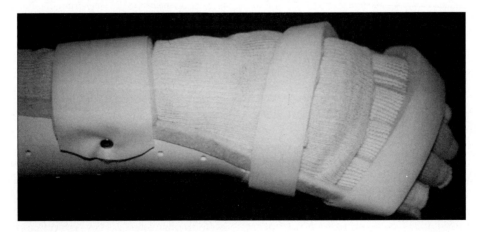

FIGURE 48-3

Photograph of a standard forearm-based resting splint constructed of thermally contoured plastic. The wrist is held in slight dorsiflexion and the fingers are supported in a resting flexion posture. Note the antiedema measures that have been instituted for the digits.

Hodgson et al.[44] categorizes rheumatoid arthritis of wrist into one of four grades.

Grade I: The majority of the wrist architecture is preserved, with the exception of early periarticular erosions and mild rotatory instability of the scaphoid.

Grade II: One or more of the following: 1) ulnar translocation of the carpus, 2) palmar flexion of the lunate, 3) palmar flexion of the scaphoid, or 4) radiolunate articular involvement.

Grade III: One of the following: 1) involvement of the articular surfaces between the carpal bones, 2) involvement of the radioscaphoid joint, or 3) palmar subluxation of the carpus.

Grade IV: Characterized by gross loss of bone stock from the distal radius.

Their recommendation was synovectomy for grade I involvement. Most agree with this approach.[24,48,56,79] Nalebuff[63] pointed out that the term "rheumatoid arthritis" is a misnomer because the disease is one of the synovium. He stressed that most synovectomies were performed too late and cautioned that there is little gain from performing synovectomies on wrists with radiographic evidence of joint destruction. Brumfield et al.[13] followed, for an average of 11 years, 102 wrist tenosynovectomies, wrist synovectomies, and Darrach resections in 78 patients. Pain was less in 83%, but 44% displayed progressive intra-articular destruction and there was a significant decrease in motion.

Other studies examined the combination of wrist synovectomy and extensor tenosynovectomy. Thirupathi et al.[90] concluded that dorsal wrist synovectomy along with tenosynovectomy of the extensor tendons, excision of the distal ulna, ulnar-sided stabilization of the wrist, and translocation of the extensor retinaculum were effective procedures. They performed surgery on 38 wrists in 27 patients with an average follow-up of 7.4 years. Ninety-five percent had pain relief. Carpal height was maintained in 70% of the wrists, but 44% displayed ulnar translocation. Kessler and Vainio[48] stressed that synovectomy of the wrist was productive only when done early in the disease process. Ishikawa et al.[46] followed, for 11 years, 43 rheumatoid wrists treated with wrist synovectomy and extensor tenosynovectomy combined with a Darrach procedure. The results in these patients were compared with the contralateral untreated wrists. They found pain was generally decreased, forearm rotation improved, and wrist dorsiflexion and palmar flexion were relatively unchanged. Progressive ulnar translation of the carpus did not occur (Fig. 48-4).

Yet, there is continued concern regarding the increased tendency toward ulnocarpal translocation in the operated wrist.[46] Most authors recommend ECU to extensor carpi radialis longus (ECRL) tendon transfer, as described by Clayton and Ferlic.[18] The biomechanical efficacy of this transfer was confirmed by Berger et al.[8] This study showed that releasing the ECRL tendon helps alleviate the ulnarly directed force responsible for the rheumatoid deformities about the wrist, including supination of the wrist and ulnar translocation of the carpus. Further, the study demonstrated that release of the ECRL tendon was the key to the procedure described by Clayton and Ferlic and that transfer of the ECRL to the ECU added little to its efficacy.

Other authors[71,89] have stressed the importance of recognizing palmar tenosynovitis and synovitis about the wrist. Taleisnik[89] recommended palmar joint synovectomy along with palmar tenosynovectomy and carpal tunnel decompression (when indicated) when palmar wrist joint involvement is suspected either clinically or radiographically. Ranawat and Straub[71] suggested early palmar tenosynovectomy in patients with rheumatoid arthritis who have progressive loss of active finger flexion as a result of palmar tenosynovitis of the wrist (Fig. 48-5).

No discussion of rheumatoid synovitis of the wrist would be complete without some mention of tendon rupture as a result of synovitis of the wrist. As mentioned previously, synovitis involving the ulnar side of

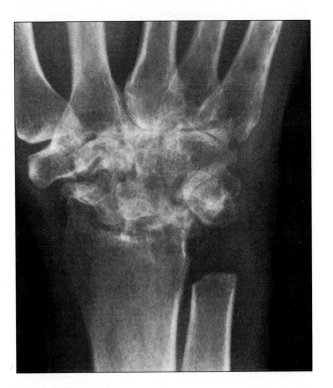

FIGURE 48-4

Posteroanterior radiograph of a wrist after a Darrach resection of the head of the ulna. Postresection ulnar translation of the carpus is not a concern here because of the ankylosis of the radiolunate articulation. Note how the radial edge of the osteotomy site has been contoured toward the radius metaphysis. An attempt to further stabilize the distal ulna is generally made by securing it with the pronator quadratus muscle and the triangular fibrocartilage complex.

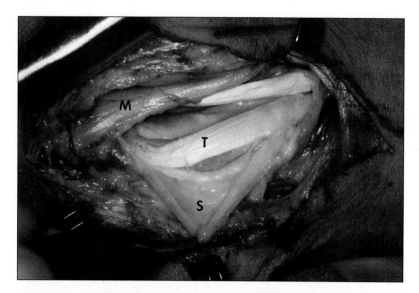

FIGURE 48-5

Intraoperative photograph of a flexor tenosynovectomy through the region of the carpal tunnel. The median nerve (*M*) is protected throughout the procedure. The tenosynovium (*S*) is stripped off of each flexor tendon (*T*) sequentially. This allows for an efficient and effective tenosynovectomy, with final resection of the residual tenosynovium at the end of the procedure. Obvious intratendinous extensions of the abnormal tenosynovium and cysts are excised at this time.

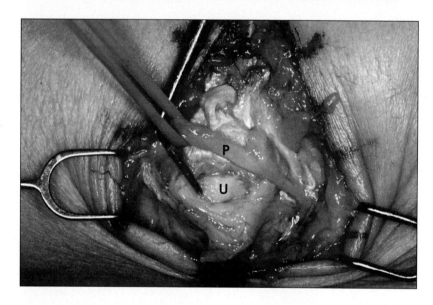

FIGURE 48-6

Intraoperative photograph of a pseudotendon (*P*) resulting from rupture of the extensor digiti minimi tendon in a patient with "caput ulnae syndrome." Note the prominence of the exposed ulnar head (*U*).

the wrist may destroy the soft–tissue stabilizers of the DRUJ, resulting in destabilization of that joint with subsequent rupture of the extensor digitorum quinti and extensor digitorum communis (EDC) to the ring finger, EDC to the long finger, EDC to the index finger, and extensor pollicis longus (EPL) (Fig. 48-6).[91,92] Direct repair or tenodesis is indicated at the time of wrist synovectomy. Moore et al.[61] found that isolated tendon rupture had a higher percentage of good results, whereas the number of favorable results decreased sharply with multiple tendon ruptures. Although abrasion of the extensor tendons over bony processes may account for the majority of attritional extensor tendon ruptures in rheumatoid arthritis, direct synovial invasion and devascularization may also play a role.

Open synovectomy of the wrist has been the standard technique of surgical synovectomy for the rheumatoid wrist, allowing access to the extensor tendons. However, the advent of arthroscopy has created another

surgical option. Adolfsson and Nylander[1] arthroscopically treated 18 wrists in 16 patients who had synovitis from rheumatoid arthritis. Motorized shavers measuring 3.5 mm and 2 mm in diameter were used to accomplish a radical synovectomy. Although follow-up was limited to 6 months, all patients experienced a decrease in pain and an increase in grip strength and range of motion. The long-term efficacy of arthroscopic synovectomy of the wrist is still not known.

AUTHORS' PREFERRED METHOD OF TREATMENT

We recommend early, open wrist synovectomy (Fig. 48-7), with extensor tenosynovectomy and extensor tendon repair as indicated, for patients with rheumatoid arthritis having grade I involvement of the wrist unresponsive to a 3- to 6-month trial of medical therapy. In patients with an unstable DRUJ along with early ulnar drift of the digits, the ECRL to ECU

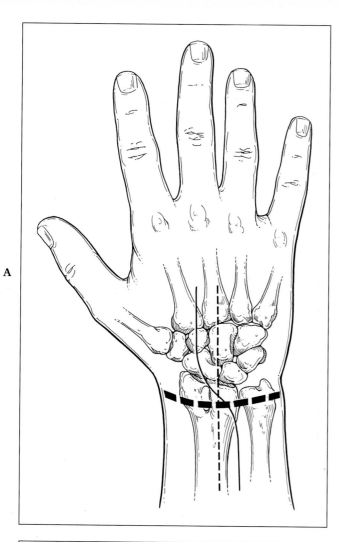

A

FIGURE 48-7

A, The skin incision can be a curvilinear incision (*solid line*), transverse along the dorsal wrist extension crease (*heavy dotted line*), or a straight longitudinal incision, which is generally preferred in the rheumatoid patient (*light dotted line*). **B,** The extensor retinaculum is freed of all soft tissue and the wrist and finger extensor tendons are identified proximal and distal to the retinaculum. *ECRB,* extensor carpi radialis brevis; *ECRL,* extensor carpi radialis longus; *ECU,* extensor carpi ulnaris; *EDC,* extensor digitorum communis; *EDM,* extensor digiti minimi; *EPL,* extensor pollicis longus.

Continued.

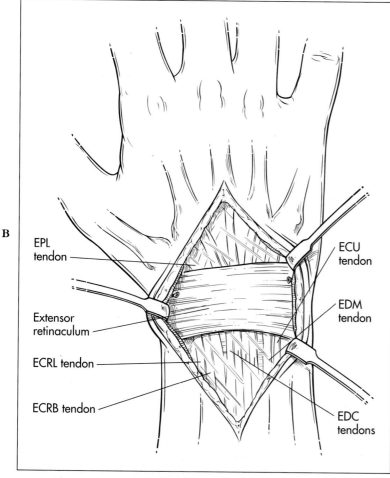

B

EPL tendon

Extensor retinaculum

ECRL tendon

ECRB tendon

ECU tendon

EDM tendon

EDC tendons

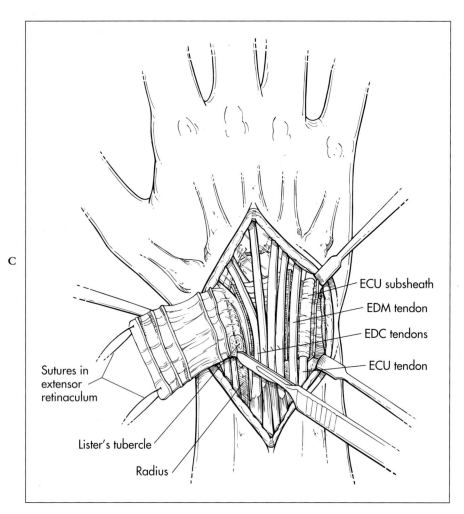

C

ECU subsheath

EDM tendon

EDC tendons

ECU tendon

Sutures in
extensor
retinaculum

Lister's tubercle

Radius

FIGURE 48-7, CONT'D.

C, The extensor retinaculum is reflected ulnar to radial from the side of the ECU tendon sheath across to the first dorsal extensor compartment. Surgical excision of the extensor tendon synovium is performed at this stage, usually with a scalpel. ECU subsheath represents a separate extensor compartment over the ECU tendon and it is not released with the extensor retinaculum. **D,** With retraction of the extensor tendons, the synovial reaction and the hyperemic vascular response along the branches of the posterior interosseous artery are noted. By sharp dissection, the intervals between the dorsal intercarpal ligament and the dorsal radiocarpal ligaments are identified.

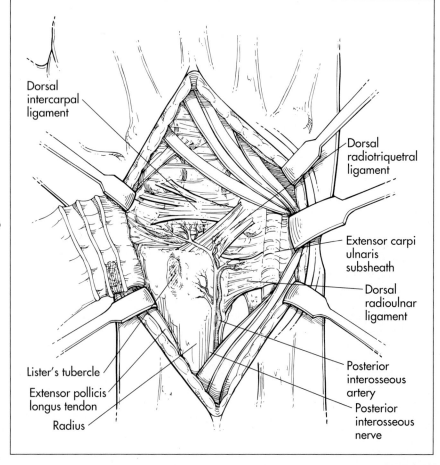

D

Dorsal
intercarpal
ligament

Dorsal
radiotriquetral
ligament

Extensor carpi
ulnaris
subsheath

Dorsal
radioulnar
ligament

Lister's tubercle

Extensor pollicis
longus tendon

Radius

Posterior
interosseous
artery

Posterior
interosseous
nerve

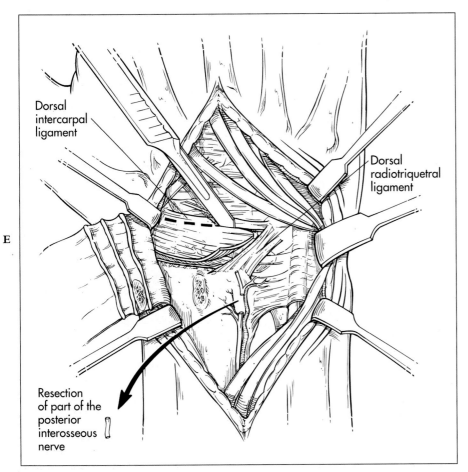

Dorsal
intercarpal
ligament

Dorsal
radiotriquetral
ligament

E

Resection
of part of the
posterior
interosseous
nerve

FIGURE 48-7, CONT'D.

E, Capsular incision outlining a radially based capsular flap between the dorsal intercarpal and dorsal radiotriquetral ligaments. **F,** Dorsal wrist synovectomy with a rongeur.

Continued.

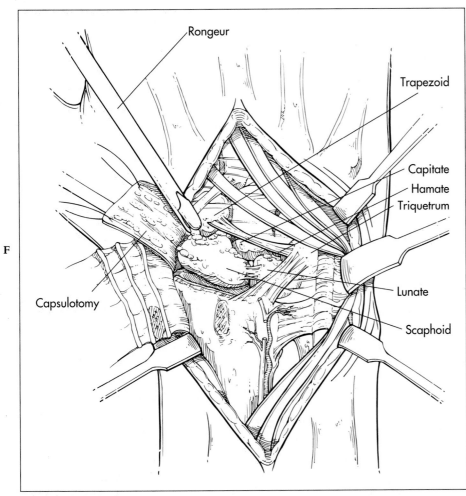

Rongeur

Trapezoid

Capitate
Hamate
Triquetrum

F

Lunate

Capsulotomy

Scaphoid

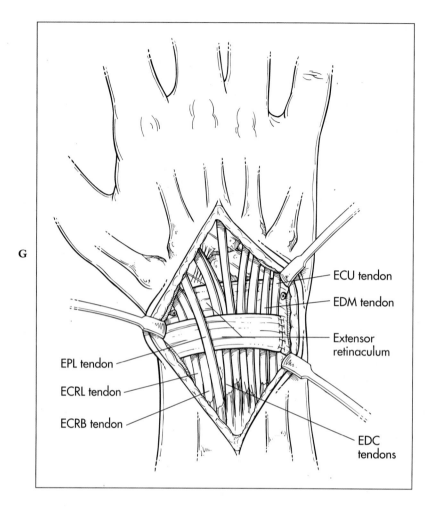

G

ECU tendon

EDM tendon

Extensor
retinaculum

EPL tendon

ECRL tendon

ECRB tendon

EDC
tendons

FIGURE 48-7, CONT'D.

G, Closure of the capsule and transfer of the extensor retinaculum. The distal half of the retinaculum is placed deep directly over the wrist capsule, providing reinforcement and protecting the overlying extensor tendons, while the proximal half is placed superficial to the extensor tendons to prevent tendon bowstringing.

transfer (Figs. 48-8 and 48-9), as described by Clayton and Ferlic,[18] is indicated along with reconstruction of the DRUJ using a distal radioulnar fusion with proximal pseudarthrosis. Patients are also carefully screened for palmar tenosynovitis and are followed clinically for signs and symptoms of carpal tunnel syndrome and diminished finger flexion. A palmar wrist synovectomy is performed when little or no response in palmar synovitis and tenosynovitis is seen from 3 to 6 months of medical therapy.

OSTEOARTHRITIS

Wrist synovitis due to osteoarthritis may occur as a result of scapholunate advanced collapse (SLAC), the most common form of osteoarthrosis of the wrist.[95] This form of synovitis creates a boggy, painful circumferential swelling of the wrist, causing the loss of the surface landmarks. It can lead to loss of integrity of the scapholunate ligament and extrinsic radiocarpal ligaments, producing advanced carpal collapse (SLAC wrist).[95] Treatment includes nonoperative measures such as the use of oral nonsteroidal anti-inflammatory

drugs and rest in a palmar, forearm-based Orthoplast splint with the wrist in a prehensile position. Typically episodic, this form of synovitis waxes and wanes, with episodes of inflammation probably due to the release of certain inflammatory mediators.[76] The vast majority of cases are responsive to oral administration of nonsteroidal anti-inflammatory drugs and rest. Occasionally, chronic recurrent painful synovitis of the wrist and extensor tendons from osteoarthrosis requires operative débridement. Arthroscopic synovectomy can be considered when the disease is limited to the radiocarpal or midcarpal joints. Biopsy of the synovium is also occasionally necessary to eliminate inflammatory arthritides or infection as possibilities. In advanced cases of osteoarthrosis with painful synovitis, limited or total wrist fusion is necessary.

CRYSTALLINE-INDUCED SYNOVITIS

In gout, supersaturation within the extracellular fluids by monosodium urate crystals results in recurrent attacks of articular and periarticular inflammation.[76] Humans lack the enzyme uricase, creating an inability

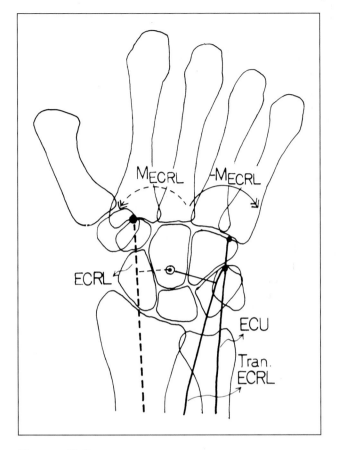

FIGURE 48-8

Schematic presentation of the Clayton-Ferlic procedure. The extensor carpi radialis longus (*ECRL*) transfer to the extensor carpi ulnaris (*ECU*). Because the direction of the moment arm changes, the deforming force of the ECRL is removed and the direction of the ECRL moment is reversed. *m*, moment arm of ECRL. *(From Boyce T, Youm Y, Sprague BL, et al.: Clinical and experimental studies on the effect of extensor carpi radialis longus transfer in the rheumatoid hand,* J Hand Surg *3:390-394, 1978. Copyright, American Society for Surgery of the Hand, by permission of Churchill Livingstone.)*

to oxidize uric acid (the end product of purine catabolism) to the more soluble allantoin. Tissue deposition of urate results (Fig. 48-10). The wrist is less often involved in acute attacks, but when involvement of the wrist does occur, the patient awakens from sleep with sudden pain and a warm, red, and tender joint. More than 25% of acute attacks occur after medical illness or operation. As attacks recur, a chronic destructive arthritis (Fig. 48-11) may develop with the deposition of tophi in the synovium and within carpal bones. A case of median nerve compression secondary to gout has been reported.[64] Additionally, two cases of scapholunate ligament disruption have been reported, suggesting the possibility of an aggressive synovitis similar in character to that seen in rheumatoid arthritis.[41] The histopathology of tophi finds a chronic granulomatous

reaction around uric acid crystals, potentially leading to a chronic synovitis.

Gout typically can be controlled by medical therapy consisting of colchicine and nonsteroidal anti-inflammatory drugs as well as prophylactic therapy with allopurinol and colchicine. Splinting of the wrist during acute or acute on chronic attacks is often helpful. In most cases, synovectomy is not indicated. If symptoms of median nerve compression occur that do not dissipate with medical therapy, flexor tenosynovectomy with median nerve decompression is indicated.

Pseudogout attacks of the wrist are a result of an inflammatory response to calcium pyrophosphate crystals shed from articular surfaces (Fig. 48-12).[9,22,76] Polymorphonuclear leukocytes phagocytize the crystals and then release lysosomal enzymes that ultimately create synovitis of the wrist (Fig. 48-13). Differentiation of pseudogout of the wrist from septic arthritis of the wrist is often difficult, and misdiagnosis resulting in complications may occur.[70] Aspiration of the wrist and identification of positive birefringent crystals located within white blood cells generally secure the diagnosis. Acute synovitis of the wrist and tenosynovitis of the flexor tendons with acute median nerve compression have required carpal tunnel release and flexor tenosynovectomy.[72] As in gout, a case of scapholunate ligament disruption in a patient with pseudogout has been reported.[41]

In most cases, acute wrist pain from pseudogout is successfully treated with nonsteroidal anti-inflammatory drugs and a palmar, forearm-based Orthoplast splint. If palmar wrist synovitis, flexor tenosynovitis, and median nerve compression occur and are unresponsive to medical treatment, palmar tenosynovectomy with palmar wrist synovectomy and median nerve decompression are indicated.

JUVENILE RHEUMATOID ARTHRITIS

Juvenile rheumatoid arthritis (JRA) is a condition of uncertain origin that causes chronic synovial inflammation of single or multiple joints (see Chapter 40). According to the American Rheumatism Association, three subtypes of JRA exist: systemic, polyarticular, and pauciarticular.[11,76] In the systemic variety, systemic manifestations occur along with a chronic polyarticular arthritis. In polyarticular JRA, a chronic debilitating arthritis occurs in up to 50% of children who test positive for rheumatoid factor.[76] In the pauciarticular variety, fewer than four joints are affected, with the wrist being commonly affected. Antinuclear antibodies may be detected in up to 40% of patients with JRA, whereas only 15% of patients will be positive for rheumatoid factor. Diagnosis of this disorder is made on clinical and radiographic grounds.

Text continued on p. 1152.

A

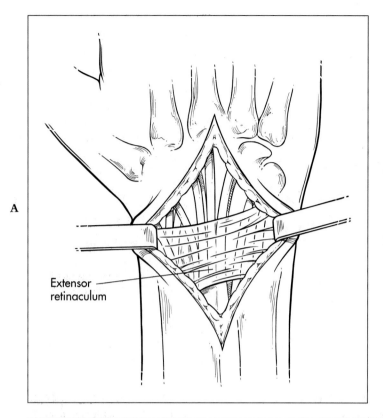

Extensor
retinaculum

FIGURE 48-9

Clayton-Ferlic procedure. **A,** Dorsal longitudinal incision
is made over the back of the wrist. Dorsal veins are ligated
and the extensor retinaculum is identified and freed of soft
tissue. The distal 2 cm of the ulna is resected if indicated.
B, The extensor retinaculum is reflected ulnar to radial and
synovectomy is performed.

B

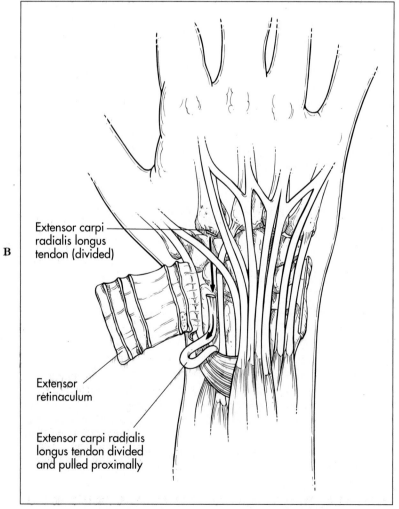

Extensor carpi
radialis longus
tendon (divided)

Extensor
retinaculum

Extensor carpi radialis
longus tendon divided
and pulled proximally

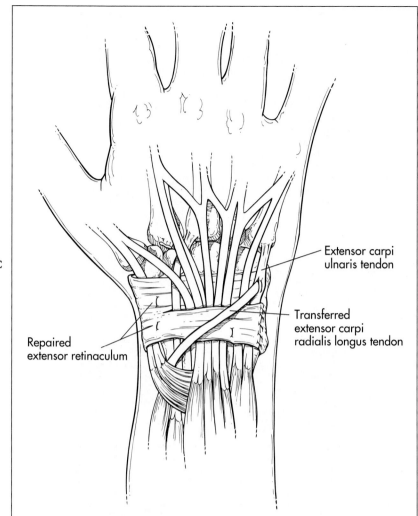

C

Repaired
extensor retinaculum

Extensor carpi
ulnaris tendon

Transferred
extensor carpi
radialis longus tendon

FIGURE 48-9, CONT'D.

C, The distal half of the extensor retinaculum
is passed beneath the extrinsic tendons and
sutured to the base of the fifth metacarpal
and distal ulna. (Pronator quadratus muscle
interposition may also be selected if the distal
ulna is unstable.) Extensor carpi radialis
longus is released from the base of the second
metacarpal and passed across the dorsal aspect
of the wrist and sutured to the insertion of
the extensor carpi ulnaris.

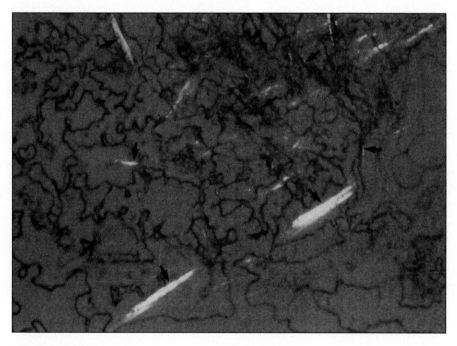

FIGURE 48-10

Photomicrograph of monosodium urate crystals (*arrows*) suspended in aspirated synovial fluid.
The long, needle-shaped profile is typical and may exhibit different coloration, depending on
orientation under polarized light. The crystals may also be found phagocytized by leukocytes.
(Courtesy of Dr. Eric Matteson, Department of Rheumatology, Mayo Clinic Rochester.)

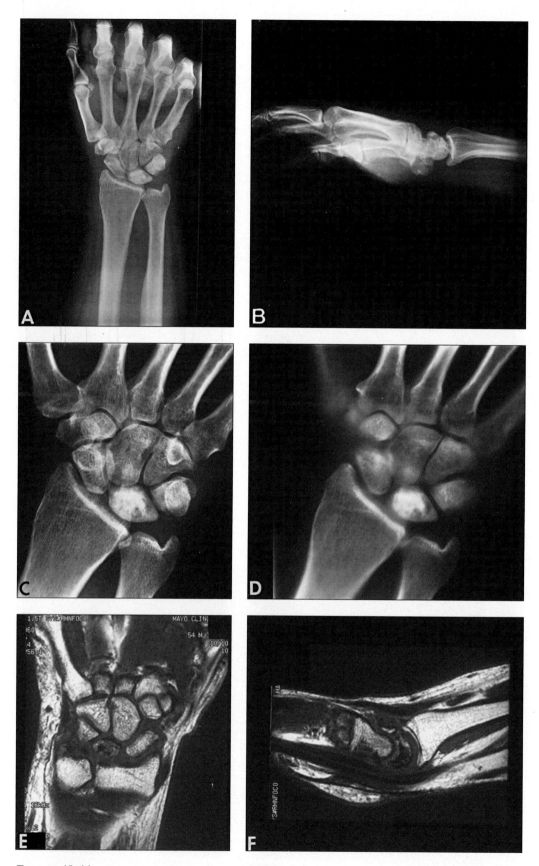

FIGURE 48-11

Painful right wrist in a patient with a history of gout. **A,** Posteroanterior radiograph of wrist shows narrowing of radiolunate joint and cystic degeneration of the lunate. **B,** Lateral radiograph of wrist shows dorsal lunate cyst and bone formation beneath the dorsal wrist capsule. **C** and **D,** Tomographic cuts show crystalline deposits within the lunate associated with cystic degeneration. **E** and **F,** Magnetic resonance imaging (posteroanterior and lateral) with large cyst within the lunate. At biopsy, the material was urate deposits compatible with gouty arthritis of the wrist.

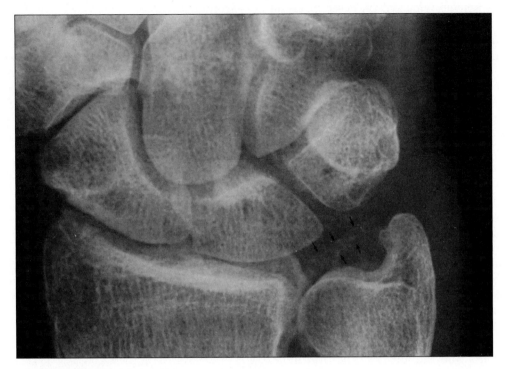

FIGURE 48-12

Posteroanterior radiograph of a wrist with pseudogout. Calcium pyrophosphate dihydrate (CPPD) crystals have been deposited near the surface of the triangular fibrocartilage (*arrows*) and appear radiodense. Another typical location for CPPD crystal deposition in the wrist is in the scapholunate ligament complex.

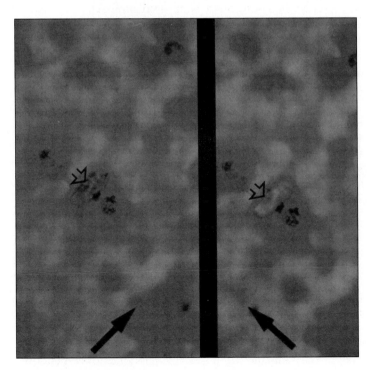

FIGURE 48-13

Photomicrograph of an aspirated synovial fluid sample with a calcium pyrophosphate crystal (*open arrows*) phagocytized by a leukocyte. Note the more thickened and blunted appearance of this crystal compared with the monosodium urate crystal illustrated in Figure 48-10. The arrows at the bottom of the field designate the direction of light polarization, which influences the color emanating from the crystal. (*Courtesy of Dr. Eric Matteson, Department of Rheumatology, Mayo Clinic Rochester.*)

Treatment depends on early recognition so that early medical therapy can be instituted. Medications used include aspirin or nonsteroidal anti-inflammatory drugs as well as penicillamine and, on occasion, corticosteroids given orally. Patients with JRA are particularly hindered by periods of inactivity and typically experience morning wrist stiffness and contracture. Nevertheless, our experience finds nighttime wrist and hand splinting helpful. The preferred splint is a forearm-based Orthoplast splint with the wrist in a slightly dorsiflexed or prehensile position and the digits in the resting position. Wrist pain itself (compared with synovitis or loss of motion), however, is generally not a significant problem in the JRA patient. Therefore, although synovectomy is helpful in adult rheumatoid arthritis patients, the efficacy of synovectomy of the wrist in JRA is controversial.

Eyring et al.[27] recommended synovectomy in JRA in any joint with active synovitis beyond 18 months, in any joint with radiographic destruction, or when loss of motion occurred despite medical therapy. Kvien et al.[52] studied 30 patients with JRA in whom 30 joints (18 wrists) were randomly selected to be treated with either synovectomy or nonoperative measures. Subjectively, the patients treated with synovectomy of the wrist in this series had less pain and joint swelling than those treated nonoperatively. Hanff et al.[38] performed 20 wrist synovectomies without ulnar head resections in 15 patients for JRA; on average, grip strength improved. Furthermore, Fink et al.[30] found that synovectomy in general was a worthwhile procedure in the child with JRA. They reported a 50% increase in range of motion after 39 synovectomies in 23 patients, including 5 wrist joints. Jacobsen et al.,[47] however, retrospectively reviewed the results of 41 synovectomies (including 4 wrist synovectomies) in 30 children and found, aside from relief of joint swelling, little if any benefit from synovectomy as judged by pain or range of motion.

It is our view that most cases of synovitis of the wrist from JRA can be treated nonoperatively. However, in cases with recurrent, significant, limiting wrist-joint swelling, synovectomy may be indicated. It is essential that the surgeon, patient, and family be aware of the potential for limited success in synovectomy of the wrist in patients with JRA.

OTHER FORMS OF SYNOVITIS

Amyloid is an extracellular protein that can accumulate in the connective tissues and may be associated with conditions such as multiple myeloma, chronic infection, tuberculosis, rheumatoid arthritis, ankylosing spondylitis, heredofamilial amyloidosis, or long-term hemodialysis.[76] Involvement of the flexor tendons may cause a flexor tenosynovitis and resultant median nerve

neuropathy at the wrist. Treatment is generally surgical, requiring a flexor tenosynovectomy, median nerve decompression, and culture of the synovium to confirm the diagnosis.

A detailed discussion of various infections that might cause synovitis about the wrist is beyond the scope of this chapter. However, in chronic or recurrent septic arthritis of the wrist or in acute fungal or mycobacterial infection, treatment is not complete without incision, drainage, and synovectomy of the affected joint. Particularly important is synovectomy in acute or chronic infections from atypical mycobacteria,[51] such as *Mycobacterium marinum,* an infection often contracted in fish handlers. Without synovectomy, *Mycobacterium marinum* can be indolent and recurrent as organisms harbor in the synovium. Cuts, punctures, and abrasions in the outdoors may inoculate the wrist to such unusual fungal infections as sporotrichosis and brucellosis. Chronic infection of the wrist with these fungi may cause rapid destruction of the joint. Once diagnosed, treatment is both medical and surgical and includes wrist synovectomy.

SILICONE SYNOVITIS

Silicone synovitis is an inflammatory process with an autoimmune component that results from a destructive foreign body. Silicone synovitis occurs in response to silicone-rubber debris and perhaps should be termed "particulate-debris synovitis" because it is a wear-debris phenomenon. Silica is an ambiguous element that is most commonly in the form of silicon dioxide or sand. Besides silicon dioxide, more than 60,000 compounds contain silica.[32] Polydimethylsiloxane is the most common Silastic polymer produced and is a chain of carbon, oxygen, hydrogen, and silica.[32] The length of the polymeric chain determines whether the compound is in a solid or liquid phase.[32,82,85] Cross-linking of polydimethylsiloxane results in the production of silicone rubber.[32] Silastic is a proprietary name of the medical-grade silicone rubber produced by the Dow Corning Company.[36]

The production of medical-grade silicone rubber is initiated by the extraction of silica in a high-temperature electric furnace followed by polymerization and repolymerization with organic agents.[32,82] The material is then vulcanized and molded and finally milled and strained to produce medical-grade silicone rubber.[32] Medical-grade silicone rubber is heat stable and has few adhesive properties.[32,84] Swanson[84] showed medical-grade silicone rubber appears to have excellent flexibility and dampening properties because it is able to withstand up to 600 million flexion repetitions. Furthermore, silicone rubber has been shown to be an inert substance and therefore very stable.[32] The tensile

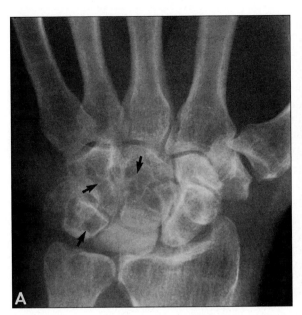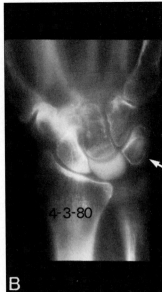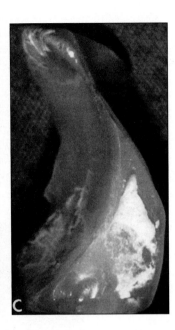

FIGURE 48-14

A, Posteroanterior radiograph of a wrist with signs of silicone synovitis, resulting from previous implantation of a silicone lunate prosthesis. Note the large cystic erosions in the capitate, hamate, and triquetrum (*arrows*). **B,** Tomogram shows large cyst within the triquetrum (*arrow*) associated with silicone lunate and reactive synovitis. **C,** Silicone lunate implant shows extreme wear and deformity.

strength of medical-grade silicone rubber is approximately 2,000 pounds/in.[2], and its elongation potential is greater than 1,000%.[84]

Silicone chemicals were first prepared by Kipping in 1907.[32] The modern process of silicone synthesis was developed in 1930 by Hyde, Oric, and MacGregor.[32] It was not until World War II that silicone rubber was first used clinically—as a lubricant for glass syringes in combat areas.[32] In 1955 Holter developed a hydrocephalus shunt using silicone rubber.[32] Also during this time, silicone rubber was first used in the tubing for renal dialysis and the heart-bypass machine.[45] In 1963, silicone breast implants were first introduced, and since that time more than one million implantations have been performed.[31] In 1966, Swanson[82] developed the lower extremity amputation stump implant that was used to cap the distal tibia in below-knee amputations. This device had an intramedullary stem and its sole purpose was cushioning the bony end within the amputation stump. Between 1963 and 1970, Swanson[82,83] developed silicone implants for replacement of the metacarpophalangeal joint, proximal interphalangeal joint, carpal trapezium, scaphoid, and lunate. In 1973, Swanson[84] developed the rubber implant for capping the ulna for radial head replacement. Durability of these implants was tested both in vitro[81] and in vivo.[86]

Despite the relatively inert structure of silicone, its use on the wrist has produced problems related to silicone-debris particles and concern regarding controversial application of silicone implants within the

wrist.[53] The clinical presentations of patients who have a reaction to silicone implants, however, are varied. The patient in whom particulate-debris synovitis develops may have a particular silicone implant in place from 10 months to 17 years.[35,36,40,65,78] The clinical features of particulate-debris synovitis can first be heralded by pain with motion of the affected joint as well as tenderness over the retained implant.[2,78] There is typically a dramatic loss of motion with concomitant soft-tissue swelling, which occurs abruptly. Radiographically, the surrounding bone may show well-defined marginal erosions with subchondral cysts (Figs. 48-14, *A* and *B*).[2,25,78] There is typically normal mineralization of the surrounding and involved bone in contradistinction to the osteopenia of rheumatoid arthritis and osteoporosis.[2] Deformity of the retained implant develops (Fig. 48-14, *C* and see Fig. 48-16, *A*) and associations exist among the deformity, the amount of particulate debris, the resultant number and size of cysts formed, and the time in service of the implant.[2,67,68,94] There is a notable loss of carpal height as deformity of the implant develops.[2] Peimer and others[69] have reported that pathologic fractures can occur through the bony cysts of particulate-wear synovitis.

Histologically, particulate-wear synovitis is a hypertrophic villous synovitis with a thickened synovial membrane that can contain lymphocytes, plasma cells, eosinophils, and multinucleated giant cells (Fig. 48-15, *A*).[15,36,42,68,94] Also, histiocytes or macrophages may be found containing refractile but nonbirefringent silicone particles (Fig. 48-15, *B*).[36,75] Also commonly noted are extracellular silicone particles.[36,68] Silicone particles in the range of 20 to 100 microns[2,4,49] typically are engulfed by macrophages and are found in the cytoplasm of the cells, whereas silicone particles greater than 100 microns are walled off by giant cells.[94] The overall histologic process is that of a pannus formation, which may invade trabecular or cortical bone and produce articular cartilage erosions.[15,16] This process is not

characterized by the presence of neutrophils, and this helps distinguish it from an acute infectious process.

The differential diagnosis for silicone synovitis includes infection, inflammatory arthritis, and pigmented villonodular synovitis. Infection may be distinguished from particulate-wear synovitis by the presence histologically of neutrophils and radiographically by generalized osteopenia. Likewise, inflammatory arthritis typically shows characteristic patterns of joint involvement, including periarticular erosions and osteopenia.

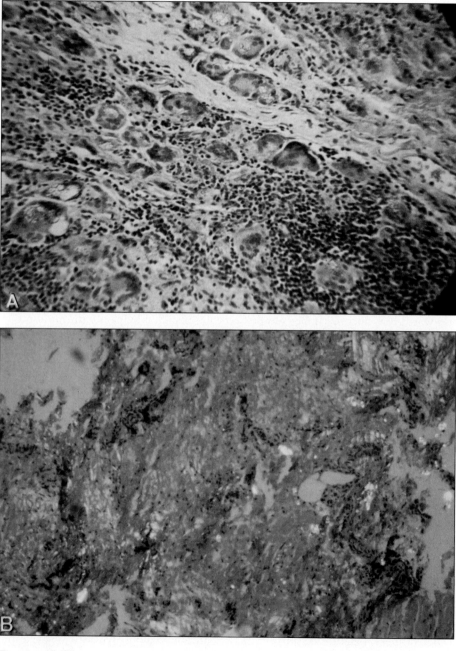

FIGURE 48–15

Photomicrograph of silicone synovitis. **A,** Histocytes, lymphocytes, eosinophils, and multinucleated giant cells with intracellular silicone particles. (See Color Plate 63.) **B,** Nonbirefringent silicone particles in the synovium of a patient with silicone synovitis. (See Color Plate 64.)

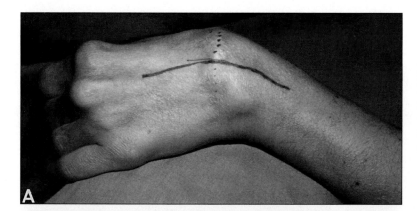

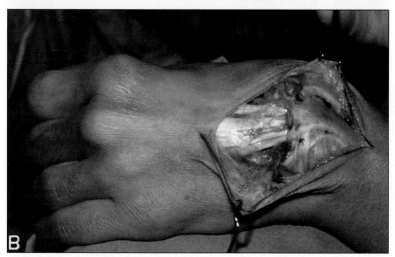

FIGURE 48-17

Dorsal wrist synovectomy. **A,** Straight surgical incision for wrist synovectomy. **B,** Reflection of the skin and soft tissues exposes the extensor retinaculum, which has been released and repaired after extensor tenosynovectomy.

the surgeon's discretion. Variations include a "lazy S" or transverse, but a straight incision (Figs. 48-7 and 48-17, *A*) is preferred to avoid necrosis at the skin margin. In patients with rheumatoid arthritis, we recommend a longitudinal incision because of the recognized complication of skin slough from curved incisions about the wrist in patients with rheumatoid arthritis.[13,56] Care is taken to elevate the skin edges in the plane between the dorsal retinaculum and the subcutaneous fat. The superficial branches of the radial and ulnar nerves are identified and protected, and dorsal veins are preserved whenever possible. The extensor retinaculum is then identified and is carefully elevated from ulnar to radial after it is divided just ulnar to the sixth extensor compartment (Figs. 48-7, *C* and 48-18, *C*). The edges of the incised retinaculum are tagged with a stay suture to prevent further trauma to the edge and to assist in retraction. The retinaculum is then elevated through the second extensor compartment. This requires division of the 5-6, 4-5, and 3-4 intercompartmental septa and subperiosteal elevation of the retinacular attachment across the 2-3 interval at Lister's tubercle. Lister's tubercle may be resected at this time, flush with the dorsal cortex of the distal radius (Fig. 48-7, *C*). Care should be exercised to preserve the integrity of the ECU tendon subsheath. The ECRL, extensor carpi

radialis brevis, EPL, extensor indicis proprius, and EDC tendons are systematically inspected and then cleaned of synovium with a Stevens' scissors (Fig. 48-18). Each tendon is elevated by the assistant with a Ragnell retractor while the surgeon carefully strips the synovium from distal to proximal. Frequently, the synovium on the extensor tendons of the wrist is quite tenacious and adherent to the tendons, and care must be exercised to avoid damage to these tendons. The EDC tendons, especially to ring and small fingers, are carefully inspected for rupture, typically identified by pseudotendon formation. Pseudotendon formation is resected and tendon ends are tagged with 4-0 Prolene for repair.

Once the tenosynovectomy is complete, the dorsal wrist capsule is exposed (Figs. 48-7, *D* and 48-18). By gently sweeping the wrist capsule with a latex sponge, the dorsal radiocarpal ligament and the dorsal intercarpal ligament can be identified and preserved.[33] The dorsal wrist capsule is then recognized, forming a "V" between these two ligaments.[7] The capsule can be incised by splitting these ligaments longitudinally and dividing the radiocarpal joint capsule from the dorsal rim of the radius, reflecting the entire flap radially (Fig. 48-7, *E*). In the rheumatoid patient, the ligamentous sparing capsulotomy may be impossible, and a longitudinal capsulotomy may be more practical.

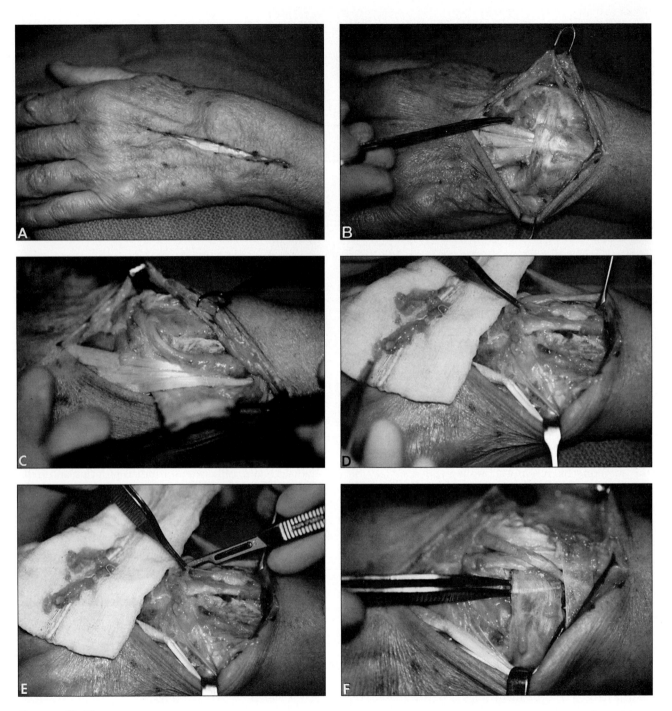

Figure 48-18

Dorsal tenosynovectomy of the wrist. **A,** Dorsal longitudinal incisions in line with the third metacarpal. **B,** Exposure of the dorsal tendons. Note extensive tenosynovitis ulnar to the finger extensor tendons and about the common wrist extensor tendons. **C,** Extensor retinaculum has been reflected and extensor tendons are visible with large area of extensor tenosynovial involvement. **D** and **E,** During extensor tenosynovectomy, each extensor tendon is retracted (with a Ragnell retractor) and the tenosynovium is sharply resected down to the dorsal joint capsule. **F,** The extensor retinaculum is split, with the distal half placed beneath the wrist and finger extensor tendons as a protective barrier and the proximal half placed over the extensor tendons to prevent bowstringing. Forceps in place beneath the distal half of the extensor retinaculum.

Once the dorsal wrist capsule is exposed, a complete synovectomy is accomplished sharply with a scalpel and bluntly with a small rongeur (Figs. 48-7, *F* and 48-18), carefully sparing the dorsal wrist joint capsule as well as the scapholunate and lunotriquetral interosseous ligaments. Tissue is sent for histologic examination and for culture to confirm the diagnosis. Typically, the synovectomy is limited to the radiocarpal joint but the midcarpal joint should be examined. The articular surfaces of the distal radius, proximal carpal row, and capitolunate articulation are inspected before closure of the capsule.

Silicone Synovitis. With silicone synovitis, we feel that an aggressive débridement is necessary along with carpal implant removal. This must include curettage of cystic bony lesions to ensure that all of the silicone debris is removed. Cauterization or applications of phenol and alcohol to the base of the cyst may be considered. We now routinely advocate bone grafting to the remaining defect, particularly when more than 50% of the bone is involved, in which case a pathologic fracture is more likely. When bone grafting is indicated, ipsilateral anterior iliac crest bone graft is harvested to fill these defects. Complete or limited wrist arthrodesis may be indicated in most circumstances. After synovectomy and partial fusion, the wrist joint capsule is closed by suturing the distal and proximal borders of the reflected capsule to their respective bordering dorsal wrist ligaments.

Wrist Joint Closure and Retinaculum Transfer. After completion of the dorsal wrist synovectomy, capsule closure and attention to the extensor tendons (EDC and EPL) are required.[57] If tendon rupture is present and direct repair of the EDC tendons is impossible, side-to-side tenodesis may be performed or extensor indicis proprius tendon transfer may be considered. With respect to the EPL rupture or significant involvement with synovitis, tenodesis to the extensor indicis proprius tendon may be performed, an interposition tendon graft considered, or a direct tendon transfer, extensor indicis proprius to EPL, may be appropriate. In addition to the radiocarpal joints and extensor tendons, it is important to inspect the DRUJ. The first step is to incise the DRUJ capsule longitudinally just proximal to the triangular fibrocartilage complex, avoiding the dorsal radioulnar ligament. Synovium, if present, is débrided with a small rongeur. The joint is evaluated for stability. If instability is present with palmar subluxation of the radius relative to the ulna and if supination deformity of the carpus exists, we recommend stabilization of the DRUJ by a limited fusion (Sauvé-Kapandji) procedure.

With respect to the extensor retinaculum, it is important to have a precise closure in the patient with rheumatoid arthritis and also to protect the extensor tendons from synovial infiltration and rupture. We recommend splitting the retinacular flap (Fig. 48-18, *F*) and passing the distal segment deep to the extensor tendons and the proximal flap superficial to the extensor tendons. At the junctions between the extensor compartments, the retinacular flaps may be sutured together as well as to the deep fascia of the forearm and hand. This may serve to protect the extensor tendons from underlying synovitis and bony prominences. We prefer leaving the EPL tendon in an "extraretinacular" plane (Fig. 48-7, *F*). Bowstringing and weakness of the EPL have not been problems. Before closure, the tourniquet is released and hemostasis is carefully achieved. After skin closure, a soft dressing is applied along with a palmar, forearm-based plaster splint with digits free and the wrist extended. If tendon repair, transfer, or tenodesis is performed, a forearm-based, dorsal extension block splint is applied and standard rehabilitation measures are instituted when the patient and the wound are stable.

PALMAR TENOSYNOVECTOMY IN CARPAL TUNNEL RELEASE

Carpal tunnel release, palmar tenosynovectomy, and palmar wrist synovectomy must be performed through a generous palmar exposure and cannot be accomplished through a small palmar incision or with an endoscopic technique. With tourniquet control, we prefer an incision beginning just proximal to Kaplan's Cardinal line and coursing proximally in a curved fashion, parallel to or within the thenar flexion crease. The incision then crosses the distal palmar crease in a zigzag fashion, tending ulnarly to avoid branches of the palmar cutaneous branch of the median nerve. The incision may extend 3 to 4 cm proximally into the distal forearm to ensure adequate exposure of the flexor tendons. The palmar fat is sharply incised down to the palmar fascia. We have not separately dissected out branches of the palmar cutaneous branch of the median nerve under direct vision, although we feel it is important to be mindful of its location when planning skin incisions. In the proximal extent of the wound, the antebrachial fascia is incised and released, and distally the palmar fascia and the transverse carpal ligament are released. When deep palmar fat is encountered distally in the wound, blunt dissection is used to locate the superficial palmar arch by gently spreading the fat in a transverse direction relative to the axial line of the forearm and hand. After identification of the superficial palmar arch, the surgeon can release all remaining bands of the palmar fascia and transverse carpal ligament that could cause continued compression on the median nerve.

At this juncture, systematically, each flexor tendon is retrieved from the forearm with a blunt retractor and the tenosynovium is excised. The tenosynovium often surrounds the flexor tendon as one large mass. The tenosynovium should be incised longitudinally about each tendon, then one-by-one each flexor tendon can be delivered from the mass and captured into a 0.25-in. Penrose drain, enabling retraction from the palmar forearm, the tenosynovium, and the median nerve. After each tendon of the carpal tunnel has been identified, the dissected tenosynovium is freed from the median nerve and then excised. A specimen may be sent for histologic examination and culture if confirmation of the diagnosis is desired. If necessary, the palmar wrist capsule may be accessed through this approach by gently retracting the flexor tendons and median nerve ulnarward.

After the flexor tenosynovectomy is performed and the carpal tunnel is completely released, the tourniquet is deflated and meticulous hemostasis obtained. A suction drain is recommended to prevent formation of a hematoma. Cortisone should *not* be placed about the flexor tendons. The combination of flexor tenolysis, cortisone, and surgical drain has an increased incidence of postoperative sepsis.[39] Tenosynovectomy alone has been implicated in increased postoperative infection rates in carpal tunnel release and probably warrants, especially in the patient with rheumatoid arthritis, the use of preoperative prophylactic antibiotics, such as 1 g of cefazolin delivered intravenously.[39] A soft dressing is applied along with a forearm-based, palmar plaster splint, with the wrist extended and the digits free.

ARTHROSCOPIC SYNOVECTOMY

In certain circumstances, arthroscopic synovectomy may be considered a safe and effective alternative to open synovectomy (see Chapter 14). The advantages of arthroscopic synovectomy include the ability to carefully evaluate the surfaces of the radiocarpal and midcarpal joints in a minimally invasive fashion. Culture and biopsy specimens are easily obtained from multiple sites through the arthroscope. Evaluations of soft tissues, such as intra-articular ligaments and the triangular fibrocartilage, can be made and documented.

There are limitations to the procedure, however, and several points should be considered before embarking on an arthroscopic synovectomy. First, the surgeon should be comfortable with the procedure, must be aware of the intra-articular anatomy of the wrist and the areas most likely to be involved with the synovitic process, and must stand ready to convert to an open procedure if the arthroscopic procedure is thought to be inadequate. Second, if arthroscopic débridement is considered, it is ideal if the inflammatory condition is in a mild-to-moderate stage of involvement. This relates specifically to the surgeon's ability to visualize the important intra-articular structures. If a florid synovitis is present, it is likely that the arthroscopist will have substantially impaired visualization. Related to this is the direct relationship between the volume of synovitic tissue to be débrided and the degree of difficulty in achieving a satisfactory synovectomy arthroscopically. Finally, arthroscopic synovectomy may limit the surgeon's ability to control intra-articular hemorrhage; a "mini arthrotomy" may be necessary to place a drain to prevent problems associated with a hemarthrosis.

Equipment. To establish appropriate distraction of the wrist, finger traps are used with application of 12 to 15 pounds of countertraction force to the index and long fingers, applied either in a vertical or horizontal orientation. A 2.4- to 2.7-mm arthroscope is used with inflow established through the arthroscope sheath. Large-bore outflow is necessary for joint lavage and to minimize intra-articular edema during the procedure. The arthroscopist should have available a full-radius and end-cutting shaver, a suction punch, a banana-blade scalpel, and various manual grabbers. There may be a good indication for using a holmium:YAG (yttrium-aluminum-garnet) laser for arthroscopic synovectomy, but this has not clearly been established as an advisable technique at this time.

Procedure. Patient preparation is identical to that for standard wrist arthroscopy (see Chapters 8 and 14). Regional or general anesthesia is induced and the longitudinal traction is applied. The procedure is generally done under the control of a pneumatic tourniquet. Standard arthroscopic portals are established, generally using the dorsal 3-4, 4-5, and 6-U radiocarpal joint portals and the radial and ulnar dorsal midcarpal joint portals. Additional portals used to switch the arthroscope and outflow portals may be needed, such as the 1-2 and the 6-R radiocarpal joint portals. As always, caution is needed when preparing the sites by blunt dissection to access the joint capsule to minimize the risk of iatrogenic cutaneous nerve injury.

Although synovitis may involve virtually any synovial membrane, there are several locations in the wrist where the most intense reactions are likely to be found. In the radiocarpal joint, the region of the radioscapholunate ligament and the prestyloid recess are the most commonly involved sites. In the midcarpal joint, the most common locations for synovitis are the ulnar joint recess, just ulnar to the triquetrohamate joint, and the dorsal capsule of the scapho-trapezium trapezoid joint. Secondary involvement of the palmar and dorsal midcarpal joint capsule in the region of the lunocapitate joint may occur, but the severity of synovitis in this situation may preclude the safe use of arthroscopy and would perhaps be better treated with an open synovectomy.

In a methodical fashion, the entire radiocarpal and midcarpal joints are initially inspected and a plan for débridement is established. With the shavers, punches, and grabbers, the abnormal synovial tissue is débrided; care is taken to avoid damage to the substrate. Samples of the débrided tissue can often be retrieved and sent to a pathologist for histologic diagnosis. It is often necessary to switch portals for the arthroscope, the débridement equipment, and even the outflow cannula, and the surgeon is encouraged to do this. It is quite common for a region of synovitis to be present immediately around the initial arthroscopic portal, but not visible until the arthroscope is moved to an adjacent portal. If excessive bleeding occurs or if the degree of soft-tissue swelling precludes safe visualization, the arthroscopic procedure should be aborted and converted to an arthrotomy.

When the débridement is completed, arthroscopic assessments of the joints are repeated, with notations made regarding the status of the joint surfaces and the supportive soft tissues. This helps immeasurably in the estimation of a prognosis.

Postoperative Management. Postoperative management must be tailored to each specific surgical condition. For patients having dorsal tenosynovectomy and dorsal wrist synovectomy without a DRUJ reconstruction, we encourage wrist and digital motion early in the postoperative period. The dressing and drain are removed within the first 48 to 72 hours and a new dressing is applied. We believe that a wound stabilization period of approximately 5 days is necessary before motion of the wrist is initiated. A removable Orthoplast splint with the wrist in dorsiflexion and the digits free is used to support the wrist and hand and is placed at 5 to 7 days postoperatively and worn for a total of 4 weeks. The sutures are removed 2 weeks postoperatively. If a hematoma develops or bloody drainage persists, motion is restricted and consideration is given to hematoma drainage. If a DRUJ reconstruction such as a Sauvé -Kapandji procedure is performed in conjunction with a dorsal wrist synovectomy and an extensor tenosynovectomy, a long arm cast with the elbow at 90°, the forearm at neutral rotation, and the wrist in extension is applied to immobilize the wrist for 6 weeks while digital motion is encouraged. At 6 weeks postoperatively, wrist motion and forearm rotation are initiated after cast removal. A long arm Orthoplast splint is applied to hold the elbow at 90°, the forearm at neutral, and the wrist in extension for an additional 6 weeks. At 3 months postoperatively, if radiographs confirm union of the fused DRUJ, no impingement of the ulnar osteotomy, and no complications of the DRUJ hardware, return to full activity is allowed.

In patients with flexor tenosynovectomy and carpal tunnel release, wound inspection, drain removal, and early digit rotation are performed during the 48- to 72-hour period. Sutures are removed at 2 weeks. If a capsular incision is made, we recommend the use of a short arm cast, placing the wrist at neutral or slight palmar flexion for approximately 3 weeks. Otherwise, patients having flexor tenosynovectomy with carpal tunnel release but no capsular incision may use an over-the-counter removable Velcro splint for approximately 4 weeks, removing it only for hygienic purposes. Excessive range of motion early and lack of splintage in patients with palmar flexor tenosynovectomy and carpal tunnel release can result in painful translocation of the flexor tendons out of the carpal canal, which occasionally has led to a wrist flexion contracture. Finally, careful attention must be paid to the wound during the early postoperative period and a significant hematoma should be evacuated.

REFERENCES

1. Adolfsson L, Nylander G: Arthroscopic synovectomy of the rheumatoid wrist, *J Hand Surg [Br]* 18:92-96, 1993.
2. Alexander AH, Turner MA, Alexander CE, et al.: Lunate silicone replacement arthroplasty in Kienbock's disease: a long-term follow-up, *J Hand Surg [Am]* 15:401-407, 1990.
3. Aptekar RG, Davie JM, Cattell HS: Foreign body reaction to silicone rubber. Complication of a finger joint implant, *Clin Orthop* 98:231-232, 1974.
4. Atkinson RE, Smith RJ: Silicone synovitis following silicone implant arthroplasty, *Hand Clin* 2:291-299, 1986.
5. Barnes CG, Currey HL: Carpal tunnel syndrome in rheumatoid arthritis. A clinical and electrodiagnostic survey, *Ann Rheum Dis* 26:226-233, 1967.
6. Beckenbaugh RD, Linscheid RL: *Arthroplasty in the hand and wrist.* In Green DP, editor: *Operative hand surgery,* ed 3, vol 1, New York, 1993, Churchill Livingstone, pp 143-187.
7. Berger RA, Bishop AT, Bettinger PC: New dorsal capsulotomy for the surgical exposure of the wrist, *Ann Plast Surg* 35:54-59, 1995.
8. Berger RA, Blair WF, Andrews JG: Resultant forces and angles of twist about the wrist after ECRL to ECU tendon transfer, *J Orthop Res* 6:443-451, 1988.
9. Berger RA, Buckwalter JA: Calcium pyrophosphate dihydrate crystal deposition patterns in the triangular fibrocartilage complex, *Orthopedics* 13:75-80, 1990.
10. Brase DW, Millender LH: Failure of silicone rubber wrist arthroplasty in rheumatoid arthritis, *J Hand Surg [Am]* 11:175-183, 1986.

11. Brewer EJ Jr, Bass J, Baum J, et al.: Current proposed revision of JRA Criteria. JRA Criteria Subcommittee of the Diagnostic and Therapeutic Criteria Committee of the American Rheumatism Section of The Arthritis Foundation, *Arthritis Rheum* 20 Suppl:195-199, Mar 1977.

12. Brown FE, Brown ML: Long-term results after tenosynovectomy to treat the rheumatoid hand, *J Hand Surg [Am]* 13:704-708, 1988.

13. Brumfield R Jr, Kuschner SH, Gellman H, et al.: Results of dorsal wrist synovectomies in the rheumatoid hand, *J Hand Surg [Am]* 15:733-735, 1990.

14. Buckland-Wright JC, Walker SR: Incidence and size of erosions in the wrist and hand of rheumatoid patients: a quantitative microfocal radiographic study, *Ann Rheum Dis* 46:463-467, 1987.

15. Carter PR, Benton LJ, Dysert PA: Silicone rubber carpal implants: a study of the incidence of late osseous complications, *J Hand Surg [Am]* 11:639-644, 1986.

16. Christie AJ, Pierret G, Levitan J: Silicone synovitis, *Semin Arthritis Rheum* 19:166-171, 1989.

17. Christie AJ, Weinberger KA, Dietrich M: Silicone lymphadenopathy and synovitis. Complications of silicone elastomer finger joint prostheses, *JAMA* 237:1463-1464, 1977.

18. Clayton ML, Ferlic DC: Tendon transfer for radial rotation of the wrist in rheumatoid arthritis, *Clin Orthop* 100:176-185, 1974.

19. Coleman DL, King RN, Andrade JD: The foreign body reaction: a chronic inflammatory response, *J Biomed Mater Res* 8:199-211, 1974.

20. de Jager LT, Jaffe R, Learmonth ID, et al.: The A1 pulley in rheumatoid flexor tenosynovectomy. To retain or divide? *J Hand Surg [Br]* 19:202-204, 1994.

21. Donahue WC, Nosanchuk JS, Kaufer H: Effect and fate of intra-articular silicone fluid, *Clin Orthop* 77:305-310, 1971.

22. Dossick PH, Bansal M, Figgie MP, et al.: Intramedullary deposits of hydroxyapatite crystals in a patient with rheumatoid arthritis, *Clin Orthop* 298:240-245, 1994.

23. Eiken O, Ekerot L, Lindstrom C, et al.: Silicone carpal implants: risk or benefit? *Scand J Plast Reconstr Surg* 19:295-304, 1985.

24. Eiken O, Haga T, Salgeback S: Volar tenosynovectomy in the rheumatoid hand, *Scand J Plast Reconstr Surg* 10:59-63, 1976.

25. Ekfors TO, Aro H, Maki J, et al.: Cystic osteolysis induced by silicone rubber prosthesis, *Arch Pathol Lab Med* 108:225-227, 1984.

26. el-Khoury GY, Larson RK, Kathol MH, et al.: Seronegative and seropositive rheumatoid arthritis: radiographic differences, *Radiology* 168:517-520, 1988.

27. Eyring EJ, Longert A, Bass JC: Synovectomy in juvenile rheumatoid arthritis. Indications and short-term results, *J Bone Joint Surg Am* 53:638-651, 1971.

28. Fatti JF, Palmer AK, Mosher JF: The long-term results of Swanson silicone rubber interpositional wrist arthroplasty, *J Hand Surg [Am]* 11:166-175, 1986.

29. Feldon P, Millender LH, Nalebuff EA: *Rheumatoid arthritis in the hand and wrist.* In Green DP, editor: *Operative hand surgery,* ed 3, vol 2, New York, 1993, Churchill Livingstone, pp 1587-1690.

30. Fink CW, Baum J, Paradies LH, et al.: Synovectomy in juvenile rheumatoid arthritis, *Ann Rheum Dis* 28:612-616, 1969.

31. Fisher JC: The silicone controversy—when will science prevail? *N Engl J Med* 326:1696-1698, 1992.

32. Frisch EE: *Technology of silicones in biomedical applications.* In Rubin LR, editor: *Biomaterials in reconstructive surgery,* St. Louis, 1983, CV Mosby, pp 73-90.

33. Garcia-Elias M, Cooney W: Ligaments of the wrist, *Surgical Rounds in Orthopedics,* September 1989.

34. Goldner JL: Tendon transfers in rheumatoid arthritis, *Orthop Clin North Am* 5:425-444, 1974.

35. Goldring SR, Schiller AL, Roelke M, et al.: The synovial-like membrane at the bone-cement interface in loose total hip replacements and its proposed role in bone lysis, *J Bone Joint Surg Am* 65:575-584, 1983.

36. Gordon M, Bullough PG: Synovial and osseous inflammation in failed silicone-rubber prostheses, *J Bone Joint Surg Am* 64:574-580, 1982.

37. Groff GD, Schned AR, Taylor TH: Silicone-induced adenopathy eight years after metacarpophalangeal arthroplasty, *Arthritis Rheum* 24:1578-1581, 1981.

38. Hanff G, Sollerman C, Elborgh R, et al.: Wrist synovectomy in juvenile chronic arthritis (JCA), *Scand J Rheumatol* 19:280-284, 1990.

39. Hanssen AD, Amadio PC, DeSilva SP, et al.: Deep postoperative wound infection after carpal tunnel release, *J Hand Surg [Am]* 14:869-873, 1989.

40. Hausner RJ, Schoen FJ, Pierson KK: Foreign-body reaction to silicone gel in axillary lymph nodes after an augmentation mammaplasty, *Plast Reconstr Surg* 62:381-384, 1978.

41. Helfgott SM, Skoff H: Scapholunate dissociation associated with crystal induced synovitis, *J Rheumatol* 19:485-487, 1992.

42. Hernandez-Jauregui P, Esperanza-Garcia C, Gonzalez-Angulo A: Morphology of the connective tissue grown in response to implanted silicone rubber: a light and electron microscopic study, *Surgery* 75:631-637, 1974.

43. Hindley CJ, Stanley JK: The rheumatoid wrist: patterns of disease progression. A review of 50 wrists, *J Hand Surg [Br]* 16:275-279, 1991.

44. Hodgson SP, Stanley JK, Muirhead A: The Wrightington classification of rheumatoid wrist X-rays: a guide to surgical management, *J Hand Surg [Br]* 14:451-455, 1989.

45. Irving IM, Castilla P, Hall EG, et al.: Tissue reaction to pure and impregnated silastic, *J Pediatr Surg* 6:724-729, 1971.

46. Ishikawa H, Hanyu T, Tajima T: Rheumatoid wrists treated with synovectomy of the extensor tendons and the wrist joint combined with a Darrach procedure, *J Hand Surg [Am]* 17:1109-1117, 1992.

47. Jacobsen ST, Levinson JE, Crawford AH: Late results of synovectomy in juvenile rheumatoid arthritis, *J Bone Joint Surg Am* 67:8-15, 1985.

48. Kessler I, Vainio K: Posterior (dorsal) synovectomy for rheumatoid involvement of the hand and wrist. A follow-up study of sixty-six procedures, *J Bone Joint Surg Am* 48:1085-1094, 1966.

49. Kircher T: Silicone lymphadenopathy: a complication of silicone elastomer finger joint prostheses, *Hum Pathol* 11:240-244, 1980.

50. Kleinert JM, Lister GD: Silicone implants, *Hand Clin* 2:271-290, 1986.

51. Kozin SH, Bishop AT: Atypical Mycobacterium infections of the upper extremity, *J Hand Surg [Am]* 19:480-487, 1994.

52. Kvien TK, Pahle JA, Hoyeraal HM, et al.: Comparison of synovectomy and no synovectomy in patients with juvenile rheumatoid arthritis. A 24-month controlled study, *Scand J Rheumatol* 16:81-91, 1987.

53. Lazaro MA, Garcia Morteo O, de Benyacar MA, et al.: Lymphadenopathy secondary to silicone hand joint prostheses, *Clin Exp Rheumatol* 8:17-22, 1990.

54. Linscheid RL, Dobyns JH, Beabout JW, et al.: Traumatic instability of the wrist. Diagnosis, classification, and pathomechanics, *J Bone Joint Surg Am* 54:1612-1632, 1972.

55. Martel W, Hayes JT, Duff IF: The pattern of bone erosion in the hand and wrist in rheumatoid arthritis, *Radiology* 84:204-214, 1965.

56. Millender LH, Nalebuff EA: Preventive surgery—tenosynovectomy and synovectomy, *Orthop Clin North Am* 6:765-792, 1975.

57. Millender LH, Nalebuff EA, Albin R, et al.: Dorsal tenosynovectomy and tendon transfer in the rheumatoid hand, *J Bone Joint Surg Am* 56:601-610, 1974.

58. Millender LH, Nalebuff EA, Hawkins RB, et al.: Infection after silicone prosthetic arthroplasty in the hand, *J Bone Joint Surg Am* 57:825-829, 1975.

59. Mirra JM, Amstutz HC, Matos M, et al.: The pathology of the joint tissues and its clinical relevance in prosthesis failure, *Clin Orthop* 117:221-240, 1976.

60. Mirra JM, Marder RA, Amstutz HC: The pathology of failed total joint arthroplasty, *Clin Orthop* 170:175-183, 1982.

61. Moore JR, Weiland AJ, Valdata L: Tendon ruptures in the rheumatoid hand: analysis of treatment and functional results in 60 patients, *J Hand Surg [Am]* 12:9-14, 1987.

62. Morrey BF, Askew L, Chao EY: Silastic prosthetic replacement for the radial head, *J Bone Joint Surg Am* 63:454-458, 1981.

63. Nalebuff EA: Rheumatoid hand surgery—update, *J Hand Surg [Am]* 8:678-682, 1983.

64. Ogilvie C, Kay NR: Fulminating carpal tunnel syndrome due to gout, *J Hand Surg [Br]* 13:42-43, 1988.

65. Paplanus SH, Payne CM: Axillary lymphadenopathy 17 years after digital silicone implants: study with x-ray microanalysis, *J Hand Surg [Am]* 13:399-400, 1988.

66. Peimer CA: Long-term complications of trapeziometacarpal silicone arthroplasty, *Clin Orthop* 220:86-98, 1987.

67. Peimer CA: Arthroplasty of the hand and wrist: complications and failures, *Instr Course Lect* 38:15-30, 1989.

68. Peimer CA, Medige J, Eckert BS, et al.: Reactive synovitis after silicone arthroplasty, *J Hand Surg [Am]* 11:624-638, 1986.

69. Peimer CA, Taleisnik J, Sherwin FS: Pathologic fractures: a complication of microparticulate synovitis, *J Hand Surg [Am]* 16:835-843, 1991.

70. Radcliffe K, Pattrick M, Doherty M: Complications resulting from misdiagnosing pseudogout as sepsis, *Br Med J [Clin Res]* 293:440-441, 1986.

71. Ranawat C, Straub LR: Volar tenosynovitis of wrist in rheumatoid arthritis, *Arthritis Rheum* 13:112-117, 1970.

72. Rate AJ, Parkinson RW, Meadows TH, et al.: Acute carpal tunnel syndrome due to pseudogout, *J Hand Surg [Br]* 17:217-218, 1992.

73. Revell PA, Weightman B, Freeman MA, et al.: The production and biology of polyethylene wear debris, *Arch Orthop Trauma Surg* 91:167-181, 1978.

74. Sasaki Y, Sugioka Y: The pronator quadratus sign: its classification and diagnostic usefulness for injury and inflammation of the wrist, *J Hand Surg [Br]* 14:80-83, 1989.

75. Sazy JA, Smith DJ Jr, Crissman JD, et al.: Immunogenic potential of carpal implants, *Surg Forum* 37:606-608, 1986.

76. Schumacher HR: *Primer on the rheumatic diseases,* ed 9, Atlanta, GA, 1988, Arthritis Foundation.

77. Smith DJ Jr, Sazy JA, Crissman JD, et al.: Immunogenic potential of carpal implants, *J Surg Res* 48:13-20, 1990.

78. Smith RJ, Atkinson RE, Jupiter JB: Silicone synovitis of the wrist, *J Hand Surg [Am]* 10:47-60, 1985.

79. Stanley JK: Conservative surgery in the management of rheumatoid disease of the hand and wrist, *J Hand Surg [Br]* 17:339-342, 1992.

80. Straub LR, Ranawat CS: The wrist in rheumatoid arthritis. Surgical treatment and results, *J Bone Joint Surg Am* 51:1-20, 1969.

81. Swanson AB: Improving end bearing characteristics of lower extremity amputation stumps. New York University Post-Graduate Medical School, *Intern Clin Inform Bull* 5:1-7, 1966.

82. Swanson AB: Silicone rubber implants for replacement of arthritis or destroyed joints in the hand, *Surg Clin North Am* 48:1113-1127, 1968.

83. Swanson AB: Silicone rubber implants for the replacement of the carpal scaphoid and lunate bones, *Orthop Clin North Am* 1:299-309, 1970.

84. Swanson AB: Implant arthroplasty for disabilities of the distal radioulnar joint. Use of a silicone rubber capping implant following resection of the ulnar head, *Orthop Clin North Am* 4:373-382, 1973.

85. Swanson AB, de Groot Swanson G: *Implant arthroplasty in the carpal and radiocarpal joints.* In Lichtman DM, editor: *The wrist and its disorders,* Philadelphia, 1988, WB Saunders, pp 404-438.

86. Swanson AB, Meester WD, Swanson GG, et al.: Durability of silicone implants—an in vivo study, *Orthop Clin North Am* 4:1097-1112, 1973.

87. Swanson AB, Swanson GG, Maupin BK, et al.: Failed carpal bone arthroplasty: causes and treatment, *J Hand Surg [Am]* 14:417-424, 1989.

88. Swett PP: Synovectomy in chronic infectious arthritis, *J Bone Joint Surg* 5:110-121, 1923.

89. Taleisnik J: Rheumatoid synovitis of the volar compartment of the wrist joint: its radiological signs and its contribution to wrist and hand deformity, *J Hand Surg [Am]* 4:526-535, 1979.

90. Thirupathi RG, Ferlic DC, Clayton ML: Dorsal wrist synovectomy in rheumatoid arthritis—a long-term study, *J Hand Surg [Am]* 8:848-856, 1983.

91. Vaughan-Jackson OJ: Rupture of extensor tendons by attrition at the inferior radio-ulnar joint, *J Bone Joint Surg Br* 30:528-530, 1948.

92. Vaughan-Jackson OJ: Rheumatoid hand deformities considered in the light of tendon imbalance. I., *J Bone Joint Surg Br* 44:764-775, 1962.

93. Vistnes LM, Ksander GA, Kosek J: Study of encapsulation of silicone rubber implants in animals. A foreign-body reaction, *Plast Reconstr Surg* 62:580-588, 1978.

94. Wanivenhaus A, Lintner F, Wurnig C, et al.: Long-term reaction of the osseous bed around silicone implants, *Arch Orthop Trauma Surg* 110:146-150, 1991.

95. Watson HK, Ballet FL: The SLAC wrist: scapholunate advanced collapse pattern of degenerative arthritis, *J Hand Surg [Am]* 9:358-365, 1984.

96. White RE Jr: Resection of the distal ulna with and without implant arthroplasty in rheumatoid arthritis, *J Hand Surg [Am]* 11:514-518, 1986.

97. Withrington RH, Seifert MH: Predominant wrist disease in rheumatoid arthritis associated with high concentration of IgA rheumatoid factor, *Br Med J [Clin Res]* 291:1388, 1985.

98. Worsing RA Jr, Engber WD, Lange TA: Reactive synovitis from particulate silastic, *J Bone Joint Surg Am* 64:581-585, 1982.

99. Wright CS, Wilgis EF: Erosive silicone synovitis, *Can J Surg* 29:45-47, 1986.

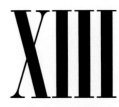

XIII
SOFT-TISSUE PROBLEMS AND NEOPLASMS

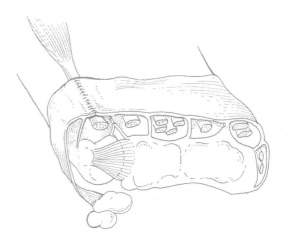

49

GANGLIONS OF THE WRIST

Scott H. Kozin, M.D.
Allen T. Bishop, M.D.

ETIOLOGY
DIAGNOSIS
    MEDICAL HISTORY
    PHYSICAL EXAMINATION
    TRANSILLUMINATION
    RADIOGRAPHS
    DIAGNOSTIC AND THERAPEUTIC ASPIRATION
    DIAGNOSTIC TESTS
NONOPERATIVE TREATMENT
OPERATIVE TREATMENT

DORSAL WRIST GANGLION
    PREFERRED APPROACH
    SPECIAL CONSIDERATIONS
PALMAR WRIST GANGLION
    PREFERRED APPROACH
    SPECIAL CONSIDERATIONS
POSTOPERATIVE TREATMENT AND REHABILITATION
DORSAL CARPAL GANGLION COMPLICATIONS
PALMAR CARPAL GANGLION COMPLICATIONS

Ganglions are the most frequent tumors seen around the wrist. They occur in predictable locations, in decreasing order of prevalence: the dorsal scapholunate area, the palmar radiocarpal region, the dorsal retinaculum of the first dorsal compartment, within the carpal tunnel, within Guyon's canal, and the ulnocarpal and second metacarpal trapezial joint (Table 49-1). They account for 50% to 70% of all soft-tissue lesions involving the hand.[5]

ETIOLOGY

Dorsal ganglions are more prevalent in women in the 2nd, 3rd, and 4th decades; radiocarpal palmar ganglions are more common in women in the 5th, 6th, and 7th decades. They are uncommon in children.[33,48] There is no social or occupational predisposition. Dorsal radiocarpal ganglions arise from the scapholunate ligament dorsally where the multidimensional motion between the scaphoid and lunate is concentrated. It is thought that joint fluid is pumped through a weak area between collagen bundles during carpal motions.[3] A one-way valve mechanism prevents the joint fluid from reentering the joint.[2] Repeated extrusion causes the development of a cyst with a pseudocapsule filled with mucinous joint fluid. Absorption during restricted activity results in diminution in size. The ganglion may protrude from the scapholunate ligament but be trapped under the radiocarpal capsule, producing an occult ganglion.[17] This may be painful even if small because of compression with wrist extension or flexion. Protrusion through the weak dorsal capsule results in a visible and palpable firm, smooth, and occasionally multilobular mass. This is often located where the dorsal interosseous nerve branches into the wrist capsule,[10,17] a possible explanation for the unique painful presentation often seen.

A ganglion may be uniloculated or multiloculated. The cyst is composed of clear, viscous, jellylike mucinous fluid surrounded by a capsule. The capsule wall is lined by compressed collagen fibers and flat nonendothelial cells that appear unlikely to have originated from the synovium[2,5,14,30,43] (Fig. 49-1). The cyst narrows to a tortuous stalk that usually connects with the underlying joint capsule or tendon sheath.

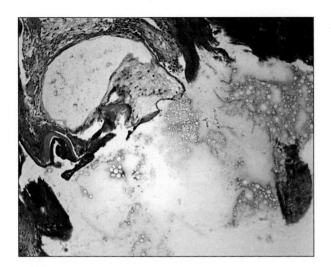

FIGURE 49-1

Photomicrograph of a ganglion cyst. Amorphous material is filling a cystic cavity that is lined by a thin layer of flattened cells.[43] (×100.)

Table 49-1. Ganglions in the Hand and Wrist

Ganglion	Incidence (%)
Dorsal wrist ganglion	60–70
Palmar wrist ganglion	18–20
Palmar retinacular cyst	5–10
Mucous cyst	5–10
Carpometacarpal ganglion	—
PIP joint ganglion	—
Extensor tendon ganglion	—
Intraosseous ganglion	—
Carpal tunnel ganglion	—
Guyon's canal ganglion	—
Intratendinous ganglion	—

PIP, proximal interphalangeal.

The exact origin and pathogenesis of a ganglion are debated.[1,3,12,35,48] Ganglions are not neoplasms and malignant degeneration has never been reported.[5] Whether the cyst originates from the synovial-capsular interface and extends into the soft tissue or results from mucoid degeneration of connective tissue with secondary joint communication remains controversial. Despite this confusion, ablation of the joint or tendon sheath connection is imperative to prevent recurrence after surgical excision.

A palmar radiocarpal ganglion may arise by a similar mechanism at or near the origin of the radiocarpal ligaments at the radial styloid and from the scaphotrapezial ligaments at the scaphotrapezial joint. Andren and Eiken[1] showed that dye injected into the scaphotrapezial joint would flow into some of these ganglions, implicating a valvular mechanism in the scaphotrapezial joint. Protrusion can follow the path of least resistance along the sheath of the flexor carpi radialis (FCR), and the ganglion often becomes prominent just proximal to the thickened band of antebrachial fascia that defines the proximal extent of the tendon sheath.

Retinacular ganglions at the first dorsal compartment are usually associated with a thickened hypertrophic retinaculum over the site of a stenosing tenosynovitis (de Quervain's disease); tenosynovial fluid in this instance is forced through a small slit on the deep retinacular surface that is easily seen when the retinaculum is cut.

Guyon's canal ganglions and ulnocarpal ganglions arise from a weak area in the pisohamate ligament or ulnocarpal capsule.[49] The former may be occult except for the presentation of a low ulnar motor palsy. Intracarpal canal ganglions occasionally are responsible for carpal tunnel syndrome.[19,27,42] Small ganglions also arise occasionally from the dorsal weak area between the V-shaped limbs of the second metacarpal trapezial ligaments. Ganglions in other locations can usually be traced to one of the above origins, although occasionally by a more circuitous route.

DIAGNOSIS

Accurate diagnosis of these common soft-tissue tumors of the hand is not always straightforward. A mass, localized pain, and weakness are the usual presenting complaints. A history of antecedent trauma may be present. The mass may fluctuate in size and degree of discomfort in accordance with level of activity. Neurologic complaints are uncommon except in carpal tunnel and Guyon's canal ganglions.[27,49]

Physical examination should demonstrate the typical location and findings of a ganglion cyst. Palpation reveals a variable consistency ranging from soft to firm. The cyst should remain stationary with tendon excursion unless the ganglion is intratendinous. Transillumination is a useful finding and helps confirm the diagnosis. Radiographs of the wrist should be obtained but are usually unremarkable for osseous abnormalities. A scapholunate dissociation may be the exception (wide scapholunate interval). Underlying osteoarthritis may be present and suggests the origin of the cyst. Such information may help plan the surgical approach. In addition, intraosseous carpal ganglions are apparent on radiographs. After initial evaluation, additional studies are usually not necessary if clinical suspicion and physical findings indicate a ganglion.

The term "occult ganglion" refers to a ganglion that is suspected by history but undetectable on examination.[17,46] High-resolution ultrasonography is

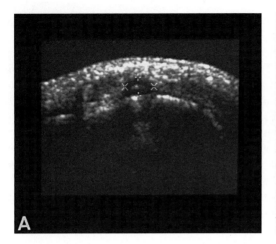 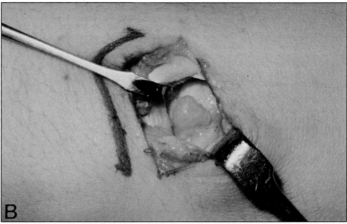

FIGURE 49-2

A, Transverse, high-resolution ultrasonogram of the right wrist demonstrates an occult dorsal ganglion. **B,** Surgical confirmation of occult dorsal wrist ganglion.

useful to confirm the diagnosis in these equivocal cases (Fig. 49-2, *A*), and magnetic resonance imaging can be considered if the ultrasonogram is equivocal.[9,21,28,33,39] Surgical exploration can be necessary to confirm the presence of an occult ganglion (Fig. 49-2, *B*).

The differential diagnosis of a ganglionlike mass in the wrist includes neoplasms, infections, localized inflammation, anomalous muscles, and vascular malformations (Table 49-2). Unusual symptoms or atypical physical findings should arouse suspicion of an alternative diagnosis. Excessive pain or pain at rest (night) suggests a more serious problem than a ganglion cyst.

Preoperative planning includes medical history, physical examination (including transillumination), radiographs, and, frequently, diagnostic or therapeutic aspiration. Additional tests such as ultrasonography or magnetic resonance imaging may be indicated (Fig. 49-3).

Patients are informed of the possible need for postoperative hand therapy. If loss of wrist or finger motion is present preoperatively, evaluation by the hand therapist is warranted.

MEDICAL HISTORY

Salient medical history includes the circumstances of the origin of the mass (spontaneous or after trauma); duration; changes in size, shape, or consistency; and the nature, degree, and fluctuations of symptoms. Information relevant to treatment includes the degree of discomfort or dysfunction, symptoms of nerve compression, and previous aspiration or excision.

Ganglions are somewhat unique in their ability to change size or symptoms. They usually become more symptomatic after activity or spontaneously resolve after direct trauma. Other mass lesions such as neoplasms rarely change size or shape.

Table 49-2. Differential Diagnosis of Common Wrist Ganglions

Cysts and Neoplasms	
Lipoma	Gout tophi
Xanthoma	Inflamed bursae
Fibroma	
Hemangioma	**Bone**
Synovial sarcoma	Carpal instability
Osteochondroma	Avascular necrosis
Malignant fibrous	Osteophyte
histiocytoma	
Lymphangioma	**Vascular**
Chondrosarcoma	Aneurysm
	Arteriovenous
Infections	malformation
Mycobacterium	
Fungi	**Muscle**
Inflammation	Anomalous muscle
Rheumatoid nodule	Extensor digitorum
	brevis manus

Additional diagnostic considerations are inclusion cyst, foreign body granuloma, inflammatory arthritis, tenosynovitis, or infectious granuloma. From an epidemiologic standpoint, ganglions have been shown to be slightly more prevalent in women and occur most often in the 2nd, 3rd, and 4th decades.[2-4,14,16,37]

PHYSICAL EXAMINATION

The ganglion is examined for location, size, extension, and loculations. Results of palpation for tenderness, consistency, fluctuance, and adherence to other structures are noted. Ballottement may help reveal the extent of the lesion and the direction of the pedicle.

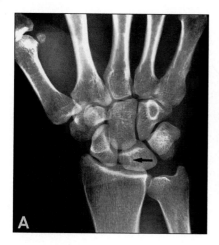
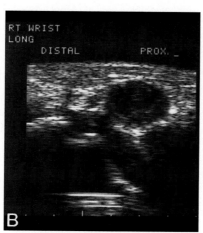
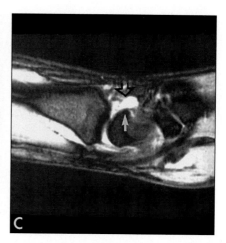

FIGURE 49-3

Imaging of the wrist. **A,** An intraosseous carpal ganglion of the lunate (*arrow*). **B,** Transverse, high-resolution ultrasonogram. **C,** Magnetic resonance image of dorsal ganglion cyst palmar to extensor tendons (*open arrow*) and dorsal to lunate and scaphoid (*white arrow*).

Ganglions on the dorsum of the wrist (70% of all hand and wrist ganglions) are usually located dorsal to and originate from the scapholunate joint (Fig. 49-4).[2-4,11,31] Palmar flexion of the wrist accentuates the boundaries of the dorsal ganglion or may reveal an occult ganglion. Careful palpation helps avoid confusion with extensor tenosynovitis, dorsal carpal synovitis, or a carpal effusion.[25,47]

Preoperative functional hand and wrist evaluations include range of motion, muscle testing, grip and pinch strength, sensibility evaluation, vascular examination, and instability testing.

Ganglions on the palmar aspect of the wrist are usually located in the vicinity of the FCR tendon adjacent to the radial artery or at the junction of the radiocarpal joint and the scaphotrapezial joint (Fig. 49-5). Dorsiflexion of the wrist may accentuate the boundaries of a small or occult palmar ganglion. Functional examination is as described above. Patency of the radial artery is determined by palpation, Allen's test, and, if needed, Doppler examination. Ganglions on the ulnar side of the wrist warrant similar evaluation of the ulnar artery and nerve.

TRANSILLUMINATION

Transillumination with a small light placed against the lesion can confirm the diagnosis or help identify solid tumors such as fibromas, granulomas, or fibrous xanthomas.[35]

RADIOGRAPHS

Although radiographs do not usually demonstrate osseous pathology, standard anteroposterior, lateral, and oblique projections may demonstrate a soft-tissue shadow and show carpal abnormalities that may be

related to the development of the ganglion, such as a concomitant intraosseous ganglion.[*] Arthritic changes may be observed at the scaphotrapezial joint or radioscaphoid articulation. A scapholunate diastasis may occasionally be found in association with a dorsal ganglion cyst.

DIAGNOSTIC AND THERAPEUTIC ASPIRATION

Aspiration is useful as a diagnostic and therapeutic procedure.[11,22] In sterile conditions, the skin is anesthetized. Aspiration of mucinous material with a large-bore needle (18 G) is usually diagnostic. If aspiration is performed for treatment as well, multiple cyst-wall punctures are placed by using digital palpation to direct the needle and to decompress the mass.[22] Multiple punctures through the scapholunate ligament may deactivate the one-way valve mechanism. After aspiration, the carpus is immobilized for 3 weeks in a cast or splint in 10° of extension.[26]

Aspiration or injection of a steroid (or both) has been shown to be effective in 27% of dorsal carpal ganglions.[†] Immobilization after aspiration significantly improved the results of dorsal aspiration to 40% compared with 13%.[44] Therefore, immobilization is recommended after aspiration and cyst-wall puncture of most carpal ganglions.

DIAGNOSTIC TESTS

In the thick-walled, firm, deeply seated or small-sized lesion, the diagnosis may be obscured.[49] Ultrasonography[33,39] is helpful in assessing the proximity and the patency of the radial artery in palmar carpal

---

* References 6,23,32,34,36,51.
† References 2,3,22,34,35,37,44,55.

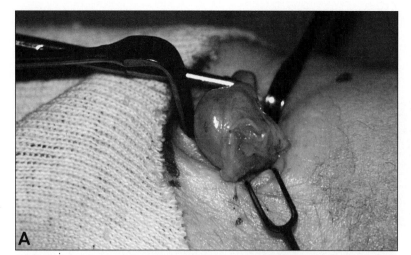

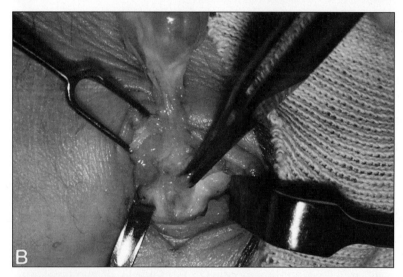

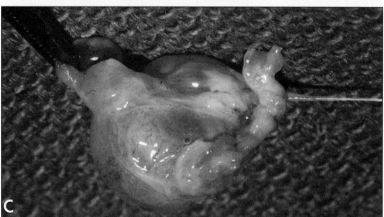

FIGURE 49-4

Dorsal carpal ganglion. **A,** Appearance of dorsal ganglion cyst. Excision through a transverse incision. **B,** Connection to the scapholunate ligament by an elongated pedicle. **C,** Excision of ganglion; stalk to the right.

ganglion and in locating a dorsal occult ganglion (Fig. 49-2, *A*). Magnetic resonance imaging is helpful in establishing the diagnosis in deeply seated or occult ganglions, such as those within the carpal canal or within Guyon's canal, but because of the cost it is indicated only for diagnostic dilemmas (Fig. 49-3, *C*).[15,49]

Arthrograms of the wrist have demonstrated the one-way valve mechanism and connection of the pedicle to the main cyst, but routine use is not warranted.[1,37] Arteriograms can assess compression of the radial artery but are usually unnecessary if careful palpation, Allen's test, and Doppler evaluation are performed.

The differential diagnosis[2] should include inflammatory (rheumatoid) or infectious (tuberculous) synovitis, tenosynovitis, inclusion cysts, rheumatoid nodules, foreign body granulomas, giant cell tumors of a

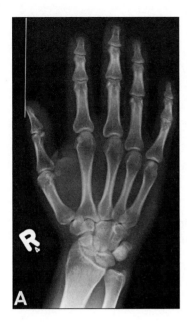
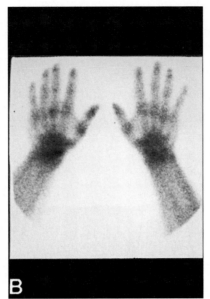
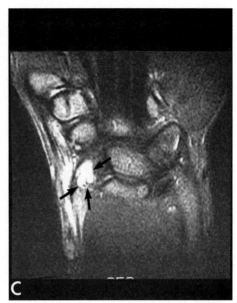

FIGURE 49-5

Palmar ganglion cyst. **A,** Posteroanterior view of wrist. Early arthritis at the scaphotrapezial joint, right wrist. **B,** Positive bone scan confirms the diagnosis of scaphotrapezial arthritis. **C,** Magnetic resonance imaging demonstrates an early (occult) ganglion on the radial palmar aspect of the wrist (*arrows*).

tendon sheath, lipomas, fibromas, neurilemomas, neurofibromas, carpal boss, osteochondromas, and, less likely, lymphangiomas, aneurysms, arteriovenous malformations, leiomyomas, aberrant muscle belly, and chronic abscesses (Table 49-2). Occasionally, the small thick-walled ganglion will be firm and nonmovable or resemble a bony deformity, and the diagnosis may be difficult.

NONOPERATIVE TREATMENT

Indications for the treatment of a ganglion include pain, weakness, nerve compression, and cosmetic deformity (Fig. 49-6). Many patients seek medical attention for fear of potential malignancy. Reassurance about the benign nature and the potential for spontaneous resolution is usually adequate treatment for the asymptomatic individual. Resolution rates without treatment range from 38% to 58%.[22,23,35,48]

There are many conservative regimens proposed for the treatment of ganglions. These methods include manual rupture, cyst-wall puncture, aspiration, and injection with steroids or sclerosing agents.[5,37,44,53,55] Sclerotherapy has been shown to be unsafe and is no longer advocated.[32] The remaining techniques have been used alone or in combination and have had variable results. Recurrence rates after conservative treatment range from 14% to 74%.[11,35,49,52,55] Repeated aspiration and immobilization of an aspirated dorsal wrist ganglion appear to decrease the recurrence

rate.[44,55] In addition, flexor tendon sheath ganglions respond better to conservative treatment. On the other hand, palmar ganglions are apt to have a high recurrence rate when treated by aspiration and injection; one study[52] found a 100% recurrence of palmar ganglion cysts.

If aspiration is selected as initial treatment, sterile technique is required.[38] The skin is anesthetized with 1% lidocaine injected through a 25-G needle. A large-bore needle (16 or 18 G) is required for aspiration because of the high viscosity of the cyst contents. The needle is directed into the cyst and its contents are evacuated. After decompression, the cyst wall can be multiply punctured or steroid may be instilled (or both). Many different steroid compounds have been advocated; we use betamethasone and vary the amount according to the cyst size.

OPERATIVE TREATMENT

Surgical excision is the most definitive treatment for hand and wrist ganglions.[4,7,28,52] The procedure should be performed in a surgical suite, with tourniquet control, and with loupe magnification. Regional or general anesthesia is required for a wrist ganglion, because local infiltration may obscure the surgical field and limit the time of tourniquet application. Neurovascular structures should be carefully protected and complete excision down to and including the wrist capsule is essential. During excision, diligent

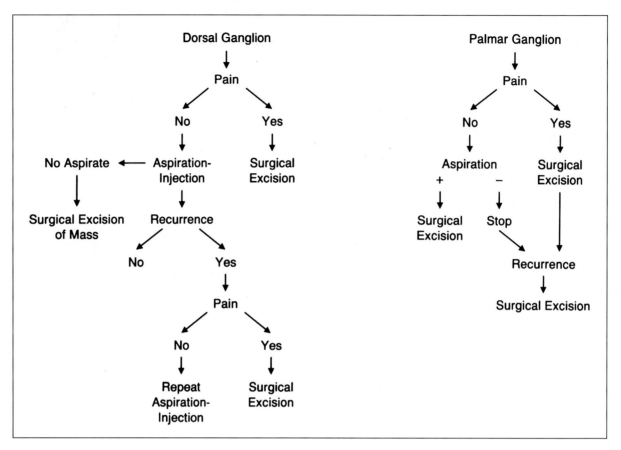

FIGURE 49-6

Treatment of ganglions and related masses.

search for and identification of the ganglion stalk are necessary. The tortuous stalk should be traced to its origin at the joint capsule or tendon sheath. The cyst, stalk, and a small portion of the joint capsule or tendon sheath origin should be excised. Closure of the capsular or tendon sheath defect may result in joint stiffness or loss of excursion and in general is not necessary. The tourniquet should be deflated and meticulous hemostasis obtained before wound closure. With proper excision, the recurrence rate is only 3% to 5% compared with 24% without stalk removal.[18,35,41]

Potential complications from surgical treatment are infection, ganglion recurrence, neurovascular injury, carpal instability, residual loss of motion, and hypertrophic scar formation. Careful surgical technique and postoperative management minimize the complication rate.

DORSAL WRIST GANGLION

The typical dorsal wrist ganglion originates from the scapholunate articulation (Fig. 49-7).[3,7,12] Vague dorsal wrist pain or a palpable mass dominates the presenting complaints. The pain is often increased by repetitive

or forceful wrist motion, especially dorsiflexion. Visualization of a dorsal wrist ganglion is accentuated by wrist flexion. Deep palpation elicits discomfort and may reveal the orientation of the pedicle. The cyst may be located directly over the scapholunate joint or at any location on the dorsal aspect of the hand. These distant ganglions are usually connected to the dorsal scapholunate ligament by an elongated pedicle.

A small ganglion may cause persistent pain and tenderness, but it may not be appreciated on physical examination.[17,46] The occult ganglion produces pain by either a pressure phenomenon or a direct compression of the posterior interosseous nerve.[10,17] High-resolution ultrasonography and magnetic resonance imaging are useful methods to delineate these small ganglions (Figs. 49-3, *B* and *C*).[9,15,33] We have had excellent success at diagnosis with ultrasound techniques.[33]

Standard wrist radiographs should be taken on all wrist ganglions to assess underlying bone and ligament integrity. Carpal instability, arthritis, or avascular necrosis can be confused with a painful wrist ganglion. Other diagnostic considerations include infectious or inflammatory tenosynovitis and an anomalous extensor digitorum brevis manus muscle[47] (Table 49-2).

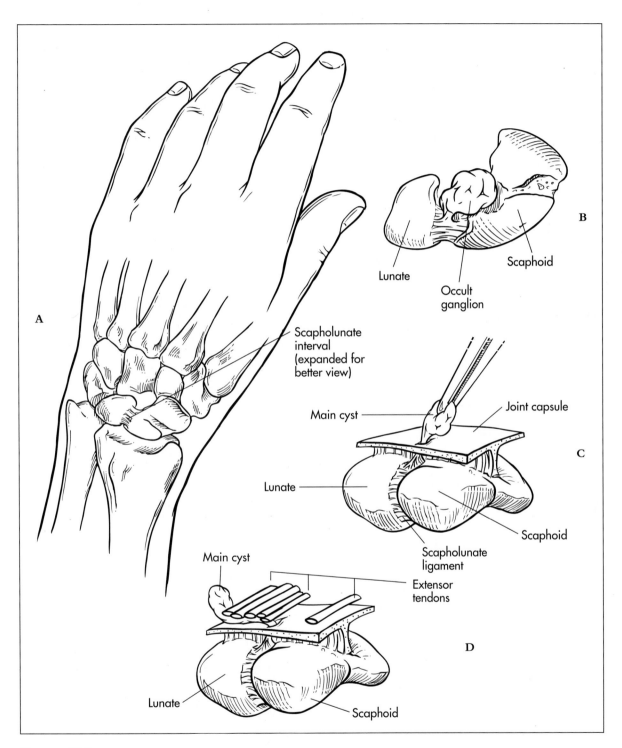

FIGURE 49-7

A, Scapholunate interval is the origin of dorsal ganglion cyst. Cyst must be traced to the scapholunate ligament. **B,** Transverse view of origin of dorsal ganglion cyst (scapholunate ligament). **C,** Distal ganglion with a long pedicle attached to scapholunate ligaments. Note stalk extending through joint capsule. **D,** Relationship of extensor tendons and stalk to a long pedicle of dorsal ganglion cyst that arises from the scapholunate ligament. *(Modified from Angelides AC and Wallace PF.[3] Copyright, American Society for Surgery of the Hand, by permission of Churchill Livingstone.)*

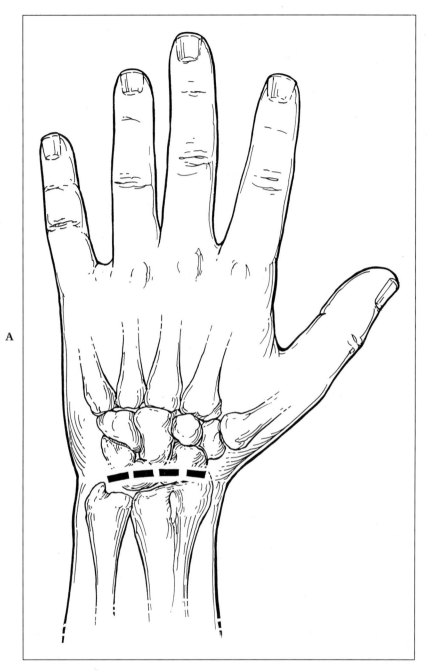

A

FIGURE 49-8

A, Transverse incision along Langer's lines for ganglionectomy and access to scapholunate ligament.

Preferred Approach. Operative excision of a dorsal wrist ganglion requires regional or general anesthesia, tourniquet control, and loupe magnification. A transverse incision along Langer's lines is planned to allow for ganglionectomy and access to the probable origin of the ganglion: the scapholunate ligament (Fig. 49-8). After the skin incision, sensory nerve branches are isolated and preserved. The cyst is identified usually between the extensor pollicis longus and the extensor digitorum communis tendons. Division of a portion of the extensor retinaculum distally between the third and fourth compartments facilitates exposure. The extensor pollicis longus and wrist extensors are retracted radially and the extensor digitorum communis is retracted ulnarly. The ganglion is mobilized circumferentially, avoiding cyst rupture. A blunt-tipped scissors or small curved hemostat helps prevent inadvertent cyst decompression. The stalk is identified and traced toward the wrist capsule. The stalk usually is located between the dorsal radiocarpal and dorsal intercarpal ligaments en route to the scapholunate articulation (Figs. 49-7 and 49-8, *B*). A circumferential excision of the capsular base of the cyst is performed with preservation of the dorsal wrist ligaments. The stalk is tangentially excised from the dorsal scapholunate ligament without violation of

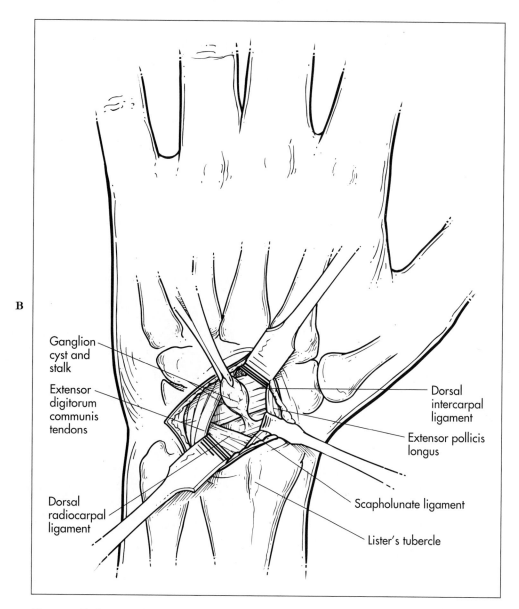

B

Ganglion
cyst and
stalk

Extensor
digitorum
communis
tendons

Dorsal
radiocarpal
ligament

Dorsal
intercarpal
ligament

Extensor pollicis
longus

Scapholunate ligament

Lister's tubercle

FIGURE 49-8, CONT'D.

B, Ganglion stalk originates from the dorsal scapholunate ligament and is between the dorsal radio-carpal and dorsal intercarpal ligaments.

the ligament's integrity. The defect in the capsule is not closed. The tourniquet is deflated and hemostasis is attained. The divided extensor retinaculum is reapproximated, and the incision is closed in a sub-cuticular fashion.

A bulky compressive hand dressing and palmar plaster forearm splint are applied. Finger motion is encouraged immediately in the postoperative period. The wound is inspected, and the dressing is replaced within a week. The sutures and splint are removed at 2 weeks. Hand therapy to regain normal wrist motion, especially flexion, is initiated at the 2-week period and may be necessary for a total of 6 weeks.

Special Considerations
1. Verify the presence and location of the ganglion on the day of operation before induction of anesthesia because it may have resolved temporarily.
2. If a ganglion is encountered away from the usual sites, one should suspect a long stalk that leads to the wrist capsule. The incision may need to be extended.
3. A curved longitudinal incision may be preferred for a multiloculated ganglion.
4. If during operation the ganglion on a long pedicle ruptures and cannot be adequately traced to its site of origin, excision of the capsule attachments to the scapholunate ligament is recommended.[2,3]

Table 49-3. Treatment of Anterior Wrist Ganglion in 84 Patients

Index Treatment	No.		Second Treatment	No.	
Aspiration		24	Aspiration and surgery		12
Recurrence	20		Recurrence	2	
No recurrence	4		No recurrence	10	
Surgery		60	Failed surgery with a second surgery		4
Recurrence	12		Recurrence	2	
No recurrence	48		No recurrence	2	

From Wright TW et al.[52] Copyright, American Society for Surgery of the Hand, by permission of Churchill Livingstone.

5. After removal of the ganglion, inspect the site of origin for adjacent small ganglion pedicles or satellite cysts.
6. If a large ganglion near the wrist is found to contain caseous material, tuberculous synovitis should be considered. Specimens are taken for culture and changes to appropriate treatment are made.

PALMAR WRIST GANGLION

Palmar wrist ganglions usually originate from the radioscaphoid or scaphotrapezial joints.[16,24,52] A palpable mass, pain along the course of the radial artery or FCR sheath, and median nerve symptoms are potential presenting complaints. The cyst is usually palpated in the vicinity of the palmar wrist crease, radial to the FCR tendon, often displacing or surrounding the radial artery. Careful palpation may reveal the direction of the cyst origin. The mass may appear pulsatile because of its close proximity to the radial artery.[24,26,29] Examination should include Allen's test or Doppler ultrasonography to assess the relative contributions of the radial and ulnar arteries to hand circulation. Signs and symptoms of carpal tunnel syndrome are uncommon, but a palmar ganglion cyst can potentiate median nerve compression.[27,50] Differential diagnosis includes an aneurysm of the radial artery, lipoma, and fibroma within soft tissues. Doppler ultrasonography can identify the presence of an aneurysm and clarify the relationship of a cyst to the artery.

Standard anteroposterior and lateral radiographs may provide evidence of ganglion origin. The presence of scaphotrapezial trapezoid arthritis may signify the source of stalk formation. Magnetic resonance imaging is usually not necessary in the evaluation of a palmar wrist ganglion. Ultrasonography can be helpful if aspiration and injection are considered. Both studies are useful to demonstrate an occult ganglion and to determine recurrent cyst formation and the relationship to the radial artery (Doppler ultrasonography) (Fig. 49-9).

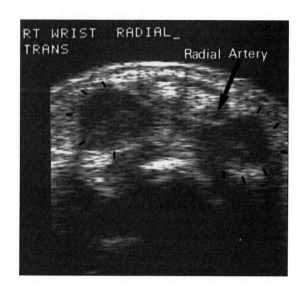

FIGURE 49-9

Doppler ultrasonogram of palmar ganglion cyst; note radial artery bright signal (*arrow*) to right of ganglion cyst.

Preferred Approach. We prefer not to aspirate, inject, or multiply puncture palmar wrist ganglions. The close proximity of the radial artery and frequent multiloculation limit the success of these conservative measures.[29,52] In addition, the recurrence rate exceeds 80% (Table 49-3). Operative intervention is the procedure of choice. It is performed during general or regional anesthesia, tourniquet control, and loupe magnification. A palmar, radial curvilinear or zigzag incision is recommended to allow access to the ganglion and periscaphoid articulations. Skin flaps are elevated and the incision is deepened through subcutaneous tissue to identify the dome of the cyst (Fig. 49-10). The palmar cutaneous branch of the median nerve and the lateral antebrachial cutaneous nerve are isolated and protected. These nerves course deep to the forearm fascia between the palmaris longus and FCR (palmar cutaneous nerve) and FCR tendon and radial artery (lateral cutaneous).[20]

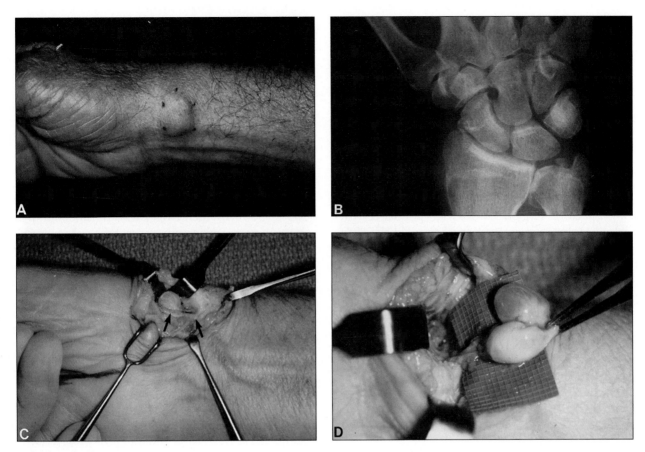

FIGURE 49-10

A, Clinical appearance of a right palmar ganglion cyst. **B,** Arthritis at scaphotrapezial trapezoid joint. **C,** Palmar wrist ganglion adjacent to radial artery (*arrows*). **D,** Excision of palmar carpal ganglion, stalk, and capsular base from the scaphotrapezial trapezoid joint.

Special care is exercised in mobilizing the cyst wall from the radial artery and FCR tendon. Adherence to the radial artery is common and dissection with a blunt-pointed scissors or small curved hemostat with loupe magnification decreases the chance of vessel injury and cyst rupture. The underlying stalk is traced to its site of origin, usually the radioscaphoid or scaphotrapezial joint (Table 49-4). The ganglion cyst, stalk, and a capsular base are excised. Any satellite cysts or extensions of the ganglion are removed. The tourniquet is deflated, and hemostasis is attained. The joint capsular defect is not closed. A subcuticular skin closure, bulky hand dressing, and palmar splint complete the procedure.

The bulky dressing is reduced within a week, and the splint is discarded at 2 weeks. Finger range of motion is encouraged throughout the postoperative period. Therapy to restore wrist motion is performed after immobilization has been discontinued.

Special Considerations

1. A bilobular palmar ganglion may involve the radial artery, dividing it into two lobules. Careful identification of the artery during dissection in a proximal

Table 49-4. Origin of Anterior Wrist Ganglion Determined at Surgery

Origin	Patients (no.)	Recurrences* (no.)
Radiocarpal joint	25	3
Scaphotrapezial joint	25	5
Ulnocarpal joint	5	2
Flexor carpi radialis sheath	6	1
Scaphotrapezial radiocarpal joint	4	0
Flexor carpi radialis tendon sheath or radiocarpal joint	1	1
Unknown	6	2
TOTAL	72	14

*$P = 0.24$, Fisher's exact test for association between site of original cyst and rate of recurrence.
From Wright TW et al.[52] Copyright, American Society for Surgery of the Hand, by permission of Churchill Livingstone.

to distal direction avoids inadvertent injury to or resection of the artery.

2. In a series of 654 patients with carpal tunnel syndrome, a ganglion was the causative factor in 3%.[42] Careful inspection of the carpal canal should be performed routinely after carpal tunnel release.

3. The FCR tendon goes deep within a fibro-osseous tunnel to reach its insertion. It passes the ulnar aspect of the scaphotrapezial joint. Opening of the tunnel and retraction of the tendon usually reveal the origin of the pedicle at the radiocarpal or scaphotrapezial joints.

4. Preoperative surgical consent for possible carpal tunnel release is recommended, because the pedicle may originate from the joints within the carpal tunnel.

POSTOPERATIVE TREATMENT AND REHABILITATION

Postoperative elevation of the upper extremity for 24 hours is recommended. Dressings are changed between the second and fifth postoperative days. If swelling permits, a commercial or custom-molded short arm splint is applied. For dorsal ganglion cysts, the wrist is immobilized in 30° of extension and the digits and elbow are left free. For a palmar ganglion, the wrist is placed in neutral flexion-extension. Hand therapy is initiated, including active finger motion. Sutures are removed in 10 to 14 days.

The period of immobilization of the wrist after dorsal carpal ganglion excision is controversial and ranges from none to 3 or 4 weeks. Those who advocate immobilization feel that removal of the portion of wrist capsule during ganglion excision warrants immobilization to allow for healing of the defect. They recommend that the wrist be immobilized for 3 weeks. After 3 weeks, more aggressive hand therapy is initiated until motion and strength have been regained. We believe that 2 weeks of splint immobilization yields satisfactory results. Because it is not uncommon for workers to require up to 6 weeks of rehabilitation before being able to return to strenuous work, preoperative discussions of the recovery period are desirable.[3,4]

DORSAL CARPAL GANGLION COMPLICATIONS

Complications after dorsal carpal ganglion excision include recurrence, continued pain or tenderness, wrist stiffness or weakness, neuroma formation, wound infection, and scar contracture or keloid formation. Carpal instability (including scapholunate dissociation), although possible, does not seem to be a common problem unless the scapholunate ligament is compromised.[8,13,51] Avascular necrosis of the scaphoid or lunate is rare.

Early recurrence, the most common complication, is usually the result of inadequate resection of the

valvular mechanism at the base of the ganglion. When this is adequately excised, the recurrence rate has been between 1% and 6%.[2-4,17,28,37] However, when only the main cyst was excised without adequate pedicle resection, recurrence rates have been between 24% and 40%.[2,3,25,35,46] A cluster of satellite ganglions is occasionally present at the base of the pedicle, indicating the site of origin. A recurrent ganglion can be difficult to manage, especially when the patient's confidence is decreased. Repeat aspiration and steroid injection can be performed; however, repeat surgical excision is usually required.[14,18,52] Dissection is done as described above; however, increased scar and adhesions make repeat surgery and identification of the stalk and origin of the ganglion more difficult. Cutaneous nerve damage is more frequent during reoperation for a recurrent ganglion, and care must be taken to identify cutaneous nerves before cyst excision.

Continued discomfort in the area of excision can be from a painful scar contracture, adhesions to neighboring structures, small neuromata, recurrent ganglion, or underlying carpal instability. Painful scar or adhesions are treated symptomatically with local injections of steroid combined with anti-inflammatory medication. Hand therapy for desensitization, heat, and rest, followed by mobilization and intermittent splinting, are often needed. Hand therapy is indicated for mobilization of painful contracture. Observation for early signs of reflex sympathetic dystrophy and appropriate treatment are warranted.

Continued wrist pain after ganglion excision may be secondary to underlying scaphoid instability.[8] Evaluation for static or dynamic instability includes the scaphoid shift maneuver[51] and standard and provocative radiographs (see Chapters 12 and 13).

Scapholunate instability has occurred from over-aggressive resection of the scapholunate ligament,[8,13] and instability may result from extensive resection of the dorsal scapholunate ligament.[8,13,17,40,45] However, the ganglion may be a manifestation of a preexisting underlying periscaphoid ligamentous instability,[51] and the ganglion excision may not cause scapholunate instability. The controversial aspects of this question have not been resolved.

Neuroma formation is avoided by identification and protection of sensory nerves during dissection. Superficial branches of the radial and of the dorsal ulnar nerves are at risk, particularly during reoperation. A longer incision in scar-free zones is recommended to avoid painful neuroma.[2-4] When neuroma occurs, steroid injection and desensitization are initiated. For refractory neuromata, surgical excision or burial of the neuroma in muscle or bone proximally is suggested.

Persistent neuropathy can occur from a long-standing ganglion that had caused preoperative nerve compression. The deep branch of the ulnar nerve has been involved occasionally.[4,5,7,50]

PALMAR CARPAL GANGLION COMPLICATIONS

Complications after palmar carpal ganglion excision are similar to those for the dorsal ganglion, with the additional potential for injury to the radial artery and the terminal branch of the lateral antebrachial cutaneous or the palmar cutaneous branch of the median nerve. The postoperative recurrence rate is much higher for palmar ganglion (30% to 33%) compared with adequately excised dorsal ganglion (1% to 24%) because of the more variable sites of origin of palmar ganglions.* Careful identification of the origin of the ganglion from the scaphotrapezial joint or radiocarpal joint is essential to prevent recurrence. Complications associated with excision of a palmar ganglion include injury to the radial artery and its branches, adhesions in the FCR tendon sheath limiting wrist extension, and hypertrophic scars on the palmar aspect of the wrist.

---

* References 2,3,11,21,35,54.

REFERENCES

1. Andren L, Eiken O: Arthrographic studies of wrist ganglions, *J Bone Joint Surg Am* 53:299-302, 1971.
2. Angelides AC: *Ganglions of the hand and wrist.* In Green DP, editor: *Operative hand surgery,* ed 2, New York, 1988, Churchill Livingstone, pp 2281-2299.
3. Angelides AC, Wallace PF: The dorsal ganglion of the wrist: its pathogenesis, gross and microscopic anatomy, and surgical treatment, *J Hand Surg [Am]* 1:228-235, 1976.
4. Barnes WE, Larsen RD, Posch JL: Review of ganglia of the hand and wrist with analysis of surgical treatment, *Plast Reconstr Surg* 34:570-578, 1964.
5. Bogumill GP: *Tumors of the hand.* In Evarts CM, editor: *Surgery of the musculoskeletal system,* ed 2, New York, 1990, Churchill Livingstone, pp 1197-1250.
6. Bowers WH, Hurst LC: An intraarticular-intraosseous carpal ganglion, *J Hand Surg [Am]* 4:375-377, 1979.
7. Clay NR, Clement DA: The treatment of dorsal wrist ganglia by radical excision, *J Hand Surg [Br]* 13:187-191, 1988.
8. Crawford GP, Taleisnik J: Rotatory subluxation of the scaphoid after excision of dorsal carpal ganglion and wrist manipulation—a case report, *J Hand Surg [Am]* 8:921-925, 1983.
9. De Flaviis L, Nessi R, Del Bo P, et al.: High-resolution ultrasonography of wrist ganglia, *J Clin Ultrasound* 15:17-22, 1987.
10. Dellon AL, Seif SS: Anatomic dissections relating the posterior interosseous nerve to the carpus, and the etiology of dorsal wrist ganglion pain, *J Hand Surg [Am]* 3:326-332, 1978.
11. Derbyshire RC: Observations on the treatment of ganglia with a report on hydrocortisone, *Am J Surg* 112:635-636, 1966.
12. de Villiers CM, Birnie RH, Pretorius LK, et al.: Dorsal ganglion of the wrist—pathogenesis and biomechanics. Operative v. conservative treatment, *S Afr Med J* 75:214-216, 1989.
13. Duncan KH, Lewis RC Jr: Scapholunate instability following ganglion cyst excision. A case report, *Clin Orthop* 228:250-253, 1988.
14. Eaton RG, Dobranski AI, Littler JW: Marginal osteophyte excision in treatment of mucous cysts, *J Bone Joint Surg Am* 55:570-574, 1973.
15. Feldman F, Singson RD, Staron RB: Magnetic resonance imaging of para-articular and ectopic ganglia, *Skeletal Radiol* 18:353-358, 1989.
16. Greendyke SD, Wilson M, Shepler TR: Anterior wrist ganglia from the scaphotrapezial joint, *J Hand Surg [Am]* 17:487-490, 1992.
17. Gunther SF: Dorsal wrist pain and the occult scapholunate ganglion, *J Hand Surg [Am]* 10:697-703, 1985.
18. Gurin J, Jakab G: Results of our operations for carpal ganglion, *Acta Chir Hung* 29:299-304, 1988.
19. Harvey FJ, Bosanquet JS: Carpal tunnel syndrome caused by a simple ganglion, *Hand* 13:164-166, 1981.
20. Hobbs RA, Magnussen PA, Tonkin MA: Palmar cutaneous branch of the median nerve, *J Hand Surg [Am]* 15:38-43, 1990.
21. Hollister AM, Sanders RA, McCann S: The use of MRI in the diagnosis of an occult wrist ganglion cyst, *Orthop Rev* 18:1210-1212, 1989.
22. Holm PC, Pandey SD: Treatment of ganglia of the hand and wrist with aspiration and injection of hydrocortisone, *Hand* 5:63-68, 1973.
23. Hvid-Hansen O: On the treatment of ganglia, *Acta Chir Scand* 136:471-476, 1970.
24. Jacobs LG, Govaers KJ: The volar wrist ganglion: just a simple cyst? *J Hand Surg [Br]* 15:342-346, 1990.
25. Janzon L, Niechajev IA: Wrist ganglia. Incidence and recurrence rate after operation, *Scand J Plast Reconstr Surg* 15:53-56, 1981.
26. Kelly GL: Radical artery occlusion by a carpal ganglion. Case report, *Plast Reconstr Surg* 52:191-193, 1973.
27. Kerrigan JJ, Bertoni JM, Jaeger SH: Ganglion cysts and carpal tunnel syndrome, *J Hand Surg [Am]* 13:763-765, 1988.

28. Leung P-C: *Tumors.* In Boswick JA Jr, editor: *Current concepts in hand surgery,* Philadelphia, 1983, Lea & Febiger, pp 32-42.

29. Lister GD, Smith RR: Protection of the radial artery in the resection of adherent ganglions of the wrist, *Plast Reconstr Surg* 61:127-129, 1978.

30. Loder RT, Robinson JH, Jackson WT, et al.: A surface ultrastructure study of ganglia and digital mucous cysts, *J Hand Surg [Am]* 13:758-762, 1988.

31. MacCollum MS: Dorsal wrist ganglions in children, *J Hand Surg [Am]* 2:325, 1977.

32. Mackie IG, Howard CB, Wilkins P: The dangers of sclerotherapy in the treatment of ganglia, *J Hand Surg [Br]* 9:181-184, 1984.

33. Mayo JG, Bishop AT, Reading CC: Ultrasonographic diagnosis of soft tissue lesions in the hand. Read at the 47th annual meeting of the American Society for Surgery of the Hand, Phoenix, 1989.

34. McEvedy BV: Simple ganglia, *Br J Surg* 49:585-594, 1962.

35. McEvedy BV: The simple ganglion. A review of modes of treatment and an explanation of the frequent failures of surgery, *Lancet* 266:135, 1965.

36. Mogan JV, Newberg AH, Davis PH: Intraosseous ganglion of the lunate, *J Hand Surg [Am]* 6:61-63, 1981.

37. Nelson CL, Sawmiller S, Phalen GS: Ganglions of the wrist and hand, *J Bone Joint Surg Am* 54:1459-1464, 1972.

38. Nield DV, Evans DM: Aspiration of ganglia, *J Hand Surg [Br]* 11:264, 1986.

39. Ogino T, Minami A, Fukada K, et al.: The dorsal occult ganglion of the wrist and ultrasonography, *J Hand Surg [Br]* 13:181-183, 1988.

40. Palmer AK, Dobyns JH, Linscheid RL: Management of post-traumatic instability of the wrist secondary to ligament rupture, *J Hand Surg [Am]* 3:507-532, 1978.

41. Palmieri TJ: Common tumors of the hand, *Orthop Rev* 16:367-378, 1987.

42. Phalen GS: The carpal-tunnel syndrome. Seventeen years' experience in diagnosis and treatment of six hundred fifty-four hands, *J Bone Joint Surg Am* 48:211-228, 1966.

43. Psaila JV, Mansel RE: The surface ultrastructure of ganglia, *J Bone Joint Surg Br* 60:228-233, 1978.

44. Richman JA, Gelberman RH, Engber WD, et al.: Ganglions of the wrist and digits: results of treatment by aspiration and cyst wall puncture, *J Hand Surg [Am]* 12:1041-1043, 1987.

45. Ruby LK, An KN, Linscheid RL, et al.: The effect of scapholunate ligament section on scapholunate motion, *J Hand Surg [Am]* 12:767-771, 1987.

46. Sanders WE: The occult dorsal carpal ganglion, *J Hand Surg [Br]* 10:257-260, 1985.

47. Shaw JA, Manders EK: Extensor digitorum brevis manus muscle. A clinical reminder, *Orthop Rev* 17:867-869, 1988.

48. Soren A: Pathogenesis and treatment of ganglion, *Clin Orthop* 48:173-179, 1966.

49. Subin GD, Mallon WJ, Urbaniak JR: Diagnosis of ganglion in Guyon's canal by magnetic resonance imaging, *J Hand Surg [Am]* 14:640-643, 1989.

50. Trevaskis AE, Tilly D, Marcks KM, et al.: Loss of nerve function in the hand caused by ganglions, *Plast Reconstr Surg* 39:97-100, 1967.

51. Watson HK, Rogers WD, Ashmead D IV: Reevaluation of the cause of the wrist ganglion, *J Hand Surg [Am]* 14:812-817, 1989.

52. Wright TW, Cooney WP, Ilstrup DM: Anterior wrist ganglion, *J Hand Surg [Am]* 19:954-958, 1994.

53. Young L, Bartell T, Logan SE: Ganglions of the hand and wrist, *South Med J* 81:751-760, 1988.

54. Zachariae L, Vibe-Hansen H: Ganglia. Recurrence rate elucidated by a follow-up of 347 operated cases, *Acta Chir Scand* 139:625-628, 1973.

55. Zubowicz VN, Ishii CH: Management of ganglion cysts of the hand by simple aspiration, *J Hand Surg [Am]* 12:618-620, 1987.

50

TENDINITIS OF THE WRIST

Scott H. Kozin, M.D.
Allen T. Bishop, M.D.
William P. Cooney, M.D.

ETIOLOGY
GENERAL DIAGNOSIS AND TREATMENT
  CONSIDERATIONS
    DIAGNOSIS
    TREATMENT
TENDINITIS OF THE EXTENSOR COMPARTMENTS
  DE QUERVAIN'S DISEASE
    NONOPERATIVE TREATMENT
    SURGICAL TREATMENT
    COMPLICATIONS
  INTERSECTION SYNDROME
    NONOPERATIVE TREATMENT
    SURGICAL TREATMENT
  EXTENSOR POLLICIS LONGUS TENDINITIS
    NONOPERATIVE TREATMENT
    SURGICAL TREATMENT

EXTENSOR INDICIS PROPRIUS SYNDROME
EXTENSOR DIGITI MINIMI TENDINITIS
EXTENSOR CARPI ULNARIS TENDINITIS
    NONOPERATIVE TREATMENT
    SURGICAL TREATMENT
TENDINITIS OF THE FLEXOR COMPARTMENTS
  FLEXOR CARPI ULNARIS TENDINITIS
    DIAGNOSIS
    TREATMENT
  FLEXOR CARPI RADIALIS TENDINITIS
    NONOPERATIVE TREATMENT
    OPERATIVE TREATMENT
  RESTRICTIVE THUMB-INDEX TENOSYNOVITIS
    (LINBURG'S SYNDROME)
      NONOPERATIVE TREATMENT
      OPERATIVE TREATMENT

Tendinitis and associated tenosynovitis are encountered daily by the clinician. Accurate diagnosis and early intervention often result in resolution of symptoms. Persistent tendinitis is more difficult to manage and recovery is delayed. Modification of activity and graduated therapy are mainstays of treatment. An understanding of the epidemiology, pathophysiology, and treatment options will better equip the physician to manage these difficult problems.

ETIOLOGY

Tendinitis or tenosynovitis may be a primary, frequently idiopathic, process or secondary to abnormalities of surrounding tissues. Tendon abnormality may result from a single traumatic event or, more commonly, may be the result of repetitive use. Ordinarily, tendons adapt to changing stress by increasing collagen content and cross-sectional area.[9,25,60] When subjected to excessive force or repetitive use, the capability of tendon to adapt is exceeded and damage to collagen bundles may occur. Such repetitive microtrauma may result in sufficient macroscopic injury to induce a repair reaction.

The repair response consists of three distinct stages: inflammation, proliferation, and maturation.[15,40,60] Inflammation results from the release of vasoactive and chemotactic factors from the damaged tissue. Vasodilatation, increased vascular permeability, and migration of cellular elements cause the clinical signs of swelling, warmth, and erythema. Proliferation eventually occurs if the inciting process is halted, as fibroblasts produce collagen and supporting ground substance. If not, a chronic inflammation results, with secondary adhesions and fibrosis. The new tissue is immature, weak, and susceptible to trauma. Maturation completes the healing process as collagen bundles form, increase in size, and become longitudinally aligned for effective force transmission.

Excessive force, repetition, or both in occupational or recreational activities[7,12] may provoke tendon microtrauma and an attempt at a reparative process. Interruption of the normal progression of healing by continued excessive use may affect the elite athlete, weekend athlete, laborer, computer operator, or musician.[2,31,60,66,72] Epidemiologic data[3] have demonstrated that the risk of wrist and hand tendinitis is 29 times greater in persons whose employment involves highly repetitive and forceful actions compared with those whose jobs involve low repetition and force. Ergonomic risk factors of upper extremity cumulative trauma disorders include repetition, force, posture, mechanical stress, vibration, temperature, and rest time.[2,4,21] Awkward positions of excessive shoulder abduction, wrist flexion, or wrist deviation increase the risk for tendinitis.[2,43] Vibration stimulates muscle contraction, a process referred to as the tonic vibration reflex.[4,17] In addition, persistent vibration decreases tactile sensation and increases the amount of force necessary to grasp an object. These effects of vibration combine to increase the incidence of upper extremity overuse.[4] Modification of ergonomic risk factors and regulation of activity are important considerations in the overall treatment plan. Alteration of working conditions and adaptation of equipment to fit the individual may require consideration.

GENERAL DIAGNOSIS AND TREATMENT CONSIDERATIONS

DIAGNOSIS

Accurate diagnosis begins with a careful history and physical examination. The history includes specific activities at work and recreation. The onset of symptoms and aggravating activity are important findings. A remote history of penetrating trauma or fracture should be investigated. Intratendinous foreign bodies are not rare and may provoke an inflammatory reaction.[44] Fracture malunion or prominent internal fixation may lead to mechanical irritation and tendinitis. The pain of tendinitis is characteristically described as aching and is aggravated by activity. Locking or triggering indicates sheath constriction, as in stenosing tenosynovitis, or sheath content increase, as in tendon nodule formation. A past medical history of infection or systemic illness is important. Indolent organisms

such as *Mycobacterium tuberculosis,* atypical mycobacteria, and fungi may be present with tenosynovial reaction and mimic benign inflammation.[67] Systemic conditions that accompany tendinitis include rheumatoid arthritis, diabetes mellitus, gout, pseudogout, and connective tissue diseases.[30,57,67]

Tenderness may be localized over the inflamed area or generalized throughout the upper extremity. Pain is often accentuated by passive stretching of the involved tendon or contraction of the attached muscle against resistance. Clinical examination may reveal subtle lacerations and scars indicative of previous trauma. Swelling, crepitus, and triggering of the involved tendon are classic findings. Range of motion and strength should be recorded in both extremities.

Standard radiographs should be obtained to assess for possible contributing causes such as fracture, tumor, osteophyte, or foreign body. Careful scrutiny of the radiograph may reveal calcific deposition in the area of inflammation, indicative of acute calcific tendinitis.[11,20,56,63] This condition is frequently misdiagnosed as infection and appropriate treatment is delayed. Management with immobilization, nonsteroidal anti-inflammatory medication, and occasionally with local injection of corticosteroids alleviates symptoms and may reverse the calcification findings within 2 to 3 weeks.

TREATMENT

Treatment of acute tendinitis is directed at control of inflammation. Rest, elevation, ice, immobilization, and anti-inflammatory medication are basic components. After resolution of symptoms, gradual rehabilitation consisting of stretching and strengthening begins. Recurrence or persistent symptoms imply a more recalcitrant and chronic form. Continued protection or immobilization, medications, and the addition of a local injection of steroid may be beneficial. Proper injection technique is mandatory, with avoidance of skin, intratendinous, or neurovascular injections. Excessive corticosteroid component increases the risk of skin depigmentation, fat atrophy, and tendon rupture. If in doubt, local anesthetic injection alone can be used to localize the site of inflammation. We use a mixture of 1 mL of a suspension containing 6 mg of betamethasone sodium phosphate and acetate suspension combined with 1 mL of 1% lidocaine to achieve therapeutic results. Betamethasone is water soluble and leaves no residue within the tendon sheath. Prolonged therapy and gradual return to activity may be necessary to promote tendon proliferation and maturation in these resistant cases. Modification of the inciting event or ergonomic alteration requires consideration. Failure to control tendinitis despite appropriate therapeutic measures is an indication for surgical intervention.

TENDINITIS OF THE EXTENSOR COMPARTMENTS

DE QUERVAIN'S DISEASE

de Quervain's disease is stenosing tenosynovitis of the first dorsal compartment.[19,59] This osteoligamentous tunnel is approximately 1 in. in length and is formed by an osseous groove in the radial styloid and the overlying extensor retinaculum[50] (Fig. 50-1). The abductor pollicis longus (APL) and extensor pollicis brevis (EPB) are enclosed in the first dorsal compartment en route to the thumb. Tendon structure and organization usually vary. Multiple APL tendon slips are present in 50% to 94% of wrists and septation between APL and EPB is evident in 20% to 50%.[33,36,45-47,55,66] Also, the EPB is absent in 5% to 12% of individuals.[47,54,55] Knowledge of these potential anatomic variations is necessary to optimize management and understand treatment failures.

de Quervain's disease usually affects women between the ages of 30 and 60 years.[66] A history of repetitive thumb abduction or extension or of ulnar wrist deviation may be elicited. This syndrome is more common in repetitive activities such as keyboarding, filing, carpentry, assembly-line work, and golfing.[21,50] Pain, tenderness, and swelling over the first dorsal compartment, increased with thumb motion, dominate the physical findings. The pain may radiate in a proximal or distal direction. The pain is exacerbated by passive wrist ulnar deviation with the thumb held neutral (Finkelstein's test).[28] Palpable crepitus is occasionally present over the compartment. Involvement of the EPB can be separated from the APL when there is pain associated with passive metacarpal flexion. Triggering of the thumb implies extensive stenosing

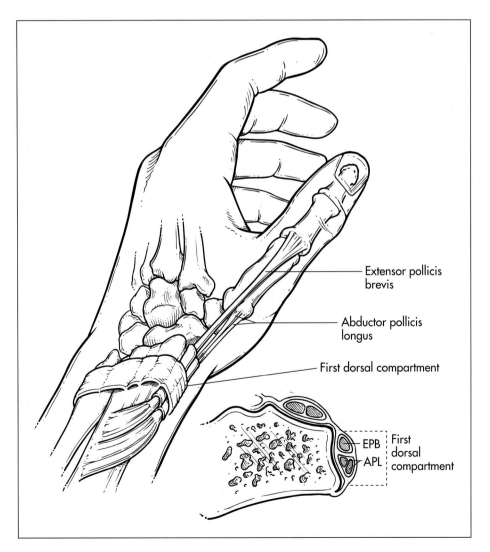

FIGURE 50-1

Anatomy of the first dorsal compartment. *APL,* abductor pollicis longus; *EPB,* extensor pollicis brevis.

A

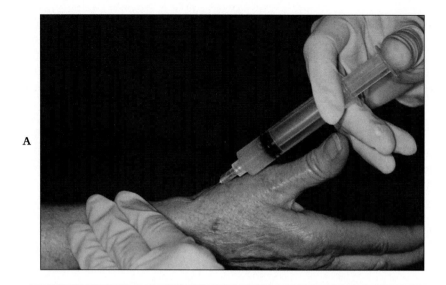

B

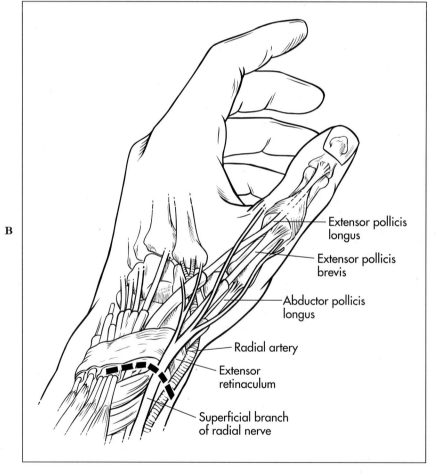

Extensor pollicis
longus

Extensor pollicis
brevis

Abductor pollicis
longus

Radial artery

Extensor
retinaculum

Superficial branch
of radial nerve

FIGURE 50–2

A, Technique of first dorsal compartment injection for de Quervain's disease. **B,** Operative release of second dorsal compartment—transverse incision. A dorsal radial curvilinear incision is preferred by some surgeons to ensure identification and protection of branching of the radial nerve.

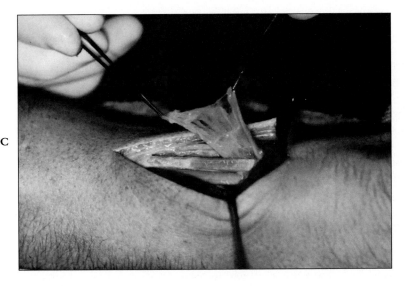

C

FIGURE 50-2, CONT'D.

C, For recalcitrant de Quervain's disease, tenosynovectomy of the abductor pollicis longus and extensor pollicis brevis, preserving the radial attachment of the extensor retinaculum, is recommended.

tenosynovitis or nodule formation on the APL or EPB and a more recalcitrant course.[68,71] Occasionally, a ganglion can be palpated over the tendon sheath at or near the distal edge of the extensor retinaculum. Affected individuals develop bilateral involvement 30% of the time.[66]

Differential diagnosis includes entrapment of the superficial branch of the radial nerve, arthrosis of the thumb axis and surrounding joints, and intersection syndrome.[18,22,67] Precise physical and sensory examination along with standard radiographic evaluation helps distinguish among these disorders.

Nonoperative Treatment. Early treatment of de Quervain's disease is directed toward control of inflammation and avoidance of aggravating activity. Forearm-based, thumb-spica-splint immobilization; oral non-steroidal anti-inflammatory medications; and direct corticosteroid injection form the basis of nonoperative treatment. Accurate injection is required to ascertain the effectiveness of the corticosteroid and to prevent complication.[36] Subcutaneous injection may cause fat atrophy and skin depigmentation. We use 1 mL of betamethasone and 1 mL of 1% lidocaine placed at a 45° angle into the distal part of the compartment (Fig. 50-2). Correct placement of the injection is indicated by filling of the proximal end of the first dorsal compartment tendon sheath. The local anesthetic should provide immediate, transient relief of symptoms. Conservative measures are effective in providing relief in up to 70% of patients.[36] Failure to respond to injection may indicate recalcitrant disease often secondary to separate compartments for the APL and EPB[36,47] tendons. A second more dorsal injection may be attempted to enter the EPB chamber.[47] Failure to abate signs and symptoms or continued recurrence despite conservative measures is an indication for surgical release.

Surgical Treatment. Surgical release is performed during local anesthesia and tourniquet control. A 2-cm transverse or gently curved incision is made just proximal to the radial styloid over the first dorsal compartment (Fig. 50-2).[49] The incision involves only the skin, and then blunt dissection is used to expose the extensor retinaculum over the compartment. Loupe magnification is used to identify and protect the branches of the radial sensory nerve. The first compartment is incised completely, maintaining a radio-palmar-based flap of retinaculum to prevent palmar subluxation of the tendons. The APL and EPB tendons are inspected and correctly identified. Bulky or adherent tenosynovium is resected to improve gliding. Atraumatic retraction of the EPB tendon should cause passive thumb metacarpophalangeal joint extension. The surgeon should not confuse multiple APL slips with EPB tendon, and a diligent search for septation should be performed, because the first compartment is commonly two separate fibro-osseous tunnels. After adequate release, the patient is instructed to move the thumb, and liberated motion of the tendons is evident. Hemostasis is attained and the skin incision is closed. The postoperative dressing is compressive and limits extensive thumb motion. This dressing is changed to a small wound dressing within a week, and graduated activity and strengthening are allowed.

Complications. Complications from operation are related to improper technique. Injury to the sensory branches of the radial sensory nerve may result from excessive retraction or direct laceration.[5,49] This most serious complication is the primary reason to avoid operation except in the chronic, unrelenting cases. Failure to release a separate EPB compartment may result in incomplete relief.[52,62] Palmar subluxation of the tendons after first compartment release has been reported and may require surgical reconstruction.[1,54,67]

Incising the compartment along the dorsal aspect maintains a palmar restraint to subluxation and prevents this complication.

INTERSECTION SYNDROME

The intersection syndrome occurs where the APL and EPB muscles obliquely traverse and intersect with the extensor carpi radialis longus and brevis tendons.[22,30,34,72] This area is located 4 to 8 cm proximal to the radial aspect of the wrist.[72] The friction of the overlying APL and EPB during repetitive motion causes the condition, which has been called APL bursitis,[73] peritendinitis crepitans,[34] and crossover tendinitis and which has been variously interpreted as a tenosynovitis of the second dorsal compartment,[34] an adventitial bursitis,[73] or a subcutaneous perimyositis.[72]

Primary presenting complaints are tenderness, pain, and swelling over the intersection area. A crepitant or squeaking sensation can often be appreciated with palpation or actually heard during wrist flexion and extension. This syndrome is common in individuals who row, weight lift, paint, or work on an assembly line that involves repetitive wrist motion.[21,72] Intersection syndrome can be differentiated from de Quervain's disease by its more proximal and dorsal location and negative result of Finkelstein's test.

Nonoperative Treatment. Nonoperative treatment of the intersection syndrome is frequently curative.[72] Cessation of the instigating cause, wrist immobilization in 20° of dorsiflexion, and anti-inflammatory medications abate the tenosynovitis. A local injection of steroid administered to the area of maximum crepitus and tenderness can supplement conservative treatment. Graduated rehabilitation is performed after control of inflammation and pain.

Surgical Treatment. Operative intervention is infrequently indicated in recalcitrant cases. A 4-cm longitudinal surgical incision is made over the intersection area. The radial sensory nerve branches are protected. Incision of the extensor retinaculum over the second dorsal compartment has been recommended[34] in addition to more proximal resection of any constrictive fascia, inflamed adventitial tissue, or bursae. The bursae,

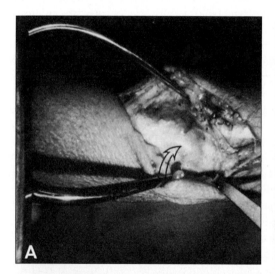

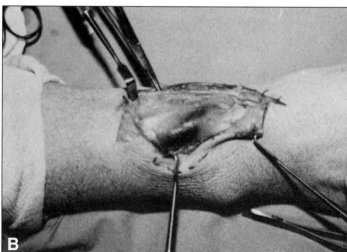

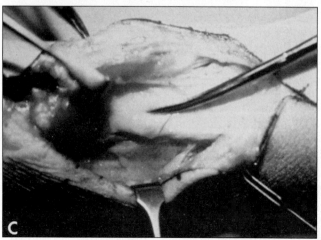

FIGURE 50-3

A, Operative approach to intersection syndrome, including dissection deep to the abductor pollicis longus (APL) and wrist extensor tendons and the APL bursa. *(From Wood and Dobyns.[72] By permission of JB Lippincott.)* **B,** Intersection syndrome and extensor carpi radialis longus and brevis tendinitis. Operative release of the second extensor compartment with synovectomy of the wrist extensor tendons. **C,** Note proximal retraction of muscle bellies of APL and wrist extensors showing tenosynovitis (end of scissors). *(From Grundberg and Reagan.[34] Copyright, American Society for Surgery of the Hand, by permission of Churchill Livingstone.)*

which may have formed between the first and second dorsal compartments, must be excised.[37] The extensor carpi radialis longus and brevis are released and inspected for potential tenosynovectomy (Fig. 50-3). Postoperative management consists of splint application with the wrist in 20° of extension for 10 to 14 days and then progressive therapy.

EXTENSOR POLLICIS LONGUS TENDINITIS

Tenosynovitis of the third dorsal compartment is not uncommon. The extensor pollicis longus (EPL) tendon is located in the third compartment around Lister's tubercle. This separate synovial compartment can become inflamed by repetitive activities such as drum playing[23] (drummer boy palsy) but usually is associated with predisposing factors such as fracture, direct trauma, or disease. Pain, swelling, and tenderness over Lister's tubercle occur with EPL tenosynovitis. The pain is accentuated with thumb flexion and extension. A careful history is needed in which one looks for inciting events.

Distal radius fractures and rheumatoid arthritis are common predisposing factors that affect the EPL tendon sheath and can lead to rupture[14,30,53] (Fig. 50-4). EPL tenosynovitis and rupture are far more common after undisplaced than displaced distal radius fractures and have been reported in wrist injuries without fracture.[26,39,41] Most ruptures occur within 8 weeks of fracture, but the rupture may be delayed for years.[26,39,41,53] The pathogenesis involves mechanical and vascular factors. Displaced fracture fragments, callus formation, or mere exposure of a bony surface can cause mechanical irritation of the EPL tendon. In addition, the vascular supply to the EPL tendon is deficient at Lister's tubercle[26,41] beneath the constrictive extensor retinaculum. A distal radius fracture can further compromise the precarious blood supply by edema,

hematoma, and bony impingement. These events can lead to primary EPL injury, secondary tenosynovitis, and eventual tendon rupture. Prodromal symptoms of swelling, tenderness, and crepitation around Lister's tubercle are frequently experienced.[41] Early operative exploration, release, and rerouting may prevent complete rupture.

Nonoperative Treatment. Initial treatment of EPL tenosynovitis is nonoperative: rest, activity modification, splint application, and anti-inflammatory medications. The splint should be forearm based and include the thumb out to distal phalanx. A local injection of corticosteroid around but not into the tendon can supplement treatment—0.5 mL betamethasone combined with 0.5 mL of 1% lidocaine. Radiographs are required after distal radius fracture to assess possible osseous contribution, but the principal clues are often clinical. Patients with rheumatoid arthritis may need medication adjustment to control the tenosynovitis. Failure to alleviate the tenosynovitis or progression of symptoms is an indication for surgical intervention to prevent EPL tendon rupture.

Surgical Treatment. Operation is performed under tourniquet control. A 3-cm longitudinal incision is made directly over Lister's tubercle. The radial sensory nerve branches are gently retracted. The EPL tendon is identified distal to the third compartment, and the retinaculum of the third compartment is then carefully incised. The EPL tendon is elevated and displaced to the radial side of the tubercle. Extensive tenosynovial formation requires a tenosynovectomy. The extensor retinaculum is then repaired deep to the tendon to prevent EPL relocation.[30] This subcutaneous rerouting alleviates symptoms with intact tendon. If tendon rupture (with fraying) is suspected, the possibility of a tendon graft or extensor indicis proprius transfer to reconstruct or

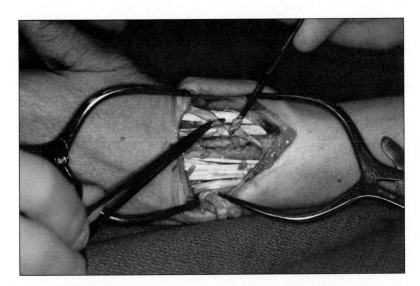

FIGURE 50-4

Extensor pollicis longus tendon rupture from rheumatoid tenosynovitis.

replace the EPL should be discussed preoperatively. Postoperative management depends on the integrity of the EPL tendon. Intact tendon does not require splintage and activity may be advanced as tolerated.

EXTENSOR INDICIS PROPRIUS SYNDROME

The extensor indicis proprius tendon is located within the fourth dorsal compartment in combination with the extensor digitorum communis tendons. Approximately 75% of individuals have the extensor indicis proprius muscle belly located *within* the fourth compartment and various anomalous extensor tendons (extensor manus brevis) have been described.[13,16,69] These anatomic features may increase the risk of fourth compartment tenosynovitis. However, symptomatic inflammation of the extensor digitorum communis or extensor indicis proprius is uncommon.[16,61]

Localized pain, tenderness, and swelling over the fourth compartment are typical findings of extensor indicis proprius tenosynovitis. The discomfort is increased with resistance to active index finger extension while maintaining the wrist in flexion.[65]

Treatment is primarily conservative: rest, protection, and anti-inflammatory medications. Local injection of corticosteroid may be beneficial in protracted cases. Splint application should hold the wrist in 20° of dorsiflexion and the index metacarpophalangeal joint in extension. After resolution of symptoms, graduated therapy is implemented. Surgical decompression of the extensor indicis proprius tendon is indicated when conservative measures fail.[61] An anatomic variation should be suspected, such as a distally located extensor indicis proprius muscle belly.

EXTENSOR DIGITI MINIMI TENDINITIS

The extensor digiti minimi courses independently in the fifth dorsal compartment. Tenosynovitis involving the extensor digiti minimi occurs rarely.[42,66,67] Swelling and pain are located over the fifth compartment. Conservative treatment—rest, immobilization, anti-inflammatory medications—and perhaps a local injection of corticosteroid usually resolve the tenosynovitis. Failure to relieve symptoms may lead to surgical exploration, retinaculum division, and tenosynovectomy. Multiple extensor digiti minimi tendon slips may be found at operation.[42]

EXTENSOR CARPI ULNARIS TENDINITIS

The sixth compartment contains the extensor carpi ulnaris (ECU) tendon and contributes to the stability of the ulnar portion of the wrist (Fig. 50-5).[64] The sixth compartment's anatomy is unique in that the extensor retinaculum contributes little to the tendon stability. Instead, a separate subsheath forms a fibro-osseous tunnel by its attachments to the ulnar styloid and head that maintains the ECU position during wrist motion. Loss of compartment integrity causes recurrent subluxation of the ECU and reactive ECU tenosynovitis. It is important to distinguish this entity from primary ECU tenosynovitis. ECU subluxation usually occurs after a discrete traumatic event

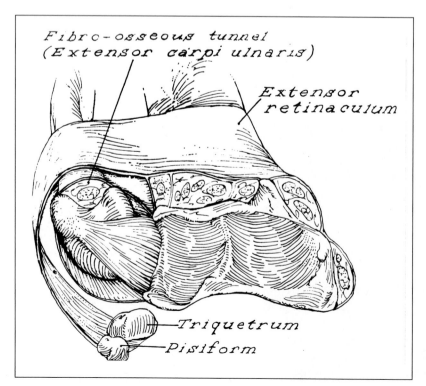

FIGURE 50-5

Anatomy of the sixth dorsal compartment. Unlike other extensor compartments, the extensor carpi ulnaris is stabilized by a separate subsheath and not primarily by the extensor retinaculum. *(From Spinner and Kaplan.[64] By permission of JB Lippincott.)*

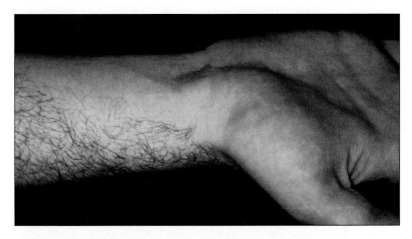

FIGURE 50-9

Swelling along the radial aspect of the wrist with flexor carpi radialis tendinitis.

A

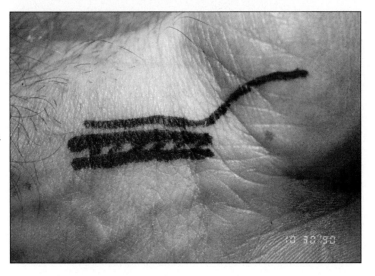

FIGURE 50-10

A, Release of the flexor carpi radialis tunnel (left wrist) showing a palmar, slightly curved longitudinal incision extending over the thenar eminence. The interneural plane between the fibers of the palmar cutaneous nerve branch of the median nerve and the lateral antebrachial cutaneous nerve and superficial branches of the radial nerve should be followed. **B,** Diagrammatic illustration of surgical incision related to tuberosity of the scaphoid and trapezium.

B

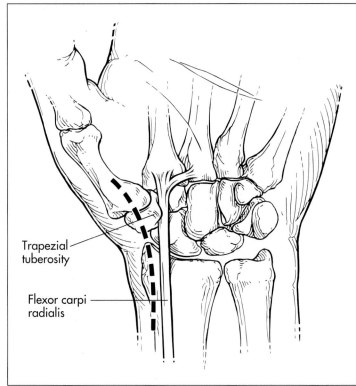

adjacent pathologic features.[32,66] Operative decompression is performed via a 5-cm palmar longitudinal incision (Fig. 50-10) over the FCR tendon, extended in a curvilinear fashion across the wrist crease. The palmar cutaneous branch of the median nerve is protected ulnarly, and the lateral antebrachial cutaneous nerve and radial nerve branches are protected radially. The origins of the thenar muscle from the transverse carpal ligament are carefully elevated to expose the FCR fibro-osseous canal. The tunnel is incised the entire length of the trapezium, with care to avoid iatrogenic tendon injury. Adjuvant procedures such as excision of a deformed or prominent trapezial tuberosity are performed as indicated by the surrounding pathologic features.

RESTRICTIVE THUMB-INDEX TENOSYNOVITIS (LINBURG'S SYNDROME)

An anatomic interconnection between the flexor pollicis longus and the index flexor digitorum profundus is present in approximately 31% of the population.[48] The connecting structure may be an anomalous tendon, musculotendinous slip, or adherent tenosynovium.[51,72] Occasionally, this interconnection can lead to restrictive thumb-index flexor tenosynovitis and pain. The pain is often vague, intermittent, and aggravated by activity. Occupational stress with forceful and repetitive pinching may be a contributing factor.[21] The discomfort is located over the radiopalmar aspect of the distal forearm and thumb. A relationship between Linburg's syndrome and carpal tunnel syndrome has been noted in some patients.

Examination reveals a positive result of the Linburg test, which is an inability to fully flex the thumb interphalangeal joint without simultaneous flexion of the index distal interphalangeal joint[48] (Fig. 50-11). When this maneuver reproduces the patient's discomfort and passive extension of the index finger increases the patient's pain, then restrictive tenosynovitis may be present.

Nonoperative Treatment. Initial treatment involves avoidance of precipitating activities of repetitive thumb or index finger flexion, nonsteroidal anti-inflammatory medications, and steroid injection within the carpal tunnel or flexor pollicis longus tendon sheath. We inject 1.0 mL of betamethasone and 1.0 mL of 1% lidocaine into the flexor pollicis longus tendon sheath at the level of the distal forearm as the first step. The injection helps confirm the diagnosis because it usually

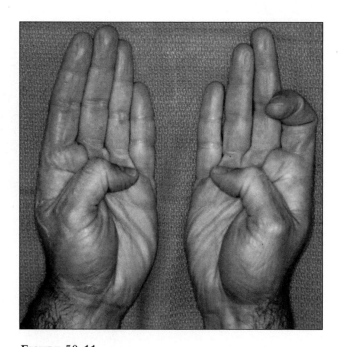

FIGURE 50-11

Positive result of Linburg test with painful simultaneous right index finger and thumb flexion.

anesthetizes the painful interconnection. With persistent symptoms, the carpal tunnel should also be injected and splints applied to immobilize the wrist. Long-term therapeutic benefit of these measures is unpredictable in many patients.[72] Failure of conservative management is an indication for operative release of the interconnection and tenosynovectomy.[51,72]

Operative Treatment. Exploration of the distal forearm provides adequate exposure for evaluation of the potential tendinous interconnection or tenosynovial hyperplasia between the flexor pollicis longus and index flexor digitorum profundus, unless carpal tunnel syndrome is also present. In this instance, the incision is prolonged into the palm to allow release of the transverse carpal ligament. The tendons are exposed and any tendon interconnections or dense tenosynovial thickenings are excised. Lombardi et al.[51] reported three patients with an anomalous second flexor pollicis longus muscle belly and tendon that inserted into the index flexor digitorum profundus, flexor digitorum superficialis, or lumbrical muscle. For such anomalies, division of the aberrant tendon is performed.

REFERENCES

1. Alegado RB, Meals RA: An unusual complication following surgical treatment of deQuervain's disease, *J Hand Surg [Am]* 4:185-186, 1979.
2. Armstrong TJ: Ergonomics and cumulative trauma disorders, *Hand Clin* 2:553-565, 1986.
3. Armstrong TJ, Fine LJ, Goldstein SA, et al.: Ergonomic considerations in hand and wrist tendinitis, *J Hand Surg [Am]* 12:830-837, 1987.
4. Armstrong TJ, Fine LJ, Radwin RG, et al.: Ergonomics and the effects of vibration in hand-intensive work, *Scand J Work Environ Health* 13:286-289, 1987.
5. Belsole RJ: DeQuervain's tenosynovitis: diagnostic and operative complications, *Orthopedics* 4:899-903, 1981.
6. Bowe A, Doyle L, Millender LH: Bilateral partial ruptures of the flexor carpi radialis tendon secondary to trapezial arthritis, *J Hand Surg [Am]* 9:738-739, 1984.
7. Brasington R: Nintendinitis (letter to the editor), *N Engl J Med* 322:1473-1474, 1990.
8. Burkhart SS, Wood MB, Linscheid RL: Posttraumatic recurrent subluxation of the extensor carpi ulnaris tendon, *J Hand Surg [Am]* 7:1-3, 1982.
9. Butler DL, Grood ES, Noyes FR, et al.: Biomechanics of ligaments and tendons, *Exer Sport Sci Rev* 6:125-181, 1978.
10. Carroll RE, Coyle MP Jr: Dysfunction of the pisotriquetral joint: treatment by excision of the pisiform, *J Hand Surg [Am]* 10:703-707, 1985.
11. Carroll RE, Stinton W, Garcia A: Acute calcium deposits in the hand, *JAMA* 157:422-426, 1955.
12. Casanova J, Casanova J: "Nintendinitis" (letter to the editor), *J Hand Surg [Am]* 16:181, 1991.
13. Cauldwell EW, Anson BJ, Wright RR: The extensor indicis proprius muscle. A study of 263 consecutive specimens, *Q Bull Northwestern Univ Med School* 17:267-279, 1943.
14. Cooney WP III, Dobyns JH, Linscheid RL: Complications of Colles' fractures, *J Bone Joint Surg Am* 62:613-619, 1980.
15. Curwin S, Stanish WD: *Tendinitis: its etiology and treatment,* Lexington, MA, 1984, DC Health and Company.
16. Cusenz BJ, Hallock GG: Multiple anomalous tendons of the fourth dorsal compartment, *J Hand Surg [Am]* 11:263-264, 1986.
17. De Gail P, Lance JW, Neilson PD: Differential effects on tonic and phasic reflex mechanisms produced by vibration of muscles in man, *J Neurol Neurosurg Psychiatry* 29:1-11, 1966.
18. Dellon AL, Mackinnon SE: Radial sensory nerve entrapment in the forearm, *J Hand Surg [Am]* 11:199-205, 1986.
19. de Quervain F: Ueber eine Form von chronischer Tendovaginitis, *Cor Bl Schweiz Aerzte* 25:389, 1985.
20. Dilley DF, Tonkin MA: Acute calcific tendinitis in the hand and wrist, *J Hand Surg [Br]* 16:215-216, 1991.
21. Dobyns JH: Cumulative trauma disorder of the upper limb, *Hand Clin* 7:587-595, 1991.
22. Dobyns JH, Sim FH, Linscheid RL: Sports stress syndromes of the hand and wrist, *Am J Sports Med* 6:236-254, 1978.
23. Dums F: Uber trommierlahmungen, *Deutsche Milit Zeitsch* 25:145, 1896.
24. Eckhardt WA, Palmer AK: Recurrent dislocation of extensor carpi ulnaris tendon, *J Hand Surg [Am]* 6:629-631, 1981.
25. Elliott DH: Structure and function of mammalian tendon, *Biol Rev* 40:392-421, 1965.
26. Engkvist O, Lundborg G: Rupture of the extensor pollicis longus tendon after fracture of the lower end of the radius—a clinical and microangiographic study, *Hand* 11:76-86, 1979.
27. Ferlic DC, Clayton ML: Flexor tenosynovectomy in the rheumatoid finger, *J Hand Surg* 3:364-367, 1978.
28. Finkelstein H: Stenosing tendovaginitis at the radial styloid process, *J Bone Joint Surg* 12:509-540, 1930.
29. Fitton J, Shea FW, Goldie W: Lesions of the flexor carpi radialis tendon and sheath causing pain at the wrist, *J Bone Joint Surg Br* 50:359-363, 1968.
30. Froimson AI: *Tenosynovitis and tennis elbow.* In Green DP, editor: *Operative hand surgery,* ed 2, vol 3, New York, 1988, Churchill Livingstone, pp 2117-2134.
31. Fry HJH: Prevalence of overuse (injury) syndrome in Australian music schools, *Br J Ind Med* 44:35-40, 1987.
32. Gabel G, Bishop AT, Wood MB: Flexor carpi radialis tendinitis. Part II: results of operative treatment, *J Bone Joint Surg Am* 76:1015-1018, 1994.
33. Giles KW: Anatomical variations affecting the surgery of de Quervain's disease, *J Bone Joint Surg Br* 42:352-355, 1960.
34. Grundberg AB, Reagan DS: Pathologic anatomy of the forearm: intersection syndrome, *J Hand Surg [Am]* 10:299-302, 1985.
35. Hajj AA, Wood MB: Stenosing tenosynovitis of the extensor carpi ulnaris, *J Hand Surg [Am]* 11:519-520, 1986.
36. Harvey FJ, Harvey PM, Horsley MW: De Quervain's disease: surgical or nonsurgical treatment, *J Hand Surg [Am]* 15:83-87, 1990.
37. Helal B: Distal profundus entrapment in rheumatoid disease, *Hand* 2:48-51, 1970.
38. Helal B: Racquet player's pisiform, *Hand* 10:87-90, 1978.
39. Helal B, Chen SC, Iwegbu G: Rupture of the extensor pollicis longus tendon in undisplaced Colles' type of fracture, *Hand* 14:41-47, 1982.
40. Herring SA, Nilson KL: Introduction to overuse injuries, *Clin Sports Med* 6:225-239, 1987.
41. Hirasawa Y, Katsumi Y, Akiyoshi T, et al.: Clinical and microangiographic studies on rupture of the E.P.L. tendon after distal radial fractures, *J Hand Surg [Br]* 15:51-57, 1990.
42. Hooper G, McMaster MJ: Stenosing tenovaginitis affecting the tendon of extensor digiti minimi at the wrist, *Hand* 11:299-301, 1979.
43. Hymovich L, Lindholm M: Hand, wrist, and forearm injuries. The result of repetitive motions, *J Occup Med* 8:573-577, 1966.

44. Jozsa L, Reffy A, Demel S, et al.: Foreign bodies in tendons, *J Hand Surg [Br]* 14:84-85, 1989.

45. Keon-Cohen B: De Quervain's disease, *J Bone Joint Surg Br* 33:96-99, 1951.

46. Leão L: De Quervain's disease: a clinical and anatomical study, *J Bone Joint Surg Am* 40:1063-1070, 1958.

47. Leslie BM, Ericson WB Jr, Morehead JR: Incidence of a septum within the first dorsal compartment of the wrist, *J Hand Surg [Am]* 15:88-91, 1990.

48. Lindburg RM, Comstock BE: Anomalous tendon slips from the flexor pollicis longus to the flexor digitorum profundus, *J Hand Surg [Am]* 4:79-83, 1979.

49. Linscheid RL: Injuries to radial nerve at wrist, *Arch Surg* 91:942-946, 1965.

50. Lipscomb PR: Stenosing tenosynovitis of the radial styloid process (De Quervain's disease), *Ann Surg* 134:110-115, 1951.

51. Lombardi RM, Wood MB, Linscheid RL: Symptomatic restrictive thumb-index flexor tenosynovitis: incidence of musculotendinous anomalies and results of treatment, *J Hand Surg [Am]* 13:325-328, 1988.

52. Louis DS: Incomplete release of the first dorsal compartment—a diagnostic test, *J Hand Surg [Am]* 12:87-88, 1987.

53. Mannerfelt L, Oetker R, Ostlund B, et al.: Rupture of the extensor pollicis longus tendon after Colles fracture and by rheumatoid arthritis, *J Hand Surg [Br]* 15:49-50, 1990.

54. McMahon M, Craig SM, Posner MA: Tendon subluxation after de Quervain's release: treatment by brachioradialis tendon flap, *J Hand Surg [Am]* 16:30-32, 1991.

55. Minamikawa Y, Peimer CA, Cox WL, et al.: De Quervain's syndrome: surgical and anatomical studies of the fibroosseous canal, *Orthopedics* 14:545-549, 1991.

56. Moyer RA, Bush DC, Harrington TM: Acute calcific tendinitis of the hand and wrist: a report of 12 cases and a review of the literature, *J Rheumatol* 16:198-202, 1989

57. Nalebuff EA, Feldon PG, Millender LH: *Rheumatoid arthritis in the hand and wrist.* In Green DP, editor: *Operative hand surgery,* ed 2, vol 3, New York, 1988, Churchill Livingstone, pp 1655-1766.

58. Palmieri TJ: Pisiform area pain treatment by pisiform excision, *J Hand Surg [Am]* 7:477-480, 1982.

59. Patterson DC: De Quervain's disease: stenosing tendovaginitis at the radial styloid, *N Engl J Med* 214:101-103, 1936.

60. Pitner MA: Pathophysiology of overuse injuries in the hand and wrist, *Hand Clin* 6:355-364, 1990.

61. Ritter MA, Inglis AE: The extensor indicis proprius syndrome, *J Bone Joint Surg Am* 51:1645-1648, 1969.

62. Rosenthal EA: Tenosynovitis: tendon and nerve entrapment, *Hand Clin* 3:585-609, 1987.

63. Shaw JA: Acute calcific tendonitis in the hand, *Orthop Rev* 15:482-485, 1986.

64. Spinner M, Kaplan EB: Extensor carpi ulnaris. Its relationship to the stability of the distal radio-ulnar joint, *Clin Orthop* 68:124-129, 1970.

65. Spinner M, Olshansky K: The extensor indicis proprius syndrome. A clinical test, *Plast Reconstr Surg* 51:134-138, 1973.

66. Stern PJ: Tendinitis, overuse syndromes, and tendon injuries, *Hand Clin* 6:467-476, 1990.

67. Thorson E, Szabo RM: Common tendinitis problems in the hand and forearm, *Orthop Clin North Am* 23:65-74, 1992.

68. Viegas SF: Trigger thumb of de Quervain's disease, *J Hand Surg [Am]* 11:235-237, 1986.

69. von Schroeder HP, Botte MJ: The extensor medii proprius and anomalous extensor tendons to the long finger, *J Hand Surg [Am]* 16:1141-1145, 1991.

70. Weeks PM: A cause of wrist pain; non-specific tenosynovitis involving the flexor carpi radialis, *Plast Reconstr Surg* 62:263-266, 1978.

71. Witczak JW, Masear VR, Meyer RD: Triggering of the thumb with de Quervain's stenosing tendovaginitis, *J Hand Surg [Am]* 15:265-268, 1990.

72. Wood MB, Dobyns JH: Sports-related extraarticular wrist syndromes, *Clin Orthop* 202:93-102, 1986.

73. Wood MB, Linscheid RL: Abductor pollicis longus bursitis, *Clin Orthop* 93:293-296, 1973.

ANATOMY

The carpal tunnel is a defined space with rigid and semirigid circumferential boundaries. The tube of space making up the carpal tunnel provides a channel for passage of all the flexor tendons of the thumb and digits from the forearm to the hand (Fig. 51-2). The median nerve also passes through this space, completing the contents of the carpal canal. In addition to providing a protected passageway for these vital structures into the hand, the transverse carpal ligament functions as a pulley to increase the power of the flexor tendons (Fig. 51-3).[38] Because of its anatomic continuity with the palmar forearm fascia and based on classic anatomic descriptions, the transverse carpal ligament is also known as the flexor retinaculum.[21,32,34]

The walls of the carpal tunnel are bounded by the internal surfaces of the carpal bones and the transverse carpal ligament (Fig. 51-3). The proximal and distal margins of the carpal canal are slightly irregular and determined by the proximal and distal borders of the flexor retinaculum (Fig. 51-4). The central third of the flexor retinaculum, the transverse carpal ligament, attaches radially to the scaphoid, trapezium, and fascia of the thenar muscles. Ulnarly, it attaches through fascia proximally to the pisiform and the hook of the hamate and more distally, to the fascia of the hypothenar muscles. The underlying bones form the floor of the carpal canal and are somewhat more distal than one tends to visualize (Fig. 51-5).

The fibers of the transverse carpal ligament are histologically transversely oriented.[21] Proximally, they tend to be contiguous on gross inspection with the thickened antebrachial fascia and overlaid by the continuation of the palmaris longus muscle and its fascia, but these structures are histologically longitudinally oriented. The transverse carpal ligament is thickest in its distal portion at the hook of the hamate, where the canal is also at its narrowest (Fig. 51-3). An additional function of the transverse carpal ligament is to stabilize the transverse carpal arch.[26,27] Occasionally, a muscle (the transverse palmaris) is present within or on the surface of the transverse carpal ligament (see section below on endoscopic release).

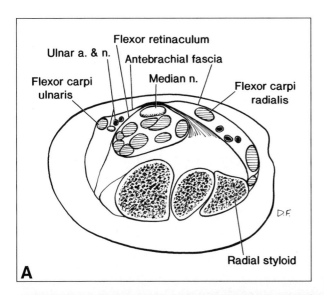

A

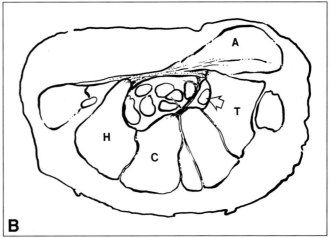

B

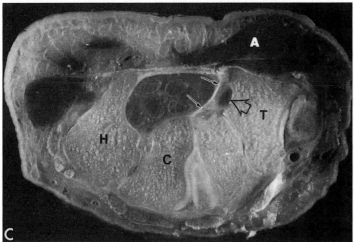

C

FIGURE 51-3

Transverse section through carpal tunnel. **A,** Proximal at level of distal radius. Note median nerve (*n.*) and flexor tendons within the carpal tunnel covered by the flexor retinaculum. *a.,* artery. Floor of carpal bones and walls of retinaculum and carpal bones. **B** and **C,** Midpalm at the level of the hook of hamate (*H*). (Arrows point to flexor carpi radialis and its sheath outside the carpal tunnel.) Flexor carpi ulnaris, ulnar artery and nerve, and flexor carpi radialis are also in a separate sheath outside the carpal tunnel. *A,* thenar muscles; *C,* capitate; *T,* trapezium. (*From Cobb et al.[21] Copyright, American Society for Surgery of the Hand, by permission of Churchill Livingstone.*)

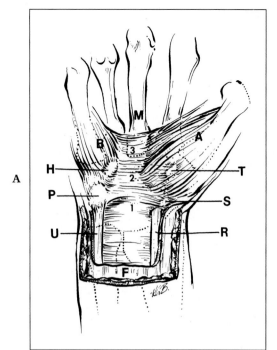

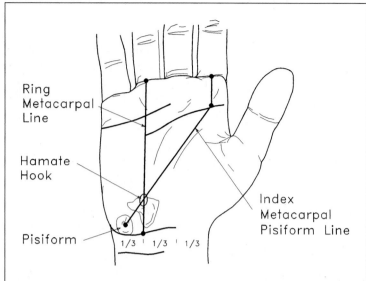

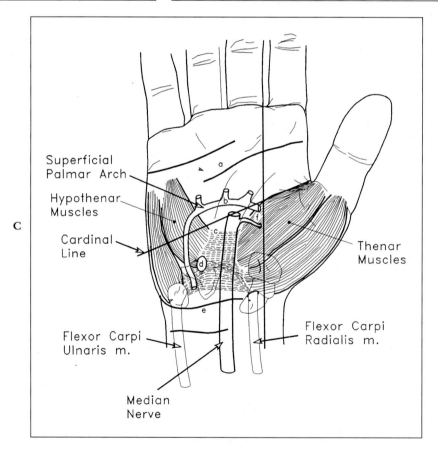

FIGURE 51-4

A, Flexor retinaculum has three components: (*1*) proximal third of distal superficial forearm fascia; (*2*) central third, the transverse carpal ligament; and (*3*) distal third, the palmar aponeurosis and organs of the hypothenar and thenar muscles. (*A,* thenar muscles; *B,* hypothenar muscles; *F,* forearm fascia; *H,* hamate; *M,* metacarpal [III]; *P,* pisiform; *R,* flexor carpi radialis; *S,* scaphoid tubercle; *T,* tubercle of trapezium; *U,* flexor carpi ulnaris.) *(From Cobb et al.²¹ Copyright, American Society for Surgery of the Hand, by permission of Churchill Livingstone.)* **B,** Topographic landmarks for safe open and endoscopic carpal tunnel release: connect ring metacarpal line with index metacarpal-pisiform line; cross at the hook of the hamate. **C,** At hook of hamate (*d*), measure 1 cm distal from distal edge of the transverse carpal ligament (*c*) and 2 cm distal for usual (but variable) location of the superficial palmar arch (*b*). *a,* metacarpal phalangeal flexion crease; *e,* wrist flexion crease; *f,* motor median nerve branch; *m.,* muscle. *(**B** and **C,** From Cobb TK, Cooney WP, An K-N: Clinical location of hook of hamate: a technical note for endoscopic carpal tunnel release,* J Hand Surg [Am] *19:516-518, 1994. By permission of Mayo Foundation.)*

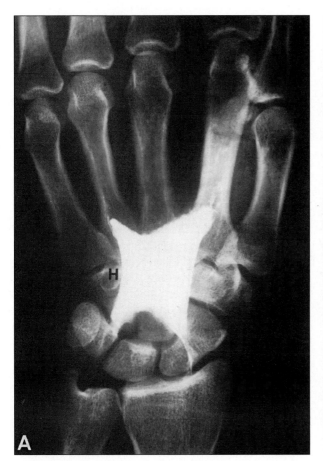 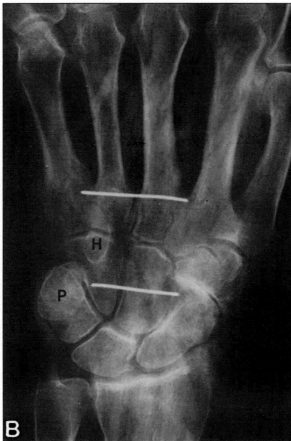

FIGURE 51-5

A, Radiographic contrast material outlining the borders of the carpal tunnel. **B,** Lines representing border of carpal tunnel superimposed on radiograph. *H,* hamate; *P,* pisiform. *(From Cobb et al.[21] Copyright, American Society for Surgery of the Hand, by permission of Churchill Livingstone.)*

PHYSIOLOGY OF CARPAL TUNNEL SYNDROME

In the condition of CTS, the median nerve becomes mechanically compressed within the fixed confines of the structures composing the walls of the carpal tunnel. The condition may occur if there is a change in the size of the canal or if there is a change in the volume of the carpal contents. Variations in wrist position additionally alter the pressure within the carpal canal.[55]

A change in the size of the carpal canal occurs with degenerative conditions of the wrist and with carpal instability problems (Fig. 51-6).[45] Fractures and dislocations of the carpus may cause impingement in the carpal tunnel, especially in perilunar dislocations. Fractures of the radius (Colles' or Smith's) are associated with an increased incidence of CTS but not because of changes in the carpal canal size. Rather, they induce an increase in the volume of the soft tissue within the carpal canal.[1]

The most common cause of CTS is an increase in the soft-tissue contents about the flexor tendons within

the fixed structure of the tunnel. Tumorous conditions including ganglions and neoplastic growths do occur, but these are quite rare.[25,83]

Thickening or enlargement of the flexor tenosynovium enveloping the flexor tendons as they pass through the carpal canal is the most commonly seen condition, but its precise cause is not always understood.[46] This thickening may occur as a result of a disease process such as the tissue edema associated with hypothyroidism or the synovial hypertrophy seen in rheumatoid arthritis. A patient who has synovial hypertrophy associated with infectious processes from bacteria, fungi, and mycobacteria may present with a clinical picture of CTS. However, the most common cause of tenosynovial thickening that results in CTS is idiopathic in nature. It appears associated with repetitive stress, which suggests an etiologic cause or event associated with certain industries. Histologically, the tissue represents a fibrosynovial noninflammatory synovium and likely represents a tissue response secondary to continuous strong frictional forces in a manner similar to the formation of a cutaneous callus on the hand.[37]

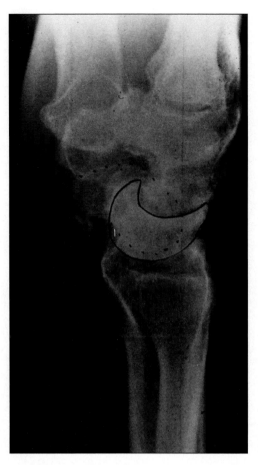

FIGURE 51-6

Dorsal intercalated segment instability pattern. The lunate (*solid line*) is displaced into proximal border of carpal canal, and the scaphoid (*dotted line*) has palmar flexed, the combination of which decreases the size (volume) of the carpal tunnel.

As previously noted, in some instances, pressures in the carpal tunnel may vary with the position of the wrist or finger in flexion or extension, and these positions appear to further increase the potential for nerve compression with tenosynovial thickening. It is also possible that wrist flexion may induce median nerve compression over the firm and narrow proximal edge of the flexor retinaculum.[38] This purely mechanical condition could cause symptoms indiscernible from those of compression of the median nerve within the carpal canal.

INCIDENCE AND CLINICAL CHARACTERISTICS OF CARPAL TUNNEL SYNDROME

In an assessment of the frequency of occurrence of the clinical symptoms of CTS, a study in a relatively stable population area indicated an increased prevalence

of CTS between 1960 and 1980.[4] Furthermore, the probability of CTS developing during a lifetime is estimated at 50% to 100%, with a peak incidence in the 5th and 6th decades.[4] The incidence of this syndrome has been seen to reach nearly 100% of persons involved in certain repetitive motion activities. Economically, the cost of caring for problems of CTS in the working population has been estimated to be greater than 10 million dollars annually in the state of Minnesota alone.[61]

Normally, the clinical history and physical findings in CTS are so characteristic and definitive that the diagnosis can be readily established. Classically, the patient describes a history of intermittent numbness and tingling in the median nerve distribution of the hand. The numbness typically occurs at night and is relieved by shaking the hand, hanging it over the bed, or flexing and extending the fingers repetitively. During the day the numbness may develop during activities requiring flexing or extending the wrist or constant grasping. Typical examples are activities such as driving a car, sewing, writing, reading a newspaper, and holding a telephone.

The condition is not generally perceived as painful. As it progresses, however, several additional complaints develop along with associated pain with the paresthesias. Weakness is experienced, although it may not be measurable. Sharp pains may occur when flexing the wrist. Numbness may become constant, and thumb weakness appears as the condition becomes a chronic nerve compression syndrome.

While the condition of CTS is caused by compression of the median nerve at the wrist, some symptoms may seem atypical from an anatomic standpoint but are nonetheless reported commonly in known CTS. These include the sense that the "whole hand is asleep" and that pain radiates up the forearm and occasionally above the elbow. Careful self-examination by the patient reveals that only the radial 3.5 digits (thumb, index, long, ½ ring) are numb. Likewise, a sense that the hand falls asleep from lying on it is a common complaint in CTS, probably from venous congestion and increased pressure in an already tight carpal tunnel. Some patients report signs of shoulder and neck or even facial pain in CTS, and these symptoms should not steer the physician away from this diagnosis.[29,64]

PHYSICAL EXAMINATION IN CARPAL TUNNEL SYNDROME

The median nerve at the wrist contains the sensory branches to the palmar surfaces of the thumb, index, long, and the radial one-half of the ring finger. In addition, it provides the motor innervation to the opponens and abductor muscles of the thumb at the thenar eminence. The motor branch is recurrent, passing

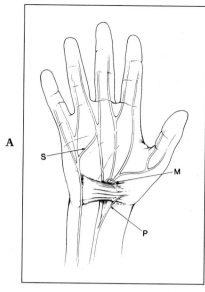

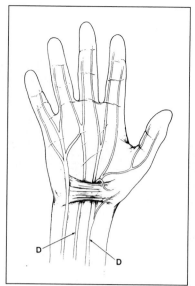

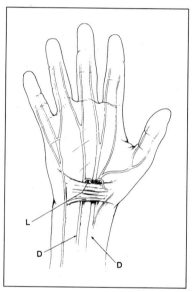

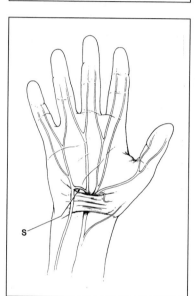

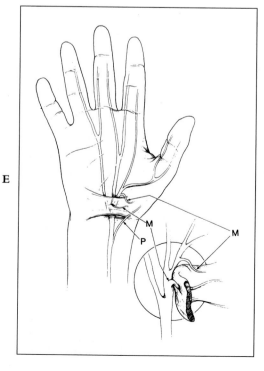

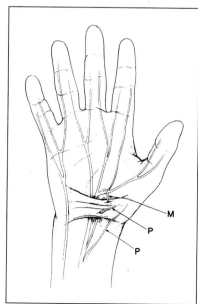

FIGURE 51-7

Proposed classification of median motor nerve distribution. **A,** Normal anatomy. **B,** High division, open branching. **C,** High division, closed loop. **D,** Proximal median-ulnar sensory ramus. *D,* division of median nerve; *L,* closed loop of median nerve; *M,* motor branch; *P,* palmar cutaneous branch; *S,* median-ulnar sensory ramus. **E,** Transligamentous motor branch. **F,** Transligamentous palmar cutaneous branch. *(From Amadio PC: Anatomic variations of the median nerve within the carpal tunnel, Clin Anat 1:23-31, 1988. By permission of Wiley-Liss, a subsidiary of John Wiley & Sons.)*

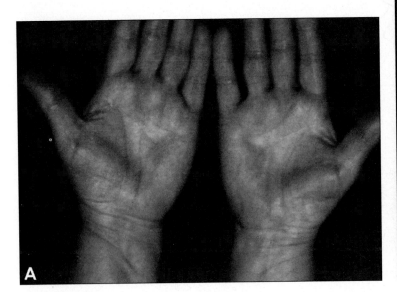
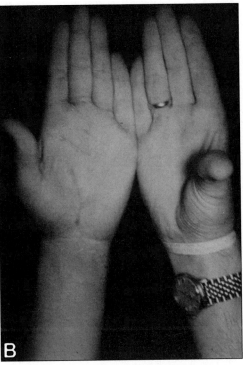

FIGURE 51-8

A, Marked opponens muscle atrophy on the right compared with normal thenar muscle size and strength in left hand. **B,** Examination for opponens pollicis muscle function. The denervated opponens muscle is unable to rotate the thumb to point at the ceiling.

through the carpal canal and therefore usually involved in CTS. Anomalies of the motor nerve distribution in the hand are not infrequent (Figs. 51-7, *A* through *D*), and occasionally this may result in an atypical clinical examination in a patient with CTS—e.g., a high take-off of the motor branch to the thenar eminence, resulting in no muscle changes in severe CTS, or a proximal median to ulnar sensory crossover (or vice versa), resulting in an atypical sensory distribution.

Sensory examination may be performed in various ways from simple light touch or temperature recognition to pinprick, vibration, two-point discrimination, and monofilament fiber testing. Although the results of all of these tests are significant, actual objective sensory loss is identified only in advanced cases of CTS, and subjective paresthesias or dysesthesias in the median nerve distribution are a significant clinical finding. In instances of advanced sensory loss, diminished sweat pattern in the median nerve distribution may be found.

Atrophy of the opponens muscle is a finding in advanced CTS (Fig. 51-8, *A*). It may be inaccurately diagnosed in the presence of thumb carpometacarpal arthritis in which metacarpal subluxation stretches the opponens muscle, leaving a flat appearance adjacent to the metacarpal. Opponens muscle weakness alone can be an earlier finding in CTS but is difficult

to identify. To test for motor weakness associated with CTS, the opponens muscle only should be examined. To do this, the patient is asked to place the back of the hands on a table and point the thumb tip at the ceiling (Fig. 51-8, *B*). The examiner then attempts to flatten the thumb on the table with two fingers. Most people with normal opponens power are able to prevent the force of the examiner's two fingers from flattening the thumb to the table. Opponens weakness is more commonly a sign of advanced CTS.

Several provocative signs for CTS have been discovered and are extremely useful in diagnosing the condition. First, the nerve should be located just ulnar to the palmaris longus tendon (Fig. 51-9, *A*). Tinel's sign demonstrates irritability of a nerve, as evidenced by direct tapping with a mallet or finger directly on the median nerve. If struck vigorously, any peripheral nerve responds by sending sensible electrical shock sensations in the distribution of the nerve. In CTS, tapping the median nerve at the wrist causes tingling or paresthesias (or both) in part or all of the distribution in the hand.[76] Occasionally, an electric shock sensation also is transmitted proximally toward the elbow or shoulder.

Phalen's test (Fig. 51-9, *B*) is performed by asking the patient to maximally palmar flex the wrist for 60 seconds (or possibly doing it yourself). The test is

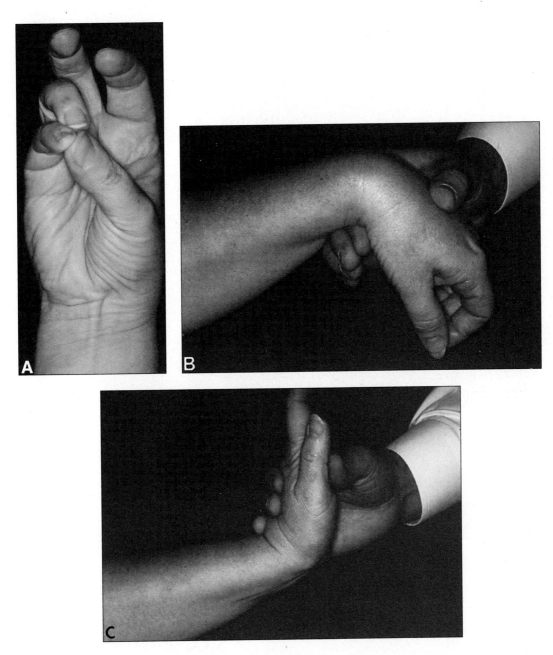

FIGURE 51-9

A, The median nerve lies on the interval between the palmaris longus and flexor carpi radialis. This space is identified by flexing the wrist and opposing the thumb. **B,** Phalen's test. **C,** Reverse Phalen's test.

Continued.

considered positive if paresthesias occur in the median nerve distribution of the hand.[63] Instant or early paresthesias are consistent with more severe CTS. Modifications of this test include placing the hand in maximum dorsiflexion with the fingers extended (reverse Phalen's) (Fig. 51-9, *C*) or holding the fingers flexed (Berger's test)[7](Fig. 51-9, *E*), which may crowd lumbrical muscles into Guyon's canal.

The carpal tunnel compression test is preferred as the most accurate provocative sign in CTS (Fig. 51-9, *D*).

The patient is asked to oppose the thumb to the small finger and flex the wrist (Fig. 51-9, *A*). This will stimulate contraction of the palmaris longus tendon and flexor carpi ulnaris tendon. The examiner's thumb then firmly compresses the area between the two tendons, indenting the skin 4 to 5 mm. In CTS, paresthesias in the median nerve distribution occur within 60 seconds. Paresthesias within 15 seconds or less indicate more advanced disease.[85]

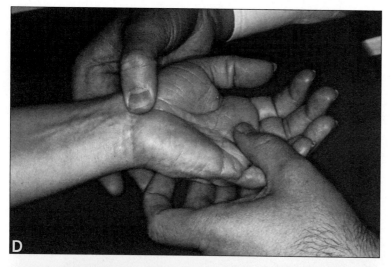

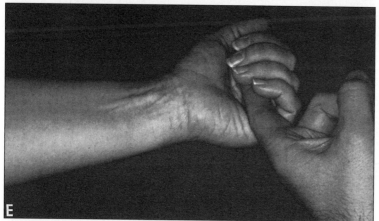

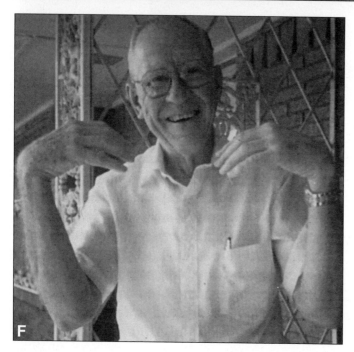

FIGURE 51-9, CONT'D.

D, Carpal tunnel compression. **E,** Berger's test (see text). **F,** Originator, Dr. George Phalen, demonstrating the test. His elbows are not resting on a table as he described for the patient examination.

LABORATORY CONFIRMATION OF CARPAL TUNNEL SYNDROME

Nerve conduction studies and electromyographic evaluations can provide definitive proof of compression of the median nerve within the carpal canal. First described in 1956, the testing methods have become specific and reliable.[72,75] Although the clinical diagnosis of CTS is generally accurate, nerve conduction velocity and electromyography studies are still routinely performed in most cases to confirm the diagnosis and to evaluate the severity of the condition in making treatment decisions. Absence of sensory responses or low sensory response amplitudes or extended values for palmar and motor nerve latencies (or both) may be considered indications for surgical treatment. Electromyography is also helpful in excluding other causes of hand numbness related to proximal nerve compression or secondary to systemic illness such as diabetic neuropathy or polyneuropathy.

Handheld devices for measuring motor latency in CTS may be effective.[6,70,74] Smaller sensory devices will also soon be available and both may be of assistance in confirming the diagnosis of CTS.

DIFFERENTIAL DIAGNOSIS AND ASSOCIATED CONDITIONS IN CARPAL TUNNEL SYNDROME

Because of the characteristic history, the accessibility of the hand for clinical examination, and the specificity of electrodiagnostic tests, the diagnosis of CTS is generally easy and accurate. Most commonly encountered mimics of CTS are cervical radiculopathy, pronator teres syndrome, and thoracic outlet syndrome. In the first diagnosis, clinical examination and electromyography can generally establish the difference, but in pronator teres syndrome and thoracic outlet syndrome the findings and history are often vague and overlap with CTS, particularly if electrical studies are nondiagnostic. In these situations a diagnostic trial of steroid injections into the carpal tunnel may be of benefit (Fig. 51-10). In the case of true nonspecific CTS, cortisone injections generally improve the symptoms, even if only temporarily. In the other conditions, there would be no expected improvement (see below for technique of cortisone injections into the carpal canal). As mentioned previously, any disease that induces synovial thickening or

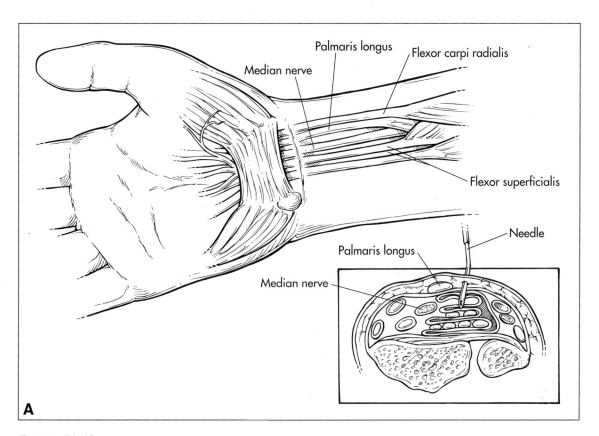

A

FIGURE 51-10

Cortisone injection into carpal tunnel, ulnar to the median nerve. **A,** Position of needle entrance and subcutaneous lidocaine infiltration ulnar to the palmaris longus. Carpal tunnel injection with steroids.

Continued.

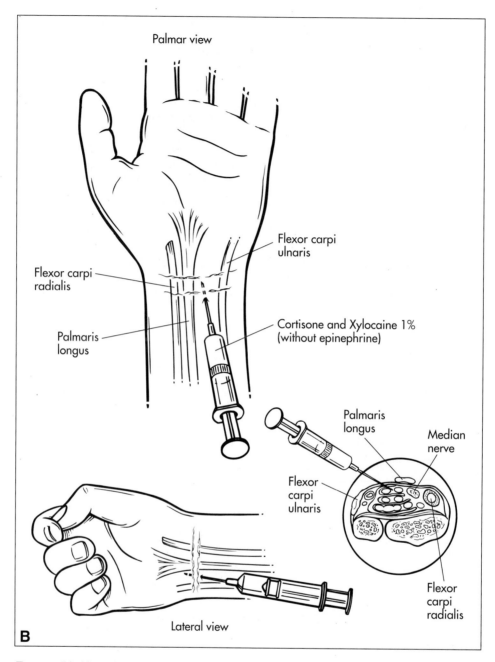

Palmar view

Flexor carpi
ulnaris

Flexor carpi
radialis

Palmaris
longus

Cortisone and Xylocaine 1%
(without epinephrine)

Palmaris
longus

Median
nerve

Flexor
carpi
ulnaris

Flexor
carpi
radialis

B

Lateral view

FIGURE 51-10, CONT'D.

B, Composite drawing of cortisone injection shows needle between palmaris longus and flexor carpi ulnaris, passing obliquely into flexor sheath with fingers flexed. Fingers are extended and flexor sheath is filled with solution.

hypertrophy can contribute to the development of CTS. Thus rheumatoid arthritis, hypothyroidism, and diabetes are associated with increased incidence of CTS. In general, though, once developed, CTS requires treatment independent of the medical treatment of these conditions. Infections with mycobacterial organisms appear to be on the increase, and the presence of a large bulky synovium should alert the physician to the need for surgical specimens for culture.

CONSERVATIVE TREATMENT OF CARPAL TUNNEL SYNDROME

Surgical release of the transverse carpal ligament has been considered the definitive treatment for CTS. However, many patients experience mild to moderate symptoms that do not progress and are not associated with evidence of disease progression or median nerve damage clinically or by electrical

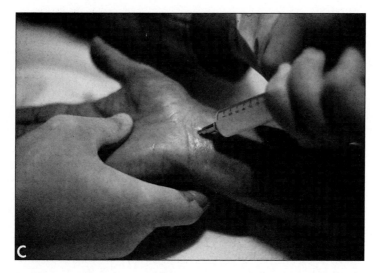

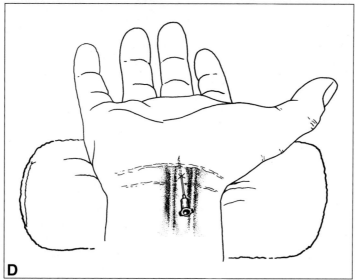

FIGURE 51-10, CONT'D.

C, Palpation of palm to determine if injection solution fills beyond the carpal tunnel. **D,** *Incorrect* needle placement between palmaris longus and flexor carpi radialis. There is danger here of direct injection into the median nerve.

studies. Conservative treatment measures are unlikely to cure the condition of CTS but may alleviate the symptoms enough to obviate the need for surgical intervention.

Oral administration of anti-inflammatory medications, including salicylates and nonsteroidal anti-inflammatory drugs, may be used to decrease the synovial inflammation and has variable success in the management of CTS. Their long-term use needs to be evaluated in a risk-benefit manner for each patient. Powerful orally administered anti-inflammatory drugs such as prednisone and methotrexate should not be used as treatment for CTS in the absence of other inflammatory systemic illnesses.

Pyridoxine or vitamin B_6 has been suggested as a therapeutic agent in CTS. Although some benefit has been observed, it has tended to be temporary.[3]

Wrist splints have been used to relieve symptoms and stop progression of CTS. Gelberman and others have shown that changes in wrist position, particularly flexion and extension, increase the pressures within the carpal canal.[11] Some employers are suggesting that daytime and work use of splints to prevent excess or repetitive wrist motion help decrease the incidence of CTS. The benefit from this method of wrist support has not been confirmed by studies, but patients have reported decreased symptoms at work. Wearing of night splints to hold the wrist in neutral position may decrease nocturnal awakenings and discomfort caused by wrist flexion or lying on an arm. Prevention of long-term progression of the disease, however, does not occur. Persons working at keyboard terminals may vary the amount of stress across the wrist and carpal tunnel area considerably by adjusting the position of the fore-arms and providing them with support. New types of tables, chairs, and armboards and new keyboard designs are currently being developed to alleviate what appears to be an epidemic increase in CTS associated with the expanded use of computer keyboards.

INJECTION OF THE CARPAL TUNNEL WITH CORTISONE

Steroid injections provide an additional nonoperative alternative for the treatment of CTS. To inject the cortisone derivative into the carpal canal, the following technique is suggested. The palmar aspect of the wrist should be cleansed and prepared in a sterile manner. A 2-mL solution of a soluble steroid such as dexamethasone is mixed with 1 mL of plain 1% lidocaine. The patient is asked to make a soft fist and a 20-G needle is inserted 1 cm proximal to the wrist flexion crease and ulnar to the palmaris longus tendon (Fig. 51-10). The needle is passed at a 45° angle distally approximately 1 cm deep. The patient is asked to extend the fingers; the needle will be felt passing distally into the carpal canal and the solution is injected, filling the flexor sheath (Fig. 51-10). Local anesthesia with lidocaine (1%) may be considered to anesthetize the skin before the cortisone injection.

Steroid injections commonly result in alleviation of CTS symptoms for 2 to 3 months but are long lasting in less than 30% of patients.[30] Their use is, therefore, generally as a temporizing measure in those persons whose work, medical condition, or other causative factor is expected to improve or in those patients who are unable to proceed with surgical correction of the syndrome because of inconvenience or other reasons. In general, steroid injections should not be repeated unless special circumstances such as pregnancy or other limited medical conditions have been encountered. A cortisone injection may occasionally be used as a diagnostic tool, as described in the section on differential diagnosis.

SURGICAL TREATMENT OF CARPAL TUNNEL SYNDROME

The definitive treatment of CTS is surgical. Traditionally and currently, the majority of surgeons believe that release of the transverse carpal ligament is the preferred method of surgical correction. Some believe that flexor tenosynovectomy frequently should

also be performed. Lluch[46] suggested that division of the carpal ligament alone results in spontaneous regression of the thickened flexor tenosynovium. Others[39,52] have suggested that removal of the tenosynovium alone without division of the flexor retinaculum is adequate and preferred treatment.

Extensive differences of opinion exist as to the proper technique of carpal tunnel ligament release. The individual methods and different incisions each have their advocates and all of the techniques will be described with the originators' thoughts on advantages of their preferred methods (Fig. 51-11). The techniques to be described are: 1) open release with the incision extending proximal to the wrist flexion crease, 2) open release through palmar only incision, 3) open release through two small incisions with direct proximal and distal visualization, 4) open release with transverse wrist incision and use of a special retinaculatome, 5) closed release with endoscopic visualization and a two-portal technique, 6) closed release with endoscopic visualization and a single-portal technique (three types), and 7) techniques including flexor tenosynovectomy.

After most forms of carpal tunnel surgery, some immobilization is required and wrist flexion should be prevented. If the condition occurs bilaterally, a decision must be made as to whether surgery should be performed on both wrists simultaneously. Simultaneous bilateral surgery can be effective and safe and decrease the total period of morbidity.[58] Some inconveniences occur in daily functional activities such as taking care of personal hygiene. Some patients have justifiable bias against having both hands "tied up." The final decision regarding simultaneous bilateral surgery is reached by the patient after descriptive consultation with the surgeon.

TECHNIQUES FOR SURGICAL TREATMENT OF CARPAL TUNNEL SYNDROME

RELEASE WITH INCISION ABOVE THE WRIST

Linscheid has preferred an incision above the wrist for better visualization and flexor tenosynovectomy[19] (Fig. 51-11, C). This incision can be outlined in the distal forearm in a lazy S-shape proximal to the wrist flexion crease and extended distally along the ring finger axis to the midpalm (Fig. 51-11, D). Keeping the incision ulnar to the palmaris longus tendon or midline of the wrist (or both) protects the median thenar cutaneous nerve, which arises 4 cm proximal to the wrist flexion crease and is located radial to the median nerve as far as the thenar eminence. The skin is perforated with a 22-G needle at the proximal incisional mark and the subcutaneous tissue is infiltrated

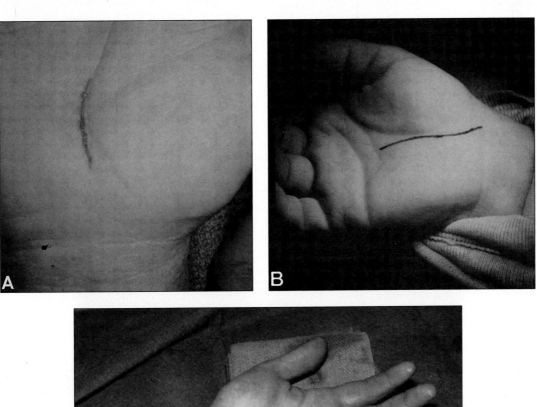

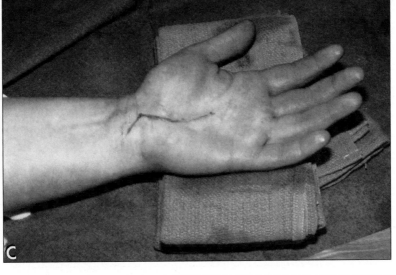

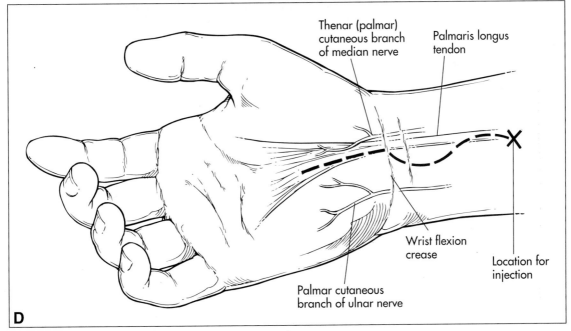

FIGURE 51-11

A, Short palmar incision. **B,** Long palmar incision. **C,** Palmar incision across the wrist flexion crease. **D,** Extended carpal tunnel incision. At the wrist flexion crease, the palm incision curves onto the forearm ulnar to the palmaris longus tendon. Note median palmar cutaneous nerve and ulnar cutaneous nerve.

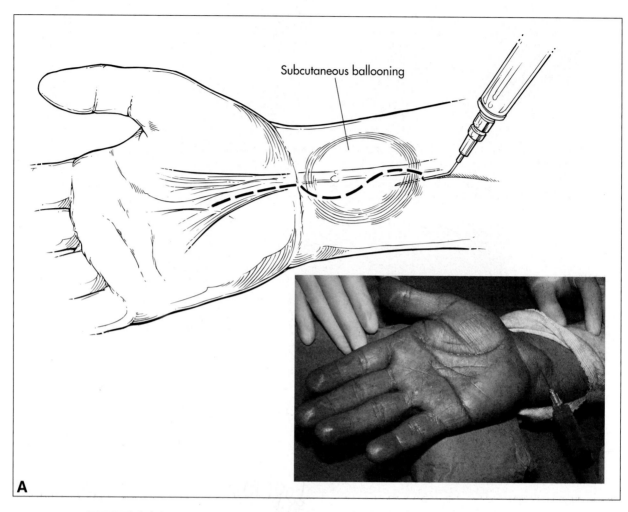

Subcutaneous ballooning

A

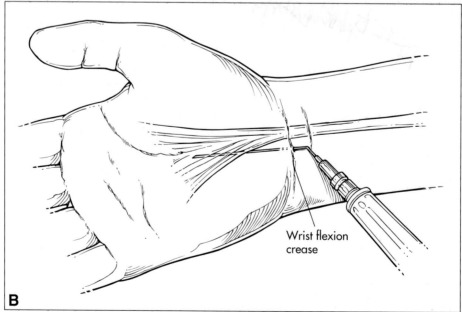

Wrist flexion crease

B

FIGURE 51-12

Local anesthesia. **A,** Local lidocaine 1% infiltration of skin and subcutaneous ballooning (*inset*) of distal forearm. **B,** Subcutaneous perforation of deep fascia and injection of flexor sheath.

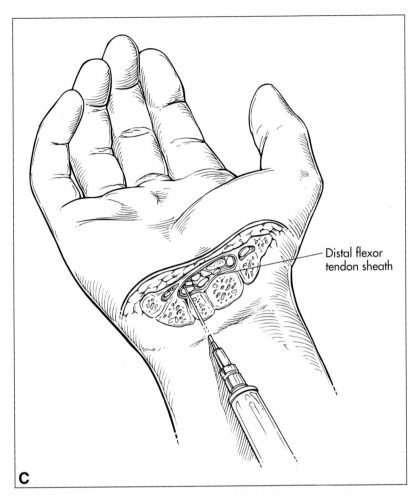

Distal flexor
tendon sheath

C

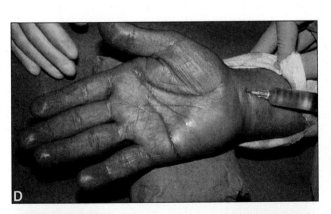

D

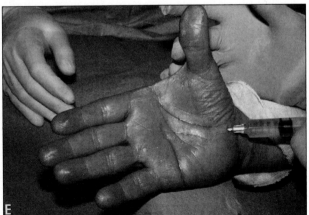

E

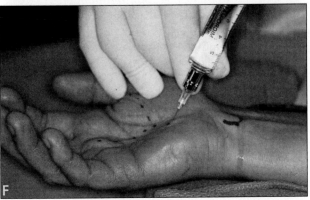

F

FIGURE 51-12, CONT'D.

C, Axial view of palm. Injection of the distal flexor sheath.
D, Clinical photograph shows skin and subcutaneous injections.
E, Palmar subcutaneous injection. **F,** Distal palmar injection;
2-portal technique.

with 5 mL of 1% lidocaine without epinephrine (Fig. 51-12, *A*). The needle is slowly advanced distally during the injection to "balloon out" the skin. The needle is then passed deep to the fascia proximally and 5 mL of lidocaine is injected into the flexor sheath (Fig. 51-12, *B*). The syringe is then filled with another 10 mL of lidocaine and the needle is passed into the already anesthetized subcutaneous area at the wrist flexion crease (Figs. 51-12, *C* and *D*). The needle is again slowly advanced, injecting 5 mL of lidocaine into the subcutaneous interthenar seam of the palm (Fig. 51-12, *E*). The needle is then withdrawn partially and passed deep and ulnarly into the distal flexor tendon sheath, where 5 mL of lidocaine is injected (Fig. 51-12, *F*). The arm is then firmly wrapped with an Esmarch bandage and the tourniquet is inflated. Using this high-volume low-pressure technique (no direct skin or ligament injection), the anesthetic administration is effective and nearly painless. It also allows mobility of the digits to assist tenosynovectomy. Patients tolerate a tourniquet for 20 to 25 min of surgery.

The incision is started in the palm and carried through the subcutaneous layer into the forearm. Two broad retractors are placed in the palm to retract the soft tissue and place tension on the transverse carpal ligament. A number 15 blade is used to incise the transverse carpal ligament and the palmar antebrachial fascia (Fig. 51-13). The carpal canal is inspected for nerve compression and tenosynovial proliferation; retraction of the flexor sheath allows visualization and palpation of the carpal canal for masses or other abnormalities. If the tenosynovium is proliferative, complete tenosynovectomy is easily accomplished with the aid of the patient's voluntary flexion of the digits (Fig. 51-14). At the completion of the procedure the tourniquet is released and the bleeding is stopped by electrocoagulation and compression. Limited anterior epineurotomy may be performed in some cases of advanced compression, but intrafascicular neurolysis is no longer favored by most surgeons.[28,51,54] Injections of cortisone solutions and use of a drain depend on the surgeon's preference.

Postoperatively, the wrist is splinted in extension for 2 weeks to prevent tendon bowstringing and median nerve adherence to the healing transverse carpal ligament. Shoulder and elbow range of motion and finger flexion and extension exercises are begun immediately. The patient is allowed to perform light activities, including dressing and feeding and limited handwriting, but no lifting or stressful activities until the splint is removed 2 weeks postoperatively. At this time, the sutures are removed and splinting is discontinued. The patient is instructed to massage the scar with an antibiotic ointment or hand lotion to decrease tenderness. Lifting of more than 10 pounds and repetitive stress activities should be restricted for

6 weeks postoperatively. At that time, unrestricted activities are allowed. Persons performing heavy work activities may require longer work restriction. It is best to advise the patient that tenderness and hardness on either side of the incision are normal and will take 3 to 4 months to diminish.

RELEASE THROUGH PALMAR INCISION

Clayton[19] and Taleisnik[80] preferred a palmar incision only for release of the transverse carpal ligament. They and others feel that the exposure is adequate for release and tenosynovectomy and that the morbidity is less.

The skin and subcutaneous tissue are infiltrated with lidocaine along both sides of the thenar crease area, as described above. The anatomy of the palmar and thenar creases varies a great deal and portions of natural skin creases may be used. In general, the incision is made ulnarly in the ring finger axis to avoid branches of the median palmar cutaneous and ulnar palmar cutaneous nerves and the motor branch of the median nerve.[80] The palmar fascia is split longitudinally to the wrist flexion crease, exposing the transverse carpal ligament. Some surgeons then prefer to insert a blunt elevator beneath the distal border of the transverse carpal ligament. It is passed beneath the ligament proximally, allowing the surgeon to cut down on the ligament with the structures of the carpal tunnel protected by the elevator (Fig. 51-15). This technique must be performed with extreme caution. If the elevator is inadvertently passed beneath the median nerve, it may inadvertently be lacerated. As in the extended incision technique, the synovium may be removed and the nerve inspected with epineurotomy or a biopsy specimen taken, as preferred. By blunt dissection, the proximal palmar carpal fascia is freed from the skin and released for 2 cm proximally with a scissors under direct vision.

The postoperative management of patients with carpal tunnel release and tenosynovectomy through the palmar incision is the same as for the extended incision technique. If the tenosynovium is not removed and the nerve not dissected free from the surrounding tissues, some surgeons may prefer not to immobilize the wrist postoperatively. If immobilization in extension is not performed, the patient should be cautioned against forceful gripping with the wrist flexed for several weeks, because bowstringing of the flexor tendons can occur postoperatively after a transverse carpal ligament release.

RELEASE WITH LIMITED-EXCISION TECHNIQUES

In 1955, Paine[60] described a technique for division of the transverse carpal ligament through a small transverse incision in the wrist. He developed a special

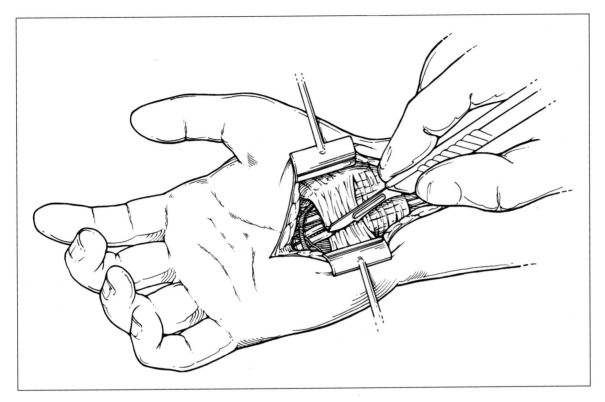

FIGURE 51-13

Open carpal tunnel release. The retractors place tension on the transverse carpal ligament, causing it to spring open after release, protecting the softer neural and tendinous tissue.

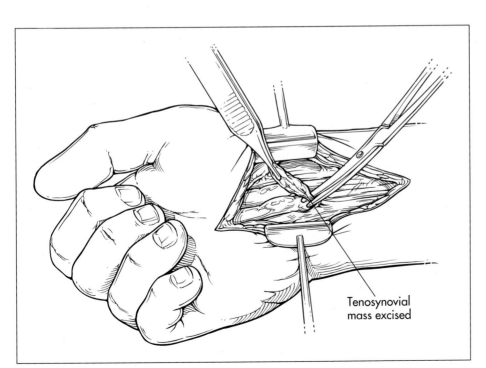

Tenosynovial
mass excised

FIGURE 51-14

The patient is asked to flex the fingers, providing for near-complete tenosynovectomy of the flexor tendons.

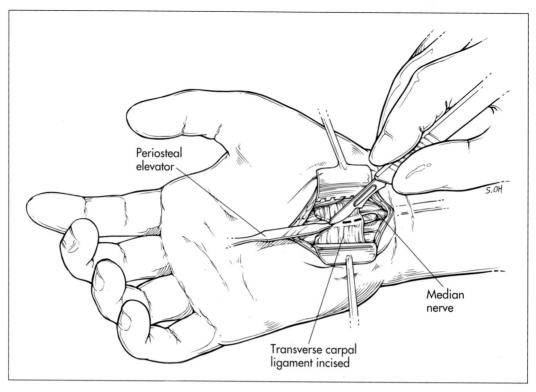

FIGURE 51-15

An elevator may be placed beneath the transverse carpal ligament and against the hook of the hamate. The elevator protects the median nerve during incision of the transverse carpal ligament and provides a guide to create a broad radial hand flap that avoids scarring directly over the median nerve.

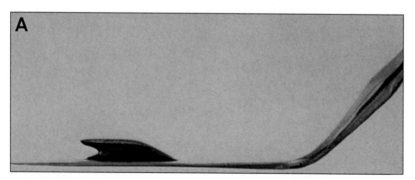

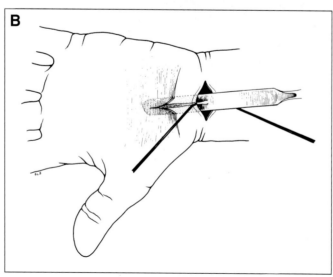

FIGURE 51-16

Limited excision release. **A,** The Paine retinaculatome. **B,** The retinaculatome is steadily advanced in a controlled manner until resistance is no longer felt. *(From Paine and Polyzoidis.[59] By permission of the American Association of Neurological Surgeons.)*

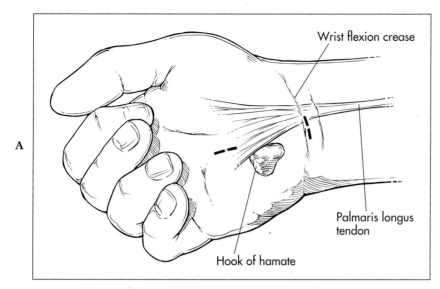

A

Wrist flexion crease

Palmaris longus tendon

Hook of hamate

FIGURE 51-17

A through **C,** Bowers exposes the ligament through proximal and distal small incisions and then releases it with a scissors under direct visualization (see text).

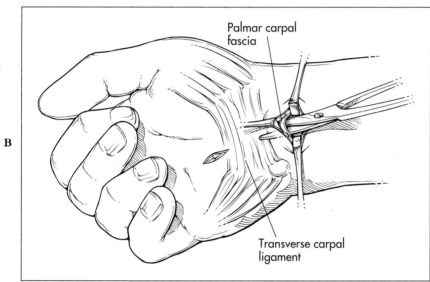

B

Palmar carpal fascia

Transverse carpal ligament

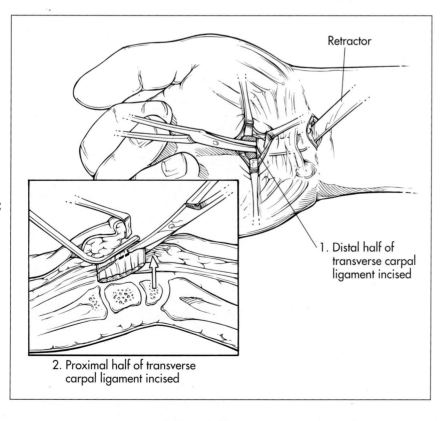

C

Retractor

1. Distal half of transverse carpal ligament incised

2. Proximal half of transverse carpal ligament incised

retinaculatome for this procedure (Fig. 51-16). The results of using this technique, as reported by the originator and others, are quite satisfactory and reportedly are associated with low morbidity and an earlier return to normal function.[57-59] Others have suggested that the technique is dangerous and associated with more complications and incomplete release.[47,48,50] As the technique of endoscopic carpal tunnel release began to be discussed in the late 1980s, the concept of performing carpal tunnel release through nonpalmar limited incisions with direct visualization has been reconsidered by others.[8,77]

PAINE RELEASE WITH TRANSVERSE LIMITED WRIST INCISION AND RETINACULATOME

Local anesthesia is injected at the level of the wrist flexion crease, with supplementary analgesia given intravenously as necessary. A transverse skin incision, 2 cm long, is made adjacent to the palmaris longus tendon at the wrist flexion crease in radial to ulnar direction. By blunt dissection, the palmar carpal fascia is identified ulnar to the palmaris longus tendon. A longitudinal 1.5-cm incision is then made in the fascia and proximal end of the transverse carpal ligament. The baseplate of the Paine retinaculatome is inserted under the proximal edge of the transverse carpal ligament. Lifting up on the instrument, the foot blade is passed into the carpal canal angled 20° ulnarly until the knife portion reaches the transverse carpal ligament. It is important to "toe-up" the blade tip toward the palm. The instrument is advanced distally using controlled pressure until the characteristic grating sound is no longer heard and resistance is no longer felt (Fig. 51-16, B). Care must be taken to avoid a more distal insertion because of risk to the superficial arch and common digital nerve branches of the median nerve.

A bulky dressing is applied for 24 hours. It is then removed, a Band-Aid is applied, and the patient is allowed full nonstrenuous use of the hand. Return to light work activities is allowed after suture removal at 1 week, but heavy lifting is restricted for 6 weeks.

RELEASE THROUGH TWO NONPALMAR INCISIONS

Regional anesthesia is injected locally. A 1-cm transverse incision is made in the wrist flexion crease ulnar to the palmaris longus tendon. The palmar carpal fascia is split proximally for 2 cm and distally to the border of the transverse carpal ligament (Fig. 51-17, A). A second 1-cm incision is made in the palm longitudinally 1 cm distal and radial to the hook of the hamate. The palmar fascia is incised, and with blunt dissection the distal ulnar border of the transverse carpal ligament is identified and the superficial palmar arch is visualized. A blunt flat periosteal

elevator is inserted into the distal and proximal incision to free the synovium and soft tissues from the internal surface of the transverse carpal ligament. A narrow blunt-tipped scissors is then passed distally, external or superficial to the transverse carpal ligament and deep to the palmar fascia; it is spread gently to form a channel *superficial* to the ligament (Fig. 51-17, B). A long narrow retractor is inserted in this channel and pulled upward. The transverse carpal ligament is incised from distal to proximal under direct vision, with the scissors switching to the proximal incision for final visualization and release of the proximal ligament (Fig. 51-17, C). The completeness of the release is confirmed by visual inspection with the long retractor.

A bulky dressing is worn for 1 to 2 days, after which a light dressing with or without any wrist support is used for 10 days. Sutures are removed and activities are allowed as tolerated.

ENDOSCOPIC VISUALIZATION FOR CARPAL TUNNEL RELEASE

Okutsu first introduced the concept of release of the transverse carpal ligament through small incisions with an endoscope.[55] In the same period in the late 1980s, Chow and Agee developed techniques for transverse carpal ligament release assisted by endoscopic visualization.[2,14] The originators' techniques have been modified by others, and the role of endoscopic visualization during carpal tunnel release is still being evaluated.[10,17,44,67] The current techniques of endoscopic carpal tunnel release are similar to those of open releases without palmar incisions, as described above, except that the endoscope is used for direct visualization of the surgical release (Fig. 51-18).

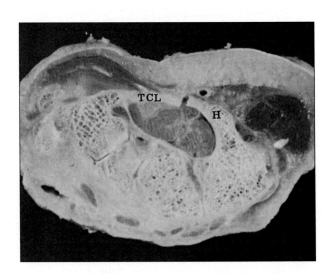

FIGURE 51-18

Transverse section in a cadaver hand demonstrates the ideal location for release of the transverse carpal ligament just radial to the hamate hook. *H,* hamate; *TCL,* transverse carpal ligament.

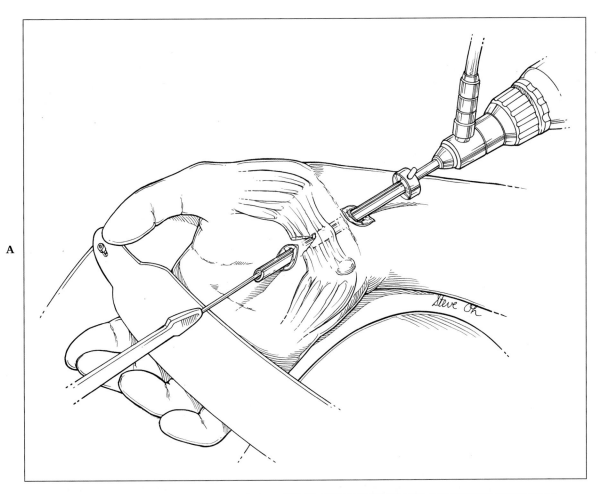

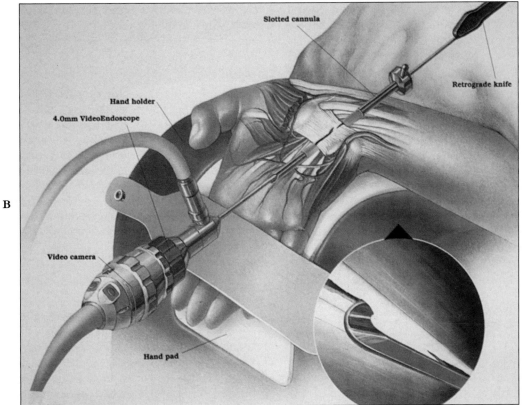

Slotted cannula

Retrograde knife

Hand holder

4.0mm VideoEndoscope

Video camera

Hand pad

Figure 51-19

A and **B,** Chow method for endoscopic visualization and release (see text). *(From Smith and Nephews Dynamics Bulletin, 160 Dascombe Road, Andover, Massachusetts 01810.)*

TWO-PORTAL TECHNIQUE OF ENDOSCOPIC RELEASE (CHOW)

Chow's original description of release of the transverse carpal ligament involved dissection to the floor of the carpal canal with retraction of the flexor tendons. This technique was modified by Chow[16] and others[67,71] to a subligamentous approach within the flexor sheath in the developed plane just beneath the transverse carpal ligament. The procedure is performed through a slotted cannula, which allows introduction of the endoscope and instruments through opposite portals. This allows visualization of the surgical instruments while they are used to divide the ligament in the slot in the cannula (Fig. 51-19). The technique and postoperative management described below are those developed by me in attempts to ensure safety and efficacy of the procedure and are slightly different from those of Chow.

AUTHOR'S PREFERRED APPROACH

A two-portal incision technique is performed during local anesthesia assisted by intravenously administered analgesia and under tourniquet control. A 1-cm incision is outlined longitudinally, proximally from the wrist flexion crease adjacent to the ulnar border of the palmaris longus tendon (or in the midline of the wrist if the palmaris longus is not present) (Fig. 51-20, A). Blunt dissection exposes the palmar carpal fascia. This is punctured with a blade. The proximal skin is elevated and with the blunt-tipped scissors the palmar carpal fascia is split longitudinally subcutaneously proximally for 2 cm (Fig. 51-20, B). Distally, the fascia is incised to the thickened proximal border of the transverse carpal ligament. A retractor is placed beneath the distal skin and pulled upward. This causes the transverse carpal ligament to slightly elevate from the flexor sheath to allow direct visualization for insertion of a blunt elevator. The blunt elevator is inserted beneath the transverse carpal ligament. The flexor sheath and nerve are freed from the ligament by sweeping the instrument back and forth beneath the "corrugated" internal surface of the transverse carpal ligament (Fig. 51-20, C). It is important to directly visualize the entrance of the elevator beneath the transverse carpal ligament. It is possible to mistake the edge of the palmar fascia for the transverse carpal ligament if it is not directly visualized, and this could cause the elevator to enter Guyon's canal. The distal end of the transverse carpal ligament can be palpated by the opposite hand as the elevator exits beneath its edge in the ulnar palm. A second 1-cm incision is made in the ulnar palm where the blade is felt to exit (Fig. 51-20, D).

An important modification at this point is dissection and inspection of the distal portal. The fatty tissues are spread and four small retractors are inserted in the distal portal. The palmar fascia is split longitudinally and distally 1 cm under direct vision. The soft deep tissues are gently spread with the small blunt-tipped scissors. This frees the superficial arch and flexor sheath-median nerve from any adherence to the adjacent soft tissues and later allows easy passage of the trocar (Fig. 51-20, E). Attention is then returned to the proximal portal and the blunt elevator is passed beneath the transverse carpal ligament under direct vision. With the wrist slightly extended, the curved elevator is passed distally through the distal portal. The elevator should pass easily as the distal palmar fascia is split and the soft tissues have been released from the distal edge of the transverse carpal ligament (Fig. 51-20, F). The elevator is removed and the trocar with the slotted cannula is passed through the track established by the elevator, with the wrist slightly extended. The trocar should again pass easily. If not, the procedure is repeated. The distal incision is inspected to confirm the absence of soft-tissue (superficial or nerve) tethering, the hand is placed in the Chow extension rack, and the trocar is removed (Figs. 51-20, E through H).

The endoscope is now inserted through the proximal cannula and a cotton swab is placed through the distal cannula. The swab is rotated toward the median nerve to cleanse the scope lens and remove fluid for better visualization. A blunt probe or brushes (or both) are used to identify the proximal and distal ends of the transverse carpal ligament, which can be clearly visualized.[14,67] Chow[14] prefers to use a three-knife system for release of the transverse carpal ligament in segments starting distally. We and others prefer to release the entire ligament with a hook knife, with visualization through the distal portal (Fig. 51-20, I).[10] The distal end of the transverse carpal ligament should be clearly visualized with the endoscope in the distal portal. The hook knife is inserted and drawn proximally. Moderate resistance will be felt. Sudden release of the blade can be prevented by stabilizing the hand controlling the blade with the index finger against the patient's wrist. The division is accomplished progressively proximally, following with the scope and visualizing the release. If fibers of the transverse palmaris muscle are encountered, they are released along with the overlying palmar fascia, in contrast to Chow. The ligament release is confirmed with the endoscope by herniation of subcutaneous fat. Longitudinal fibers of palmar fascia may be left. If excellent visualization is not achieved, the procedure should be abandoned. After release of the transverse carpal ligament, the slotted cannula generally turns quite easily within the canal. It is removed, the hand is placed back on the operating table, and an important inspection process is begun.

With the use of small retractors, the proximal portal is inspected. With the aid of a blunt elevator, the release edge of the transverse carpal ligament is visualized. The median nerve can now also be seen after release of the

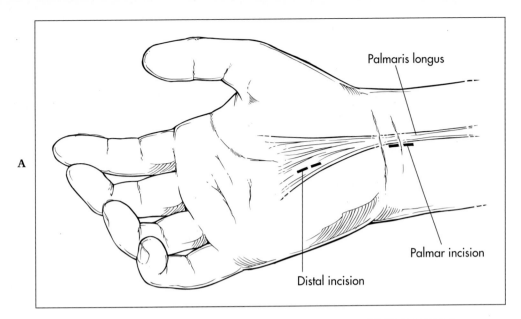

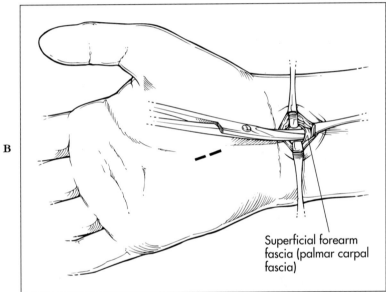

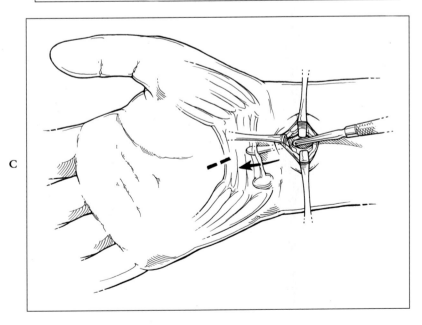

FIGURE 51-20

Author's method for two-portal endoscopic release. **A,** Incisions outlined; distal incision at radial axis of ring finger and base of thumb web. **B,** Palmar carpal fascia incised proximally. **C,** Blunt elevator sweeps through carpal canal.

Continued.

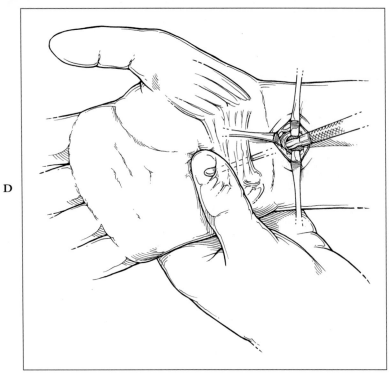

D

FIGURE 51-20, CONT'D.

D, Elevator confirms location of exit incision.
E, The scissors are gently spread to release the distal
soft tissues. **F,** Passing the elevator through distal incision to prepare the cannula tract.

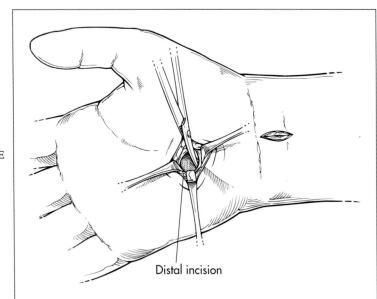

E

Distal incision

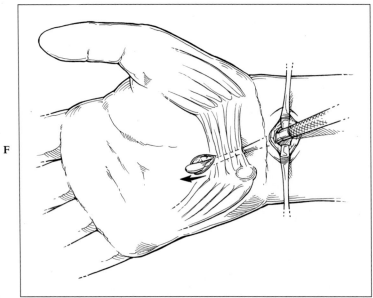

F

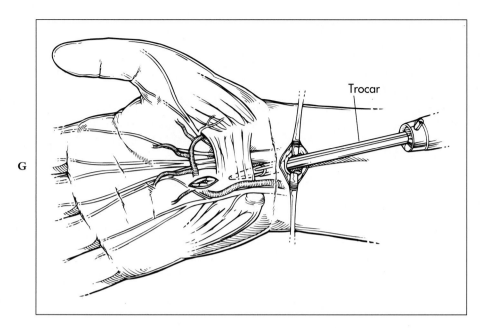

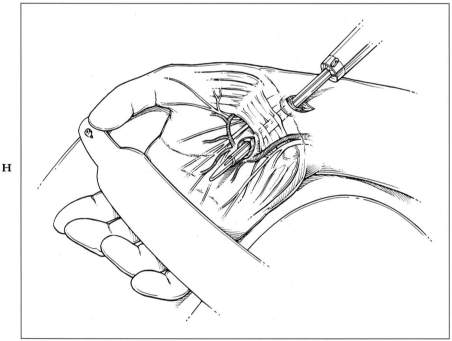

FIGURE 51-20, CONT'D.

G, The cannula is easily passed through the proximal portal. **H,** The hyperextension rack stabilizes the hand and places the transverse carpal ligament in tension. *Continued.*

ligament. The distal portal is inspected and release of the entire ligament is visually confirmed. The surgeon can also palpate the distal incision to ensure that the entire ligament has been divided. After the completion of these inspections, it should not be possible for any persistent median compression to occur (Fig. 51-20, *J*).

At this point, the tourniquet is released, hemostasis is attained, and the wounds are sutured over a drain. The wound is irrigated with 0.01% neomycin solution and the flexor sheath is injected with 3 mL of lidocaine and 1 mL of soluble dexamethasone (author's preference). A compression dressing is applied with a plaster splint to maintain the wrist in dorsiflexion.

Chow uses a minimal postoperative dressing and allows immediate movement of the hand and wrist. I prefer to remove the bulky dressing and drain at 1 day postoperatively and use a wrist extension splint for 10 days. At that time, sutures are removed and activities are allowed as tolerated, with no heavy activities until 4 to 6 weeks postoperatively.

SINGLE-PORTAL TECHNIQUE OF ENDOSCOPIC RELEASE (AGEE)

Agee developed a three-component pistol-grip device with a disposal blade and viewing channel

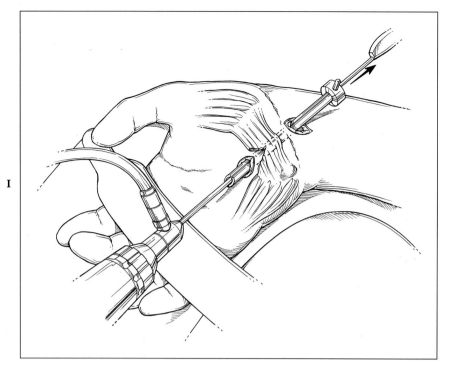

I

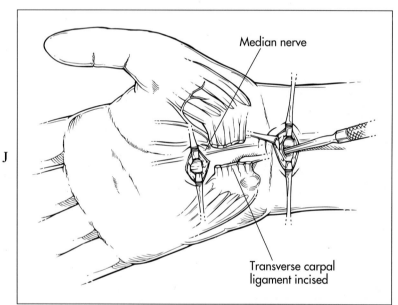

J

Median nerve

Transverse carpal
ligament incised

FIGURE 51-20, CONT'D.

I, The hook knife is used through the proximal portal to release the entire transverse carpal ligament. **J,** The ligament release is confirmed by direct visualization and palpation.

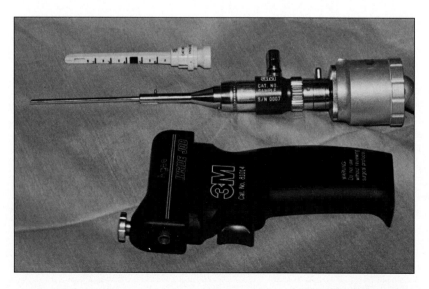

FIGURE 51-21

Agee "Inside Job Device" components: blade assembly, pistol grip handle, and endoscope. Compression of the trigger mechanism elevates the blade. The light source and endoscopic camera enter the base of the instrument and provide clear visualization of the surgical blade during endoscopic carpal tunnel release.

mechanism for single-portal endoscopic carpal tunnel release (Fig. 51-21).[2]

Regional or general anesthesia is used along with tourniquet control. A transverse incision is made at the wrist flexion crease between the palmaris longus and flexor carpi ulnaris. The subcutaneous tissues are dissected off of the palmar carpal fascia. A 1 cm² distally based flap of palmar carpal fascia (flexor retinaculum) is elevated just proximal and ulnar to the palmaris longus tendon and just radial to the pisiform. This is elevated as a tongue to function as a shoehorn to place a pathfinder instrument. This blunt instrument is passed into the carpal canal along the radial side of the

hook of the hamate to prepare a track for the blade assembly (Figs. 51-22, *A* and *B*). Dilation of the carpal tunnel ensures safe insertion of the blade assembly.

With the blade assembly device aimed at the ring finger and with the wrist in extension, the blade assembly is inserted until the distal end of the transverse carpal ligament is easily identified with the endoscope. The fat pad just distal to the transverse carpal ligament should be visualized to ensure correct depth of blade insertion. Once this is confirmed, the trigger is squeezed to elevate the blade. Upward pressure is applied, and the device is withdrawn proximally, releasing the transverse carpal ligament. The device is

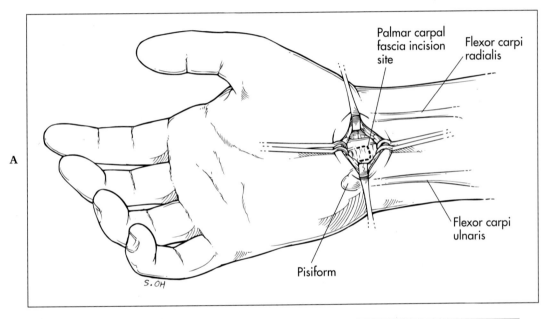

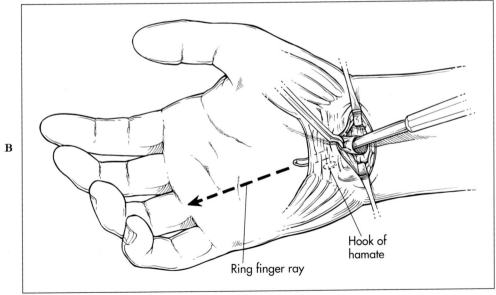

FIGURE 51-22

Agee technique for endoscopic carpal tunnel release. **A,** The palmar carpal "tongue" is prepared. **B,** All instruments and the device follow the ring finger ray. *Continued.*

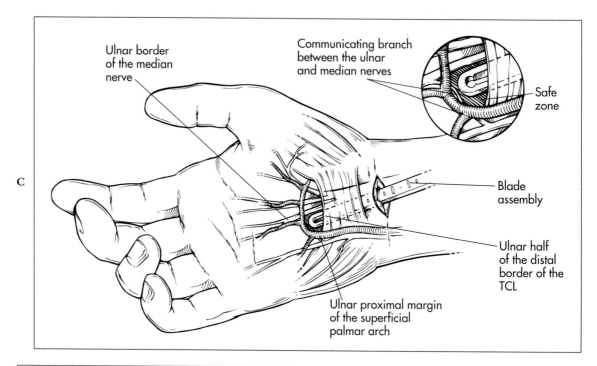

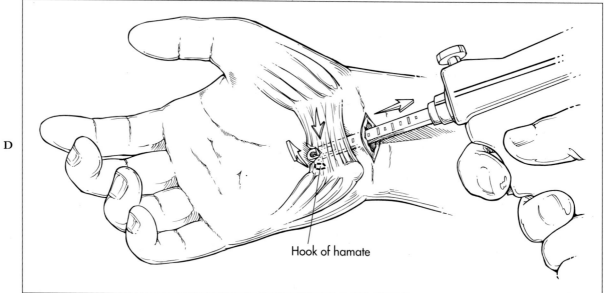

FIGURE 51-22, CONT'D.

C, Agee "safe zone" for blade elevation: a triangular area at the ulnar half of the distal border of the transverse carpal ligament (*TCL*), the ulnar border of the median nerve, and the ulnar proximal margin of the superficial palmar arch. **D,** Release of the TCL as the blade is pulled proximally.

then reinserted and one to two passes can be made until the edges of the ligament and fat are identified to confirm release (Figs. 51-22, *C* and *D*).

A dressing and splints are worn for 1 week, followed by activities as tolerated.

Other types of single-portal endoscopic release systems are being developed and will need to be evaluated for efficacy and safety (Figs. 51-23 and 51-24).

TREATMENT OF CARPAL TUNNEL RELEASE BY TENOSYNOVECTOMY ALONE

In 1989 Melvin[52] presented his work on treatment of CTS without release of the transverse carpal ligament. In

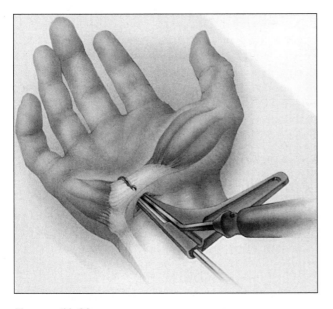

FIGURE 51-23

Uni-Cut system of endoscopic release. The device has a cannula for the endoscope and a slot for a hook knife. *(Technique designed by Terrence R. Orr, M.D., South Lake Tahoe, California; Acuflex Microsurgical, Inc., 130 Forbes Blvd., Mansfield, Massachusetts 02048.)*

this technique, the pressure on the median nerve is relieved by decreasing the bulk of the soft tissue within the carpal canal.

The distal forearm and flexor sheath are injected with local anesthetic and the tourniquet is elevated. A lazy S-shaped incision is made for 4 cm from the wrist flexion crease proximally and ulnarly to the palmaris longus tendon. The palmar carpal fascia (superficial fascia of the forearm) is incised; the median nerve is identified, freed from the synovium, and retracted radially. Individually, each of the superficialis, profundus, and flexor pollicis longus tendons is pulled into the wound and a tenosynovectomy is performed.

Light dressings are worn and full wrist and digital motion are permitted. Return to heavy work activities may be possible as early as 2 weeks postoperatively.[39]

PERSPECTIVES ON COMPLICATIONS, RESULTS, AND TECHNIQUES OF CARPAL TUNNEL SURGERY

COMPLICATIONS

Infection after carpal tunnel surgery can seriously compromise functional results through flexor tendon scarring and limited motion. Although every effort to avoid this complication is beneficial, infection is still seen occasionally.[15,33] A key factor in successful treatment may be early recognition of the condition. Recalling the normal tenosynovial anatomy is critical in evaluating this complication. The flexor tendon sheaths of the small finger and thumb are the only tendon sheaths that extend from the carpal canal to the digit tips. The ring, long, and index finger tendon sheaths stop in the palm and re-form separately in the digits. Therefore, an infection in a carpal tunnel wound is often heralded by pain, swelling, and stiffness in the thumb or small finger. If either of these conditions

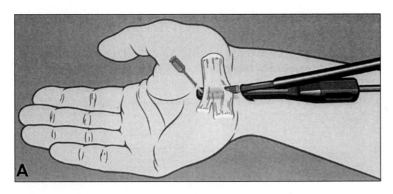
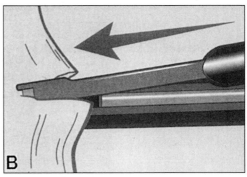

FIGURE 51-24

Menon technique of single portal release. **A,** Half open cannula provides channel for endoscopic and **(B)** pusher-type cutting blade: needle marks distal end of transverse carpal ligament. *(From Concept CTS Relief Kit, Surgical Technique, Linvatic Concept Arthroscopy, Linvatic Corporation, Largo, Florida.)*

occurs, a presumptive diagnosis of infection within the carpal canal should be made.

For infection, immediate débridement and flexor tenosynovectomy are performed, followed by loose wound closure over Penrose drains and intravenous antibiotic therapy. The wounds should not normally be packed open unless one can ensure that the nerve will not be exposed to any desiccation. After open débridement, active digital flexion and extension exercises are initiated as soon as possible. The combination of flexor tenosynovectomy, surgical drain, and local injection of cortisone within the carpal tunnel has been associated with increased incidence of post-operative infection.[33]

Injury to the median nerve can occur in carpal tunnel surgery. The most commonly reported problem is division of the palmar cutaneous nerve branch of the median nerve.[48] This should be avoidable with ulnar incisions, as outlined above, and likely will not be seen with endoscopic techniques in which the ligament is divided immediately adjacent to the hook of the hamate.[80] The possibility of damage to the main trunk of the median nerve or to its motor branch is small with open incision palmar techniques but does occur. It has been seen more frequently (including superficial palmar arch lacerations) by the author and others in limited wrist-incision techniques.[47] Some authors[2,67] have described a serious incidence of nerve injury with endoscopic techniques. Others[10,14] have reported high levels of safety with endoscopic methods, and modifications of technique, as outlined above, should eliminate nerve injury as a complication.

Incomplete release of the transverse carpal ligament is possible with any technique and reported as a significant complication of both open and closed techniques.[42,48,71] With limited incisions at the wrist, incomplete release is more likely, but with careful open techniques or double-portal endoscopic-assisted visualization, as described above, this complication should not occur.

RESULTS

Results of carpal tunnel surgery appear to be gratifying regardless of the surgical method used. Patients with classic symptoms, not involved in occupational repetitive stress, can be expected to achieve relief of symptoms even in the presence of other neuropathic diseases (e.g., diabetes, polyneuropathy) with superimposed CTS; the release of the carpal ligament provides symptomatic relief.[18] Even in patients with motor atrophy or advanced sensory disturbance, some improvement can be expected in the majority of cases.[28,54]

The major failures in carpal tunnel surgery appear to be in the worker population. Although the majority of these patients are improved with surgical treatment, relief may be incomplete, especially if they return to the same job that provoked the condition. In these patients it is likely that mechanical compression of the median nerve occurs when the patient flexes the fingers with the wrist flexed, compressing the median nerve against the firm healed transverse carpal ligament. In these situations, job modification or adaptive methods may be necessary. Recurrence of CTS is rare in the nonworker population, but it may occur with surgical procedures such as wrist prostheses, which can cause a mechanical impingement of the canal, or in a recurrent proliferative synovitis that might be seen in a mycobacterial infection.

Results of reoperations after carpal tunnel surgery have been mixed but generally successful if a specific pathologic condition is identified.[20,48] In performing reoperation, an open method of carpal tunnel surgery is recommended. One must assume that the median nerve is adherent to the transverse carpal ligament and flexor tendons. Therefore, surgery is best performed during regional or general anesthesia with loupe magnification and tourniquet control. Dissection should be initiated in the pristine proximal tissue where the normal median nerve may be identified and then proceed distally, dissecting the median nerve from scarred tissue.

SUMMARY

CTS is a common condition that is treated by many surgeons with many different techniques. Regardless of the technique used, a surgeon experienced with the technique of his or her choice will provide satisfactory results. Unfortunately, with so many surgeons performing the technique in distinctly different ways, closed camps have tended to develop that accept one technique as the only acceptable method. The surgeon and patient must keep an open mind to the various past, present, and future techniques, because the final result will likely depend on the skill of the surgeon using the technique and not the technique itself. In the future, drug therapy or physical modalities may become even more common than surgical treatment and they are being investigated now.[5,79]

RECURRENT CARPAL TUNNEL SYNDROME

After primary carpal tunnel release, there is an incidence of failure between 10% and 18%, with recurrence of symptoms.[22,24,40,48,64] The most common cause of recurrence noted by Langloh and Linscheid[40] was incomplete release of the transverse carpal ligament. Other causes are failure to release the superficial or antebrachial fascia of the forearm when part of the etiology of the CTS is fracture displacement or carpal displacement in this region, such as may occur with distal radius fractures or dislocations of the wrist.[63] A third and more difficult area to treat is scarring and fibrosis about the median nerve associated with the original pathology, such as internal injury associated with previous carpal tunnel surgical procedures.[23,36,51]

When there is evidence of recurrence after a previous carpal tunnel release, it is important to confirm the symptomatic presentation with both positive physical findings and electromyographic testing (including conduction studies). There is a group of patients who have symptoms of median neuropathy with pain that is different from CTS. These patients often have pain out of proportion to physical findings and usually have a work overuse history. In such patients, surgical intervention may not be indicated and can be harmful by contributing to nerve hypersensitivity through surgery. My colleagues and I believe that it is important to separate this group of patients with pain dysfunction from those with CTS (recurrent) where further surgical intervention may help. Positive physical findings with recurrent CTS should include not only a positive Tinel sign but other objective signs of nerve compression such as Phalen's sign, direct compression along the median nerve increasing the symptoms, evidence of objective loss of sensibility, and occasionally thenar muscle weakness. The nerve conduction studies should show decreased distal latency of sensory or motor fibers across the carpal tunnel, decreased nerve amplitude, and occasionally decreased nerve conduction velocity. Electromyography may demonstrate increased voluntary motor units, ongoing evidence of decreased muscle fiber recruitment, and fibrillations.

When recurrent CTS is present, treatment should at first be conservative. Modalities may include wrist splint support, cortisone injection of the carpal tunnel or cortisone phonophoresis, and transcutaneous electrical nerve stimulation along the median nerve. We have also used repetitive nerve blocks (see Chapter 46) to decrease median nerve hypersensitivity and pain. We also believe that an effort should be made to change the work environment or to treat any underlying systemic conditions that might be contributing to the recurrence of carpal tunnel symptoms. For the patient with persistent pain symptoms referred to the median nerve at the wrist but without localizing physical findings to suggest actual recurrence of the CTS, we recommend pain management and not surgical intervention.

When conservative (nonoperative) methods of treatment fail, several treatment modalities have been suggested. Studies to date and our own experience suggest that reoperation and neurolysis of the median nerve alone is not usually successful.[40,49,51,82] Occasionally, one finds incomplete release of the transverse carpal ligament or a space-occupying mass as reason for the recurrence, and simple further release or mass excision (or both) is sufficient. Release of the transverse carpal ligament and tenolysis also may be sufficient in those cases in which inflammatory synovitis is part of the

cause of recurrence of the carpal tunnel symptoms. It appears quite clear from the literature that neurolysis alone of the median nerve is not the treatment of choice for recurrent CTS and that other ancillary procedures should be used to increase vascular supply to the nerve and provide an improved gliding surface area.[28,36,49,82]

We have recently reviewed our experience with local flaps combined with external neurolysis in the treatment of recurrent CTS. Lumbrical flaps have been used to revascularize the distal half of the median nerve after release of the carpal tunnel, and the pronator quadratus has been rerouted to improve excursion and vascular supply to the medial nerve in the proximal portion of the carpal tunnel.[84] Our best experience is with the palmaris brevis and hypothenar fat pad, which can be rotated to cover the majority of the median nerve through the carpal tunnel.[69,78] It can be combined with the lumbrical muscles in selective cases. The other alternative used in our practice is a radial forearm fascial flap.[13,68,73,81] Here, a vascular pedicle flap based distally on the radial artery can be rotated to cover the median nerve. In our experience it is necessary, in some cases, to divide the radial artery proximally and then rotate the mid-forearm portion of the superficial fascia to cover over the median nerve proximal to and through the carpal tunnel. In other cases, the forearm fascia can be rotated on a rich vascular fascia without ligating and rotating the entire radial artery. The location of nerve compression and scarring helps to dictate the best flap for coverage of the median nerve.

OPERATIVE PROCEDURES: HYPOTHENAR FLAP

The median nerve is identified first proximally through an incision in the distal third of the forearm. The nerve is traced distally with loupe magnification through the carpal tunnel. External neurolysis (but not internal neurolysis) is performed as necessary. The re-formed transverse carpal ligament is divided and the incision is extended distally to the palmar aponeurosis. After release of the median nerve, the ulnar border of the incision is elevated deep to the subdermal plexus and carried over to the hypothenar region. Care is taken to identify and maintain vascular supply to the palmaris brevis muscle and hypothenar pad. As needed, the ulnar nerve and artery are identified proximally and retracted with a vessel loop. Beginning ulnarly, the dissection is extended deep to the fat pad and muscle and a rectangular segment of the hypothenar tissue is elevated ulnar to radial and proximal to distal. The flap is then rotated on itself ulnar to radial, maintaining a good vascular pedicle from the ulnar artery. The rotated edge of the flap is placed over the median nerve and beneath the radial edge of the transverse carpal ligament.

In some patients in whom the fat pad is particularly thick, it is possible to elevate the fat pad both superficially and deep (protecting again the neurovascular pedicle) and slide the fat pad from an ulnar to radial direction. The deep dissection of this type of flap must be performed with care taken to identify the ulnar nerve and distal common digital nerves to the ring and little finger. The elevated flap is then pulled radially to cover the palmar surface of the median nerve. This transposed flap is sutured to the radial edge of the transverse carpal ligament as described for the rotation flap. The tourniquet, which must be used in such cases, is deflated after the flap is transposed and hemostasis is achieved. Skin closure usually can be performed tension free. The wrist is splinted postoperatively but assisted wrist motion to promote gliding of the median nerve beneath the flap is started on the first postoperative day. Scar massage, assisted wrist motion, and active finger flexion and extension are performed during a 2- to 3-week rehabilitation program.

OPERATIVE PROCEDURES: RADIAL FOREARM FLAP

The radial forearm flap, which can include fascia only or skin, subcutaneous tissue, and fascia, is elevated before formal dissection of the median nerve through the carpal tunnel. Care is taken to first confirm that there is good collateral circulation through the ulnar artery and palmar arch. The flap and radial communicating branches are identified. Attention is then turned to the carpal tunnel region where the median nerve is dissected from the superficial forearm fascia. It is then traced distally through the carpal tunnel, and the length of scarred area is determined. The proximal dissection of the radial artery and forearm fascia is based on the length of flap needed. In general, one begins a pivot point 5 cm proximal to the wrist flexion crease. The forearm fascia is dissected from distal to proximal and ulnar to radial. The depth of the dissection should include the superficial fascia over the muscles of the

forearm. Cutaneous vessels are cauterized as needed ulnarly, but the radial vessels are preserved. The number of vessels within the superficial fascia determines if the radial artery needs to be divided proximally and rotated with the flap. If the number of communicating vessels is small, the radial artery is then included with the flap.

The radial fascial flap is rotated distally and the distal extent judged on the amount of median nerve to cover. It is usually possible to place part of the flap dorsal and the majority of the flap palmar to the median nerve. The flap is sutured in place with attachment to palmar fascia and the ulnar and radial borders of the carpal tunnel. The tourniquet is deflated to assess vascularity, and hemostasis is achieved. Skin closure is determined by the amount of fat associated with the flap. In some cases, we have primary skin closure, and others may require a skin graft. In general, we do not recommend completely wrapping the median nerve in the flap for fear of overcompressing the nerve. Motion after closure of the wounds is initiated the day after operation.

The principles in each of these procedures are to provide a scar-free gliding bed for the median nerve, to increase vascularity about the nerve, and to decompress the external scar. It is again important to assess the median nerve symptoms of recurrent CTS carefully and to treat associated pathology. Depending on the site and extent of the pathology (i.e., nerve compression), different types of local flaps can be considered to provide an improved nerve bed. Our experience suggests that despite these efforts at revascularization, only about 70% of the surgical cases will be successful. We have found in review of our cases that the hypothenar flap appears to work best and the lumbrical flap is the least successful. Other options include the abductor digiti minimi flap,[43,53,66] pronator quadratus flap,[23] vascularized fascia from ulnar artery,[31] and potentially a free transfer using omentum, a thoracic adventitial flap, or a serratus anterior flap.

REFERENCES

1. Abbott LC, Saunders JB deCM: Injuries of the median nerve in fractures of the lower end of the radius, *Surg Gynecol Obstet* 57:507-516, 1933.
2. Agee JM, McCarroll HR Jr, Tortosa RD, et al.: Endoscopic release of the carpal tunnel: a randomized prospective multicenter study, *J Hand Surg [Am]* 17:987-995, 1992.
3. Amadio PC: Carpal tunnel syndrome, pyridoxine, and the work place, *J Hand Surg [Am]* 12:875-880, 1987.
4. Amadio PC: The Mayo Clinic and carpal tunnel syndrome, *Mayo Clin Proc* 67:42-48, 1992.
5. Basford JR, Hallman HO, Matsumoto JY, et al.: Effects of 830 nm continuous wave laser diode irradiation on median nerve function in normal subjects, *Lasers Surg Med* 13:597-604, 1993.
6. Beckenbaugh RD, Simonian PT: Clinical efficacy of electroneurometer screening in carpal tunnel syndrome, *Orthopedics* 18:549-552, 1995.
7. Berger RA: Endoscopic carpal tunnel release. A current perspective, *Hand Clin* 10:625-636, 1994.

8. Bowers B: Perspectives on endoscopic carpal tunnel release, technique and complications. Read at 22nd annual meeting of the American Association for Hand Surgery, Washington, DC, September 17 and 18, 1992.

9. Brain WR, Wright AD, Wilkinson M: Spontaneous compression of both median nerves in the carpal tunnel: six cases treated surgically, *Lancet* 1:277-282, 1947.

10. Brown MG, Keyser B, Rothenberg ES: Endoscopic carpal tunnel release, *J Hand Surg [Am]* 17:1009-1011, 1992.

11. Brown RA, Gelberman RH, Seiler JG III, et al.: Carpal tunnel release. A prospective, randomized assessment of open and endoscopic methods, *J Bone Joint Surg Am* 75:1265-1275, 1993.

12. Cannon BW, Love JG: Tardy median palsy; median neuritis; median thenar neuritis amenable to surgery, *Surgery* 20:210-216, 1946.

13. Cavanagh S, Pho RW: The reverse radial forearm flap in the severely injured hand: an anatomical and clinical study, *J Hand Surg [Br]* 17:501-503, 1992.

14. Chow JC: Endoscopic release of the carpal ligament for carpal tunnel syndrome: 22-month clinical result, *Arthroscopy* 6:288-296, 1990.

15. Chow JC: The Chow technique of endoscopic release of the carpal ligament for carpal tunnel syndrome: four years of clinical results, *Arthroscopy* 9:301-314, 1993.

16. Chow JC: Endoscopic carpal tunnel release. Two-portal technique, *Hand Clin* 10:637-646, 1994.

17. Chow JCY: Endoscopic carpal tunnel release. Pro-Point of view, *Bull AAOS* 1:12, July 1992.

18. Clayburgh RH, Beckenbaugh RD, Dobyns JH: Carpal tunnel release in patients with diffuse peripheral neuropathy, *J Hand Surg [Am]* 12:380-383, 1987.

19. Clayton ML, Linscheid RL: Carpal tunnel surgery: should the incision be above or below the wrist? *Orthopedics* 11:819-821, 1988.

20. Cobb TK, Amadio PC, Leatherwood DF, et al.: Outcome of reoperation for carpal tunnel syndrome, *J Hand Surg [Am]* 21:347-356, 1996.

21. Cobb TK, Dalley BK, Posteraro RH, et al.: Anatomy of the flexor retinaculum, *J Hand Surg [Am]* 18:91-99, 1993.

22. Cseuz KA, Thomas JE, Lambert EH, et al.: Long-term results of operation for carpal tunnel syndrome, *Mayo Clin Proc* 41:232-241, 1966.

23. Dellon AL, Mackinnon SE: The pronator quadratus muscle flap, *J Hand Surg [Am]* 9:423-427, 1984.

24. De Smet L: Recurrent carpal tunnel syndrome: clinical testing indicating incomplete section of the flexor retinaculum, *J Hand Surg [Br]* 18:189, 1993.

25. Evangelisti S, Reale VF: Fibroma of tendon sheath as a cause of carpal tunnel syndrome, *J Hand Surg [Am]* 17:1026-1027, 1992.

26. Garcia-Elias M, An KN, Cooney WP, et al.: Transverse stability of the carpus. An analytical study, *J Orthop Res* 7:738-743, 1989.

27. Garcia-Elias M, Sanchez-Freijo JM, Salo JM, et al.: Dynamic changes of the transverse carpal arch during flexion-extension of the wrist: effects of sectioning the transverse carpal ligament, *J Hand Surg [Am]* 17:1017-1019, 1992.

28. Gelberman RH, Pfeffer GB, Galbraith RT, et al.: Results of treatment of severe carpal-tunnel syndrome without internal neurolysis of the median nerve, *J Bone Joint Surg Am* 69:896-903, 1987.

29. Gelberman RH, Rydevik BL, Pess GM, et al.: Carpal tunnel syndrome. A scientific basis for clinical care, *Orthop Clin North Am* 19:115-124, 1988.

30. Gellman H, Gelberman RH, Tan AM, et al.: Carpal tunnel syndrome. An evaluation of the provocative diagnostic tests, *J Bone Joint Surg Am* 68:735-737, 1986.

31. Gilbert A, Becker C: *A flap based on distal branches of the ulnar artery and its use in recurrent carpal tunnel syndrome.* In Tubiana R, editor: *The hand,* vol 4, Philadelphia, 1993, WB Saunders, pp 499-505.

32. Gray H, Clemente CD: *Anatomy of the human body,* ed 13, Philadelphia, 1985, Lea & Febiger, pp 531, 542, 551.

33. Hanssen AD, Amadio PC, De Silva SP, et al.: Deep postoperative wound infection after carpal tunnel release, *J Hand Surg [Am]* 14:869-873, 1989.

34. Hoppenfeld S, deBoer P: *Surgical exposures in orthopaedics: the anatomic approach,* Philadelphia, 1984, JB Lippincott, pp 162-165.

35. Hunt JR: Occupation neuritis of the thenar branch of the median nerve (a well defined type of neutral atrophy of the hand), *Trans Am Neurol Assoc* 35:184, 1910.

36. Hunter JM: Recurrent carpal tunnel syndrome, epineural fibrous fixation, and traction neuropathy, *Hand Clin* 7:491-504, 1991.

37. Kerr CD, Sybert DR, Albarracin NS: An analysis of the flexor synovium in idiopathic carpal tunnel syndrome: report of 625 cases, *J Hand Surg [Am]* 17:1028-1030, 1992.

38. Kline SC, Moore JR: The transverse carpal ligament. An important component of the digital flexor pulley system, *J Bone Joint Surg Am* 74:1478-1485, 1992.

39. Kutz JE: Synovectomy only in the treatment of carpal tunnel syndrome, *AAOS Instruct Course Lect,* December 1995.

40. Langloh ND, Linscheid RL: Recurrent and unrelieved carpal-tunnel syndrome, *Clin Orthop* 83:41-47, 1972.

41. Learmonth JR: The principle of decompression in the treatment of certain diseases of peripheral nerves, *Surg Clin North Am* 13:905-913, 1933.

42. Lee DH, Masear VR, Meyer RD, et al.: Endoscopic carpal tunnel release: a cadaveric study, *J Hand Surg [Am]* 17:1003-1008, 1992.

43. Leslie BM, Ruby LK: Coverage of a carpal tunnel wound dehiscence with the abductor digiti minimi muscle flap, *J Hand Surg [Am]* 13:36-39, 1988.

44. Linscheid RL: Endoscopic CTS. Con-point of view, *Bull AAOS* 7:13, July 1992.

45. Linscheid RL, Dobyns JH, Beabout JW, et al.: Traumatic instability of the wrist. Diagnosis, classification, and pathomechanics, *J Bone Joint Surg Am* 54:1612-1632, 1972.

46. Lluch AL: Thickening of the synovium of the digital flexor tendons: cause or consequence of the carpal tunnel syndrome? *J Hand Surg [Br]* 17:209-212, 1992.

47. Louis DS, Greene TL, Noellert RC: Complications of carpal tunnel surgery, *J Neurosurg* 62:352-356, 1985.

48. MacDonald RI, Lichtman DM, Hanlon JJ, et al.: Complications of surgical release for carpal tunnel syndrome, *J Hand Surg [Am]* 3:70-76, 1978.

49. Mackinnon SE: Secondary carpal tunnel surgery, *Neurosurg Clin N Am* 2:75-91, 1991.

50. Mackinnon SE, Dellon AL: *Surgery of the peripheral nerve,* New York, 1988, Thieme Medical Publishers, pp 149-169.

51. Mackinnon SE, McCabe S, Murray JF, et al.: Internal neurolysis fails to improve the results of primary carpal tunnel decompression, *J Hand Surg [Am]* 16:211-218, 1991.

52. Melvin M: Flexor tenosynovectomy as the only treatment for carpal tunnel syndrome. Read at the annual meeting of the American Society for Surgery of the Hand, Seattle, September, 1989.

53. Milward TM, Stott WG, Kleinert HE: The abductor digiti minimi muscle flap, *Hand* 9:82-85, 1977.

54. Nolan WB III, Alkaitis D, Glickel SZ, et al.: Results of treatment of severe carpal tunnel syndrome, *J Hand Surg [Am]* 17:1020-1023, 1992.

55. Okutsu I, Ninomiya S, Natsuyama M, et al.: Subcutaneous operation and examination under the universal endoscope [Japanese], *Nippon Seikeigeka Gakkai Zasshi* 61:491-498, 1987.

56. Paget J: *Lectures on surgical pathology,* ed 2, Philadelphia, 1854, Lindsay and Blakiston, p 42.

57. Pagnanelli DM, Barrer SJ: Carpal tunnel syndrome: surgical treatment using the Paine retinaculatome, *J Neurosurg* 75:77-81, 1991.

58. Pagnanelli DM, Barrer SJ: Bilateral carpal tunnel release at one operation: report of 228 patients, *Neurosurgery* 31:1030-1033, 1992.

59. Paine KW, Polyzoidis KS: Carpal tunnel syndrome. Decompression using the Paine retinaculatome, *J Neurosurg* 59:1031-1036, 1983.

60. Paine KWE: An instrument for dividing flexor retinaculum, *Lancet* 1:654, 1955.

61. Palmer DH, Paulson JC, Lane-Larsen CL, et al.: Endoscopic carpal tunnel release: a comparison of two techniques with open release, *Arthroscopy* 9:498-508, 1993.

62. Phalen GS: Spontaneous compression of the median nerve at the wrist, *JAMA* 145:1128-1133, 1951.

63. Phalen GS: The carpal-tunnel syndrome. Seventeen years' experience in diagnosis and treatment of six hundred fifty-four hands, *J Bone Joint Surg Am* 48:211-228, 1966.

64. Phalen GS: Reflections on 21 years' experience with the carpal-tunnel syndrome, *JAMA* 212:1365-1367, 1970.

65. Phalen GS, Gardner WJ, La Londe AA: Neuropathy of the median nerve due to compression beneath the transverse carpal ligament, *J Bone Joint Surg Am* 32:109-112, 1950.

66. Reisman NR, Dellon AL: The abductor digiti minimi muscle flap: a salvage technique for palmar wrist pain, *Plast Reconstr Surg* 72:859-865, 1983.

67. Resnick CT, Miller BW: Endoscopic carpal tunnel release using the subligamentous two-portal technique. Read at the annual meeting of the American Society for Surgery of the Hand, Orlando, October 3, 1991.

68. Reyes FA, Burkhalter WE: The fascial radial flap, *J Hand Surg [Am]* 13:432-437, 1988.

69. Rose EH, Norris MS, Kowalski TA, et al.: Palmaris brevis turnover flap as an adjunct to internal neurolysis of the chronically scarred median nerve in recurrent carpal tunnel syndrome, *J Hand Surg [Am]* 16:191-201, 1991.

70. Rosier RN, Blair WF: Preliminary clinical evaluation of the digital electroneurometer, *Biomed Sci Instrum* 20:55-62, 1984.

71. Seiler JG III, Barnes K, Gelberman RH, et al.: Endoscopic carpal tunnel release: an anatomic study of the two-incision method in human cadavers, *J Hand Surg [Am]* 17:996-1002, 1992.

72. Simpson JA: Electrical signs in the diagnosis of carpal tunnel and related syndromes, *J Neurol Neurosurg Psychiatry* 19:275-280, 1956.

73. Soutar DS, Tanner NS: The radial forearm flap in the management of soft tissue injuries of the hand, *Br J Plast Surg* 37:18-26, 1984.

74. Steinberg DR, Gelberman RH, Rydevik B, et al.: The utility of portable nerve conduction testing for patients with carpal tunnel syndrome: a prospective clinical study, *J Hand Surg [Am]* 17:77-81, 1992.

75. Stevens JC: The electrodiagnosis of carpal tunnel syndrome, *Muscle Nerve* 10:99-113, 1987.

76. Stewart JD, Eisen A: Tinel's sign and the carpal tunnel syndrome, *Br Med J* 2:1125-1126, 1978.

77. Strickland J: A minimally open Indiana Tome™ carpal tunnel release system. Biomed Inc., P.O. 587, Warsaw, Indiana 46581.

78. Strickland JW, Idler RS, Lourie GM, et al.: The hypothenar fat pad flap for management of recalcitrant carpal tunnel syndrome, *J Hand Surg [Am]* 21:840-848, 1996.

79. Sucher BM: Myofascial manipulative release of carpal tunnel syndrome: documentation with magnetic resonance imaging, *J Am Osteopath Assoc* 93:1273-1278, 1993.

80. Taleisnik J: The palmar cutaneous branch of the median nerve and the approach to the carpal tunnel. An anatomical study, *J Bone Joint Surg Am* 55:1212-1217, 1973.

81. Tham SKY, Ireland DCR, Riccio M, et al.: Reverse radial artery fascial flap: a treatment for the chronically scarred median nerve in recurrent carpal tunnel syndrome, *J Hand Surg [Am]* 21:849-854, 1996.
82. Urbaniak JR: *Complications of treatment of carpal tunnel syndrome.* In Gelberman RH, editor: *Operative nerve repair and reconstruction,* vol 2, Philadelphia, 1991, JB Lippincott, pp 967-979.
83. Weiss AP, Steichen JB: Synovial sarcoma causing carpal tunnel syndrome, *J Hand Surg [Am]* 17:1024-1025, 1992.
84. Wilgis EF: Local muscle flaps in the hand. Anatomy as related to reconstructive surgery, *Bull Hosp Jt Dis Orthop Inst* 44:552-557, 1984.
85. Williams TM, Mackinnon SE, Novak CB, et al.: Verification of the pressure provocative test in carpal tunnel syndrome, *Ann Plast Surg* 29:8-11, 1992.
86. Woltman HW: Neuritis associated with acromegaly, *Arch Neurol Psychiatry* 45:680-682, 1941.

52

TUMORS OF THE WRIST

George B. Irons, M.D.
James H. Dobyns, M.D.

TUMORS OF THE SKIN
  PRINCIPLES OF EVALUATION AND TREATMENT
  BENIGN SKIN TUMORS
    BENIGN SEBORRHEIC KERATOSIS
    ACTINIC KERATOSIS
    KERATOACANTHOMA
    DERMATOFIBROMA
    NEVI
    EPIDERMOID
  MALIGNANT SKIN TUMORS
    BASAL CELL CARCINOMA
    SQUAMOUS CELL CARCINOMA
    MELANOMA
SOFT-TISSUE TUMORS
  PRINCIPLES OF EVALUATION AND TREATMENT
  BENIGN SOFT-TISSUE TUMORS
    GANGLION
    GIANT CELL TUMOR OF TENDON SHEATH
    (XANTHOMA, VILLONODULAR TENOSYNOVITIS)
    EPIDERMOID INCLUSION CYST
    LIPOMA
    HEMANGIOMA
    FIBROUS TUMORS
    SCHWANNOMA (NEURILEMOMA)

    NEUROFIBROMA
    PERINEURIOMA
    ANEURYSM
  MALIGNANT SOFT-TISSUE TUMORS
    FIBROSARCOMA
    EPITHELIOID SARCOMA
    SYNOVIAL SARCOMA
    RHABDOMYOSARCOMA
    MALIGNANT FIBROUS HISTIOCYTOMA
    MALIGNANT SCHWANNOMA
BONE TUMORS
  PRINCIPLES OF EVALUATION AND TREATMENT
  BENIGN BONE TUMORS
    ENCHONDROMA
    OSTEOCHONDROMA
    SOLITARY BONE CYST
    OSTEOID OSTEOMA
    ANEURYSMAL BONE CYST
    GIANT CELL TUMOR OF BONE
  MALIGNANT BONE TUMORS
    OSTEOGENIC SARCOMA
    CHONDROSARCOMA
    EWING'S SARCOMA

Almost any tumor that occurs in the hand can occur in the region of the wrist. This chapter discusses general principles of evaluation and treatment for tumors involving the skin, soft tissue, and bone. Some of the more common tumors in each group will be discussed, but it is not our purpose to present a complete discussion of all tumors. In dealing with a tumor about the wrist, it is important to always consider the possibility of a malignant lesion, because if overlooked it could pose a threat to life as well as to limb. Tumors about the wrist should be broadly classified as malignant or benign.

TUMORS OF THE SKIN

PRINCIPLES OF EVALUATION AND TREATMENT

A thorough history, physical examination, and routine hand radiograph usually result in a clinical diagnosis (Table 52-1). In most cases, this is followed by an excisional biopsy. Incisional biopsy may be considered for a large lesion but is usually not required for benign skin lesions. If the lesion is malignant, an adequate margin should be achieved by frozen section control. Whether the lesion is benign or malignant, after the surgeon is satisfied that the lesion has been adequately removed, the defect should be reconstructed by the simplest and fastest method.

BENIGN SKIN TUMORS

Benign Seborrheic Keratosis. These are benign lesions of the epidermis, consisting of various elements of hyperkeratosis, papillomatosis, and acanthosis. They are common in individuals past middle age. They are brownish pigmented and may be flat or elevated. The elevated lesions may have a verrucous appearance and have been described as looking pasted on the skin. They are perhaps the most common skin lesions removed to eliminate the possibility of melanoma. The flat-type are similar in appearance to senile lentigo. Squamous cell carcinoma should also be considered in a differential diagnosis. Because these lesions are epidermal, they can be shaved off with a scalpel blade during local anesthesia. After this minor procedure, the

specimen is sent to the Pathology Department for diagnosis. The base is cauterized lightly and heals quickly with no sutures or scar.

Actinic Keratosis. Actinic keratosis is an epidermal lesion of the skin consisting of hyperkeratosis and erythema. It is most common in elderly people with a long history of sun exposure. These appear as elevated, scaly, and nonpigmented lesions (Fig. 52-1, *A*), which frequently are picked off by the patient, leaving a raw surface that forms a crust. These lesions may be premalignant, similar to actinic dermatitis (Fig. 52-1, *B*). The treatment is a shave biopsy under local anesthesia and light cautery of the base. If the lesion exhibits malignant change, it should be excised.

Table 52-1. Skin Tumors

Benign	Malignant
Seborrheic keratosis	Basal cell carcinoma
Actinic keratosis	Squamous cell carcinoma
Keratoacanthoma	Melanoma
Dermatofibroma	Malignant keratoacanthoma
Nevi	Kaposi's sarcoma
Sweat gland tumor	Sweat gland tumor
or acrospiroma	Merkel cell tumor
Glomus tumor	
Granuloma	
Epidermoid cyst	

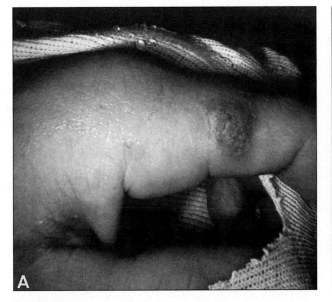
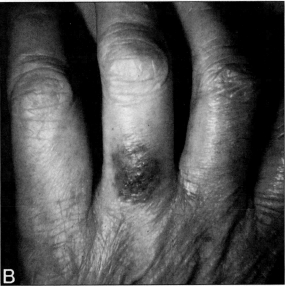

FIGURE 52-1

A, Actinic keratosis on the radial aspect of the index finger with hyperkeratosis and mild erythema surrounding the lesion. **B,** Actinodermatitis resulting from actinic radiation of ultraviolet light. At presentation, it appeared as a premalignant focus of squamous cell carcinoma (central area of carcinoma).

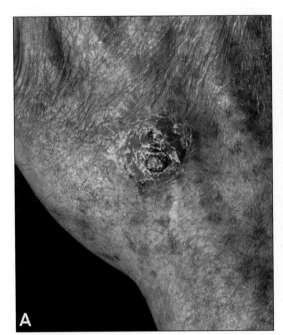 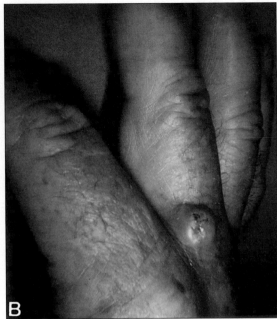

FIGURE 52-2

Keratoacanthoma. **A,** Lesion on the dorsoradial aspect of the wrist with characteristic elevated crablike appearance and central plug of keratin. **B,** Lesion on dorsoradial aspect of the long finger with prominent raised squamous cellular response and small center keratin plug.

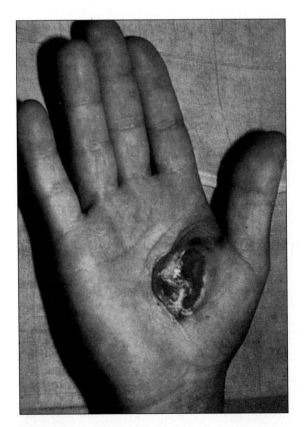

FIGURE 52-3

Basal cell carcinoma. Slightly unusual palmar location of a basal cell carcinoma with ulcerative central region in a dentist unprotected from office radiation. The lesion was treated by wide local excision and closure by rotation flap from the thenar eminence.

Keratoacanthoma. This benign, rapidly growing papular lesion with a superficial squamous hyperplasia and keratin has sometimes been called a "sheep in wolf's clothing," because it may grow rapidly in a few weeks, suggesting a malignant lesion. Typically, it appears as an elevated, craterlike lesion with a keratin plug in the center (Fig. 52-2). It is important to eliminate as a possibility squamous cell carcinoma, which may have a similar appearance. Treatment is excision during local anesthesia and examination of the lesion by the pathologist.

Dermatofibroma. Dermatofibroma is a benign nodular lesion of the dermis, consisting of various elements of collagen fibers, histiocytes, inflammatory cells, and capillary blood vessels. It appears as a firm nodular lesion within the skin. Treatment is excision under local anesthesia, with pathologic examination to eliminate the uncommon malignant dermatofibrosarcoma protuberans as a possibility.

Nevi. Nevi are lesions arising from the dermis and are variously pigmented. They may be flat or elevated and hairless or hairbearing. They may be classified as junctional, compound, or intradermal depending on their location within the skin. The junctional type are more commonly flat, whereas the intradermal are elevated, and the compound exhibit elements in between. The practical significance is that the junctional nevi are more likely to exhibit malignant transformation. The

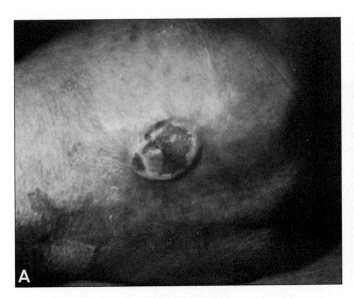

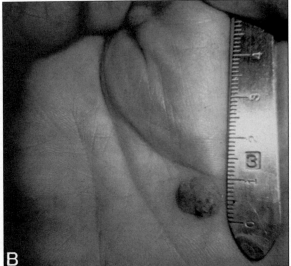

FIGURE 52-4

A, Squamous cell carcinoma on the dorsoradial aspect of the wrist. Note central ulceration and hypertrophic borders. Treatment included local excision with a 5-mm margin and skin grafting. **B,** Epithelioma. A malignant tumor consisting mainly of epithelial cells also referred to as epithelial carcinoma. The tumor appears on the palmar aspect of the hand (thenar eminence at the wrist).

indications for removal are to improve appearance or to eliminate malignancy as a possibility. Any history of change in the lesion, such as its color, size, or shape, is an indication for biopsy. Because these lesions are intradermal, they should be surgically excised; the specimen is sent to the pathologist and the defect is sutured.

Epidermoid. Epidermoids are intradermal, squamous epithelialized cysts containing a white cheesylike, musty-smelling keratin material. They can result from minor trauma trapping epithelial cells beneath the dermis. They may become infected and, if so, should be incised and drained. If not infected, they should be excised during local anesthesia. Care must be taken to remove all of the sac lining to prevent recurrence.

MALIGNANT SKIN TUMORS

Basal Cell Carcinoma. Basal cell carcinoma is a malignant skin tumor arising from the basal cell layer of the epidermis.[9] It is the most frequent malignant skin tumor. It is more common in fair-skinned individuals, with increased instances in areas exposed to ultraviolet radiation or radiation therapy. The patient typically presents with an elevated, pearly, translucent nonulcerated lesion that exhibits telangiectasia or pigmentation (Fig. 52-3). It usually has a well-defined border, but it may occasionally have a morphea-like or fibrosing appearance with an ill-defined border. Treatment is excision with a 3- to 5-mm margin and pathologic control of the margin by examination of frozen sections. Closure of the defect can usually be

accomplished primarily by simple closure or by means of a local skin flap or skin graft.

Squamous Cell Carcinoma. Squamous cell carcinoma is a malignant lesion of the epidermis of the skin with invasion into the dermis. It appears as a thickened, erythematous lesion, which often becomes ulcerated (Fig. 52-4). Treatment is excision during local anesthesia with a 5-mm margin and pathologic control of the margin by examination of frozen sections.[45] The defects may be closed primarily; however, on the back of the hand there may not be enough flexibility of the skin, and a skin flap or graft may be necessary for closure. These tumors have the potential for metastasis; the regional lymphatic drainage and lymph nodes should be examined at the time of operation and followed postoperatively.

Melanoma. Melanoma is a malignant tumor of melanin-producing cells. It is uncommon, with an incidence of about 4 per 100,000 population[13]; however, it is increasing in incidence and is potentially lethal.[10] Like the epitheliomas, it seems to be related to sun exposure; however, much is unknown about its cause, which is undoubtedly multifactorial. For the ulcerated, abnormally black-pigmented lesion with irregular borders and satellites, the diagnosis may be easy (Fig. 52-5). For other lesions, however, the diagnosis is not so apparent and may be confused with pigmented seborrheic keratosis, pigmented basal cell carcinoma, benign pigmented nevi, dermatofibroma, or pyogenic granuloma.

Varieties of melanoma, which must be confirmed by pathologic diagnosis, may in many cases be suspected

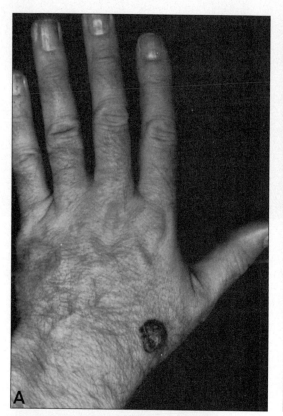

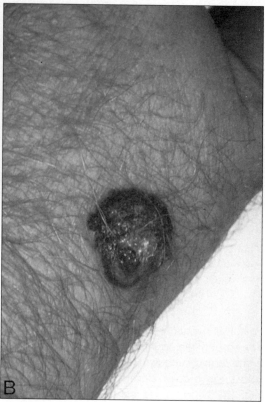

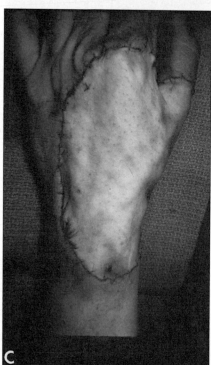

FIGURE 52-5

Malignant melanoma. **A** and **B,** Dorsal wrist melanoma with irregular highly pigmented border and central necrosis extending through the dermis. **C,** Treatment required a wide local excision down to superficial fascia and thumb and wrist extensor tendons; coverage of the defect was obtained with full thickness skin graft coverage.

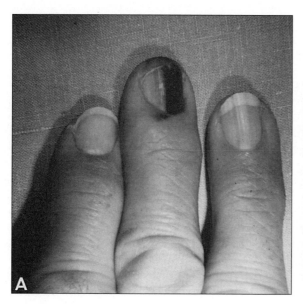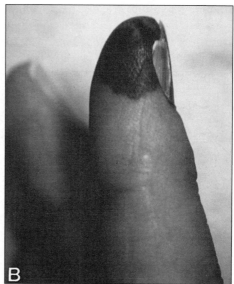

FIGURE 52-6

Melanoma. **A,** Acral melanotic whitlow—subungual melanoma. **B,** Acral-lentiginous melanoma.

clinically. Patients who have lentigo maligna melanoma present with a slow-growing, flat, irregularly pigmented, brownish black lesion. Superficial spreading melanoma, so called because it tends to spread laterally, is the most common variety and frequently develops in a preexisting lesion. It has a prognosis intermediate between lentigo maligna and nodular melanoma. Nodular melanoma grows in a more vertical direction, thus appearing as a more nodular lesion. It is less frequent than the two previous types, but has a worse prognosis. Acral-lentiginous melanoma indicates a melanoma arising on the palm of the hand, sole of the foot, or under the nail bed (Fig. 52-6) and clinically resembles lentigo maligna melanoma.

Pathologically, melanomas have been graded by Clark[10] according to their level of invasion into the skin on a scale of 1 to 5 and by Breslow[5] according to their thickness as measured by a micrometer. This pathologic information is helpful in prescribing treatment and also in predicting prognosis. The treatment of a lesion suspicious for melanoma should be excision biopsy, during local anesthesia, followed by pathologic examination and classification of permanent sections.

If the lesion is diagnosed as a melanoma, the patient should have a thorough oncologic evaluation and clinical staging: stage I, local disease; stage IA, local disease with recurrence or satellites; stage II, metastasis to regional lymph nodes; and stage III, distant metastasis. Reexcision of the biopsy site should be performed, but the extent of effective margins of the reexcision is unclear and awaits further long-term studies. It is generally accepted, however, that a margin of 1 to 3 cm should be achieved if possible (Fig. 52-5, C). This

should include the underlying fascia. Patients with stage II disease, who have clinically positive regional nodes or in whom positive regional nodes develop on follow-up, should have lymphadenectomy. Stage II disease generally has a poor prognosis, because adjuvant treatment using chemotherapy, immunotherapy, and radiation therapy alone or in combinations has been disappointing.

SOFT-TISSUE TUMORS

PRINCIPLES OF EVALUATION AND TREATMENT

Soft-tissue tumors about the wrist and hand present as a mass. The history, physical examination, and radiograph may give a clue to the diagnosis of a benign or a malignant lesion (Tabel 52-2).[27] Information such as onset, duration, increase in size, location, consistency, localization, mobility, bony involvement, pain, and impairment of function assists in determining the basic nature or seriousness of the mass. Most tumors about the wrist and hand are benign, but if they are malignant, they can threaten life as well as limb.

The possibility of malignancy has to be considered in all cases. A malignant tumor cannot be eliminated as a possibility without a tissue study. If the lesion is believed to be benign, either excision or incision should be done, depending on its size. If an unsuspected soft-tissue sarcoma is encountered after an incisional biopsy, the patient should have a sarcoma work-up followed by surgical treatment and irradiation, as will be discussed later. If the patient is thought to have a malignant lesion from the outset, a sarcoma work-up (Fig. 52-7) should be performed before biopsy. Excisional biopsy may be appropriate if a lesion is small and isolated from important structures and if the biopsy can be done with minimum tissue dissection that does not preclude later excision. In most other cases, it is essential that an incisional biopsy be performed through a longitudinal incision to set the stage for a formal tumor operation without violating tissue planes. If an excised lesion is found to be malignant and a sarcoma work-up has not been done, it should be done before definitive treatment.

Our present approach to treatment of these lesions is multidisciplinary and multimodal, consisting of limb-sparing surgery and irradiation, provided a functional limb can be salvaged. We try to excise the lesion to achieve tumor-free margins and only rarely accept marginal excision to preserve vital structures. The irradiation may be given preoperatively, intraoperatively, or postoperatively or by a combination of these. If the lesion has had an incisional biopsy, we give preoperative external irradiation in the range of 45 to 55 Gy. At surgery, the radiation oncologist is present to decide whether or not to treat with interstitial brachytherapy or intraoperative radiation therapy, depending on the pathologist's report and the architecture of the wound.[20] If indicated, brachytherapy is in the range of 1.5 to 2 Gy. If further radiation is needed, but could not be given interstitially, an external boost is given postoperatively.

If the patient had an excisional biopsy, the program is slightly different. At the time of reexcision, interstitial brachytherapy of 15 to 20 Gy would be given if possible, followed by postoperative external irradiation of 45 to 50 Gy. It has been our experience, as well as that of others,[37,51,54] that the results of limb-sparing surgery combined with irradiation are comparable to amputation. With this approach we have achieved good local control with a recurrence rate of 5%.[44] Metastasis of sarcomas (average 40%) remains a problem. Various experiments in chemotherapy protocols are in progress to assess the best combinations of drug treatment for the different types of soft-tissue tumors that can involve the upper extremity.

BENIGN SOFT-TISSUE TUMORS

Ganglion. This is the most common tumor occurring in the hand. These are discussed in Chapter 49.

Giant Cell Tumor of Tendon Sheath (Xanthoma, Villonodular Tenosynovitis). Giant cell tumor of the tendon sheath is a benign fibrous histiocytoma, which usually develops from tendon sheaths or joint capsule, but it may develop from muscles, tendons, and deep fibrous tissues (Fig. 52-8). This tumor is usually confined to subcutaneous tissue but invasion of carpal bones has been reported.[41] This is the second most frequent soft-tissue tumor seen in the hand after ganglion.[5] The patient presents with a soft-tissue tumor which is smooth, firm, nontender, and attached to underlying tissue but not to skin. Treatment is surgical excision, taking care to remove the tumor as completely as possible without sacrificing vital structures. The lesion has a fairly characteristic brownish yellow, encapsulated appearance. Local recurrence is infrequent, but it can produce local invasion that is difficult to treat. The lesion, however, never becomes malignant.

Epidermoid Inclusion Cyst. Epidermoid inclusion cyst is an epithelialized keratin cyst, probably caused by skin elements buried in the subcutaneous tissue as a result of trauma. It presents as a slow-growing painless mass that may be attached to the skin but not to underlying tissue. Treatment is surgical excision, taking care to remove the entire sac.

Lipoma. Lipoma is a benign soft-tissue tumor arising from fat cells. The patient presents with a nontender, smooth, and soft mass. In the wrist it may produce symptoms secondary to pressure on the median nerve.

Table 52-2. Soft-Tissue Tumors

Benign	Malignant
Ganglion	Fibrosarcoma
Giant cell tumor of tendon sheath	Malignant giant cell tumor
	Epithelioid sarcoma
Epidermoid inclusion cyst	Synovial sarcoma
	Rhabdomyosarcoma
Lipoma	Liposarcoma
Hemangioma	Hemangiopericytoma
Fibrous tumors	Hemangioendothelioma
Fibromatosis	Leiomyosarcoma
Desmoid	Malignant fibrous histiocytoma
Nodular fasciitis	
Fibrous histiocytoma	Malignant schwannoma
Schwannoma	Extraosseous chondrosarcoma
Neurofibroma	
Aneurysm	Clear cell sarcoma
Leiomyoma	Angiosarcoma
Granular cell myeloblastoma	Malignant granular cell myeloblastoma
Myxoma	
Fibrous hamartoma of infancy	
Extraskeletal chondroma	
Angiolipoma	
Fibrolipoma	
Epithelioid hemangioendothelioma	
Calcifying aponeuritic fibroma	

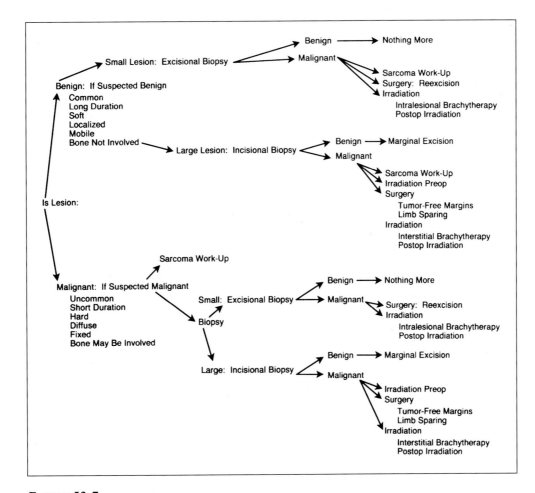

FIGURE 52-7

Algorithm for soft-tissue tumor management. *Postop.*, postoperative; *Preop.*, preoperative.

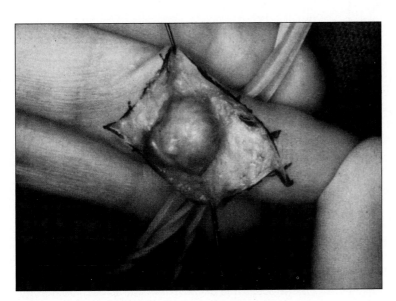

FIGURE 52-8

Giant cell tumor of tendon sheath along the palmar aspect of the long finger. It is a smooth, fibrous encapsulated lesion but may have local extension, making complete excision difficult.

On open surgical excision, the tumor has a typical yellowish fatty appearance, is well circumscribed, and tends to "shell out." It may, however, grow around tendons or nerves, so care should be exercised not to injure these structures during treatment.

Table 52-3. Biologic Classification of Vascular Tumors

Hemangiomas	Malformations
Hyperplasia of vessels	Ectasia of vessels
Proliferating phase	Capillary
Involuting phase	Venous
	Arterial
	Lymphatic
	Combined

Modified from Mulliken JB, Glowacki J: Hemangiomas and vascular malformations in infants and children: a classification based on endothelial characteristics, *Plast Reconstr Surg* 69:412-420, 1982. By permission of the American Society of Plastic and Reconstructive Surgeons.

Table 52-4. Classification of Vascular Tumors of Soft Tissue

I. Benign vascular tumors
   A. Localized hemangioma
      1. Capillary hemangioma (including juvenile type)
      2. Cavernous hemangioma
      3. Venous hemangioma
      4. Arteriovenous hemangioma (racemose hemangioma)
      5. Epithelioid hemangioma (angiolymphoid hyperplasia, Kimura's disease)
      6. Hemangioma of granulation tissue type (pyogenic granuloma)
      7. Miscellaneous hemangiomas of deep soft tissue (synovial, intramuscular, neural)
   B. Angiomatosis (diffuse hemangioma)
II. Vascular tumors of intermediate or borderline malignancy (hemangioendothelioma)
   A. Epithelioid hemangioendothelioma
III. Malignant vascular tumors
   A. Angiosarcoma (including lymphangiosarcoma)
   B. Kaposi's sarcoma
   C. Malignant endovascular papillary angioendothelioma
   D. Proliferating angioendotheliomatosis

Modified from Enzinger FM, Weiss SW: *Soft tissue tumors,* St. Louis, 1988, CV Mosby.

Hemangioma. Hemangioma is a benign hamartoma developing from blood vessels. The classification of blood vessel tumors is confused by the mixing of various terms derived from physical examination, etiology (including congenital syndromes), histology, and physiology. From a practical standpoint, these lesions cover a spectrum of vascular tumors from the benign localized, relatively asymptomatic lesion, to the seemingly uncontrollable, large expanding lesion. Mulliken[33] attempted to clarify our thinking about these vascular tumors by suggesting a biologic classification (Table 52-3). Rather than classifying all of these tumors as generic "hemangiomas," he suggested limiting the term to lesions that exhibit cellular hyperplasia. These are congenital lesions[52] that exhibit rapid growth soon after birth, followed by slow involution by age 5 to 7 years. Intralesional administration of sodium tetradecyl sulfate,[56] systemic administration of steroids[17] given cyclically, and pressure[32] have been reported to be beneficial in cases that demonstrate a rapid proliferative phase or that compromise hand function. If the lesions are well localized and amenable to surgical excision, this may be expedient. Most hemangiomas, however, do *not* require any surgical treatment and by age 4 to 5 years, the majority involute and simply disappear, leaving little if any residual.

Vascular malformations represent cellular ectasia or structural abnormality (Table 52-4). It is extremely important to distinguish them from a hemangioma. They are often progressive and do not regress on their own. These may involve capillaries, veins, arteries, lymphatics, or combinations. From a practical standpoint, it is important to distinguish between low-flow and high-flow vascular malformations. The low-flow lesions generally are easier to treat than high flow and include capillary, venous, lymphatic, and combinations. These can usually be diagnosed clinically. Computed tomographic scan with dye enhancement may be helpful. Arteriography for low-flow malformations is not routine but may be necessary to eliminate an arterial component to the lesion as a possibility. Burrows et al.[7] described the differential diagnosis of vascular tumors by angiographic studies. Sclerotherapy[25] by direct injection into the lesion with arterial inflow and venous outflow occluded has had variable success. Riché and Merland[46] reported good results with the use of Ethibloc injected intralesionally. Surgical excision is a definitive treatment, and debulking may be beneficial to improve appearance or function. Total excision may be difficult because of the diffuse nature of the lesion. Among the vascular malformations, lymphangiomatosis may be the most difficult to treat. Lymphatic malformations can produce extensive extremity overgrowth with massive soft-tissue malformations, limb edema, and large cystic communications. Debulking of the extremity in stages combined with limited appendage amputations may be required (Fig. 52-9).

High-flow vascular malformations exhibit a more "malignant" behavior. These are either arterial or arteriovenous malformations. The overlying skin has an increased temperature. There is a palpable thrill and an audible bruit. The recommended treatment of embolization[2,28] followed by surgical excision has yielded good results, but total excision is difficult and any residual will regrow in time. Low-dose radiation (15-20 Gy) may help control recurrence and, in some cases, obliterate residual tumor. There may be hypertrophy of soft tissue and bone associated with arteriovenous malformations. This combination presents a difficult management problem for which there is no good treatment. Peled and associates[42] reported intraneural hemangioma involving the median nerve and patients presenting with a mass at the wrist and symptoms of carpal tunnel syndrome.

Fibrous Tumors. Fibrous tumors and tumorlike proliferations manifest in a confusing array of tumors including fibroma, fibromatosis, benign fibrous histiocytoma, synovial fibromatosis (Fig. 52-10), desmoid, and fasciitis. Additionally, tumors originating from fat or nerve may contain large amounts of fibrous tissue. Because the fibrocyte is so ubiquitous, the services of a good pathologist are all important in identifying these benign lesions of fibroblasts.

Fibroma is a tumor formed by proliferative fibroblasts in the subcutaneous tissue. The patient presents with a firm soft-tissue mass. Treatment is excision, which presents no problem because the tumor is usually encapsulated and does not recur.

Fibromatosis refers to a benign fibrous growth that tends to be infiltrative and nonencapsulated. It covers a spectrum of growth ranging from the benign palmar fibromatosis of Dupuytren's disease to the more aggressive fibromatosis, which is difficult to remove and thus recurs and is sometimes confused with fibrosarcoma. Desmoid tumors are included in the fibromatoses.

Nodular fasciitis is a benign proliferative fibrous lesion that can be distinguished from other fibrous lesions because it contains inflammatory cells and no collagen. There is usually a history of trauma to the area.

Benign fibrous histiocytoma is a benign fibrous lesion with many lipid-containing histiocytes. These include the tumorlike xanthomas and the true neoplasm fibroxanthomas. Because of the close relationship of the histiocyte and the fibroblast, fibrous histiocytoma could be viewed as a fibroma arrested in its early stage of development. The patient usually presents with an asymptomatic soft-tissue mass. Treatment is wide local excision. These are not well encapsulated, so wide excision should be performed to minimize recurrence.

Schwannoma (Neurilemoma). Schwannoma is the most common benign nerve tumor and originates from the Schwann cells. The patient presents with a

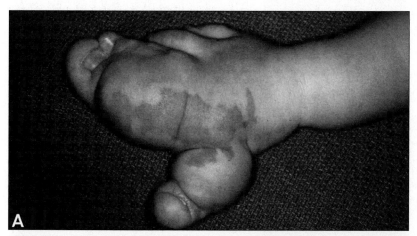

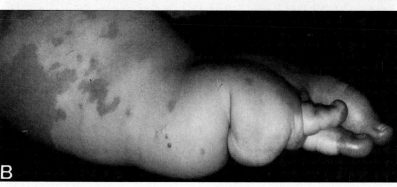

FIGURE 52-9

A, Bilateral lymphangiomatosis malformation demonstrates a port-wine stain with hypertrophic overgrowth of the thumb, index, and long fingers with extension down to the wrist (right hand) and extensive involvement of the wrist, forearm, and above the elbow on the **(B)** left upper extremity. Surgical treatment included amputation of the index and long fingers with debulking of the thumb (right hand) and staged palmar and dorsal excision of tumor on left forearm and elbow and ulnar aspect of the wrist.

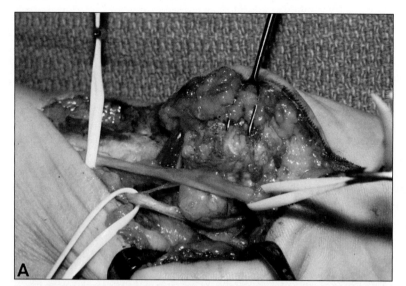

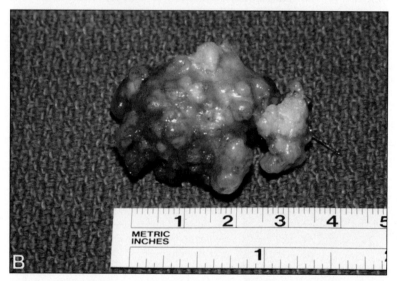

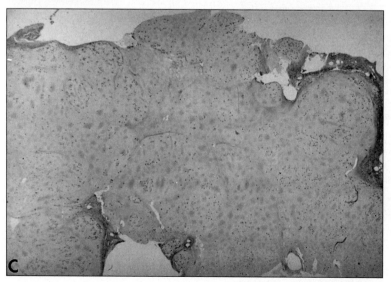

FIGURE 52-10

A, Synovial fibromatosis. Synovial enlargement of palmar capsule of the wrist produces compressive lesions of both the median nerve (between two Penrose drains) and ulnar nerves (lower Penrose drain). **B,** Excised specimen. **C,** Photomicrograph of specimen demonstrates low cellular and loose fibroblastic background with cells arranged in whorled bundles associated with a lipidization. Few giant cells. (×4.)

soft-tissue mass, which may or may not be painful and may or may not cause paresthesia. Owen and associates[38] described the use of computed tomography in making the diagnosis. Treatment is surgical excision, which can often be performed without interrupting fascicles.

Neurofibroma. Neurofibroma is a nerve tumor arising from the Schwann cells and fibrocytes. This tumor is usually intertwined with the nerve fascicles, and complete removal requires a segmental resection of the nerve and reconstruction with a nerve graft (Fig. 52-11). Neurofibrolipoma is a benign nerve tumor with elements of fibrous and lipomatous hyperplasia. Like the neurofibroma, it tends to be intimately associated with the nerve and removal requires segmental nerve resection (Fig. 52-12). If these benign tumors involve a major nerve and cannot be removed without interrupting nerve fibers, one has to seriously consider the cost/benefit ratio. If they are not large and symptomatic, it may be better to leave them intact and maintain nerve function.

Perineurioma. This is a rare peripheral nerve tumor that can affect the median and ulnar nerves of the wrist. It is similar to neurilemomas and schwannomas in gross appearance, but the cell of origin is from the perineurium covering of fascicle (or funiculus) and not the epineurium (Fig. 52-13). As such, the tumor growth, although benign, is perineural and limits the surgeon's ability to resect the tumor without doing permanent damage to the nerve. As a result, complete excision of the tumor has been necessary, with interposition nerve grafting.

Aneurysm. The wrist is the most common site for aneurysms in the hand that arise from the ulnar or the radial artery. This may be a true aneurysm, a dilatation of the vessel wall, or a false aneurysm (an organizing hematoma adjacent to the artery). In the wrist, a false aneurysm is usually caused by a needle stick. Aneurysms may create vascular disturbances from thromboses or embolization. Diagnosis can usually be made clinically and confirmed by angiography if necessary. A true aneurysm should be resected and the artery should be repaired. In some cases, a false aneurysm may be removed without a segmental resection of the artery.

MALIGNANT SOFT-TISSUE TUMORS

Fibrosarcoma. Fibrosarcoma is a malignant tumor arising from fibroblasts and containing collagen reticulum fibers and interlacing bundles of spindle cells with mitoses (Fig. 52-14). A review of the biologic nature of this tumor is difficult because the term "fibrosarcoma" has been used to include many different fibrosarcomatous tumors. Also, benign fibromatosis must be considered in the differential diagnosis. Fibrosarcoma is most frequently seen in middle-aged adults. The tumor is infiltrative and metastasis is by way of the blood stream.

Epithelioid Sarcoma. Epithelioid sarcoma was named in 1970 by Enzinger,[18] who described it as a sarcoma simulating a granuloma or a carcinoma and containing the characteristic epithelioid cell. The cell of origin is unclear, although synovioblasts, fibroblasts, and histiocytes have all been implicated[6,48] (Fig. 52-15). This tumor develops insidiously in the subcutaneous tissue as a painless nodule. It spreads relentlessly to regional soft tissues, lymph nodes, and distant sites.[21] It may involve the skin; the nodules may be multiple and may ulcerate. With surgical excision it is important to note any extension along longitudinal tissue

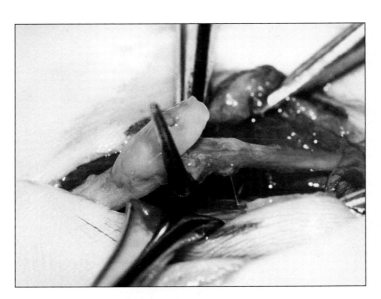

FIGURE 52-11

Myxomatous neurofibroma. Intraneural neurofibroma appeared to be carpal tunnel syndrome at presentation. The encapsulated lesion is dissected from the median nerve.

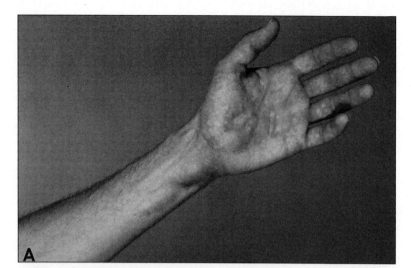

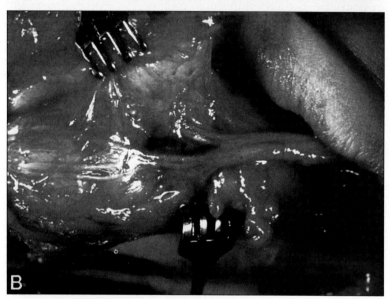

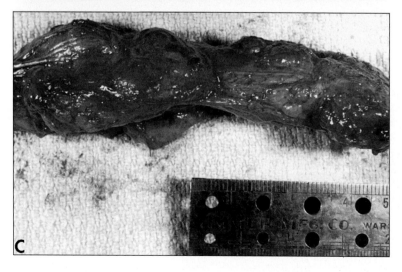

FIGURE 52-12

Neurofibrolipoma. **A,** Locally invasive neural tumor appeared to be progressive median neuropathy at presentation. Failed carpal tunnel incision with progressive enlargement proximal and distal to the wrist flexion crease. **B,** At exploration, the tumor displaced nerve fascicles. The lesion is seen within the palm. **C,** Excision of the median nerve (shown). Reconstruction with a sural nerve graft.

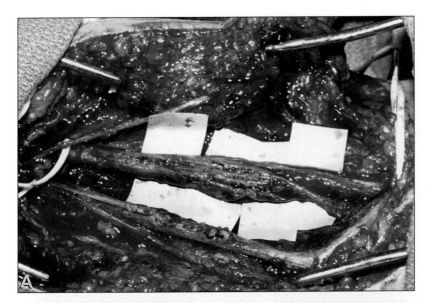

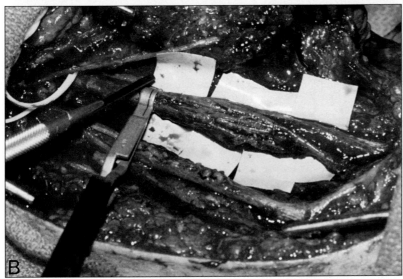

FIGURE 52-13

Perineurioma is an intraneural tumor arising from the perineurium. **A,** Expansion of the median nerve in the midforearm from intraneural perineurioma. **B,** Resection of the tumor with a neurotome was followed by sural nerve grafting.

planes, especially longitudinal extension along muscles and tendons, the frequent direction of spread. A review of 51 cases at the Mayo Clinic[4] and 42 cases at the MD Anderson Cancer Center[55] demonstrated no difference in the results of wide local excision with tumor-free margins compared with amputation. The MD Anderson study demonstrated no advantages for elective regional node excision, although this has been recommended by others. Regarding prognosis, Hoopes and associates[22] accumulated data on 112 cases of epithelioid sarcoma from the literature followed for an average of 6 years and found a recurrence rate of 71% and a metastasis rate of 40%.

Synovial Sarcoma. Synovial sarcoma originates around joints and tendon sheaths. It may contain both synovioblastic and fibroblastic cells. Characteristics of synovial sarcoma are fibrosarcomatosis spindle cells and epithelioid cells lining glandlike spaces.[8] This tumor is highly malignant, tends to grow slowly, and may metastasize through the blood stream or the lymphatics. It is more frequent in early adult life.

Rhabdomyosarcoma. Rhabdomyosarcoma is a tumor that develops from muscle and may be classified as adult pleomorphic or juvenile. The juvenile type rarely occurs in the extremities. This tumor may be confused with fibrosarcoma and malignant fibrous histiocytoma, as discussed by Linscheid and associates[30] in their review of 87 cases at the Mayo Clinic. Rhabdomyosarcoma spreads diffusely and may metastasize via the blood stream or the lymphatics.

Malignant Fibrous Histiocytoma. Malignant fibrous histiocytoma was described by O'Brien and Stout[36] in 1964, ending its confusion with other sarcomas,

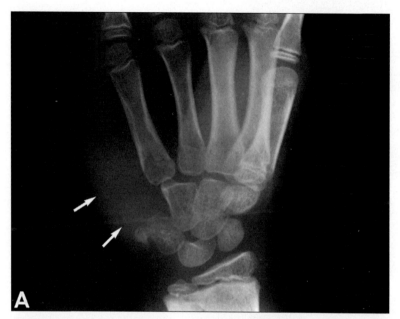

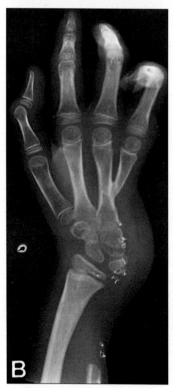

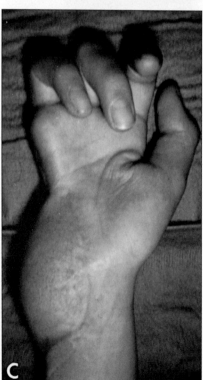

FIGURE 52-14

Fibrosarcoma. **A,** Anteroposterior radiograph of wrist. Soft-tissue swelling noted over the ulnar aspect of the wrist (*arrows*) with resorptive lesion involving the bone of the fifth metacarpal. **B,** Wide local excision includes the entire fifth ray, hamate, triquetrum, pisiform, and distal ulna. **C,** Soft-tissue closure with free groin flap; intrinsic minus position of the fingers secondary to sacrifice of the ulnar nerve.

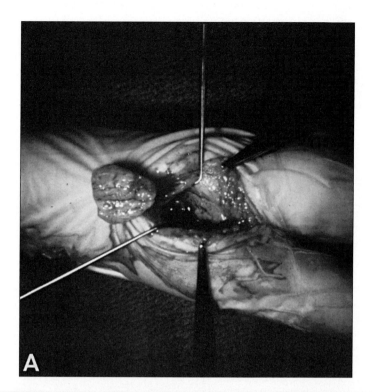

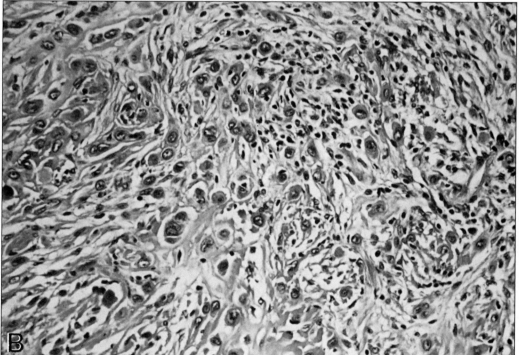

FIGURE 52-15

Epithelioid sarcoma. **A,** Recurrent palmar mass of the wrist in patient originally diagnosed as having fibroma who presented with proximal extension and increasing size of mass; appearance at time of deep excision from distal forearm. **B,** Histologic appearance of whorling clusters of histiocytes, fibroblasts, and synovioblasts. (×100.)

including fibrosarcoma, liposarcoma, and rhabdomyo-sarcoma. Ultrastructural studies have confirmed the histiocyte as the cell of origin.[50] These tumors are nonencapsulated and they spread through the blood stream or the lymphatics. Weiss and Enzinger[53] found no difference in the rate of metastasis between patients treated by wide local excision and those treated by amputation, but there was local recurrence in 58% of those treated by local excision.

Malignant Schwannoma. Malignant schwannoma develops from the Schwann cells in the nerve sheath. It develops as a fusiform enlargement of the nerve with a pseudocapsule. It may progress and spread directly along the nerve or through lymphatics, producing satellite nodules and metastasis. At the time of resection, the nerve of origin must be dissected proximally and distally and checked on frozen sections. If satellite lesions are found, amputation should be considered.

Table 52-5. Bone Tumors

Benign	Malignant
Enchondroma	Osteosarcoma
Osteochondroma	Chondrosarcoma
Solitary bone cyst	Ewing's sarcoma
Aneurysmal bone cyst	Adamantinoma
Giant cell tumor	Angiosarcoma
Osteoblastoma	Giant cell sarcoma
	Lymphoma of bone

Table 52-6. Sarcoma Work-Up in Soft Tissue and Bone

History and physical examination
Radiographs
   Routine hand and wrist
   CT hand and wrist
   CT chest
Magnetic resonance images
Laboratory tests
   Complete blood cell count
   Fasting blood sugar
   Blood urea nitrogen
   Erythrocyte sedimentation rate
   Alkaline phosphatase
   Calcium
   Phosphorus

CT, computed tomography.

BONE TUMORS

PRINCIPLES OF EVALUATION AND TREATMENT

The evaluation of a bony lesion should be similar to that of a soft-tissue tumor (Table 52-5). Because the majority of tumors in the wrist area are benign and usually appear benign on plain films, one may proceed with biopsy. Most benign lesions can be adequately managed by curettement and bone graft. If malignancy is suspected, a more thorough work-up is indicated (Table 52-6). Computed tomography may more clearly show cortical destruction. Magnetic resonance imaging may better demonstrate intramedullary or soft-tissue involvement. Malignant tumors of small bones in the hand generally necessitate removal of the involved bone plus any involved adjacent soft tissue. In a single digit or metacarpal this results in ray amputation. In the wrist, resection of multiple carpal bones, which could be reconstructed with bone graft if adequate margins can be achieved, may preserve a functional limb. After resection, malignant bone tumors are considered for a chemotherapy protocol. If the resection has not resulted in good tumor-free margins, irradiation is

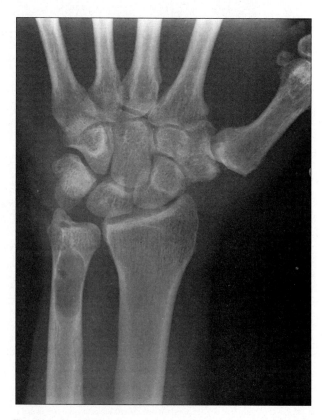

FIGURE 52–16

Enchondroma. Radiopaque lesion in metaphyseal central location in the distal ulna; curettage and bone grafting were performed.

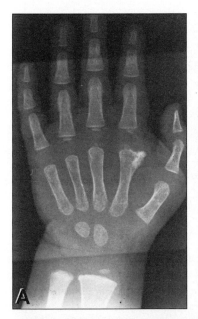
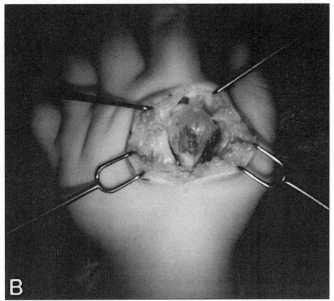
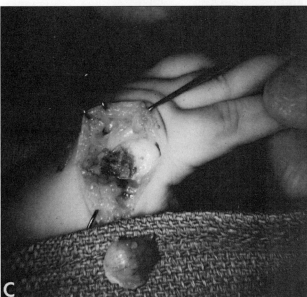

FIGURE 52-17

Osteochondroma. **A,** Exostotic lesion involves the index metacarpal; the cartilage-capped exostosis projects from the cortex. **B,** Surgical exposure of the exostosis shows the prominent cartilage cap. **C,** Excision of osteochondroma proximal to the physeal growth plate; the base is cauterized and covered with bone wax.

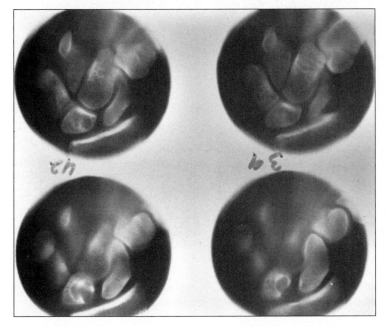

FIGURE 52-18

Solitary bone cyst within the lunate is demonstrated by polytomography. It appears to communicate with the radiocarpal joint. When the cyst is painful, curettage and bone grafting (cancellous) are recommended.

added at the operative site. Most malignant bone tumors of the wrist require an amputation through the distal forearm.

BENIGN BONE TUMORS

Enchondroma. Enchondroma is the most common benign tumor of the hand and wrist. It is a neoplasm of cartilaginous origin, located most often in small bones. The phalanges are the most common location, followed by the metacarpals and less frequently the carpals.[3] This tumor usually appears in early adult life. It is often an incidental finding on a routine radiograph or a component of a fracture. Multiple enchondromatosis of the hand has been reported.[19] Radiographs reveal a characteristic lucent area (Fig. 52-16) resembling a bubble that may contain specks of calcification, with expansion and thinning of the cortex. Treatment is by curettage and bone grafting.

Osteochondroma. Osteochondroma develops from cartilaginous rests in the periosteum, resulting in a cartilage-capped exostosis. This is a tumor of early life, appearing before maturity. On radiographs, it appears as a bony mass projecting on the cortex. Osteochondroma may be solitary, but when it is multiple (Fig. 52-17), there is often a familial history. The hereditary type may occur in the distal ulna or radius. At any site it can appear as a painless mass or as an incidental radiographic finding. Treatment should be delayed until epiphyseal closure, unless there is significant angular deformity or impairment of motion.

Solitary Bone Cyst. Solitary bone cyst is a benign cystic lesion composed of fibrous connective tissue and a brownish yellow fluid (Fig. 52-18). It appears as a swelling within or on the bone, and radiographically it is a radiolucent area with thinning of the cortex. It may resemble an enchondroma. It occurs commonly in the distal radius. Treatment is curettage and bone graft.

Osteoid Osteoma. Osteoid osteoma, first described by Jaffe and Mayer,[24] is made up of osteoid osteoblasts and fibrovascular connective tissue. This benign bony lesion occurs most frequently in the first two decades of life. Pain and swelling are the presenting symptoms. Radiographically, it has a characteristic "target" appearance, with a central lucency surrounded by a sclerotic ring. Angiography may demonstrate increased vascularity (Fig. 52-19, *C*). In a review of 19 cases, Ambrosia and associates[1] reported four involving carpal bones. Treatment is excision and bone graft. If the articular surface is involved in the carpal bones, fusion may be necessary.

Aneurysmal Bone Cyst. Aneurysmal bone cyst, as described by Jaffe and Lichtenstein in 1942,[23] is a benign expansive lesion of bone. It consists of multicystic blood-filled spaces and solid areas of osteoid,

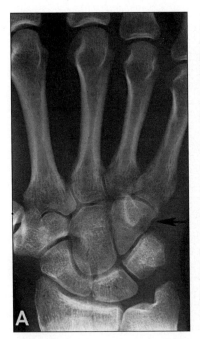
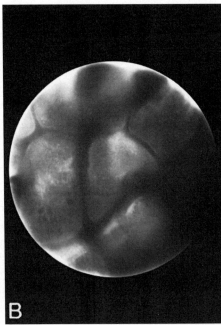
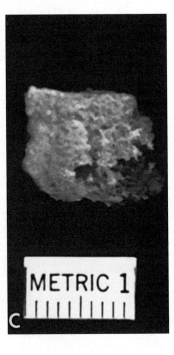

FIGURE 52-19

Osteoid osteoma. **A,** Lesion of the wrist involves the hamate; note small resorptive lesion along medial cortex (*arrow*). **B,** Tomography confirms the central lucent lesion with a small sclerotic area. **C,** Excision of lesion shows the bone defect and reactive bone sclerosis.

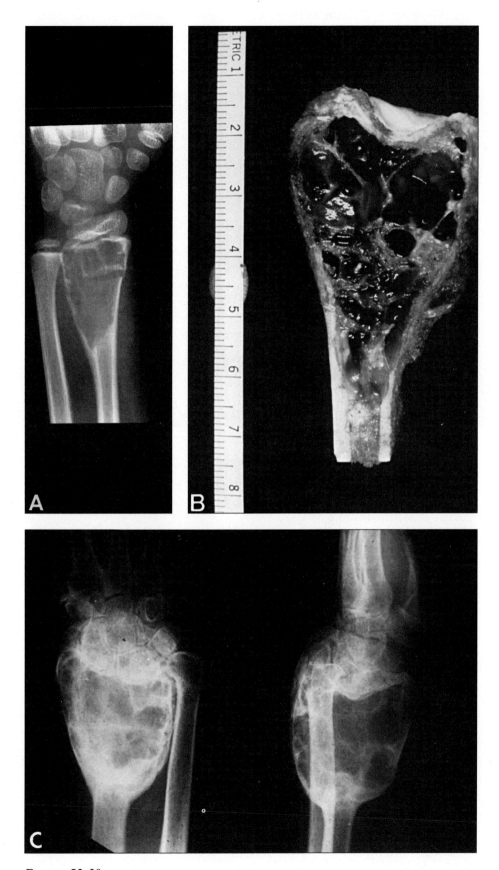

FIGURE 52-20

Aneurysmal bone cyst. **A,** Expansile lesion involves the distal metaphyseal region of the radius. The central margin, although thin, has not been penetrated by the lesion. **B,** Surgical specimen demonstrates the broad extent of the aneurysmal bone cyst that occupies the entire intramedullary canal of the distal radius. **C,** Anteroposterior and lateral radiographs demonstrate a well-advanced aneurysmal bone cyst expanding toward the distal ulna and compromising the radiocarpal joint articular surface.

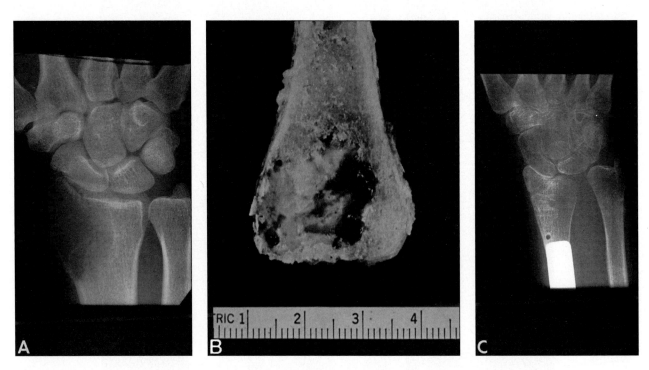

FIGURE 52-21

Giant cell tumor. **A,** Posteroanterior radiograph of distal radius. Radiolucency of radial two-thirds of the epiphyseal region of the distal radius. **B,** Pathologic specimen after excision of the entire distal radius. **C,** Fibular replacement of the distal radius; plate fixation.

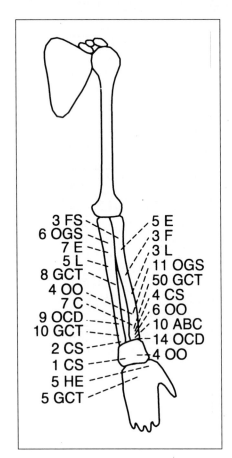

FIGURE 52-22

Incidence of aggressive benign and malignant tumors about the wrist and forearm. The most common lesions about the distal radius and ulna and the carpus are noted in the schematic presentation updated from the work of Dahlin DC and Unni KK, *Bone tumors: general aspects and data on 8,542 cases,* ed 4, Springfield, Illinois, 1986, Charles C Thomas. *ABC,* aneurysmal bone cyst; *C,* chondroma; *CS,* chondrosarcoma; *E,* Ewing's sarcoma; *F,* fibroma; *FS,* fibrosarcoma; *GCT,* giant cell tumor; *HE,* hemangioendothelioma; *L,* lymphoma; *OCD,* osteochondroma; *OGS,* osteogenic sarcoma; *OO,* osteoid osteoma.

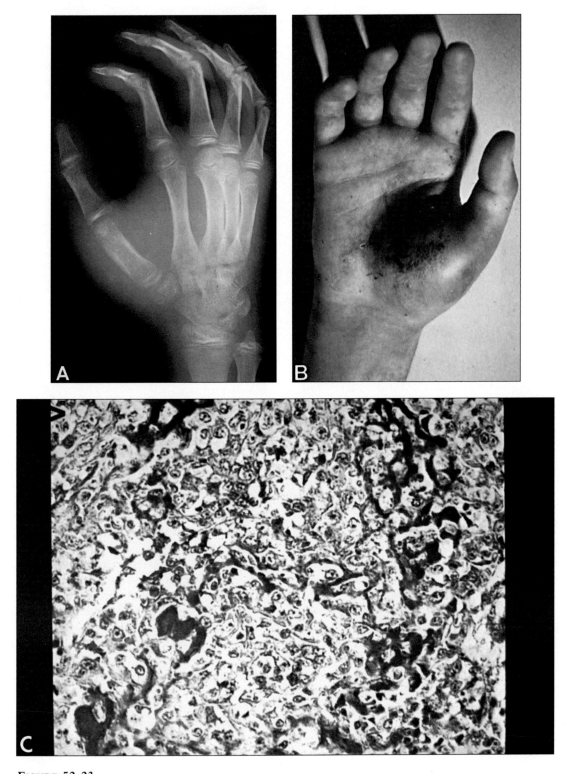

FIGURE 52-23

Osteogenic sarcoma. **A,** Oblique radiograph of the hand and wrist shows extensive soft-tissue swelling and osteoid formation on the soft tissues of the thenar or adductor pollicis muscles. **B,** Appearance of the hand and wrist with markedly advanced, high-grade osteogenic sarcoma. Amputation was performed at the radiocarpal level for treatment. **C,** Histopathologic section of grade 4 osteogenic sarcoma with irregular-shaped black masses of osteoid produced by highly anaplastic cells. (×100.)

multinucleated giant cells, and a spindle stroma. This tumor is rare in the hand and the patient presents with pain, swelling, or tenderness. Radiographs show a cystic lesion of bone in a faint lacy pattern with expansion of the cortex (Fig. 52-20). Treatment is by curettage or resection and bone graft. For lesions of the distal radius that extend outside of bone, complete excision of bone and a fibular bone graft may be considered. If not treated adequately, aneurysmal bone cyst has a tendency to recur. Lichtenstein[29] advised using radiation therapy for lesions uncontrolled by surgery.

Giant Cell Tumor of Bone. The giant cell tumor is of uncertain origin, but it probably arises from mesenchymal cells of the connective tissue framework of bone. These cells differentiate into mononuclear cells and multinucleated osteoclastlike cells, which are fibroblasts and osteoclasts. This tumor has also been termed an "osteoclastoma." This tumor has a vascular stroma containing spindle- or ovoid-shaped cells and many multinucleated giant cells. One of the largest reviews of giant cell tumors, consisting of 407 cases, was reported by Dahlin.[12,13] The most frequent location in the upper extremity was the distal radius. Most tumors occurred in the 3rd, 4th, and 5th decades of life and were more common in women. Symptoms are pain and swelling. On radiographic examination, there is a radiolucency in the epiphysis, with expansion and thinning of the cortex and no sclerosis (Fig. 52-21). The tumor may break through the cortex. There is nothing characteristic about the radiographic appearance to distinguish this tumor from others with a similar appearance, such as fibrosarcoma.[25] At operation, the covering over the tumor is thin. The tumor is reddish brown, as opposed to the gray-white tissue found in enchondroma. Some of these tumors may be cured by curettage and bone grafting or by use of bone-cement implantation if they are small, low grade, and have not broken through the periosteum. However, because of the high recurrence rate and possibility of malignant change, resection and reconstruction with bone graft is the best form of treatment. Reconstruction after resection of the distal radius may be with fibula autograft,[31,34,35,40] distal radius allograft,[47,49] or vascularized fibular bone graft.[43] These tumors can appear as multiple giant cell tumors of bone or even as benign metastatic pulmonary lesions. In both diagnoses, skeletal surveys are indicated.

MALIGNANT BONE TUMORS

Osteogenic Sarcoma. Osteogenic sarcoma is a malignant bone tumor consisting of malignant stroma and osteoid. In Dahlin's series,[11] osteosarcoma represented 21% of malignant bone tumors (Fig. 52-22). It is a

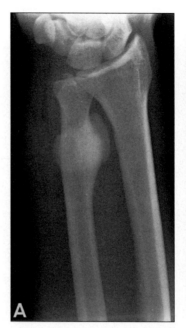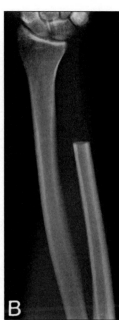

FIGURE 52-24

Chondrosarcoma. **A,** Apparent osteochondroma of the distal ulna; note widening of the proximal periosteal sleeve of the ulna. **B,** After frozen section histopathology demonstrated malignant changes of chondrosarcoma, excision of the distal third of the ulna was performed.

rare bone tumor in the hand or wrist area and is more common in the 2nd and 3rd decades of life and in males. Clinically, patients who have these tumors present with pain and swelling and there may be a palpable mass and tenderness. The alkaline phosphatase concentration is often increased. Radiographic findings indicate a destructive bony lesion (Fig. 52-23). Treatment is wide resection of bone and involved soft tissue. Amputation of the involved extremity may also be required because wide local resection within the wrist may be impossible. Metastasis is by way of the blood stream. Chemotherapy may be helpful in controlling metastasis; treatment involves amputation.

Chondrosarcoma. Chondrosarcoma is a malignant bony tumor arising from cartilage (Fig. 52-24). In Dahlin's series,[11] it was the second most frequent malignant bone tumor (17%). It rarely appears in the hand at presentation,[14,39] there is no predisposition to sex, and it usually occurs after the 4th decade of life.[15] Clinically, the patient presents with pain and swelling. Laboratory data are not helpful. Radiographs demonstrate a lobulated mass with bony destruction, including the cortex, and speckled calcification. Treatment is wide excision of bone and involved soft tissue, which often involves amputation. Metastasis is by way of the blood stream. Chemotherapy has not been helpful.[15]

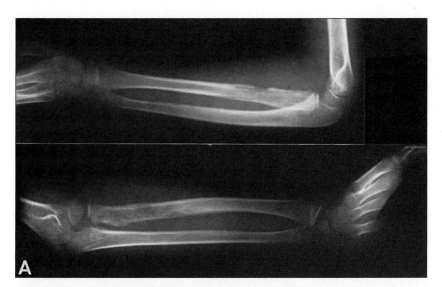

FIGURE 52-25

Ewing's sarcoma. **A,** Anteroposterior
(*bottom*) and lateral (*top*) radiographs of the
forearm demonstrate a destructive lesion of
the mid to proximal third of the radius. At
presentation the patient had dorsoradial
wrist pain from pressure on the radial sensory nerve. **B,** Planning of surgical incision.
Note previous incisional biopsy site, which
must be included in the surgical procedure.
Excision of skin, radial sensory nerve, and
cuff of muscle of wrist and finger extensor
tendons was done. **C,** Surgical pathologic
specimen, which on gross observation suggested a Ewing's sarcoma that was confirmed
histopathologically.

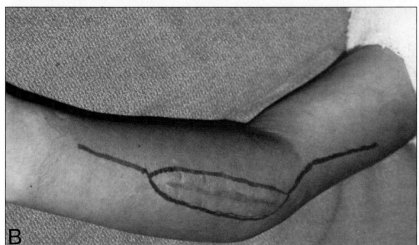

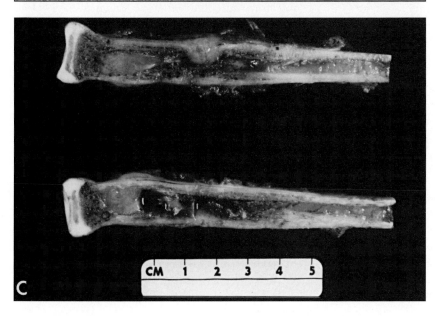

Ewing's Sarcoma. Ewing's sarcoma is a malignant bone tumor arising from the primitive mesenchyme of the medullary cavity. In Dahlin's series,[11] it accounted for 7% of malignant bone tumors. It is rare in the hand.[16,39] It occurs primarily in the 1st and 2nd decades of life. Clinically, the patient presents with pain and swelling and the tumor may compromise function. Laboratory studies may demonstrate anemia and increased sedimentation rate. The results of radiologic examination are not specific, although there may be a detectable onion-skin pattern of subperiosteal bone formation that is fairly characteristic. There is a destructive lesion with a varying amount of sclerosis (Fig. 52-25). Pathologic study shows diffuse anaplastic, small round cells. Treatment may be with a combination of surgery, radiation, and chemotherapy.[26] We recommend surgical excision when the lesion is confined to the intramedullary canal of the involved bone.

REFERENCES

1. Ambrosia JM, Wold LE, Amadio PC: Osteoid osteoma of the hand and wrist, *J Hand Surg [Am]* 12:794-800, 1987.
2. Azzolini A, Bertani A, Riberti C: Superselective embolization and immediate surgical treatment: our present approach to treatment of large vascular hemangiomas of the face, *Ann Plast Surg* 9:42-60, 1982.
3. Bogomill GP: *Tumors of the hand.* In Evarts CM, editor: *Surgery of the musculoskeletal system,* ed 2, vol 2, New York, 1990, Churchill Livingstone, p 1208.
4. Bos GD, Pritchard DJ, Reiman HM, et al.: Epithelioid sarcoma. An analysis of fifty-one cases, *J Bone Joint Surg Am* 70:862-870, 1988.
5. Breslow A: Prognosis in cutaneous melanoma: tumor thickness as a guide to treatment, *Pathol Annu* 15:1-22, 1980.
6. Bryan RS, Soule EH, Dobyns JH, et al.: Primary epithelioid sarcoma of the hand and forearm. A review of thirteen cases, *J Bone Joint Surg Am* 56:458-465, 1974.
7. Burrows PE, Mulliken JB, Fellows KE, et al.: Childhood hemangiomas and vascular malformations: angiographic differentiation, *AJR* 141:483-488, 1983.
8. Cadman NL, Soule EH, Kelly PJ: Synovial sarcoma: an analysis of 134 tumors, *Cancer* 18:613-627, 1965.
9. Casson PR, Robins P: *Malignant tumors of the skin.* In McCarthy JG, editor: *Plastic surgery,* vol 5, *Tumors of the head & neck and skin,* Philadelphia, 1990, WB Saunders, pp 3614-3662.
10. Clark WH Jr, From L, Bernardino EA, et al.: The histogenesis and biologic behavior of primary human malignant melanomas of the skin, *Cancer Res* 29:705-727, 1969.
11. Dahlin DC: *Bone tumors: general aspects and data on 3,987 cases,* ed 2, Springfield, IL, 1967, Charles C Thomas, pp 156-175.
12. Dahlin DC: Giant cell tumor of bone: highlights of 407 cases, *AJR* 144:955-960, 1985.
13. Dahlin DC, Cupps RE, Johnson EW Jr: Giant-cell tumor: a study of 195 cases, *Cancer* 25:1061-1070, 1970.
14. Dahlin DC, Salvador AH: Chondrosarcomas of bones of the hands and feet—a study of 30 cases, *Cancer* 34:755-760, 1974.
15. Dick HM: *Bone tumors: chondrosarcoma.* In Green DP, editor: *Operative hand surgery,* ed 2, vol 3, New York, 1988, Churchill Livingstone, pp 2358-2359.
16. Dick HM, Francis KC, Johnston AD: Ewing's sarcoma of the hand, *J Bone Joint Surg Am* 53:345-348, 1971.
17. Edgerton MT: The treatment of hemangiomas: with special reference to the role of steroid therapy, *Ann Surg* 183:517-532, 1976.
18. Enzinger FM: Epithelioid sarcoma. A sarcoma simulating a granuloma or a carcinoma, *Cancer* 26:1029-1041, 1970.
19. Fatti JF, Mosher JF: Treatment of multiple enchondromatosis (Ollier's disease) of the hand, *Orthopedics* 9:512-518, 1986.
20. Gunderson LL, Nagorney DM, McIlrath DC, et al.: External beam and intraoperative electron irradiation for locally advanced soft tissue sarcomas, *Int J Radiat Oncol Biol Phys* 25:647-656, 1993.
21. Halling AC, Wollan PC, Pritchard DJ, et al.: Epithelioid sarcoma: a clinicopathologic review of 55 cases, *Mayo Clin Proc* 71:636-642, 1996.
22. Hoopes JE, Graham WP III, Shack RB: Epithelioid sarcoma of the upper extremity, *Plast Reconstr Surg* 75:810-813, 1985.
23. Jaffe HL, Lichtenstein L: Solitary unicameral bone cyst, with emphasis on the roentgen picture, the pathologic appearance and the pathogeneses, *Arch Surg* 44:1004-1025, 1942.
24. Jaffe HL, Mayer L: An osteoblastic osteoid tissue-forming tumor of metacarpal bone, *Arch Surg* 24:550-564, 1932.
25. Jones FE, Soule EH, Coventry MB: Fibrous xanthoma of synovium (giant-cell tumor of tendon sheath, pigmented nodular synovitis). A study of one hundred and eighteen cases, *J Bone Joint Surg Am* 51:76-86, 1969.
26. Kedar A, Bialik V, Fishman J: Ewing sarcoma of the hand: literature review and a case report of nonsurgical management, *J Surg Oncol* 25:25-27, 1984.

27. Lattes R: Tumors of the soft tissues. Atlas of tumor pathology, 2nd series, *Fascicle* 1:219-227, 1982.

28. Leikensohn JR, Epstein LI, Vasconez LO: Superselective embolization and surgery of noninvoluting hemangiomas and A-V malformations, *Plast Reconstr Surg* 68:143-152, 1981

29. Lichtenstein L: Aneurysmal bone cyst. Observations on fifty cases, *J Bone Joint Surg Am* 39:873-882, 1957.

30. Linscheid RL, Soule EH, Henderson ED: Pleomorphic rhabdomyosarcomata of the extremities and limb girdles. A clinicopathological study, *J Bone Joint Surg Am* 47:715-726, 1965.

31. Mack GR, Lichtman DM, MacDonald RI: Fibular autografts for distal defects of the radius, *J Hand Surg* 4:576-583, 1979.

32. Miller SH, Smith RL, Shochat SJ: Compression treatment of hemangiomas, *Plast Reconstr Surg* 58:573-579, 1976.

33. Mulliken JB: *Cutaneous vascular anomalies.* In McCarthy JG, editor: *Plastic surgery,* vol 5, *Tumors of the head & neck and skin,* Philadelphia, 1990, WB Saunders, pp 3191-3274.

34. Murray JA, Schlafly B: Giant-cell tumors in the distal end of the radius. Treatment by resection and fibular autograft interpositional arthrodesis, *J Bone Joint Surg Am* 68:687-694, 1986.

35. Noellert RC, Louis DS: Long-term follow-up of non-vascularized fibular autografts for distal radial reconstruction, *J Hand Surg [Am]* 10:335-340, 1985.

36. O'Brien JE, Stout AP: Malignant fibrous xanthomas, *Cancer* 17:1445-1455, 1964.

37. Okunieff P, Suit HD, Proppe KH: Extremity preservation by combined modality treatment of sarcomas of the hand and wrist, *Int J Radiat Oncol Biol Phys* 12:1923-1929, 1986.

38. Owen RS, Fishman EK, Healy WL, et al.: Schwannoma of wrist, *Skeletal Radiol* 15:69-71, 1986.

39. Palmieri TJ: Chondrosarcoma of the hand, *J Hand Surg [Am]* 9:332-338, 1984.

40. Parrish FF: Treatment of bone tumors by total excision and replacement with massive autologous and homologous grafts, *J Bone Joint Surg Am* 48:968-990, 1966.

41. Patel MR, Zinberg EM: Pigmented villonodular synovitis of the wrist invading bone—report of a case, *J Hand Surg [Am]* 9:854-858, 1984.

42. Peled I, Iosipovich Z, Rousso M, et al.: Hemangioma of the median nerve, *J Hand Surg [Am]* 5:363-365, 1980.

43. Pho RW: Malignant giant-cell tumor of the distal end of the radius treated by a free vascularized fibular transplant, *J Bone Joint Surg Am* 63:877-884, 1981.

44. Pritchard DJ, Nascimento AG, Petersen IA: Local control of extra-abdominal desmoid tumors, *J Bone Joint Surg Am* 78:848-854, 1996.

45. Rayner CR: The results of treatment of two hundred and seventy-three carcinomas of the hand, *Hand* 13:183-186, 1981.

46. Riché M-C, Merland J-J: *Embolization of vascular malformations.* In Mulliken JB, Young AE, editors: *Vascular birthmarks: hemangiomas and malformations,* Philadelphia, 1988, WB Saunders, pp 436-453.

47. Smith RJ, Mankin HJ: Allograft replacement of distal radius for giant cell tumor, *J Hand Surg [Am]* 2:299-308, 1977.

48. Soule EH, Enriquez P: Atypical fibrous histiocytoma, malignant fibrous histiocytoma, malignant histiocytoma, and epithelioid sarcoma. A comparative study of 65 tumors, *Cancer* 30:128-143, 1972.

49. Szabo RM, Thorson EP, Raskind JR: Allograft replacement with distal radioulnar joint fusion and ulnar osteotomy for treatment of giant cell tumors of the distal radius, *J Hand Surg [Am]* 15:929-933, 1990.

50. Taxy JB, Battifora H: Malignant fibrous histiocytoma. An electron microscopic study, *Cancer* 40:254-267, 1977.

51. Tepper JE, Suit HD: Radiation therapy of soft tissue sarcomas, *Cancer* 55 Suppl 9:2273-2277, 1985.

52. Walsh TS Jr, Tompkins VN: Some observations on the strawberry nevus of infancy, *Cancer* 9:869-904, 1956.

53. Weiss SW, Enzinger FM: Malignant fibrous histiocytoma: an analysis of 200 cases, *Cancer* 41:2250-2266, 1978.

54. Wexler AM, Eilber FR, Miller TA: Therapeutic and functional results of limb salvage to treat sarcomas of the forearm and hand, *J Hand Surg [Am]* 13:292-296, 1988.

55. Whitworth PW, Pollock RE, Mansfield PF, et al.: Extremity epithelioid sarcoma. Amputation vs local resection, *Arch Surg* 126:1485-1489, 1991.

56. Woods JE: Extended use of sodium tetradecyl sulfate in treatment of hemangiomas and other related conditions, *Plast Reconstr Surg* 79:542-549, 1987.

XIV

REHABILITATION OF THE WRIST

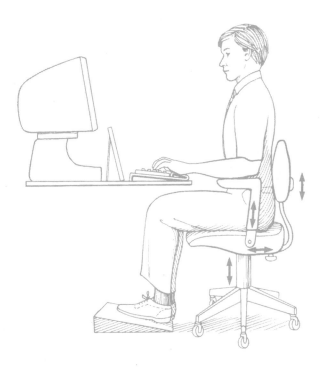

53

PHYSICAL THERAPY MODALITIES

Steven D. Bogard III, M.A., P.T.

CONTINUOUS PASSIVE MOTION
CRYOTHERAPY
THERAPEUTIC HEAT
HOT PACKS
PARAFFIN BATH
FLUIDOTHERAPY
DEEP HEAT
ULTRASOUND

PHONOPHORESIS
HYDROTHERAPY
ELECTROTHERAPY
PAIN CONTROL
MUSCLE STIMULATION
BIOFEEDBACK
SUMMARY

Patients with wrist injuries of various severities are frequently seen at upper extremity rehabilitation centers. A significant number of these injuries are the result of trauma from a direct striking force or a fall.[17] Trauma associated with surgical treatment must also be considered because of the tissue dissection necessary to allow access to the injury site and for the repair or reconstruction of the damaged tissues.

The initial period of wrist rehabilitation is usually limited by the immobilization necessary to allow tissues to heal.[11] If surgical fixation (or other considerations) allows for early mobilization, the recovery period is shorter.[16] Owing to the complexity of the wrist joint and the variable involvement of wrist structures in an injury,[8,9] cooperation among the patient, referring surgeon or physician, and therapist is paramount during the patient's rehabilitation.

This chapter presents various physical therapy modalities that may be used to enhance a patient's response to rehabilitation. Treatment options for patients with injuries of the wrist (fractures or dislocations), after surgical reconstruction, or who have rheumatoid disease or minor problems such as tendinitis or neuritis are discussed. The goal of treatment is to hasten the patient toward maximal recovery of functional range of motion and strength. Various modalities are suggested and

discussed. The clinician is advised to seek specific modality-related literature before application of these modalities to the patient.

CONTINUOUS PASSIVE MOTION

With the goal of attaining as functional a wrist as possible, motion plays a vital role in the rehabilitation process. The timing (initiation, repetition, duration) and type (active or passive) of motion have various effects on the tissues and the ultimate recovery of the patient.

The use of a continuous passive motion (CPM) device to augment the patient's formal rehabilitation as well as home therapy programs has been shown to provide many clinical benefits, including the reduction of pain and edema, the promotion of wound healing, the preservation of joint range of motion, the restoration of tissue gliding, and a decrease in total rehabilitation time.[7,10-12,28]

The clinical benefits are the result of the application of Wolff's law. As stress is applied to the tissues through motion, the tissues accommodate to that stress with remodeling and elongation. Regular motion with controlled stress helps to maintain joint and tissue elasticity, ensuring that healing is accomplished in an

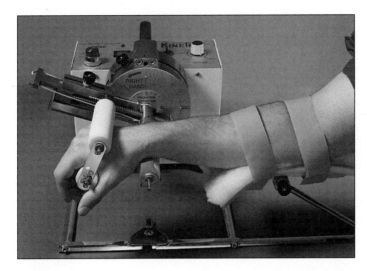

FIGURE 53-1
Kinetic continuous passive motion for wrist flexion and extension.

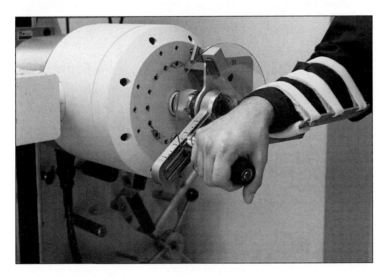

FIGURE 53-2
LIDO Workset in continuous passive motion mode for the wrist.

elongated position and thus preventing adhesions and contractures.[12]

Joint motion enhances the nutrition of articular cartilage by increasing the hydrodynamic movement of the synovial fluid and allowing for proper diffusion of nutrients. This permits the cartilage to remain healthy and potentially to heal—a fact demonstrated in laboratory animals.[12,28] CPM has the additional benefit of producing a decrease in adhesion formation,[29] which is essential if rehabilitation is to achieve the most functional wrist for the patient.

The use of CPM devices in rehabilitation is appropriate for stable fractures, burns, ligament reconstruction, after release of adhesions, synovectomy, capsulotomy, arthroplasty, tenolysis, and any situation in which controlled CPM may enhance patient recovery.[11,12]

The current modalities my colleagues and I use for continuous passive wrist motion are the Kinetic Wrist CPM, the Toronto Wrist CPM, the LIDO Workset, and the Danninger Wrist CPM (Figs. 53-1, 53-2, and 53-3). Our program is to use CPM during waking hours 50% to 75% of the time available, combining it with active assisted motion. We do not advise passive motion (or any type of passive stretch) at night. In our clinic, contraindications to CPM include the presence of active infection, active joint inflammation, unstable fractures, questionable tendon quality, a compromised vascular status, lack of sensibility, and inability of the patient to operate or tolerate the CPM device.

CRYOTHERAPY

The acronym PRICE (protection, rest, ice, compression, elevation) has long been associated with the acute care of patients with mild trauma. Ice or cold may be used therapeutically in the rehabilitation of the wrist from acute problems and chronic injuries. Ice (cold) has many positive biologic effects: decrease in tissue temperature concurrent with a decrease in metabolic rate, release of histamine, and decrease in inflammation and edema from the outward flow of

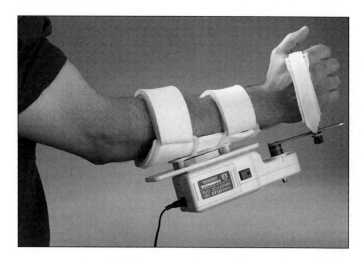

FIGURE 53-3

Danninger portable continuous passive motion.

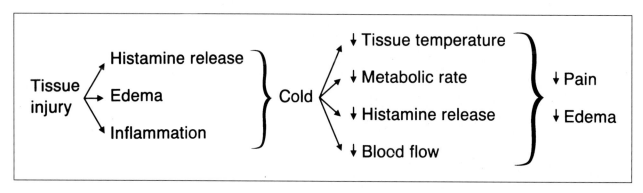

FIGURE 53-4

Effects of cold on injured tissue.

fluid into the tissue space. Arteriolar constriction limits potential bleeding. As a result of the decrease in initial blood flow and its associated body core heat, the deeper tissue temperatures are effectively lowered. If the tissue is significantly cooled, to 18°C or lower, periodic episodes of vasodilation occur. These events were termed the "hunting reaction" by T. Lewis.[20] The reaction was postulated to be an axon reflex. It is believed that severe cooling causes pain and the release of a neurotransmitter that causes vasodilation and tissue warming. As the tissue temperature increased, the ice again became an effective vasoconstrictor. Another beneficial effect of cooling is the elevation of the pain threshold, allowing patients more comfort during their rehabilitation program (Fig. 53-4).[23a,31]

Muscle strength is also affected by cold. Short-duration cooling enhances strength, whereas cooling for a long duration decreases strength. Spasticity, when present, can also be inhibited by cold and this factor further assists in the patient's rehabilitation. Spasticity appears to be influenced by two mechanisms: reflex inhibition of the muscle spindle via the spinal cord and direct cooling of the muscle.[23a] Ice is thus recommended for muscle spasticity and muscle cocontraction.

The clinical indications for cryotherapy are most often seen after acute musculoskeletal trauma. Cold therapy has been effective in minimizing edema and inflammation and decreases post-trauma pain. Cold, when used with exercise (cryokinetics), decreases muscle soreness and increases the range of joint motion.

In our Hand Center, the most popular methods of application of cold to the wrist are ice massage, cold or ice packs, and cold baths. The cold baths are used for general cooling: water temperature range of 4° to 18°C for 10 to 20 min. Ice packs (cold packs) are used for more localized cooling, depending on pack size. Clinical application usually involves a damp-towel interface between the pack and the body to enhance cold transfer and additional insulating towels over the pack on the treatment site (Fig. 53-5). Treatment is for 20 to 30 min, with skin checks every 10 min. If the area being treated turns noticeably white or blue, it is best to discontinue treatment immediately to avoid frostbite damage to the skin. Another modality is ice massage. Ice massage is performed over an area no bigger than 10 × 15 cm. The ice is applied directly to the skin in circular or stroking motions. The patient should experience sensations of cold, burning, or aching and, after

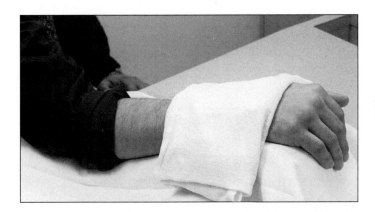

FIGURE 53-5

Cold pack application to elevated wrist.

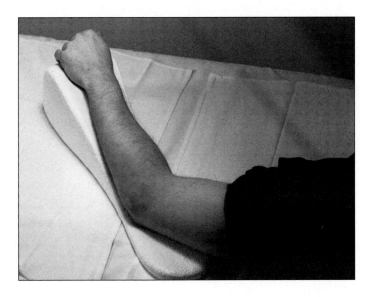

FIGURE 53-6

Infrared heat application allows visualization of the treated wrist. An additional benefit is no weight related to the application of the heat source.

approximately 3 to 5 min of application, cutaneous anesthesia.[31] Again, care should be taken to prevent cold-induced skin and soft-tissue damage.

Clinical precautions or contraindications to the use of cryotherapy involve patients with Raynaud's disease, neurovascular injury, tissue previously injured by cold, or various cold allergies (cold urticaria, paroxysmal cold hemoglobinuria, syncope, or any sudden excessive increase or decrease in blood pressure). Other considerations include an increased potential for delay in wound healing or a decrease in tissue extensibility.[23a,31]

THERAPEUTIC HEAT

Therapeutic heat used in the treatment of wrist problems can be divided into two subgroups: *superficial* and *deep*. Superficial-heating agents raise the superficial tissue and skin temperature. They affect deep structures through reflex action. Deep-heating agents are able to increase tissue temperatures to a depth of 3 to 5cm.[23b,31]

The physiologic effect of heating local tissue is an increase in tissue temperature, producing local analgesia and sedation. The temperature increase also causes increased metabolism and arteriolar dilatation, which improve capillary flow. This leads to a further increase of local temperature with a clearing of metabolites. In addition, there is an increase in nutrients, oxygen, and blood products at the treated site. The greater arteriolar dilatation that results has a negative effect of increasing capillary pressure and producing edema in the tissues.[31] The magnitude of these changes is affected by total temperature increase, the state at which the energy is added, and the total surface area of treated tissue.[23b]

Superficial heat may be added to the tissues about the wrist by *radiation, conduction,* or *convection,* depending on the modality chosen.

The use of heat lamps (infrared radiation) allows energy penetration of up to 3 mm with 95% of the radiation absorbed by the skin. Dosage depends directly on application duration and the angle of incidence of application. The infrared radiation intensity varies inversely with the square of the distance from the source to the treatment area.[31] In our clinic, typical treatment application with a 250-W infrared lamp is for 20 to 30 min at a distance of 18 to 20 in. from the source (Fig. 53-6). Repeated treatment with infrared radiation can result in mottled erythema that may become erythema ab igne (without heat).

Conduction is a second effective way of transmitting heat. The use of conduction for raising tissue temperatures is mainly with paraffin and hot packs. The heat transferred to the patient's tissues depends on the temperature of the source and the specific heat of the source, defined as the amount of heat required to raise 1 g 1°C, measured in calories. The use of these modalities allows heat to be added to the tissues about the wrist in a nondependent position, thus decreasing the possibility of position-related edema.

HOT PACKS

In clinical application, hot packs usually contain a hydroscopic material and, when applied to the wrist, provide a superficial moist heat. Six to eight layers of towels are placed between the pack and the heated body part and additional towels or blankets are used for insulation against heat loss over the pack. The treatment duration is 20 to 30 min, and the initial hot pack temperature is 160°F (Fig. 53-7).

PARAFFIN BATH

Paraffin for heating the wrist may be applied by a dipping or a brushing technique. The most frequently used paraffin is actually a mixture of seven parts paraffin to one part mineral oil.[27] Clinical application of paraffin is at a temperature of 126° to 128°F, with 7 to 10 layers either dipped or brushed on the body part. A thin towel is placed over the wax, followed by a plastic wrap and more towels for insulation. The duration of heat application is 20 to 30 min. An additional advantage to the use of paraffin as a superficial heat source is its ability to increase the compliance of superficial tissue in the area of application.[1]

The disadvantages of these conductive heat sources are the lack of visibility of the affected area during treatment, the susceptibility to spreading infection, and the difficulties in the appropriate application to large open wounds.

FLUIDOTHERAPY

Fluidotherapy is the only convective heating unit currently available for clinical use. It uses circulating warm air to suspend ground cellulose particles and is occasionally referred to as a dry whirlpool. The manufacturer recommends a treatment temperature between 110° and 125°F. Care must be taken to prevent dependent edema. If edema is present, the treatment temperature should be lowered. Additional benefits of treatment include various levels of desensitization and minimal resistance exercise made possible by the low-viscosity, air-particle system (Fig. 53-8).[4] Cross contamination is a concern for patients with wounds. The use of a plastic bag over the body part is recommended to minimize this risk.[23b] Treatment is usually for 20 to 30 min. Poor circulation and insensitive skin require precautions or are contraindications to Fluidotherapy as well as all the superficial heats.

DEEP HEAT

Of the deep heats available for use by the clinician, ultrasonography and short wave diathermy are the two most frequently used for wrist treatment. Short wave diathermy produces electromagnetic radiation by means of an oscillating electromagnetic field with a frequency between 10 and 100 MHz and a wavelength between 3 and 30 m.[27,29] Various machines are available that deliver this electromagnetic radiation with either inductive or capacitance applicators. The technique of application affects the electromagnetic field intensity and

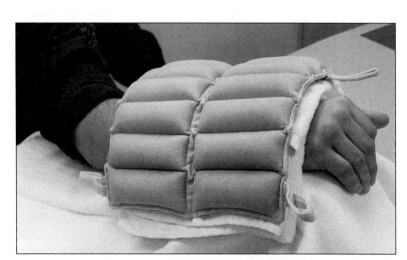

FIGURE 53-7

Hot pack application to elevated wrist.

density, thus affecting the temperature increases in the radiated tissue. Increase in tissue temperature has been reported to depths of 2 cm.[19] Because of the potential for current concentration, sweat accumulation should be avoided through the use of towels. No metal, either jewelry or implant material, should be allowed in or around the area of treatment. The benefits of short wave diathermy for distal upper extremity heating include increases in blood flow and tissue compliance to stretch and decreases in joint stiffness, muscle spasm, and pain.[18] It is contraindicated in areas of neurologic and vascular compromise and where tumor or infection is present.

ULTRASOUND

The Hand Center's most commonly used deep heat source is ultrasound. When used at a frequency of 1.0 MHz, ultrasound can increase tissue temperatures to a depth of 5 cm. If the ultrasound source is a 3.0-MHz unit, most of the energy absorption and temperature increase occur within the initial 1 to 2 cm of tissue. Duration of treatment is from 5 to 10 min per site. Selective heating of different tissues in the same treatment field is possible because of the higher rate of energy absorption by tissues of greater collagen content. A 40° to 45°C tissue temperature is the goal for treatment.[34] This temperature increase is associated with an increased tissue compliance and blood flow; both are therapeutically useful (Fig. 53-9).

PHONOPHORESIS

Phonophoresis is another common modality used in our Hand Center. It involves the use of ultrasound to drive medications across the skin to target tissues and may be of significant benefit for patients apprehensive about needle delivery of drugs about the wrist.[13] Various explanations for the increase in drug delivery

with ultrasound are changes in tissue permeability with heating, changes in diffusion rate, and radiation pressure of the ultrasound beam.[34] However, some investigators think that phonophoresis is ineffective for intra-articular conditions.[24] The use of ultrasound is contraindicated in areas of decreased sensation and circulation, areas of infection or malignant growth, children's epiphyseal areas, and the bone-cement interfaces of joint replacements. Metal-only implants do not restrict ultrasound usage because they disperse the sound and do not cause increased temperatures in the area.[23a] Phonophoresis and ultrasound may also be used around joints replaced with silicone material or prostheses.

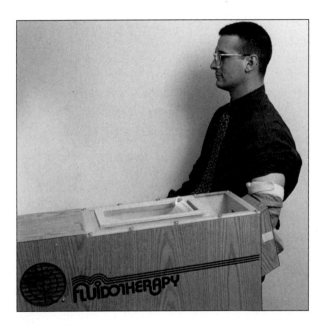

FIGURE 53-8

Fluidotherapy to the wrist. The hand, wrist, and forearm are placed through a sleeve into the convective heat unit. Warm air circulates dry cellulose particles. Benefits include desensitization and minimal resistance to active movement.

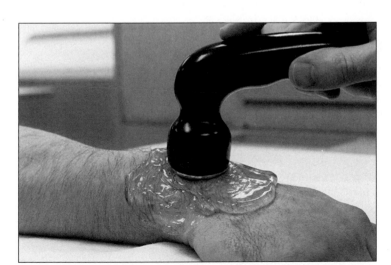

FIGURE 53-9

Ultrasound application to the wrist with aquasonic gel medium.

HYDROTHERAPY

Water has many properties that make it a valuable tool in the treatment of wrist injuries. The buoyancy of water helps to support the body part with a force equal to the weight of water displaced. The viscosity and cohesive property of water allow the therapist to use hydrotherapy as a mild resistive exercise. Water's high specific heat causes it to release heat at a slow rate and makes it an effective therapeutic tool for heating or cooling extremities. Therapeutic temperature ranges are defined as cold, 55° to 65°F (13° to 18°C); cool, 65° to 80°F (18° to 27°C); tepid, 80° to 92°F (27° to 33.5°C); neutral, 92° to 96°F (33.5° to 35.5°C); warm, 96° to 98°F (35.5° to 36.5°C); hot, 98° to 104°F (36.5° to 40°C); and very hot, 104° to 115°F (40° to 46.1°C).[35] Temperature selection depends on the degree of heating or cooling desired. Wound contamination by pathogens from the use of hydrotherapy is controlled by using one of the many bactericidal agents available to the therapist.

Whirlpools are effective in assisting with wound care. The agitation helps with wound débridement and the stimulation of new granulation tissue. Regulation of water temperature and extremity position help to control swelling but allow local circulation increase, with its benefits of increased nutrition and metabolite removal.[32,33]

Contrast baths are a type of hydrotherapy used to stimulate peripheral circulation in the treated extremity. In our clinic, water temperatures in the baths are 110°F (43.3°C) and 65°F (18.3°C). After the initial 10 min in the very hot water, the patient alternates between 1 min in cool and 4 min in very hot water, always finishing in very hot water. The extremity is best kept elevated to prevent edema during the whirlpool process.

The main contraindications to hydrotherapy are poor circulation and extreme hypersensitivity to cold.

ELECTROTHERAPY

There are many uses for electrical current in the treatment of musculoskeletal problems about the wrist. Electrical stimulation for drug delivery, neuromuscular reeducation, and pain control are discussed briefly. More details can be found in standard texts on rehabilitation.*

Iontophoresis is the use of direct current to move free ions into the skin-subcutaneous target tissues.[14] This relatively old treatment[25] has gained in popularity with the clinical availability of new treatment units.[3,26] Our present units and electrodes are designed for efficient application of lidocaine hydrochloride or dexamethasone sodium phosphate (or both) after the drug

---

* References 19,21,27,29,30,34.

ion polarity is determined.[26,32] Indications for use include the desire for local anesthesia or local anti-inflammatory therapy (or both), acute and subacute bursitis, epicondylitis, acute nonspecific tenosynovitis, and situations where needle and infiltration tissue trauma are not wanted. Contraindications for wrist area treatment include damaged skin, recently formed scar tissue, patient sensitivity to the drugs to be administered or to electricity, and patients with electrically sensitive pacemakers.[26]

PAIN CONTROL

Since Melzack and Wall[22] published their gate theory of pain, transcutaneous electrical nerve stimulation (TENS) has been used to assist in controlling patient discomfort. Research has advanced our understanding of pain and modified the machines we use to attempt to control it. Therapeutic units are designed for production of one or more of the types of stimulation listed in Table 53-1.[6,21,25,27,30]

TENS is indicated for wrist pain that is related to peripheral nerves and musculoskeletal structures and for reflex sympathetic dystrophy. Precautions that should be taken include avoiding skin irritation, electrical burns, and patients with demand pacemakers.

Other sources of electrical stimulation involve interferential current and high-voltage galvanic stimulation, which are applied to treat pain, decrease edema, and produce muscle contractions. The different therapeutic effects depend on the current frequency, duration, and wave induced in the patient. Interferential current has a sine waveform with a duration of 250 μs, a frequency of 4,000 Hz, and an intensity of up to 70 to 90 mA. High-voltage galvanic stimulation has a twin-peak waveform, a duration of 5 to 65 μs, a frequency of 1 to 150 Hz, and an average current of 1.2 to 1.5 mA, with peak intensity of 2,000 to 2,500 mA.[27] Modality selection depends on available units, patient's wrist condition, treatment goals, and the patient's tolerance of electrical stimulation.

MUSCLE STIMULATION

The clinical use of electrical stimulation for muscle contraction offers an adjunct to the patient's own ability to control muscle.[2] There are basically two types of therapeutic currents available to the therapist: direct (galvanic) and alternating currents.

Direct or *galvanic current* is often used to treat denervated muscle. The rationale for galvanic stimulation is to maintain muscle in as healthy a state as possible until there is reinnervation. Keeping the muscle as healthy as possible allows faster return to functional use by slowing muscle fiber degeneration and fibrosis.

Thus, stimulation should decrease the effects of prolonged intramuscular stasis, minimize edema, and maintain flexibility. Concerns related to the stimulation of denervated muscle are increased muscle degeneration, delayed reinnervation, and accentuated atrophy of type I muscle fibers. Currently, there are no conclusive studies that resolve these issues.[25,30] The therapist must consider this when deciding on its use. Recently, we have *not* advocated galvanic stimulation of muscle in cases of muscle denervation secondary to peripheral nerve injury because there is no apparent therapeutic benefit.

Alternating current, with its pulse duration adjusted to less than 300 ms, is effective for stimulating innervated muscle. For a comfortable stimulation, a pulse duration of 200 to 300 μs should be used. Applications for its use in the upper extremity include preventing disuse atrophy, decreasing spasticity by stimulating the antagonist muscles, reeducating muscle, conditioning and strengthening of muscle groups, and providing an active stretch to assist in decreasing joint contracture or increasing tendon pull-through. Care should be taken to prevent irritation at the stimulation site. The method should not be used on patients who have a cardiac pacemaker. It is important to adjust current outputs to levels that do not cause pain, fainting, or ventricular fibrillation.[5]

BIOFEEDBACK

Inappropriate muscle function can interfere with the recovery from wrist injury. Biofeedback can be helpful in the reeducation of a patient by decreasing unwanted muscle activity and cocontraction and by increasing wanted muscle activity and coordination in the performance of a desired movement. This is possible because of the electrochemical gradient associated

Table 53-1. Application of Transcutaneous Electrical Nerve Stimulation

Stimulation Parameter	Conventional High TENS	Low TENS Acupuncture-like	Pulsed TENS Acupuncture-like	Hyperstimulation
Frequency (rate)	50-500 Hz (high)	1-4 Hz (low)	2-3 Hz carrier with 70-100 Hz internal frequency	2-4 Hz (low)
Pulse duration (width)	50-100 μs (narrow)	100-400 μs (wide)	100-200 μs (wide)	10 ms to 0.5 s (wide)
Intensity	Perceptible paresthesia (low) sensory	To tolerance (high) motor	As tolerated (high) motor	As tolerated (high) pain

TENS, transcutaneous electrical nerve stimulation.

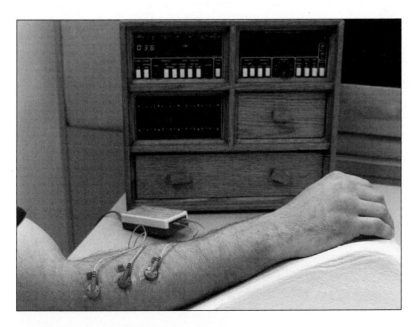

FIGURE 53-10

Surface electromyographic biofeedback is valuable for reeducation and relaxation of the muscles that affect the wrist.

with muscle activity. An electrode located in the area of the contracting muscle detects this electrochemical gradient or action potential. The muscle action potential activity is amplified and quantified in a visual or audio format (or both). The patient who needs to improve function of the muscle is asked to increase the output format activity. If the patient needs to decrease the monitored muscle activity, the patient is taught to lower the output activity and the muscle relaxes (Fig. 53-10). Treatment quality can be enhanced by using the smallest electrodes possible to decrease any artifact activity of adjacent muscles and by proper site preparation to lower the electrode-tissue interface impedance. This may be accomplished with the use of alcohol or abrasive rubs and by shaving the hair from the electrode site.[15] Biofeedback is indicated in any treatment plan where reeducation or relaxation of muscle activity is a goal.

SUMMARY

There are many physical therapy modalities available to the medical team to enhance the patient's recovery from traumatic, systemic, or surgical problems about the wrist. The optimal use of these modalities depends on good communication between patient and therapist. Good communication enhances the utilization of professional expertise and allows timely and appropriate rehabilitation goals. This ultimately enhances the patient's functional outcome and the clinical practice of the involved professionals.

REFERENCES

1. Askew LJ, Beckett VL, An KN, et al.: Objective evaluation of hand function in scleroderma patients to assess effectiveness of physical therapy, *Br J Rheumatol* 22:224-232, 1983.
2. Benton LA, Baker LL, Bowman BR, et al.: *Functional electrical stimulation, a practical clinical guide,* Downey, California, 1980, Rancho Los Amigos Rehabilitation Engineering Center.
3. Bogard SD, Fanton GS, Figgie MP, et al.: Elbow: keep the whole arm in focus, *Patient Care* 26(4):108-131, 1992.
4. Borrell RM, Henley EJ, Ho P, et al.: Fluidotherapy: evaluation of a new heat modality, *Arch Phys Med Rehabil* 58:69-71, 1977.
5. Bruner JM: Hazards of electrical apparatus, *Anesthesiology* 28:396-425, 1967.
6. Castel JC: Management of pain with non invasive acupuncture therapy. A medical research laboratory seminar manual, April 11 to 13, 1980. Medical Research Laboratories, Inc., 7450 Natchez Avenue, Niles, Illinois 60648.
7. Cohen EJ: Adjunctive therapy devices: restoring ROM outside of the clinic, *Physical Therapy Products* 6(2):10-13, 1995.
8. Cooney WP, Agee JM, Hastings H, et al.: Symposium: management of intra-articular fractures of the distal radius, *Contemp Orthop* 21:71-104, 1990.
9. Cooney WP, Schutt AH: *Rehabilitation of the wrist.* In Nickel VL, Botte MJ, editors: *Orthopaedic rehabilitation,* ed 2, New York, 1992, Churchill Livingstone, pp 711-731.
10. Coutts RD, Craig EV, Mooney J, et al.: Symposium: the use of CPM in the rehabilitation of orthopaedic problems, *Contemp Orthop* 16:75-106, Mar 1988.
11. Covey MH, Dutcher K, Marvin JA, et al.: Efficacy of continuous passive motion (CPM) devices with hand burns, *J Burn Care Rehabil* 9:397-400, 1988.
12. Diehm SL: The power of CPM: healing through motion, *Continuing Care* 8:28; 30; 32; 34; 36; 50, Nov 1989.
13. Griffin JE, Echternach JL, Price RE, et al.: Patients treated with ultrasonic driven hydrocortisone and with ultrasound alone, *Phys Ther* 47:594-601, 1967.
14. Harris PR: Iontophoresis: clinical research in musculoskeletal inflammatory conditions, *J Orthop Sports Phys Ther* 4:109-112, 1982.
15. Hayes KW: *Manual for physical agents,* ed 4, Norwalk, Connecticut, 1993, Appleton & Lange.
16. Herbert TJ, Fisher WE: Management of the fractured scaphoid using a new bone screw, *J Bone Joint Surg Br* 66:114-123, 1984.
17. Johnson RP: The acutely injured wrist and its residuals, *Clin Orthop* 149:33-44, 1980.
18. Kloth LC, Ziskin MC: *Diathermy and pulsed electromagnetic fields.* In Michlovitz SL, editor: *Thermal agents in rehabilitation,* Philadelphia, 1990, FA Davis, pp 170-199.
19. Lehmann JF: *Diathermy.* In Krusen FH, editor: *Handbook of physical medicine and rehabilitation,* ed 2, Philadelphia, 1971, WB Saunders, pp 273-345.
20. Lewis T: Observations upon reactions of vessels of human skin to cold, *Heart* 15:177-208, 1930.
21. Mannheimer JS, Lampe GN: *Clinical transcutaneous electrical nerve stimulation,* Philadelphia, 1984, FA Davis.

22. Melzack R, Wall PD: Pain mechanisms: a new theory, *Science* 150:971-979, 1965.

23. Michlovitz SL, editor: *Thermal agents in rehabilitation,* Philadelphia, 1990, FA Davis, a, pp 63-87; b, pp 88-108.

24. Muir WS, Magee FP, Longo JA, et al.: Comparison of ultrasonically applied vs. intra-articular injected hydrocortisone levels in canine knees, *Orthop Rev* 19:351-356, 1990.

25. Nelson RM, Currier DP: *Clinical electrotherapy,* Norwalk, Connecticut, 1987, Appleton & Lange.

26. Phoresor II, Model PM 700: Product insert instructions (treatment guidelines), Salt Lake City, Iomed Incorporated.

27. Rothstein JM, Roy SH, Wolf SL: *The rehabilitation specialist's handbook,* Philadelphia, 1991, FA Davis, pp 627-646.

28. Salter RB: *Regeneration of articular cartilage through CPM: past, present and future.* In Strauts LR, Wilson PD, editors: *Clinical trends in orthopedics,* New York, 1982, Thieme-Stratton, pp 101-107.

29. Shriber WJ: *A manual of electrotherapy,* ed 4, Philadelphia, 1975, Lea & Febiger.

30. Snyder-Mackler L, Robinson AJ: *Clinical electrophysiology: electrotherapy and electrophysiologic testing,* Baltimore, 1989, Williams & Wilkins.

31. Stillwell GK: *Therapeutic heat and cold.* In Krusen FH, editor: *Handbook of physical medicine and rehabilitation,* ed 2, Philadelphia, 1971, WB Saunders, pp 259-272.

32. Taylor Mullins PA: *Use of therapeutic modalities in upper extremity rehabilitation.* In Hunter JM, Schneider LH, Mackin EJ, et al., editors: *Rehabilitation of the hand: surgery and therapy,* ed 3, St. Louis, 1990, CV Mosby, pp 195-220.

33. Walsh M: Relationship of hand edema to upper extremity position and water temperature during whirlpool, *J Hand Surg [Am]* 9:609, 1984.

34. Ziskin MC, McDiarmid T, Michlovitz SL: *Therapeutic ultrasound.* In Michlovitz SL, editor: *Thermal agents in rehabilitation,* Philadelphia, 1990, FA Davis, pp 134-169.

35. Zislis JM: *Hydrotherapy.* In Krusen FH, editor: *Handbook of physical medicine and rehabilitation,* ed 2, Philadelphia, 1971, WB Saunders, pp 346-362.

54

WRIST REHABILITATION AND SPLINTING: OCCUPATIONAL THERAPY

Ann H. Schutt, M.D.

PREOPERATIVE EVALUATION OF THE WRIST
POSTOPERATIVE MANAGEMENT
SPLINTING
   GENERAL PRINCIPLES OF SPLINTING
   TYPES OF SPLINTING

STATIC SPLINTING
DYNAMIC SPLINTING
COMMERCIALLY AVAILABLE SPLINTING
CONCLUSION

The overall approach to rehabilitation of the wrist after fractures, fracture dislocations, ligamentous injuries such as scapholunate dissociation, and surgery for stabilization of the wrist or rheumatoid arthritis requires meticulous evaluation and therapy to maximize the residual functional capacity of the patient who has sustained a wrist injury, has been operated on, or is diseased. Rehabilitation is a team approach that requires evaluation of the patient's condition and then a prescribed and coordinated program of rehabilitation by the occupational therapist, hand therapist, physical therapist, or orthotist that can provide the required therapy for the wrist. The rehabilitation team may also include social workers, psychologists, vocational counselors, and qualified rehabilitation counselors of an insurance company or employer.[33] Good coordination among the surgeon, the physiatrist, the psychologist, and the therapists is essential for efficient and effective rehabilitation.[78,79,93]

PREOPERATIVE EVALUATION OF THE WRIST

The therapist must have precise knowledge of the anatomy, kinesiology, and physiology of the muscles, tendons, nerves, and joints of the wrist and the upper extremity. It is essential in the evaluation of functional status of the upper extremity and wrist. Measurements must be well defined, precisely executed in the standard manner, and reproducible by other evaluators.* Where possible, measurement of the volume and circumference of the digits is important if edema is present. A volumometer and specifically devised measurement tapes are helpful. Small goniometers are used to measure active and passive range of motion and these measurements should be recorded. Computerized goniometers have been developed as well as computerized vibration measurements, and static and dynamic grip and pinch measurements are available (NK Biotechnical Engineering, Greenleaf, Baltimore Therapeutics Equipment, Cybex [Product Index 19]).[2,4,13,36] These computerized instruments are helpful in standardized recordings of the data. Simpler tools can be used to get these data without added cost. It is important that these data be gathered and recorded accurately. Most occupational and hand therapy departments have special forms and graphs to record a patient's initial evaluation and progress, such as range of motion and grip strength. The patient should be reevaluated and measured at least weekly during the initial treatment program and more often if necessary.

Reproducibility of the measurements is essential, and measurements of the digits in flexion and extension,

---

* References 22,35,42–44,59,67,69.

abduction and adduction, wrist flexion and extension, radial and ulnar deviation, and pronation and supination; range of motion of the shoulder flexion, abduction, and internal and external rotation; and elbow flexion and extension should be noted and recorded. Strength is measured with a dynamometer. Measurements for opposition (tip pinch), apposition (lateral pinch), and grip in several positions are important.* Sensory evaluation should include touch, moving touch, two-point discrimination, proprioception, temperature perception, and vibration for the evaluation of sensation.[14-17,73,92,96,97]

Nylon monofilaments of various diameters, two-point calipers, needles, tuning forks, vibrometers, test tubes of various temperatures, and objects of various sizes, shapes, and weights are used to test sensation and functional discrimination in upper extremities.† Muscle testing of all muscles in the hand and wrist innervated by the median, ulnar, and radial nerves is important. Electromyographic examinations are always helpful in carpal tunnel syndrome and ulnar nerve compression injuries at the wrist, elbow, or forearm and the radial nerve involving the wrist extensors and thumb extensors. All of these evaluations should be done preoperatively if possible, and postoperatively these evaluations are necessary to formulate a treatment plan. Many functional evaluations for activities of daily living and homemaking are available.[79] The Jebsen objective standardized test[39] and the Moberg objective method[62] for determining the functional sensibility of the hand are helpful. Assessment of recorded observations is essential during the initial treatment and follow-up examinations. Serial evaluations are essential in quantifying the outcome of the therapy.[2,4,13,36]

The treatment goals may include prevent and decrease edema; assist tissue healing; relieve pain; allow relaxation; prevent misuse, disuse, and overuse of the muscles; avoid jamming and further injury of the joints; desensitize areas of hypersensitivity; reeducate for sensation; and redevelop motor and sensory functions.[79] Complications can be prevented by early evaluation and treatment. These complications include edema, pain, loss of range of motion, loss of strength, adhesions, hypersensitivity, misuse, disuse, and overuse of the extremity. Overuse and repetitive use of the upper extremity before and during rehabilitation are counterproductive. Work hardening and endurance training should not be undertaken until the patient is relatively free of pain while using the upper extremity.[4,79] Conservative management of wrist problems consists of relative rest, splinting, modalities that may decrease pain, reeducation of the muscles, and the improvement or maintenance of range of motion of the wrist and upper extremity. Other modalities include Fluidotherapy, paraffin wax and hydrotherapy, transcutaneous electrical nerve stimulation, therapeutic heat and cold, diathermy, and iontophoresis.*

POSTOPERATIVE MANAGEMENT

Edema often occurs following limb overuse and following wrist injuries or after fractures and surgical procedures. Prevention and treatment of edema are essential to effective hand, wrist, and upper extremity rehabilitation. Lasting edema caused by immobilization of the upper extremity decreases lymphatic and venous drainage.[11,26,34,66] Also the loss of pumping action of the hand that moves the lymph fluid contributes to the edema.[11,26,34,66] After tourniquet use in surgery, its release may overwhelm the lymph circulation by the rapid return of circulation to the extremity, particularly the dorsum of the hand and wrist, and result in secondary hyperemia and edema.[11,64-66] Edema that persists and becomes chronic may cause fibrosis of the joints and muscles and loss of movement of the muscle planes, vessels, and nerves. Chronic edema also promotes infection.

In the early stages, elevation and range of motion are effective as preventive measures for edema control.[84,86] In joints that can be moved, range of motion should be started as soon as possible after fixation of the fracture, surgery, trauma, or burns. Even the smallest movements of the muscles assist in removing the lymph from the hand, wrist, and upper extremity. If possible, the extremity should be elevated with the elbow above the level of the shoulder and the hand above the level of the elbow. The elbow should be relatively extended if possible. This position allows for two-thirds more circulation than if the upper extremity is held at the level of the waist.[84,86] Patients should be instructed to keep the hand and upper extremity elevated 24 hours per day or whenever possible. Initial postoperative edema is prevented by the bulky dressing, with gentle even compression while the hand and wrist are splinted. If postoperative edema is present, the extremity usually should be elevated for at least 3 to 5 days.

Edema is also detrimental after fractures and can occur in and after protective casting is removed. It is essential that edema of the upper extremity be decreased as quickly as possible. Elastic wraps such as Coban (3M [Product Index 6]) (Fig. 54-1), Cowrap, Tubigrip, dental rubber dam, or a thick string wrap around the fingers from distal to proximal can be helpful.[25] Elastic wraps and elastic dressings also are used. These materials are inexpensive and effective in decreasing edema [Product Index 1, 2, 3, 4, 5]. Active range of motion exercises can be performed during

---

* References 22,35,42-44,59,67,69.
† References 16,20,28,29,58,87.

* References 6,7,27,30,38,52,57,88.

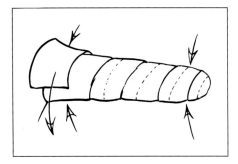

FIGURE 54-1

Elastic paper wrapping. Begin at the tip of the finger and wrap in a spiral direction toward the base of the finger. Overlap each turn by ½ width of the wrap. Pressure should be firm but not painful and should decrease as you wrap toward the base of the finger.

and after wrapping of the hands and wrists and are helpful in decreasing the swelling through the pumping action of the active muscle contraction. Elastic gloves (Isotoner [Product Index 5]) and elastic sleeves (Jobst) with graded pressure distal to proximal are also helpful in decreasing edema.[3,40] Decongestant massage should be performed before the elastic gloves or garments are applied.[48] Elastic garments are available from the Jobst Institute or Barton-Carey, Medi, and Segvaris [Product Index 1, 2, 3, 4]. These elastic garments help to enforce fluid dynamics of the upper extremity.[32,89] They can be worn during activities of daily living.

Intermittent pneumatic compression pumps are useful in decreasing edema that is caused by soft-tissue injury or reflex dystrophy or postoperatively if the wounds are healed and no open wounds are present. It is important that the extremity is not painful during the use of the intermittent pump. The intermittent pneumatic compression devices can apply even pressure to the upper extremity. It is helpful to place the hand and wrist in a plastic bag of Styrofoam beads and then insert the extremity into the pneumatic pump so that the pumping action can be equal between the fingers and at the wrist creases.[40,79,84] The sleeve in the pump is intermittently inflated to about 50 mm Hg and then deflated as tolerated.

Control of edema is vital for tissue healing.[31,78] Continued active range of motion of the shoulder, elbow, forearm, wrist, and digits is important. Reeducation of the wrist flexion and extension synergistic patterning is vital. Immobilization of the joints results in capsular and ligamentous tightness that causes loss of range of motion.[1] Bones and soft-tissue structures that have been repaired require immobilization for healing, but for any joint that does not require immobilization, range of motion exercises should begin as soon as possible.[20,68,79,90] Gentle,

active-assisted range of motion exercises should be done without force. Tightness and contractures may result from prolonged immobilization.[1]

Immobilization also decreases muscle power, and this loss of muscle power or innervation of the muscles can lead to decreased range of motion, tightness, and contractures. The shoulder can become stiff and painful when the hand, wrist, and forearm are immobilized and the extremity is not used in a normal fashion. Specific range of motion exercises are needed to help the patient maintain shoulder range, elbow range, and finger range when immobilization is necessary at the wrist.[79] The patient can be taught to do these exercises in a supine, sitting, or standing position.[78] The patient is often more comfortable in a supine position and can relax and avoid guarding and muscle misuse and overuse.[78] Active-assisted and passive-relaxed range of motion of the shoulder and elbow in these cases are important. The exercises should be assisted until the patient can do the range of motion actively and correctly. Elbow, forearm, and wrist range of motion should begin when appropriate. The surgeon must specify the degree of permissible range of motion on the basis of the operative procedures.[21,37,47]

It is important to know the goals to be achieved and the degree of protection needed for the structures after operation. Tendon and nerve repairs, ligament or capsular repairs or releases, and stability of the joint fractures should be clarified with the surgeon before the hand rehabilitation is attempted.[90] Active-assisted range of motion exercises are done without stretch and applied so that the patient can coordinate and produce the muscle contractions through the available range of motion. When the purpose is to increase the arc of motion, active-assisted or active range of motion with stress can be used as long as it does not cause pain, guarding, cocontraction, and jamming of the joints.[79,90] Stretching should be gentle and prolonged. Stretching and active force help mobilize adhesions of the tendon or move planes restricted by proximal motion of the tendon. When adhesions of the tendons or movable planes restrict the proximal range of motion, gentle stretching is necessary by gradually and gently increasing the range of motion of the digits and wrist and by gentle prolonged contraction of the muscles. These two mechanisms are the only forces that can move the tendons with adhesions and overcome joint contracture.

After stretching, active range of motion can effectively mobilize and maintain motion of scarred, adherent tendons. Passive range of motion implies motion by an external force applied to produce motion. Passive range of motion may be used after operation or in a patient who is paralyzed, where there is muscle weakness present, or if neurologic lesions are present [Product Index 9, 10, 11, 12, 13].[78] Continuous passive range of motion machines, dynamic splinting [Product Index 8 and 14], an occupational physical or hand therapist, and the patient's own contralateral hand can be used to perform the required passive motion.[78] The patient must be fully relaxed to prevent harm and undesirable force on the extremity. Passive range of motion is not stretching and must be done without muscle contraction.[78] These exercises are done slowly with fully relaxed muscles to increase the available range of motion.

Gentle and prolonged passive stretching by external force can also be prescribed. Stretches can be as brief as 1 min or as long as 20 min. Usually after operation, connective tissue needs about 6 weeks to regain adequate tensile strength.[21,38,78,90] Therefore, gentle prolonged stretching should be delayed until the tensile strength is adequate. The prolonged gentle stretching force is much more effective and safer than high-deforming forces for short periods.[21] Repetitions with rest intervals can increase the recovery process. The patient should tolerate these procedures without pain, swelling, or fatigue.

Various passive range of motion devices are on the market: Toronto Portable Wrist and Hand CPM, Staniger Portable Wrist and Hand, Kinetek, and Dynasplints are a few of the helpful devices. The clinical use of these machines requires careful monitoring.[78] They must be properly fitted and should be well tolerated by the patient. They can aid healing of cartilage, tendons, and ligaments by producing continuous motion and can prevent adhesions and joint stiffness without interfering with the healing process. However, patients often become dependent on the device and do not use their own muscles for specific range.[78]

Specific guidelines must be given to the patient for the use of the passive range of motion, such as when and at what speed the machine should be used and at what angle and force the joint should be moved. These machines can never take the place of active motion, and when healing tissues are stressed, the movements must be carefully controlled and repetitive. In properly selected cases, passive range of motion devices can be used, particularly if there is fatigue of the skeletal muscles during the active movement and lack of control over active movement.[36] Proper alignment and motion must be carefully monitored. These devices should not achieve the extremes of joint motion. These machines are expensive to rent and time is needed to initiate the treatment, to educate the patient, and to fit the extremity. When time is limited, the devices can be more frustrating than helpful. Excessive cost is also a factor when using passive range of motion machines, so their application must be carefully selected. However, the final result may be cost effective and should be documented to justify the cost factor. The patient must be comfortable with using the machine and be warned against improper stretching from poor alignment, which can occur if the machines are not fitted properly.[36,78]

Joint mobilization techniques performed properly by the therapist can help to gain capsular motion and full joint movement in the extremity. With proper technique, overstretching or injury to the joint capsule does not occur. Friction massage can be helpful to improve range of motion of the skin that is tight over scar tissue. This massage softens scar tissue to allow better range of motion. Lotions such as Lubriderm, Eucerin cream, Alpha-Keri lotion, white Vaseline Intensive Care lotion, lanolin creams, and Vanicream or cocoa butter can be used during the massage.[78] Elastomer pads, iodoform pads, silo pads [Product Index 16 and 17], or elastic wraps and elastic garments can be used to apply constant firm pressure to help soften scars.[78]

Activities of daily living should be increased gradually as the patient's range of motion, strength, endurance, and comfort increase. Exercises and activities for strengthening and endurance must not cause pain. There is usually some muscle discomfort, but it should be tolerated and not painful. There should be no signs of overuse or muscle misuse when these activities are increased or when strengthening exercises are done.[78,79] Techniques to train the nondominant hand to take over activities from the dominant hand have been helpful in patients with permanent disability of the dominant hand. Long-term follow-up is essential for patients with severe injuries.[78,79] When the patient is first injured, it is often necessary to prescribe assistive devices to help activities of daily living. It is often difficult when the patient is first injured, however, to determine which assistive devices may need to be permanent. Often patients are resistant to these assistive devices when first injured. These devices may be quite helpful to get the patients back into functional activities and activities of daily living.

Often special devices such as finger traps, web-space dressing, flexion gloves, and rubber-band strapping for stretching can afford prolonged passive stretching and be used to increase range of motion. With prolonged immobility, however, dense adhesions and rigid capsular tightness can occur, resulting in loss of joint motion of the fingers and wrist, and decrease functional activities when the wrist is involved. In these circumstances, joint jacks, knuckle benders, and reverse knuckle benders can be effective in stretching joint contractures and directing proper joint motion. The joint motion must be in the proper plane and performed without cutting off circulation, injuring the skin, or compressing peripheral nerves. These devices must be fitted properly and worn effectively to avoid soft-tissue damage and to avoid increased pain. The angle of pull must be effective and not compromise the adjacent circulation.

SPLINTING

An integral part of wrist rehabilitation is the use of appropriate splinting.[23,50,60,61,63] Splints are applied to the external surface to support or immobilize the segment in a certain position, prevent deformities, maintain correction, relieve pain, mobilize joints, exercise parts, and assist or support weakened and paralyzed parts.* Different splints can be used to substitute for absent motor power, stretch contracted parts, provide and allow motion, and supply correct forces to increase directional control.[54-56,77,78] Often these splints can provide traction to improve deformities and increase function. Thus, splinting can be used for either individual joints or an entire region such as the elbow, wrist, hand, or any portion of the upper extremity. Low-temperature thermoplastics, such as neoprene [Product Index 7], lightweight orthotic material (Kydex [Product Index 15]), and metal-like casting material can be used to fabricate these splints. The newer thermoplastic splint materials allow quick molding onto the patient and give the physician, hand therapist, physical therapist, and occupational therapist an innovative and comfortable material with which to design the orthosis. Many prefabricated splints of plastic, thermoplastic, canvas, and elastic are available, but they usually do not fit as well as the custom-made splints.[77,79,81,82]

---

* References 54,56,61,71,77,79.

GENERAL PRINCIPLES OF SPLINTING

The splint for the wrist must be prescribed by a physician who must indicate if the basis of the splint is to be palmar, dorsal, radial, or ulnar and the general purpose of the splint. The position of the segments to be splinted should be indicated in the prescription. The splint must be needed and meet the purpose of the prescription. Fabrication of the splint can be done by a physical therapist, occupational therapist, hand therapist, or orthotist.

The orthopedist or physiatrist should evaluate the finished orthosis to determine proper fit and outline the goals and purposes of the splint to the patient as well as to the therapist. The length of time that the orthosis should be worn and the precautions to be observed should be outlined by the physician and the therapist and understood by the patient. Often, more than one splint is ordered for the patient, and the sequence of wearing must be given to the patient with specific details. Occasionally, the patient may be permitted to develop a tolerance to the wearing of the orthosis.[54-56,77] The patient must know how to apply the splint, how long it should be worn, how to care for the splint, and why the splint is prescribed. The splint needs to be evaluated periodically for proper fit. The return or loss of muscle bulk or function, increasing or decreasing edema, continuation or lessening of muscle spasms, and arthritic changes or growth in the case of children often alter the fit of the splint.[10,49,54,75] The

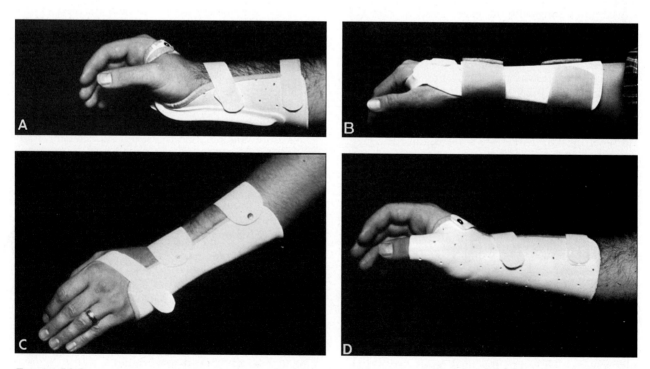

FIGURE 54-2

Common static wrist splints. **A,** Palmar splint; wrist extension. **B,** Dorsal splint. **C,** Ulnar splint. **D,** Radial splint.

splint must inhibit sensation as little as possible. The splint should avoid damage to the underlying parts, avoid pressure areas and insensate skin areas, and avoid compression of the digital arteries and nerves.[78,79,90]

The successful use of the splint depends in large part on acceptance by the patient as well as the patient's ability to use the splint effectively. The splint must be of good design, lightweight material, and yet capable of extended wear. The patient must also be capable of learning how to use the device, and it must not be more trouble than it is worth or the splint will be rejected.[20,77] The patient must find the splint's appearance acceptable. The splint should not cause rashes, pressure sores, pressure neuropathies, or circulatory problems. The cost/benefit ratio of the orthosis needs to be considered. The orthosis must be able to be cleaned and maintained. The team of therapists, orthopedist, and physician must work together to make suggestions, modify the device, and train the patient in acceptance and use of the orthosis.[77]

Dynamic splinting materials may be made of high-temperature plastics, light casts, thermoplastic mesh rolls, metal strips and wires, neoprene, low-temperature thermoplastics, fiberglass, leather, elastomer, and fabrics.[77,85,95] They can be held on with hooks, loop tapes, webbing, self-adhesive tapes, loop-type composites, Ace wraps, and elastics.[76] The direction, magnitude, and point of application of forces applied by the splint are important in the fabrication.[5,23,77,90] The orthosis should be positioned to maintain the normal arches of the hand. Effectiveness of these forces depends on the point of application, the distance from the axis of rotation, and the magnitude of the forces. Motion of the joint can be in rotation, translational, or a combination

of these two.[5] Rotation is angular motion, translation is motion without change of angulation orientation, and torque is the strength of the rotation tendencies. To reduce the pressure over the areas of the hand or wrist, the area to which force is applied should be maximized. When necessary, leverage can be used to amplify the forces. Optimal rotational forces can be increased by dynamic traction when a joint needs to be mobilized.[23]

In the wrist, the splint crosses successive joints within the longitudinal segment and passive mobility of the successive joints must be considered. This may be necessary to block or restrain some motions in some joints to mobilize a successive joint.[23] As the distance between the joint axis and the attachment of the dynamic assistance increases, the amount of torque on the joint increases. This dynamic assist must be placed at a 90° angle to the joint being stretched to maximize the angle of pull fully. The greater the flexion deformity, the less effective the orthosis becomes in its ability to correct the deformity.[23] Effective reciprocal parallel forces must be considered when designing the orthosis and the placement of the strapping. Contouring the splint and rounding the inner corners of the splint increase the durability.[23] Any strenuous movement between a splint and the skin should be eliminated to prevent maceration and skin irritation. The correct alignment is important to prevent nonperpendicular pull and abnormal rotational forces. The splint must be padded and accurately contoured.[23]

TYPES OF SPLINTING

Static Splinting. There are two general types of splints: static and dynamic. Some splints are a combination of

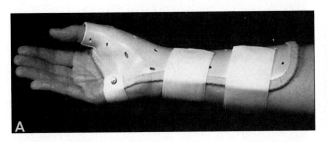
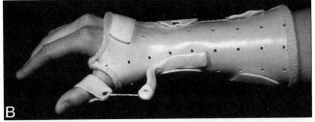
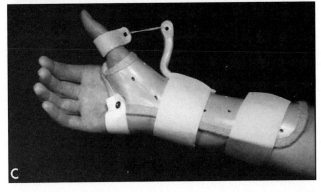

FIGURE 54-3

A, Radial thumb shell splint; palmar view. **B,** Radial wrist dynamic thumb extension splint; radial view. **C,** Radial wrist dynamic thumb extension splint; palmar view.

static and dynamic principles. The static splint does not allow motion (Fig. 54-2).[78,79] It is prescribed according to the *joint* it is to hold (i.e., wrist splint, thumb abduction splint). It is used to support weakness, afford immobilization in a desired position, prevent deformities, and maintain a certain correction of posture during

healing.[54,61,77] Static splinting can be used as an added support for external fixation and comfort of the patient and for special accessories. It is also used to rest inflamed joints and tendons, after injury or during healing[70-72] or arthroplasty,[53] for protection of a healing fracture, or after tendon or peripheral nerve repair. The static splint can be used to relieve pain, particularly in the case of arthritic changes of the joint.[24,41]

Progressive stretching of a contracted joint can be helped with serial splinting. A thumb shell splint, for example, can be used for the treatment of degenerative

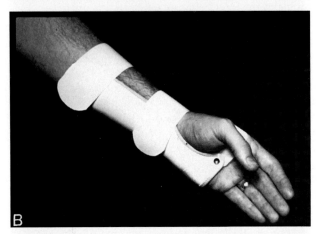

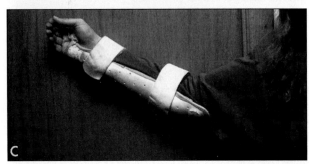

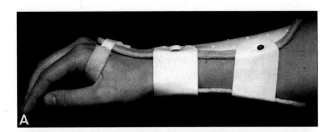

FIGURE 54-4

Ulnar gutter splint. **A,** Radial view; Velcro straps. **B,** Palmar view. **C,** Extended to elbow, with added pronation and supination control.

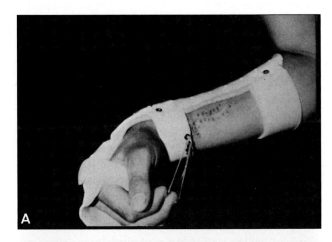

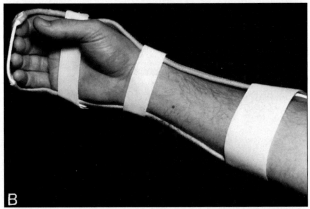

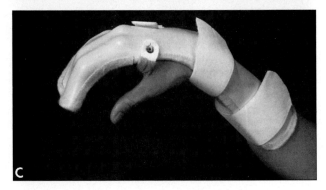

FIGURE 54-6

"Shepherd's crook" wrist splints with wrist flexion and finger flexion post flexor tendon repair. **A,** Dynamic finger flexion assist. **B,** Static dorsal shell, palmar view. **C,** Dorsal shell, dorsal view.

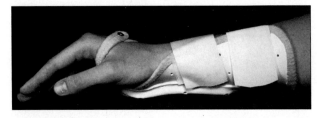

FIGURE 54-5

Palmar wrist extension resting splint; wrist neutral.

arthritis, rheumatoid arthritis, tenosynovitis,[91] and scaphoid fractures (Fig. 54-3) and also to maintain the thumb web space. It can also be used to support a subluxation of the metacarpal joint, stabilize an injured carpometacarpal thumb joint, or hold support after fusion of an interphalangeal, metacarpophalangeal, or thumb basal joint. Stabilization of the wrist with a long trough is preferable up to at least two-thirds of the forearm.

A radial-based splint is used in metacarpal arthritis, tendinitis of the thumb, tenosynovitis of the wrist, intersection syndrome, and fracture of the scaphoid and carpal bones.[61,77,78,91] This allows movement of the fingers and occasionally the interphalangeal joint of the thumb. It can be used for tendon repairs and transfers, after a surgical procedure of the carpal bones, for wrist stabilization or fusion, and for thumb carpometacarpal arthrosis.[80]

An ulnar-based wrist splint is used in arthritis of the ulnar carpal bones as well as in ulnar styloid fracture, subluxation or dislocation of the distal radioulnar joint, subluxation of the fourth and fifth metacarpal heads, or fractures of the distal or ulnar carpal bones (Fig. 54-4).[24,41,78,79] It can also be used in triangular fibrocartilage repair and sprains.

A static palmar splint supports the wrist in a resting position and is often used in carpal tunnel syndrome, allowing the proximal transverse arc of the hand to be cupped (Fig. 54-5).[19,76,79] The fingers should be allowed to move freely. This palmar-based splint is used for functional stabilization of the wrist.

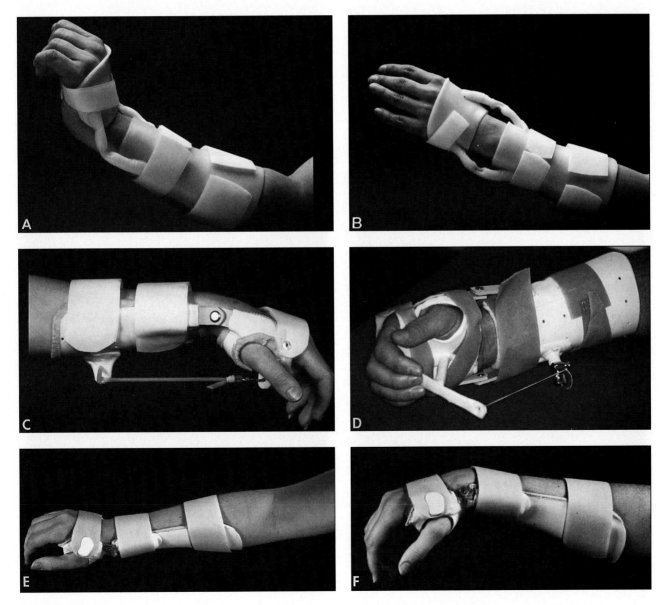

FIGURE 54-7

Dynamic wrist splint. **A,** Plastic hinge splint, extension. **B,** Plastic hinge splint, neutral position. **C,** Dynamic flexion hinge. **D,** Static pull flexion hinge. **E,** Extension-flexion metal hinge; extension. **F,** Extension-flexion metal hinge; flexion.

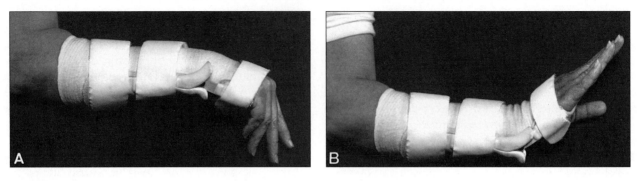

FIGURE 54-8

Controlled motion. **A,** Neutral wrist flexion block. **B,** Wrist extension block.

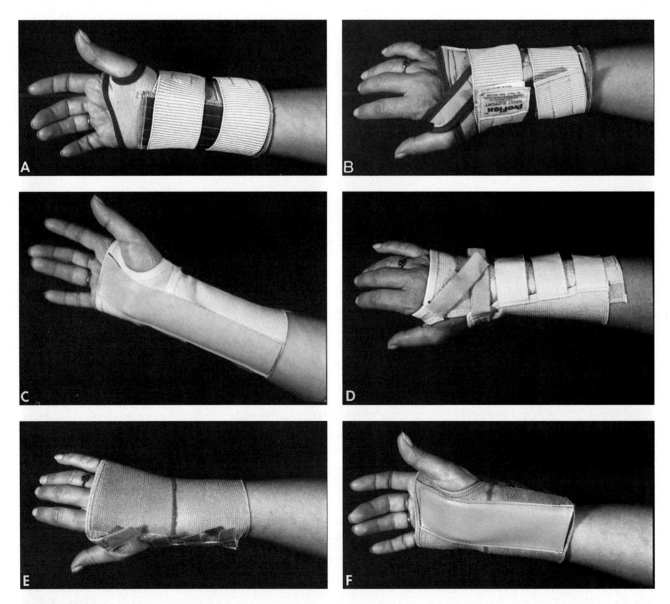

FIGURE 54-9

Commercially made splints. **A,** ProFlex palmar view. **B,** ProFlex dorsal view. **C,** AOA long; palmar view. **D,** AOA short; dorsal view. **E,** Elastic, semirigid; dorsal view. **F,** Elastic, semirigid; palmar view.

If it is used during function, the wrist should be placed in approximately 20° to 40° of wrist extension, whereas a resting wrist splint should be in 0° to 15° of extension.[54,77,79] A static palmar splint of the wrist can be used in healing carpal fractures,[47] after soft-tissue injuries of the wrist (e.g., a sprain to the wrist), in tendinitis of the wrist flexors or extensors, after burns about the wrist, after arthroplasty, and after ligamentous repairs of the wrist.[54,77-79]

The dorsal wrist splint stabilizes the wrist, allowing fingers and thumb motion and also allowing the palmar areas to be free for enhanced sensation. This also allows the palmar surfaces to be free for inspection and sensory input. After nerve and tendon repair, the extremity is splinted to prevent traction on the repaired nerves and tendons.[8,83] This can be the "shepherd's crook"-type flexor splint (Fig. 54-6) in the case of flexor tendon repair and nerve repair at or about the wrist and fingers or the reverse extensor splint can be used in repair of the extensor tendons or joint capsule about the wrist (Fig. 54-7).*

Dynamic Splinting. When movement is desired but protection of the extremity is needed, a dynamic splint is prescribed.[54,61,77,79] The dynamic splint can be used to substitute for paralyzed muscles and allow assisted motion in weakened muscles, supply a corrective force around the wrist, pull against impending contractures, or increase function. The dynamic splint can be used for strengthening opposing muscles.[77] The dynamic splint can be made of orthotic material, metal, spring wire, or elastic.[54,77-79] Springs, elastic thread, or rubber bands are often used for the dynamic motors of the splint. The dynamic orthosis is used to align, resist, assist, and simulate movement.[77,90] Dynamic attachments to the splint

---
* References 18,21,46,74,77,83.

can give continuous prolonged stretch for contractures of the joint in a flexed or extended position (Fig. 54-7). Dynamic pull should be gentle and not cause pain, swelling, or undue pressure. Dynamic attachments should give a continuous prolonged stretch for contracture of the joint. The tension depends on the length of the rubber bands or the elastic threads.[78] Dynamic splinting can be used to increase range of motion.

A dynamic orthosis can be used with weakened extensor muscles, to support healing fractures where motion is desirable, and after extensor or flexor tendon repair and after wrist arthroplasties where motion is desired but must be a controlled motion in a desired plane (Fig. 54-8). The dynamic splint can be used to resist abnormal or undesirable movements.[78,79] Also, dynamic forearm splints aid in spinal cord and brachial plexus injuries to correct or prevent wrist contractures. The dynamic wrist splint allows support of the wrist while controlling flexion and extension and radial and ulnar deviation motions. Assisted flexion or extension can be provided. This type of dynamic orthosis can be used after wrist arthroplasty,[53] synovectomy, and proximal row carpectomy (Fig. 54-8). These splints are particularly helpful in instances of tightness in wrist flexion and extension after surgery or to gain useful motion after carpal fractures, Colles fractures, and carpal ligament repairs. Often a dorsal- or palmar-based dynamic splint is used in our practice after major carpal reconstructive surgery when motion is desirable and necessary. Functional movements can be simulated in the presence of paralysis by specially made dynamic splinting that can be activated by the patient's own muscles, as in a myoelectric orthosis or external power orthosis.[61,77,78] When the patient's own wrist extensor muscles are present but the wrist flexor muscles are paralyzed or weak, as in spinal cord injury, a flexor tenodesis orthosis can be helpful.

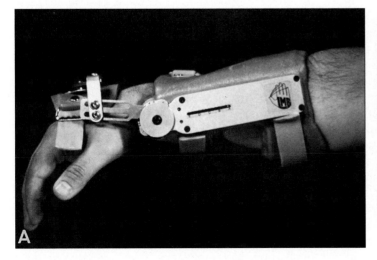
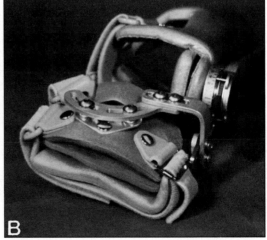

FIGURE 54-10

LMB splint with prolonged dynamic stretch. **A,** Radial view. **B,** Forward view.

Commercially Available Splinting. There are many commercially available splints [Product Index 7, 9, 14, 18]. Excellent articles have compared them.[19,81,82] Most of the available hinges can be added to the wrist splints and can be used to block or enhance dynamic immobilization of the wrist (Fig. 54-9).[45] Partial splints can often make fitting a problem.[81,82] The fit of a ready-made orthosis may be sacrificed for convenience and cost; unfortunately, it often allows some motion despite the intended support of the wrist (Fig. 54-9).[77] The inflatable air splints have been used for controlled contact immobilization to decrease spasm and to control edema after a mastectomy, amputation, or major trauma. These air splints can be used to support the extremity in emergency fracture management.[77] A proper fit is often difficult to achieve and the fit must be evaluated. The LMB orthosis for the wrist can be helpful because it can be set at a certain pressure, but it must be fitted properly (Fig. 54-10). Wire-form splints are helpful for bathing and hygiene of the wrist. There are also commercially made dynamic splints with a motor drive for both the fingers and the wrist (Fig. 54-11). Finally, the Thomas suspension splint has been used in radial nerve palsies and does allow dynamic thumb extension and wrist extension, and the Openheimer spring splint supports both wrist and thumb in extension. However, the potential malalignment and pull of these dynamic single-bar supports leave much to be desired in mechanically supporting areas.[77]

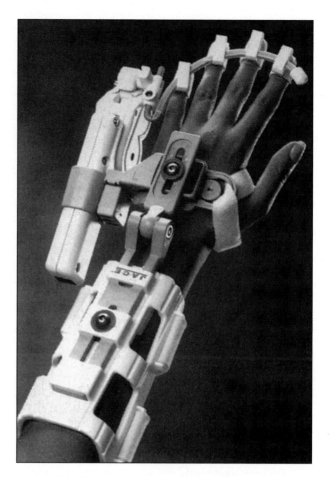

FIGURE 54-11

Toronto dynamic wrist and finger motion splint.

CONCLUSION

The primary goal of rehabilitation of the wrist is to maximize the residual functional capacity of a patient with an injured, operated, or diseased wrist, hand, or upper extremity.[94] The second and equal goal is to return the patient quickly and efficiently to appropriate levels of employment and activities. The patient is usually referred for rehabilitation shortly after diagnosis of a disease entity or completion of a surgical procedure or casting of fractures. As soon as disease is recognized in the wrist, therapy is recommended at the earliest possible stage so that rehabilitation can be maximized and management of residual contractures and complications is minimized.[12] The goals of therapy are to prevent or decrease edema; assist in tissue healing; relieve pain; assist in relaxation; prevent misuse, disuse, or overuse of the muscles; avoid muscle spasms; improve coordination; and provide proper tendon and muscle reeducation.[9,12,51] At appropriate times, desensitization of hypersensitive areas and sensory reeducation are important. Rehabilitation measures can maintain an increased range of motion and provide independence, endurance, and improved performance of activities of daily living.

During the rehabilitation process, splints may be prescribed. These are of two types: static and dynamic.[12] Static splints for the wrist are used to protect soft tissues, promote stretching, prevent contractures, and support the wrist after fractures or surgical repair to facilitate healing of the bone and soft tissue. The splint can be placed in a resting position or in a position of function and can be used to maintain increased motion that has been achieved after range of motion exercises. The static splint helps to provide rest and protection.

The dynamic splint allows movement. It may be hinged or have external joints. It requires some type of power source: the patient's own muscles, rubber bands, elastic, motors, or springs. Dynamic splints help to resist, assist, or simulate movement and allow mobility of the joint in a specific direction to be controlled. The dynamic splints can be used for prolonged passive stretch, contraction of the capsule or ligaments of the wrist, or after wrist reconstruction surgery. All splints must be carefully prescribed and reviewed with the patient and therapist regarding the purpose, method of application, and limitations. Finally, review in detail explanations of wearing schedules as they are combined with physical therapy and work rehabilitation efforts.

PRODUCT INDEX

1. Barton-Carey Medical Products
   P.O. Box 421
   Perrysburg, Ohio 43552
   1-800-421-0444
   fax (419) 874-0888
2. Medi, USA, L.P.
   76 W. Seegers Road
   Arlington Heights, Illinois 60005
   (708) 640-8400
3. Segvaris Inc.; Ganzoni & Cie AG
   St. Gallen, Switzerland
4. Jobst Co.
   635 Miami Street
   Toledo, Ohio 43605
   1-800-537-1063
5. Isotoner gloves, Aris-Isotoner Glove
   New York, New York
6. Coban Medical Products Division, 3M
   St. Paul, Minnesota
7. Neoprene, North Coast Medical
   San Jose, California
8. Commercial Dynamic Wrist Splint, Ultra Flex
   St. Paul, Minnesota
9. Dyna Splint System
   Corporate Headquarters
   1300 Route 73
   Mount Laurel, New Jersey 08054
   (609) 778-1166
   fax (609) 778-8965
   or 645 Baltimore Annapolis Boulevard
   Severna Park, Maryland 21146
10. Joce W55D Wrist CPM, Thera Kinetics
    1300 Route 73
    Mount Laurel, New Jersey 08054
    (800) 234-0900
    fax (609) 778-8965
11. Danniflex™ 200, Donninger Medical Technology Inc.
    4140 Fisher Road
    Columbus, Ohio 43228-1067
    1-800-225-1814
    fax (614) 276-8271
12. Mobilimb™ WI Wrist CPM, Toronto Medical
    901 Dillingham Road
    Pickering, Ontario, Canada L1W 2Y5
    (416) 420-3303
    fax (416) 420-3970
    In USA, P.O. Box 26
    Yellow Springs, Ohio 45387
    1-800-289-5139
13. Kinetec 8080™ CPM for hand and wrist, Smith & Nephew Richards Inc.
    1450 Brooks Road
    Memphis, Tennessee 38116
14. Phoenix Outriggers and Low Profile Dynamic Outriggers and Aquaplast, WFR/Aquaplast Corp.
    P.O. Box 635
    Wycokoff, New Jersey 07481
    1-800-526-5247
15. Kydex Long Opponens Hand and Wrist Orthosis, Restorative Care of America Inc
    Corporate Headquarters
    11236 47th Street North
    Clearwater, Florida 34622
    (813) 573-1595
16. Silastic, Dow Corning Wright
    Arlington, Indiana
17. Otoform, Dreze
    Unna, West Germany
18. Basic Wrist Splint, P.M.D.
    2020 Grand Avenue
    P.O. Box 19777
    Kansas City, Missouri 64141
19. Computerized goniometers:
    a) Loredan Biomedical
       Davis, California
    b) NK Biotechnical Engineering
       Minneapolis, Minnesota
    c) Baltimore Therapeutics Equipment
       Hanover, Maryland
    d) Cybex
       Ronkonkoma, New York

REFERENCES

1. Akeson WH, Amiel D, Mechanic GL, et al.: Collagen cross-linking alterations in joint contractures. Changes in the reducible cross-links in periarticular connective tissue collagen after nine weeks of immobilization, *Connective Tissue Res* 5:15-19, 1977.
2. Anderson PA, Chanoski CE, Devan DL, et al.: Normative study of grip and wrist flexion strength employing a BTE Work Simulator, *J Hand Surg [Am]* 15:420-425, 1990.
3. Aris-Isotoner Glove, Aris Gloves, Inc.; 417 Fifth Avenue, New York, NY 10016.
4. Ballard M, Baxter P, Bruening L, et al.: Work therapy and return to work, *Hand Clin* 2:247-258, 1986.

5. Bender LF: *Upper extremity orthotics.* In Kottke FJ, Stillwell GK, Lehman JF, editors: *Krusen's handbook of physical medicine and rehabilitation,* ed 3, Philadelphia, 1982, WB Saunders, p 519.

6. Borrell RM, Henley EJ, Ho P, et al.: Fluidotherapy: evaluation of a new heat modality, *Arch Phys Med Rehabil* 58:69-71, 1977.

7. Borrell RM, Parker R, Henley EJ, et al.: Comparison of in vivo temperatures produced by hydrotherapy, paraffin wax treatment, and fluidotherapy, *Phys Ther* 60:1273-1276, 1980.

8. Bosarge J: Finger replant patient undergoing rehabilitation, *J Rehabil* 42:29-30, 1976.

9. Bunker TD, Potter B, Barton NJ: Continuous passive motion following flexor tendon repair, *J Hand Surg [Br]* 14:406-411, 1989.

10. Byron PM: *Splinting of the hand of a child.* In Hunter JM, Schneider LH, Mackin EJ, et al., editors: *Rehabilitation of the hand: surgery and therapy,* St. Louis, 1990, CV Mosby, pp 1147-1152.

11. Casley-Smith JR: The structural basis for the conservative treatment of lymphedema, *Lymphology* 10:13-25, 1977.

12. Cooney WP, Schutt AH: *Rehabilitation of the wrist.* In Nickel VL, Botte MJ, editors: *Orthopaedic rehabilitation,* ed 2, New York, 1992, Churchill Livingstone.

13. Curtis RM, Engalitcheff J Jr: A work simulator for rehabilitating the upper extremity—preliminary report, *J Hand Surg [Am]* 6:499-501, 1981.

14. Dellon AL: The moving two-point discrimination test: clinical evaluation of the quickly adapting fiber/receptor system, *J Hand Surg [Am]* 3:474-481, 1978.

15. Dellon AL: *Evaluation of sensibility and re-education of sensation in the hand,* Baltimore, 1981, Williams & Wilkins.

16. Dellon AL: The vibrometer, *Plast Reconstr Surg* 71:427-431, 1983.

17. Dellon AL, Curtis RM, Edgerton MT: Reeducation of sensation in the hand after nerve injury and repair, *Plast Reconstr Surg* 53:297-305, 1974.

18. Dovelle S, Heeter PK: The Washington Regimen: rehabilitation of the hand following flexor tendon injuries, *Phys Ther* 69:1034-1040, 1989.

19. Eberhard BA, Sylvester KL, Ansell BM: A comparative study of orthoplast cock-up splints versus ready-made Droitwich work splints in juvenile chronic arthritis, *Disabil Rehabil* 15:41-43, 1993.

20. Edinburg M, Widgerow AD, Biddulph SL: Early postoperative mobilization of flexor tendon injuries using a modification of the Kleinert technique, *J Hand Surg [Am]* 12:34-38, 1987.

21. Evans RB: Clinical application of controlled stress to the healing extensor tendon: a review of 112 cases, *Phys Ther* 69:1041-1049, 1989.

22. Fess EE: *Documentation: essential elements of an upper extremity assessment battery.* In Hunter JM, Schneider LH, Mackin EJ, et al., editors: *Rehabilitation of the hand: surgery and therapy,* ed 3, St. Louis, 1990, CV Mosby, pp 53-81.

23. Fess EE, Gettle KS, Strickland JW: *Hand splinting: principles and methods,* St. Louis, 1981, CV Mosby, pp 38-96.

24. Findley TW, Halpern D, Easton JK: Wrist subluxation in juvenile rheumatoid arthritis: pathophysiology and management, *Arch Phys Med Rehabil* 64:69-74, 1983.

25. Flowers KR: String wrapping versus massage for reducing digital volume, *Phys Ther* 68:57-59, 1988.

26. Foldi M: Physiology and pathophysiology of lymph flow, *Lymphology* 10:1-11, 1977.

27. Fried T, Johnson R, McCracken W: Transcutaneous electrical nerve stimulation: its role in the control of chronic pain, *Arch Phys Med Rehabil* 65:228-231, 1984.

28. Frohring WO, Kohn PM, Bosma JF, et al.: Changes in the vibratory sense of patients with poliomyelitis as measured by the pallesthesiometer, *Am J Dis Child* 69:89-91, 1945.

29. Frykman GK, Waylett J: Rehabilitation of peripheral nerve injuries, *Orthop Clin North Am* 12:361-379, 1981.

30. Gangarosa LP, Park NH, Fong BC, et al.: Conductivity of drugs used for iontophoresis, *J Pharm Sci* 67:1439-1443, 1978.

31. Giudice ML: Effects of continuous passive motion and elevation on hand edema, *Am J Occup Ther* 44:914-921, 1990.

32. Griffin JW, Newsome LS, Stralka SW, et al.: Reduction of chronic posttraumatic hand edema: a comparison of high voltage pulsed current, intermittent pneumatic compression, and placebo treatments, *Phys Ther* 70:279-286, 1990.

33. Grunert BK, Devine CA, Matloub HS, et al.: Flashbacks after traumatic hand injuries: prognostic indicators, *J Hand Surg [Am]* 13:125-127, 1988.

34. Guyton AC, Granger HJ, Taylor AE: Interstitial fluid pressure, *Physiol Rev* 51:527-563, 1971.

35. Heck CV, Hendryson IE, Rowe CR: *Joint motion: method of measuring and recording,* 1965, American Academy of Orthopaedic Surgeons.

36. Herbin ML: Work capacity evaluation for occupational hand injuries, *J Hand Surg [Am]* 12:958-961, 1987.

37. Hung LK, Chan A, Chang J, et al.: Early controlled active mobilization with dynamic splintage for treatment of extensor tendon injuries, *J Hand Surg [Am]* 15:251-257, 1990.

38. Hunter JM, Schneider LH, Mackin EJ, et al.: *Rehabilitation of the hand: surgery and therapy,* ed 3, St. Louis, 1990, CV Mosby.

39. Jebsen RH, Taylor N, Trieschmann RB, et al.: An objective and standardized test of hand function, *Arch Phys Med Rehabil* 50:311-319, 1969.

40. Jobst Glove, Jobst Institute Inc., 635 Miami Street, Toledo, OH 43605.

41. Johnson PM, Sandkvist G, Eberhardt K, et al.: The usefulness of nocturnal resting splints in the treatment of ulnar deviation of the rheumatoid hand, *Clin Rheumatol* 11:72-75, 1992.

42. Jones JM, Schenck RR, Chesney RB: Digital replantation and amputation—comparison of function, *J Hand Surg [Am]* 7:183-189, 1982.

43. Kellor M, Frost J, Silberberg N, et al.: Hand strength and dexterity, *Am J Occup Ther* 25:77-83, 1971.

44. Kellor M, Krondrosuk R, Iversen I: Technical manual: hand strength and dexterity test. Kenny Rehabilitation Institute, Minneapolis, MN, 1971, Research Division.

45. Kennedy JM: *Orthopaedic splints and appliances,* London, 1974, Baillière-Tindall, p 48.

46. Knapp ME: The contribution of Sister Elizabeth Kenny to the treatment of poliomyelitis, *Arch Phys Med Rehabil* 36:510-517, 1955.

47. Knapp ME: *Aftercare of fractures.* In Krusen FH, editor: *Handbook of physical medicine and rehabilitation,* ed 2, Philadelphia, 1971, WB Saunders, pp 579-582.

48. Knapp ME: *Massage.* In Krusen FH, editor: *Handbook of physical medicine and rehabilitation,* ed 2, Philadelphia, 1971, WB Saunders, pp 382-384.

49. Koman LA, Gelberman RH, Toby EB, et al.: Cerebral palsy. Management of the upper extremity, *Clin Orthop* 253:62-74, 1990.

50. Krusen FH: *Handbook of physical medicine and rehabilitation,* ed 2, Philadelphia, 1971, WB Saunders.

51. Lane C: Therapy for the occupationally injured hand, *Hand Clin* 2:593-602, 1986.

52. Lehmann JF: *Diathermy.* In Krusen FH, editor: *Handbook of physical medicine and rehabilitation,* ed 2, Philadelphia, 1971, WB Saunders, pp 316-321.

53. Linscheid RL, Beckenbaugh RD: Total arthroplasty of the wrist to relieve pain and increase motion, *Geriatrics* 31:48-52, 1976.

54. Long C, Schutt AH: *Upper limb orthotics.* In Redford JB, editor: *Orthotics etcetera,* ed 3, Baltimore, 1986, Williams & Wilkins, pp 198-277.

55. Malick MH: *Manual of dynamic hand splinting with thermoplastic materials,* ed 2, Pittsburgh, 1978, Harmarville Rehabilitation Center.

56. Malick MH: *Manual on static splinting,* ed 4, vol 1, Pittsburgh, 1978, Harmarville Rehabilitation Center.

57. Mannheimer JS, Lampe GN: *Clinical transcutaneous electrical nerve stimulation,* Philadelphia, 1984, FA Davis.

58. Markley JM Jr: The preservation of close two-point discrimination in the interdigital transfer of neurovascular island flaps, *Plast Reconstr Surg* 59:812-816, 1977.

59. Mathiowetz V, Kashman N, Volland G, et al.: Grip and pinch strength: normative data for adults, *Arch Phys Med Rehabil* 66:69-74, 1985.

60. Mayo Clinic Occupational Therapy Department. Joint protection for the arthritic person, Rochester, Minnesota, 1985, Mayo Foundation.

61. Meier RH III, Danek JC, Friedmann LW, et al.: Prosthetics, orthotics, and assistive devices (syllabus). American Academy of Physical Medicine and Rehabilitation, ed 2, Self-Directed Medical Knowledge Program, Chicago, IL 1984.

62. Moberg E: Objective methods for determining the functional value of sensibility in the hand, *J Bone Joint Surg Br* 40:454-476, 1958.

63. National Arthritis Foundation, 3400 Peachtree Road Northeast, Atlanta, GA 30326.

64. Olszewski W: Pathophysiological and clinical observations of obstructive lymphedema of the limbs, *Lymphology* 10:79-102, 1977.

65. Olszewski WL, Engeset A: Intrinsic contractility of leg lymphatics in man: preliminary communication, *Lymphology* 12:81-84, 1979.

66. Olszewski WL, Engeset A: Intrinsic contractility of prenodal lymph vessels and lymph flow in human leg, *Am J Physiol* 239:H775-H783, 1980.

67. Opitz JL: *Reconstructive surgery of the extremities.* In Kottke FJ, Stillwell GK, Lehmann JF, editors: *Krusen's handbook of physical medicine and rehabilitation,* ed 3, Philadelphia, 1982, WB Saunders, pp 815-839.

68. Opitz JL, Linscheid RL: Hand function after metacarpophalangeal joint replacement in rheumatoid arthritis, *Arch Phys Med Rehabil* 59:160-165, 1978.

69. Parkes A: Some thoughts on examination of the hand, *Hand* 7:104-106, 1975.

70. Press JM, Wiesner SL: Prevention: conditioning and orthotics, *Hand Clin* 6:383-392, 1990.

71. Prokop LL: Upper-extremity rehabilitation: conditioning and orthotics for the athlete and performing artist, *Hand Clin* 6:517-524, 1990.

72. Rettig AC: Closed tendon injuries of the hand and wrist in the athlete, *Clin Sports Med* 11:77-99, 1992.

73. Russel WR: *Percussion and vibration.* In Licht SH, editor: *Massage, manipulation and traction,* New Haven, Connecticut, 1960, E Licht, pp 113-121.

74. Saldana MJ, Chow JA, Gerbino P II, et al.: Further experience in rehabilitation of zone II flexor tendon repair with dynamic traction splinting, *Plast Reconstr Surg* 87:543-546, 1991.

75. Scherling E, Johnson H: A tone-reducing wrist-hand orthosis, *Am J Occup Ther* 43:609-611, 1989.

76. Schultz Johnson K, Stanley BG, Tribuzi SM, editors: *Concepts in hand rehabilitation,* Philadelphia, 1992, FA Davis, pp 238-271.

77. Schutt AH: Upper extremity and hand orthotics, *Phys Med Rehabil Clin North Am* 3:223-241, 1992.

78. Schutt AH: *Hand rehabilitation.* In DeLisa JA, Gans BM, editors: *Rehabilitation medicine: principles and practice,* Philadelphia, 1993, JB Lippincott, pp 1191-1205.

79. Schutt AH, Opitz JL: *Hand rehabilitation.* In Goodgold J, editor: *Rehabilitation medicine,* St. Louis, 1988, CV Mosby, pp 646-659.

80. *Static and dynamic splinting of the upper extremity with orthoplast,* ed 4, Rochester, Minnesota, 1995, Mayo Clinic Department of Physical Medicine and Rehabilitation.

81. Stern EB: Wrist extensor orthoses: dexterity and grip strength across four styles, *Am J Occup Ther* 45:42-49, 1991.

82. Stern EB, Sines B, Teague TR: Commercial wrist extensor orthoses. Hand function, comfort, and interference across five styles, *J Hand Ther* 7:237-244, 1994.

83. Stewart KM: Review and comparison of current trends in the postoperative management of tendon repair, *Hand Clin* 7:447-460, 1991.

84. Stillwell GK: Treatment of postmastectomy lymphedema, *Mod Treat* 6:396-412, 1969.

85. Stillwell GK: *Therapeutic heat and cold.* In Krusen FH, editor: *Handbook of physical medicine and rehabilitation,* ed 2, Philadelphia, 1971, WB Saunders, p 264.

86. Stillwell GK: The law of Laplace. Some clinical applications, *Mayo Clin Proc* 48:863-869, 1973.

87. Terzis JK: Sensory mapping, *Clin Plast Surg* 3:59-64, 1976.

88. Thorsteinsson G, Stonnington HH, Stillwell GK, et al.: Transcutaneous electrical stimulation: a double-blind trial of its efficacy for pain, *Arch Phys Med Rehabil* 58:8-13, 1977.

89. Tinkham RG, Stillwell GK: The role of pneumatic pumping devices in the treatment of postmastectomy lymphedema, *Arch Phys Med Rehabil* 46:193-197, 1965.

90. Weeks PM, Wray RC: *Management of acute hand injuries: a biological approach,* ed 2, St. Louis, 1978, CV Mosby.

91. Witt J, Pess G, Gelberman RH: Treatment of de Quervain tenosynovitis. A prospective study of the results of injection of steroids and immobilization in a splint, *J Bone Joint Surg Am* 73:219-222, 1991.

92. Wynn Parry CB: Painful conditions of peripheral nerves, *Aust N Z J Surg* 50:233-236, 1980.

93. Wynn Parry CB: The Ruscoe Clarke Memorial Lecture, 1979. The management of traction lesions of the brachial plexus and peripheral nerve injuries in the upper limb: a study in teamwork, *Injury* 11:265-285, 1980.

94. Wynn Parry CB: Sensory rehabilitation of the hand, *Aust N Z J Surg* 50:224-227, 1980.

95. Wynn Parry CB: *Rehabilitation of the hand,* ed 4, London, 1981, Butterworths.

96. Wynn Parry CB, Salter M: Sensory re-education after median nerve lesions, *Hand* 8:250-257, 1976.

97. Yerxa EJ, Barber LM, Diaz O, et al.: Development of a hand sensitivity test for the hypersensitive hand, *Am J Occup Ther* 37:176-181, 1983.

55

WORK REHABILITATION

Elizabeth Mohror, O.T.R.
Margaret A. Moutvic, M.D.

WORK HARDENING
   CONCEPTS AND DESIGN OF A WORK-HARDENING
     PROGRAM
   REFERRAL
   THE THERAPY TEAM
   INITIAL EVALUATION

   ELEMENTS OF A WORK-HARDENING PROGRAM
   CUMULATIVE TRAUMA DISORDER
   OTHER INJURIES
FUNCTIONAL CAPACITY EVALUATION
CONCLUSION

The rehabilitation of work skills has existed since the early 1900s. After World War I, vocational education and rehabilitation programs were initiated for the benefit of returning soldiers. During World War II, the role of occupational therapy was expanded to include medical services designed to rehabilitate disabled soldiers and facilitate their reentry into the workforce. With the passage of time and the delineation of medical practice, the occupational therapist has become a key member of the work-rehabilitation team.[3] Today, a multidisciplinary team is considered optimum for comprehensive care of the injured worker. Of utmost importance in rehabilitation of an injured worker is to keep the person working whenever possible. The work-rehabilitation team provides an excellent link between treatment of the acute injury and restoration of the worker's full work potential. Work-hardening programs, functional-capacity evaluations (FCE), and work-site visits are all helpful services that can be provided by a comprehensive work-rehabilitation team.

WORK HARDENING

In the 1980s, work hardening became a recognized treatment, as demonstrated by the increased number of publications, dedicated specialists, laws, and regulations devoted to this area. In 1992, the Commission on Accreditation of Rehabilitation Facilities (CARF) established program guidelines for accredited programs. CARF has defined work hardening as follows.

Work hardening is a highly structured, goal-oriented, individualized treatment program designed to maximize a person's ability to return to work. Work hardening programs are interdisciplinary in nature with the capability of addressing the functional, physical, behavioral, and vocational needs of the person served. Work hardening provides a transition between the initial injury management and return to work while addressing the issues of productivity, safety, physical tolerances, and work behaviors. Work hardening programs use real or simulated work activities in a relevant work environment in conjunction with physical conditioning tasks. These activities are used to progressively improve the biomechanical, neuromuscular, cardiovascular/metabolic, behavioral, attitudinal, and vocational function of the person served.[11]

To establish a recognized base of reference, this chapter discusses work hardening in the context of the CARF guidelines, which are recognized by the American Occupational Therapy Association and the American Physical Therapy Association.

CONCEPTS AND DESIGN OF A WORK-HARDENING PROGRAM

To fully meet the needs of appropriately referred patients, a structured work-hardening program should be available 5 days a week and up to 8 hours a day. General strengthening, focused limb strengthening, and work simulation all must be included in a work-hardening program. Referral and admission into a work-hardening program should be offered to persons who will benefit from such therapy or whose current capabilities do not meet the functional demands of their jobs and who have no other conditions that would prohibit participation. A commonly encountered candidate for a work-hardening program is a patient who is recovering from a wrist injury or operation. Initially, the program goals for such a patient may seem few and specific in nature. When the elements of functional endurance and activity tolerance such as repetition are introduced, however, the need for a comprehensive program is recognized. The specialized function of the wrist is evident when the functional components of range of motion, strength, coordination, sensation, and endurance are considered as required for job-specific tasks.

Program goals necessary for a safe return to work include 1) the elimination or control of pain, 2) the development of compensation and protection techniques to prevent reinjury, 3) the reestablishment of functional range of motion and strength, 4) the reestablishment of coordination and skill, and 5) the development of aerobic and muscular conditioning to ensure adequate underlying fitness. The structure and duration of the program should be tailored to fit the individual patient. Regardless of whether the patient is referred for a fully balanced program or one focused on a particular body part, the type of program needed should be clearly delineated and understood by the referring physician, the patient, and the therapy staff. All patients in a program should not and will not be doing the same tasks because limiting factors and critical job demands vary from patient to patient. The importance of this concept is especially evident in patients who are referred for rehabilitation of the wrist.

REFERRAL

The structures of the wrist can potentially be inflamed and fatigued in a work-hardening program. To minimize this risk, the principles of work hardening should be introduced early in treatment through the use of functional activities. Functional activities are used in conjunction with passive hand therapy modalities to ensure the development of mobility, stability, and strength. The use of functional activities promotes light, purposeful use of the injured wrist while avoiding the development of muscle cocontraction and guarding. Through the use of the functional tasks, numerous difficulties ranging from dysfunctional movement patterns to psychologic issues can be addressed.

Before a patient is referred to a work-hardening program, the initial medical treatment goals of pain relief, tissue healing, and improved range of motion should be met. The work-hardening program can then focus on the exploration and reestablishment of functional skills that are part of the patient's physical job demands. The success of any program depends in part on the resources and means of referral. Sound communication among the work therapy staff, the physician, the patient, and the employer is imperative and cannot be underestimated. In particular, a good working relationship with the employer facilitates a safe and smooth transition back to work. The specific indications for referral vary from program to program. The successful referrals will be those patients with appropriate work behaviors and realistic potential to return to their previous vocation. Referral to a work-hardening program should include all the information the rehabilitation team needs to make an appropriate evaluation and treatment recommendations. A complete patient background file should include vocational data and medical documentation.

The vocational information should include a description of essential functions of the job, an ergonomic job-site analysis, and possibly a vocational counselor report. If the patient does not have a specific job to return to, the work history should be reviewed and vocational testing may need to be incorporated into the program. Often the goal for such a patient is simply to maximize the functional status in a limited amount of time. Most work-hardening programs last 4 to 6 weeks as deemed necessary by comparing the patient's current capabilities to those required on the job. Factors that affect the duration of a work-hardening program include overall fitness, aerobic conditioning, and psychologic status. Delay in recovery can be seen whenever there is unresolved litigation or complicating medical, psychologic, or social difficulties. Return to work will be aided when the employer offers transitional or light duty work modifications.

The medical information in the referral file should include the results of a recent general medical examination. This information helps the rehabilitation team identify any contraindications to the program or secondary problems that may need to be monitored during therapy such as diabetes, cardiac conditions, or other musculoskeletal disorders. During the initial phase of work hardening, further testing in such areas as cardiovascular fitness, musculoskeletal strength, and functional work capacity may be required to provide a baseline for comparison as the patient progresses through the work-hardening program. Further evaluation may also be indicated in behavioral, attitudinal, cognitive, and vocational areas.

THE THERAPY TEAM

A well-organized program featuring cooperation of the patient, the employer, the physician, and the work-hardening team ensures a timely safe return to work. Depending on the needs of the individual patient, the team dedicated to work hardening may consist of an occupational therapist, a physical therapist, a psychologist, and a vocational specialist. In addition, some patients may benefit from services for dietary or nutritional counseling, drug dependency counseling, or remedial education. Also, consultation with a social worker may be needed. Team conferences held at least every other week ensure that all issues relating to a particular patient are addressed in a timely manner. Such a team approach promotes integration of the various components of the work-hardening program needed to achieve recovery efficiently.

INITIAL EVALUATION

The program should begin with an evaluation of functional status and physical fitness. Function should be considered in relationship to specific job demands such as the patient's tolerance for the number of repetitive grips that must be completed in a set time (Fig. 55-1). In addition to traditional assessment of range of motion and strength, the fitness of the entire body should be assessed to ensure that the patient has the overall physical strength and stamina needed to sustain the physical demands of the job for a full work shift. Endurance is lost when patients spend weeks away from their jobs. It must be restored as part of the return-to-work program.

A thorough description of the physical demands of the job is necessary to determine the appropriate treatment regimen and associated treatment goals. Often, the physical demands of the job are not clearly outlined in job descriptions. However, with the passage of the Americans With Disabilities Act (PL101-336) of 1990,[15] employers are becoming increasingly aware of the need to delineate the "essential functions" required for specific positions. If an outline of physical demands is not provided in the job description, a job-site analysis is required. A job-site analysis promotes clear education among the employer, the vocational specialist, the therapist, and the patient. This job-site analysis also aids in the identification of ergonomic risk factors, which, if addressed, can decrease the potential for further injury to the patient and other employees.

ELEMENTS OF A WORK-HARDENING PROGRAM

The transition from traditional therapy to work hardening may cause the patient to experience anxiety and fear of pain or reinjury. A sound program with clear objectives and protocols helps diminish many of these fears. The success of the program depends on active involvement of all disciplines with the patient. The elements of a sound work-hardening program include patient education, flexibility and strengthening exercises, and work simulation activities designed to reestablish work skills without reinjury (Fig. 55-2).

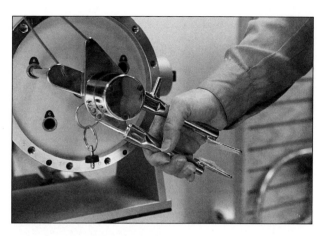

FIGURE 55-1

Strength and tolerance for repetitive gripping can be estimated using computer-assisted devices.

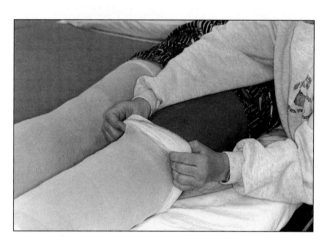

FIGURE 55-2

Work-simulation activities are helpful for this nurse recovering from a wrist injury.

As the patient progresses through the program, specific activities are monitored and graded to reestablish the physical demands and skills necessary for a safe and confident return to work.[12]

The structure of the program varies. For example, patients in the initial phase of work hardening may benefit from a combination of soft-tissue warming and flexibility exercises at the beginning of the treatment session and the use of other activities at the end of the session to control pain. The primary objective of this early phase of treatment is a smooth transition from traditional therapy to work-oriented therapy. Decreasing and eliminating the use of therapeutic modalities reinforce the concept that the patient is ultimately responsible for monitoring and controlling the condition.

Patient education should be an active part of all facets of the work-hardening program. The informed patient is able to modify tasks without interfering with productivity. Essential elements in the education of the patient include the following basic concepts: joint anatomy, use of the joint in a neutral position, avoiding extremes of pronation and supination and flexion and extension, and appropriate movement

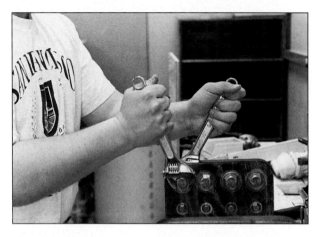

FIGURE 55-3

Work-simulation activities can be graded and progressive as they are overseen by a work therapist.

patterns as opposed to unnecessary substitution patterns. Instruction in pain-management techniques should also be offered, including muscle-use patterns, pacing techniques, preliminary and periodic stretching exercises, and the use of heat and cold. Patients who are knowledgeable about their condition and the principles and goals of work-hardening programs are more likely to participate actively in the rehabilitation program and take responsibility for their recovery.

During the initial phases of work hardening, the use of splints may be beneficial. The incorporation of a properly fitted splint into the treatment regimen can promote healing and joint stability and affords the opportunity for instruction in the correct positioning of the joint for work simulation activity. As the patient meets the initial goals of work hardening, the patient can be weaned slowly from the use of the splint as endurance, strength, and stability increase.

The selection of work simulation tasks to be incorporated into the work-hardening program requires the involvement of the employee patient, the employer, and possibly a vocational counselor. The use of work-simulation tasks graded over time allows the introduction of work-related activities in a supervised structured environment. This treatment aspect can provide

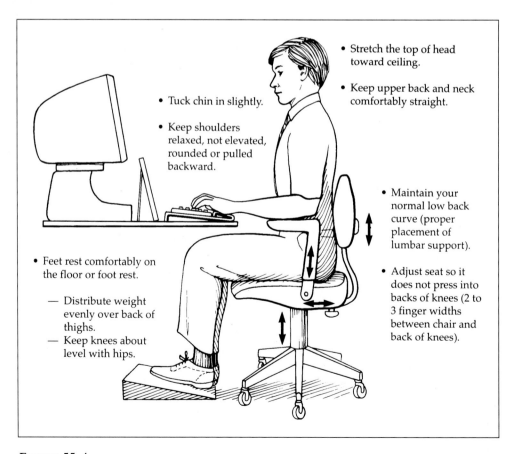

FIGURE 55-4

Proper positioning at a visual-display terminal. (*From* Care of the neck, shoulder and upper back, *Rochester, Minnesota, 1996, Mayo Press. By permission of Mayo Foundation.*)

valuable feedback regarding performance and compensation techniques, with the additional advantage of the opportunity for immediate intervention in problem areas (Fig. 55-3). Work simulation can be likened to sport-specific training so important to rehabilitating athletes. Efficiency and coordination of muscle activation are maximized with work-simulation activities.

CUMULATIVE TRAUMA DISORDER

As Workers' Compensation costs continue to increase, a problem of particular concern to work-hardening programs is the patient with wrist dysfunction. Many commonly encountered cumulative trauma disorders are conditions that affect the function of the wrist or hand.[1] One of the most frequent of these is carpal tunnel syndrome. For patients with this disorder, the goals of work hardening include 1) patient education in maintaining the wrist in a neutral position and avoiding firm gripping and pinching whenever possible, 2) assessment of the work environment for identification of ergonomic risk factors and possible modifications to equipment or pacing of job tasks, 3) reestablishment of functional range of motion and strength in relation to job demands, and 4) conditioning the wrist to sustain the physical demands of prolonged work tasks as in an 8-hour workday.

Patients who are returning to their previous jobs can be at increased risk for the redevelopment of symptoms if effective changes are not made in work method or the work environment.[4] The therapist or a knowledgeable plant safety director (or both) can address this issue. For example, proper positioning is a primary consideration for patients who use a visual-display terminal. Use of a wrist support to allow neutral positioning, adjustment of the height of the chair and desktop equipment to position the arms comfortably, and installation of a partial armrest that provides adequate support are simple but effective measures (Fig. 55-4). Work flow should be organized in a manner that encourages periodic breaks from the keyboard and allows the patient to perform simple upper extremity stretching exercises.

Similarly, a patient returning to assembly-line work involving repetitive hand motions should be cognizant of tasks that may predispose to excessive grip, direct wrist or palmar pressure, and suboptimal wrist position. Involvement of the company safety and health personnel can expedite changes needed to avoid reinjury, such as tool changes or modifications and possible task expansion and changes or rotation of tasks.

OTHER INJURIES

Limited motion is a common residual impairment resulting from forearm or wrist fractures, fusions, or adhesions. By strengthening proximal muscle groups,

the patient can use compensation techniques without developing secondary conditions (Fig. 55-5). Job-specific problem solving may involve a job-site visit by the patient, the therapist, and the employer to identify alternative techniques that will balance the patient's capacities with productivity demands.

Sensory recovery in the wrist and hand is slow compared with recovery of motor function. As in the recovery of all patients, patient education is of utmost importance. During the early phase of sensory recovery when protective sensation may be compromised, the element of safety is important. Hand function may require constant visual feedback. As sensibility improves to include the recognition and localization of moving touch, the elements of gross manipulation with vision occluded can be introduced into the work-hardening program. During the late phase of sensory regeneration, the patient can become frustrated by the feeling of "dropping objects" as a result of the lag between the fast-adapting (moving touch) fibers and the slow-adapting (constant touch) fibers. Work-simulation tasks for these patients should be graded and progress should match and challenge their capacities.

Individualized work-hardening programs for rehabilitation of patients with disability from overexposure to cold, heat, or vibration should involve the employer. The rehabilitation team can appraise and suggest the availability of personal protection equipment and possible tool alternatives. An appropriate ergonomic change can provide protection and avoid additional mechanical forces for the hand to overcome.

Regardless of the present impairment and resulting disability, employers currently have a greater incentive to accommodate injured employees because of the passage of the Americans With Disabilities Act of 1990.

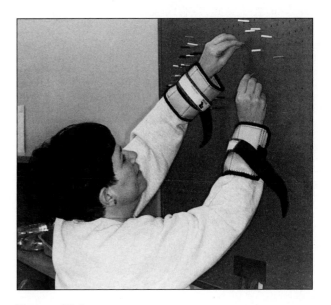

FIGURE 55-5

Proximal upper extremity strengthening using functional activities.

The knowledgeable therapist can facilitate return to work by comparing the patient's physical capacities and the demands of the job with identified potential means of accommodation. Acceptable methods of accommodation include job restructure, alternative scheduling, transfer to a new job, and purchase of special equipment. Reasonable accommodation is required by law unless it causes "undue hardship" for the employer or results in a safety risk for the patient or co-workers (or both).

FUNCTIONAL CAPACITY EVALUATION

The work therapist is often called on to perform an FCE. The purpose of such an examination is objective assessment of a patient's physical capacities in terms of ability to perform the 20 physical demands of work

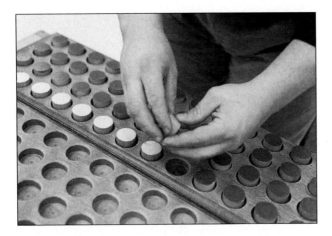

FIGURE 55-6

Minnesota Rate of Manipulation Test.

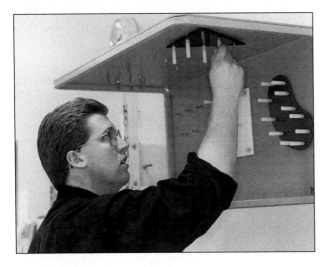

FIGURE 55-7

Valpar 9—whole body range of motion.

identified by the US Department of Labor as representative of occupational demands of labor in the *Dictionary of Occupational Titles*.[13] An FCE can be used to evaluate a patient's capacity to perform job-specific tasks, establish permanent work restrictions, and provide objective input regarding functional disability ratings.[6]

On referral for an FCE, the patient's file should contain all the information the therapist needs to perform the evaluation, including a detailed job description that delineates physical and postural demands. If the patient does not have a specific job to return to, the *Dictionary of Occupational Titles*[13] offers general descriptions of demands associated with specific types of jobs in various businesses and industries. A complete referral file enables the functional capacity evaluator to make objective comparisons between the patient's observed physical capacities and the physical demands of the job. The format for an FCE varies from facility to facility and includes the use of commercially available standardized evaluations such as the Polinsky Advantage[10] and Key[5] evaluations and others. Professional instruction in evaluation techniques and procedural manuals are also available.[2,8] Individualized facilities can develop their own format to fit their needs and coordinate with standardized evaluations. For example, a particular facility may find that the Minnesota Rate of Manipulation Test[9] (Figs. 55-6 and 55-7) used in conjunction with the West II[7] in addition to other test items coordinates optimally with their equipment and personnel. Computerized

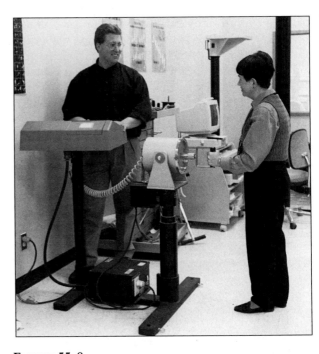

FIGURE 55-8

Baltimore therapeutic equipment machine can be helpful for determining strength and endurance for repetitive upper extremity tasks.

equipment is frequently used for comprehensive evaluation of functional activities and is being used in many work rehabilitation centers at present. Validity and reliability of test measures are required to ensure useful results.

Weight-handling activities, as part of the FCE, provide input into wrist stability and endurance as well as overall patient fitness. As a result of an FCE, patients may have identified functional limitations not related to the wrist (e.g., a patient who cannot use appropriate techniques to lift from low levels because of knee conditions or lower extremity weakness).

Upper extremity test items can be chosen to address the evaluation of specific motions, postural demands, and repetition (Fig. 55-8). The evaluator must be cautious in drawing conclusions about a patient's capacity to perform for an 8-hour workday.

Regardless of the format chosen, predetermined standards or norms are needed to ensure consistency and objectivity.[14] The use of standardized tests enables the evaluator to assess the patient's performance level within the context of established protocols. Of particular importance is the identification of such problems as limiting factors, a commonly encountered facet of disability. In discussing test items in which limiting factors may play a role, the Polinsky Advantage defines the term "functionally limited" as the degree of disability in which the patient is unable to complete an activity because of observable difficulties or completes the task but has obvious accompanying discomfort. Another term, "self-limited performance," is defined as a situation in which the patient stops an activity but no observable physical deficiencies can be documented. Such guidelines are invaluable to the therapist performing an FCE and to the referral source.

Additional studies that may be required for a complete FCE, particularly in the patient with a wrist condition, include volumetric and circumferential measurements, pretest and post-test sensibility testing with the use of monofilaments, two-point discrimination, and vibrometry. This information and data from self-reports completed by the patient assist the therapist in determining the patient's inabilities. The trained evaluator also notes compensation techniques, movement patterns associated with cocontracting and guarding, and performance consistency among activities.

The interpretation of the results of the FCE in relationship to functional capacity and the ability to perform specific work tasks for an entire work shift requires skill and insight. The wrist is a primary functioning component required for stability in many weight-handling activities. In the interpretative portion of the evaluation, the evaluator must consider how the functional limiting factors demonstrated during testing relate to anticipated or identified risk factors listed in the job description or job-site analysis. Such factors as repetition; extremes in motion; direct pressure; tight or prolonged grip and pinch; and exposure to vibration, cold, and heat may adversely influence the patient's ability to return to work. The patient's physician will find this information helpful in determining long-term prognosis and long-term work disability.

CONCLUSION

The occupational therapist is an important member of the work rehabilitation team. Through such activities as work hardening and the performance of an FCE, the work therapist has a unique opportunity to interact one-on-one with the patient in a work-oriented environment. This team relationship promotes communication with the patient and employer on a level perhaps not experienced in any other health care environment. The challenge for the future is to prove how participation in work-rehabilitation programs improves functional outcome of injured workers.

REFERENCES

1. Armstrong TJ: Ergonomics and cumulative trauma disorders, *Hand Clin* 2:553-565, 1986.
2. Blankenship KL: *Industrial rehabilitation* (procedural manual), Macon, Georgia, 1988, American Therapeutics.
3. Jacobs K: *Occupational therapy: work related programs and assessments,* ed 2, Boston, 1991, Little, Brown.
4. Joseph BS: Ergonomic considerations and job design in upper extremity disorders, *Occup Med* 4:547-557, 1989.
5. Key K: *Functional capacity testing.* In *Proceedings of the Third Annual Symposium for Physical Therapy Educators,* 1988.
6. Lechner D, Roth D, Straaton K: Functional capacity evaluation in work disability, *Work* 1:37-47, 1991.
7. Matheson LN: *West II,* Huntington Beach, California, 1982, Work Evaluations Systems Technology.
8. Matheson LN: *Work capacity evaluation* (procedural manual), Anaheim, California, 1988, Employment and Rehabilitation Institute of California.

9. *Minnesota Rate of Manipulation Test,* Circle Pines, Minnesota, American Guidance Service.

10. *Polinsky Advantage Functional Capacities Assessment* (procedural manual), Duluth, Minnesota, 1990, Polinsky Medical Rehabilitation Center.

11. Recommendation of CARFs 1991 National Advisory Committee regarding revisions for CARFs 1992 Standards Manual. CARF, 101 North Wilmot Road, Tucson, Arizona 85711.

12. Schultz-Johnson K: Work hardening: a mandate for hand therapy, *Hand Clin* 7:597-610, 1991.

13. United States Department of Labor, Employment and Training Administration: *Dictionary of occupational titles,* ed 4 (revised), Washington, DC, 1991, Government Printing Office.

14. *Valpar International Corporation* (brochure), Tucson, Arizona, 1986, Valpar International Corporation.

15. Wright M: *Americans With Disabilities Act: making the ADA work for you,* ed 2, Northridge, California, 1992. (Attention: Richard Pimental, 19151 Parthenia Street, Northridge, California 91324.)

56

OVERUSE SYNDROME

Keith A. Bengtson, M.D.
Damien C.R. Ireland, M.D.

HISTORICAL BACKGROUND
TERMINOLOGY
EPIDEMIOLOGY
INVESTIGATIONS
TREATMENT
SUMMARY

There is no agreement concerning the cause; the pathology is unknown; the clinical features are diffuse; there are no useful diagnostic investigations; and the prognosis is uncertain.
                                        —McDermott 1986

Although this may be true of many of the frustrating chronic pain conditions that physicians encounter, this passage from McDermott[33] refers to an upper extremity disorder that some authors call "upper extremity overuse syndrome" (OS). As with many vague diseases of which we know little, the terminology for this entity has evolved into a confusing array of syndromes with little consensus as to definition or classification. This chapter attempts to guide the reader through the miasma of classifications and also discusses the importance and current understanding of OS.

HISTORICAL BACKGROUND

In 1713, Ramazini[38] reported about "diseases of clerks and scribes," describing the same symptoms as modern OS, implicating "continuous sitting, repeated use of the hand and strain of the mind." In 1833, Sir Charles Bell[4] described "writer's cramp," which differs from OS only in the high incidence of hand spasm. Gowers[21] further elaborated on "writer's cramp" in 1888, calling it an "occupation neurosis" in his extensive monograph *A Manual of Diseases of the Nervous System*. He dismissed this as a peripheral condition, believing it to be of central nervous system origin. He also noted that patients who have writer's cramp frequently "are of distinctly 'nervous' temperament, irritable, sensitive, bearing over-work and anxiety badly" and that "it is a disease that is easily imagined, especially by those who have witnessed the disorder." He estimated that 50% of cases of writer's cramp occurred bilaterally.

Gowers[21] also mentioned other similar occupational neuroses of the time: pianoforte players' cramp, violin players' cramp, seamstresses' cramp, and telegraphists' cramp. The similarity of telegraphists' cramp to writer's cramp was also noted in 1882 by Robinson.[40] The incidence of telephonists' cramp steadily increased, affecting 60% of operators after its addition in 1908 to the schedule of diseases covered by the British Workmen's Compensation Act. The Great Britain and Ireland Post Office Departmental Committee of Enquiry[22] concluded that telegraphists' cramp was a "nervous breakdown" due to "nervous instability and repeated fatigue." The incidence subsequently declined, although as late as 1971, Ferguson[14] described cramp of Australian keyboard telegraphists. They used the same equipment and had the same work environment as earlier described, and the clinical presentation was similar to today's OS.

TERMINOLOGY

The term "overuse syndrome" was first popularized by Fry[17] in 1986 in describing a condition he found in more than 60% of 495 professional musicians whom he examined. He has since published a series including more than 650 musicians with OS.[19] Similar problems have been seen in musicians throughout the world. His original definition is a cogent description of the condition.

Overuse syndrome is a painful condition of the hand and arm produced by hand-use-intensive activities over long periods and use which is excessive for those individuals affected. The muscles are the structures primarily affected, but some joint ligaments which take high loading also become painful and tender to the examination and often suffer loss of function.[18]

He also proposed a grading scale[18] based largely on the symptoms and functional capacity of these patients.

Grade I: Pain in one site on causal activity

Grade II: Pain in multiple sites on causal activity

Grade III: Pain with some other uses of the hand, tender structures demonstrable, may show pain at rest or loss of muscle function

Grade IV: Pain with all uses of the hand, postactivity pain with minor uses, pain at rest and at night, marked physical signs of tenderness, loss of motor function, loss of response control, weakness

Grade V: Loss of capacity for use because of continuous pain, loss of muscle function particularly weakness, gross physical signs

At the same time that Fry was studying this condition among Australian musicians, a parallel condition was being observed in the Australian workplace. This disease was labeled "repetitive strain injury" (RSI). Other permutations include *repetition* strain injury and repetitive *stress* injury. Unfortunately, the literature on RSI is confusing because the subject being discussed is poorly defined. The Australian National Occupational Health and Safety Commission's own statement defines the disease only in relation to its cause, saying little regarding symptoms, course, or physical findings.

[RSI is defined as] a soft tissue disorder caused by the overloading of particular muscle groups from repetitive use or maintenance of constrained postures... [which] occurs among workers performing tasks involving either frequent repetitive movements of the limbs or the maintenance of fixed postures for prolonged periods, e.g. process workers, keyboard operators and machinists.[35]

The lack of consensus as to definition is illustrated by examining those articles which addressed the disease RSI. Of the 18 papers that give or imply a definition of RSI, two separate camps are formed. Seven of those papers elect for a narrow definition of RSI (stating the term in the singular) describing an entity with little or no difference from Fry's OS.* The remaining 11 papers

follow the broader definition implied by the name (stated in the plural) and use RSI as a category of diseases which are united by their etiologic roots in repetitive strain.* Most limit these to problems in the upper extremity. Included in this category are many well-known entities such as tendinitis, tenosynovitis, epicondylitis, and many other inflammatory diseases of the soft tissue which have some suggestion of strain as an etiology. Also included, but more controversial in their connection to repetitive strain, are focal dystonias and nerve entrapment syndromes such as carpal tunnel, cubital tunnel, pronator teres, and posterior interosseous syndromes. Finally, OS as described by Fry would be included in this category of RSI. Much of the confusion regarding RSI is a direct consequence of this double definition. For example, one finds criticism of Fry's work on OS as it relates to the umbrella definition of RSI and vice versa.[5]

Besides having a vague and ambiguous definition, some critics argued that the name "repetitive strain injury" was too suggestive; it implied that repeated micro-stress had been proved to cause a definite injury.[15] The word "injury" was also considered too inflammatory in the medicolegal climate of Australia. As a consequence, the Royal Australian College of Physicians issued a statement[41] in September 1986, suggesting that the term "RSI" be replaced by the term "regional pain syndrome," which is perhaps less confusing. The College did not attempt to revise the definition of this entity. Despite the attempted shift toward "regional pain syndrome," RSI continues to be used and is still a medical subject heading in the *Index Medicus*.

A third term in this maze is "cumulative trauma disorder" (CTD). This is a group of upper extremity problems all thought to be etiologically linked to "cumulative trauma." This term was first introduced by Armstrong et al.[2] in 1982 to describe the category of upper extremity problems seen in the industrial setting, in this case a poultry processing plant. This, in essence, is the American term for the broad definition of RSI and includes OS and all forms of upper limb tendinitis, tenosynovitis, muscle pain, and nerve entrapment syndromes. CTDs tend to occur at work as the result of continuous and repetitive use of the body in performing certain tasks. The wrist is a common location for CTDs.

Other less common terms used in this context are "occupational arm pain," "occupational cervicobrachial disorder," "occupational stress syndrome," "occupational cramp,"[13] and "regional musculoskeletal illness of the upper extremity."[24]

The term "RSI" was expanded to include patients suffering from clearly defined and recognized overuse conditions. Similarly, the original problem of organic

CTD was expanded to CTDs of repetitive strain, which confused nonorganic disease with the diagnosis of true traumatic overuse conditions.

EPIDEMIOLOGY

The prevalence of OS is only well studied among musicians. Fry[17] studied professional orchestra members in eight orchestras in Australia, Britain, and the United States. After interviewing and examining all but 29 of the members of these orchestras, he found that 301 of the 485 musicians (62%) had some degree of OS. Those with grade II or worse OS showed a 42% prevalence. Fry[20] also looked at Australian music students. Again using interview and examination methods, he found 116 of 1,249 students (9.3%) had OS. In the United States, Newmark and Lederman[36] surveyed 79 amateur musicians participating in an intensive 2-week chamber music conference. With the necessary increase in playing time, 53 of the musicians (67%) developed symptoms of OS. They also surveyed 48 nonclassical musicians. Thirteen of these (27%) had experienced symptoms of OS at some time.

The incidence of OS among industrial workers and other sectors of the population can only be inferred (Fig. 56-1). In the United States, government statistics report the incidence of broad categories of ailments, usually CTDs. The National Institute of Occupational Safety and Health[9] estimated the incidence of CTDs to be approximately 6% of all workers (Fig. 56-1). The Occupational Safety and Health Administration[27] estimated that there were 78,000 new cases of "disorders associated with repeated trauma" in 1988. In 1990, the Bureau of Labor Statistics[9] reported that CTDs accounted for more than 50% of all occupational illnesses reported in the United States.

Silverstein et al.[45] examined the prevalence of CTDs in seven investment casting plants in 1983. Of 152 employees surveyed and examined, 12.5% had some type of CTD. Armstrong et al.[2] studied the incidence of CTDs in a poultry processing plant and found an incidence of 12 cases/200,000 hours worked. Interestingly, this categorization excluded nerve entrapment disorders and therefore more closely approximated the incidence of OS than other statistics.

In Australia, RSI was reported to be present in epidemic proportions by the lay press. Several authors charted the epidemiology of this phenomenon. Gun[23] reported the incidence of what the Australian Bureau of Statistics termed "repetitive movement injuries classified as accidents" and "repetitive movement injuries classified as diseases." Only accidents and diseases resulting in absence from work of 1 week or more were included. Gun also limited reporting to upper limb disorders but added to this the category called "rheumatism excluding the back." Unfortunately this also included other soft-tissue problems such as tendinitis, tenosynovitis, and the rheumatoid diseases. The study found that the number of cases in South

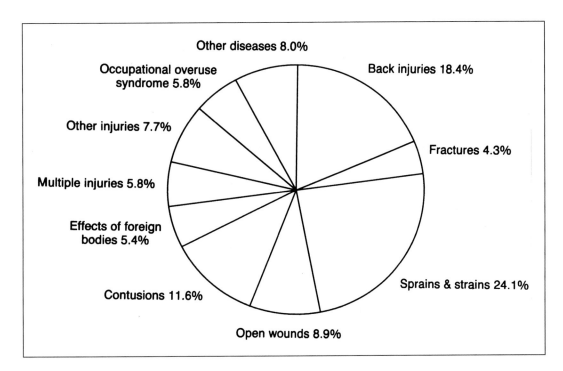

FIGURE 56-1

Breakdown of conditions for new claims received by ComCare (1.12.88 to 30.6.89). This reveals claims for repetitive strain injury (occupational overuse syndrome) represented only 5.8% of the total.

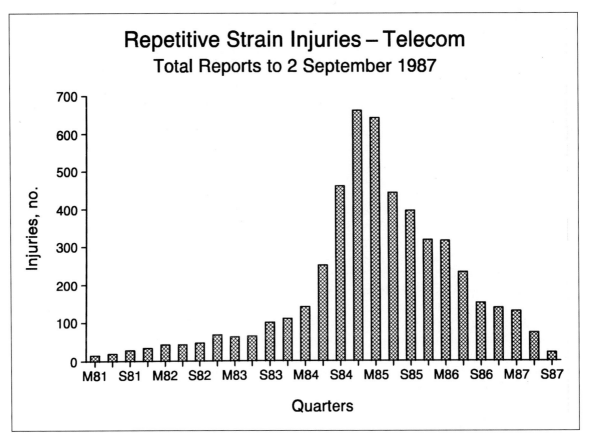

FIGURE 56-2

The incidence of repetitive strain injury increased steadily from 1981 to peak in early 1985. The rapid decline thereafter has been more precipitous than the steady increase before 1985.

Australia gradually increased until 1984–1985, after which they began to decline. In men, there were 262 cases in 1980–1981, increasing to a peak of 366 cases in 1984–1985, and decreasing to 326 cases in 1986–1987. Among women, 214 cases were reported in 1980–1981, 590 in 1984–1985, and 314 in 1986–1987. The occupational categories with the highest frequency among men with RSI were farmers, fishermen, and timber getters, with 46 cases/1,000 persons per year. Among women, the highest incidence was 4.1 cases/1,000 persons per year in service, sport, and recreation workers. The next highest was 2.5 cases/1,000 persons per year among clerical workers.

Hocking[26] similarly charted the course of "RSI" (broadly defined) in the company Telecom Australia (the Australian analog of AT&T in the United States) from 1981 to 1985 (Fig. 56-2). A steadily increasing number of cases was reported in this period. There were 109 cases reported in 1981, increasing to 1,783 cases in 1985. A total of 3,976 cases were reported for these 5 years. Studying only those individuals who worked at keyboards (telegraphists, telephonists, and clerical workers), Hocking found an incidence of 302 cases/1,000 workers during the 5 years, or 60 cases/1,000 persons

per year. In all workers at Telecom Australia, the average lost time per case was 74 days. The total cost for medical treatment and for lost production was 15.5 million Australian dollars during 5 years.

In reaction to the epidemic of upper extremity pain disorders in Australia during the 1980s, a plethora of articles and editorials were published in the medical and lay press. This perhaps reflected the great financial impact the malady had on the Australian business and industrial communities. By the mid 1980s, RSI was one of the highest causes of work time lost in Australia, second only to low back problems.[35] However, many physicians claim that the disease does not even exist. Bell,[5] for example, labeled RSI as "an iatrogenic epidemic of simulated injury" and related the cause of the epidemic to "mass motor hysteria." Ferguson[15] called the increase in incidence of RSI "a complex psychosocial phenomenon with elements of mass hysteria, that were superimposed on a base of widespread discomfort, fatigue, and morbidity." He criticized the very term "RSI," which he claimed "implies injury and cause where neither may exist." Cleland[11] related the cause of RSI to "social iatrogenesis" by which "otherwise trivial discomfort may become transformed into a protracted, painful, disabling condition which precludes effective work and degrades the quality of life." Ireland[29] believed RSI should be classified as a "socio-political phenomenon, rather than a medical condition" because "the symptoms fail to respond to any form of treatment other than psychological counseling." Lucire[32] termed RSI a "functional," "conversion," or "somatization" disorder. She also believed it to be "predominantly manual astasia–abasia" secondary to "epidemic hysteria."

Miller and Topliss[34] presented a more moderate view of this phenomenon in their review of 229 patients referred to them with the diagnosis of RSI. By carefully eliminating other neurologic and rheumatologic diagnoses, they narrowed the group to 200 patients with apparent OS or what they call "a local chronic rheumatic pain syndrome." All patients had physical findings of "nonspecific soft tissue tenderness" and an average of four Smythe tender points in the upper limb. If they had seven or more Smythe points, they fulfilled the criteria for fibrositis syndrome and were excluded from this group. A majority of the patients also had general symptoms related to fibrositis syndrome such as anxiety, irritability, sleep disturbance, chronic fatigue, and frequent tension headaches.

As Smythe tender points are uncommon in healthy subjects, in nonrheumatic populations, and in rheumatic disease clinic patients, the finding of tender points in persons who do not even know of the existence of these points let alone their precise locations is objective evidence that they *are* different from normal subjects.... By analogy we suggest that the combination of persistent localized pain or aching and a smaller number of Smythe tender points in the region of pain should be considered sufficient to establish the existence of a local chronic rheumatic pain syndrome....The epidemic suggests that social acceptability (fashion) may shape the clinical expression of chronic rheumatic pain syndromes.[34]

INVESTIGATIONS

The first investigation into the underlying pathology of OS was published by Dennett and Fry[12] in 1988. They obtained muscle biopsy specimens of the first dorsal interosseous muscles of 29 women keyboard operators with OS of grade III or worse on Fry's scale. Each had involvement of one or both of their first dorsal interosseous muscles. These biopsy specimens were compared with biopsy specimens from eight normal controls and six contralateral specimens from study patients with unilateral symptoms. Their specimens showed changes similar to myofascial pain syndrome patients studied by Bengtsson et al.[7]: namely, increased Type I fiber counts, decreased Type II fibers, and Type II fiber hypertrophy as well as various changes in mitochondria and nuclei. The significance of these changes has been argued in subsequent journal editorials.

Sandow et al.[43] suggested that OS may be a form of upper extremity chronic compartment syndrome (CCS). OS has many similarities to CCS. Both are related to overexertion of the involved muscle group, and pain in the affected muscle is the primary symptom. There are only three cases of upper extremity CCS reported in the literature.[28,31,37] Each case report mentions the rarity of this condition. Perhaps it is not surprising that it is rarely diagnosed because the diagnosis must be confirmed by intracompartmental pressure monitoring, a study that few physicians are willing to perform on patients who are already suffering from an ill-defined painful condition. Nonetheless, one group of authors[31] suggested that "the diagnosis should be considered in any patient who describes nonspecific aching hand pain precipitated by repetitive hand use."

In 1985, with the possible connection between CCS and OS in mind, Sandow et al. embarked on a study to look at the forearm compartment pressure of typists with and without OS. The pressure was to be monitored during typing exercise and at rest. In 1987 they reported[43] difficulty finding subjects for the study, presumably due to the sharp decline in incidence of OS. At this time, no completed study has been published by this team on this subject.

Another analogous entity is delayed onset muscle soreness (DOMS). Again, the primary symptom is diffuse muscle pain temporally related to exertion of that muscle group. Biopsy studies[16] have shown significant histologic changes in muscles with DOMS. Although the tissues showed no signs of ischemic fiber necroses or of fiber rupture, there was significant Z-band disorganization in biopsy specimens obtained 2 days after exercise.

Magnetic resonance imaging studies have also shown significant findings both in CCS and DOMS. T2 signal intensity was shown to vary linearly with intracompartment pressure in patients with CCS.[1] This suggests that magnetic resonance imaging could be used in place of intracompartmental pressure monitoring, eliminating the need for invasive testing in these patients. T2 signal intensities were also shown to peak 3 days after exercise in the muscle and muscle-tendon junction of subjects with DOMS.[44] Increased T2 signal is closely correlated with increased water content, thus implying the presence of edematous tissues in these patients. These findings suggest that magnetic resonance imaging could be a powerful tool in studying the analogous entity of OS.

Bengtson et al.[6] measured compartment pressures with the use of magnetic resonance imaging in musicians with overuse syndrome. They postulated that not only CCS and DOMS could be seen with magnetic resonance imaging but also any edematous process that might be present such as tendinitis or tenosynovitis. They imaged the patients' forearms before activities as well as after exercising to the point of fatigue or severe pain. Their results were negative in the small number of patients that they studied.

Electrophysiologic studies have likewise been unsuccessful in demonstrating any abnormalities in these patients. Unlike the sympathetic nervous system, where hyperactive disorders such as reflex sympathetic dystrophy syndrome can be inferred by concomitant abnormalities in sudomotor or autonomic functions, hyperactivity of the somatic nervous system is undetectable.

TREATMENT

Treatment of OS tends to be more of an art than a science (Fig. 56-3). Perhaps this reflects the lack of understanding of the disease's underlying pathophysiology. Many of the treatment principles have developed from empirical experience, others from what seems like common sense. None of the treatments have been proved in scientific trials. The suggestions for treatment discussed below reflect only our opinion and experience.

When evaluating a patient with OS, one must look at the inciting activity. In industrial or clerical workers this is often assembly line work or keyboard activity. In musicians, this is playing their instrument. Many times there is also an initial injury that is not related to the patient's day-to-day tasks. Ergonomic modification of the incriminated activity is one way of decreasing the stress and strain that this activity causes

the patient's upper extremity. These modifications may be costly and are often met with resistance by the employer and insurance provider. One must decide how much modification is reasonable given the severity of the patient's complaints.

Rest is also a mainstay of treatment for OS. Again, one must determine how much rest is reasonable given the severity of the complaint. In the more limited cases, regular breaks from the task involved (e.g., 5 minutes every 30 minutes) may be sufficient to calm the symptoms. In more severe cases, not working or discontinuing instrument practice sessions is necessary for 1 to 2 weeks in order to reach a pain-free state. Again, this may be met with considerable resistance from the employer and the patient as well.

Light aerobic exercise and regular stretching of upper extremity muscles are recommended to maintain general fitness and flexibility. This is largely borrowed from the treatment protocols for fibromyalgia. However, it also stems from the observation that many of these patients are in poor physical condition and tend to have tight forearm muscles. The latter is likely secondary to prolonged cocontraction of upper extremity muscles in response to painful tasks. Aerobic conditioning is most easily accomplished by a walking program consisting of 30 or more minutes 3 to 4 times a week at a moderate pace. This is usually well tolerated by the patients and requires minimal equipment

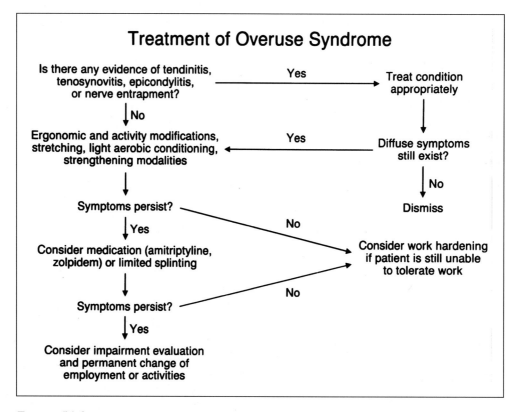

FIGURE 56-3

Treatment of overuse syndrome.

XV
THE FUTURE

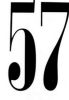

57

ANTICIPATIONS AND NEEDS

James H. Dobyns, M.D.
William P. Cooney, M.D.
Ronald L. Linscheid, M.D.

ANTHROPOLOGIC ADAPTATIONS
SOURCES OF WRIST INJURY—PRESENT AND FUTURE
ASSESSMENT OF STRUCTURE AND FUNCTION
   STRUCTURE
   FUNCTION
FUTURE ANTICIPATIONS
DIAGNOSTIC METHODS
MANAGEMENT OF DAMAGE

FUTURE DIRECTIONS
EDUCATION
TECHNICAL TRAINING
ATTENTION TO DETAIL
EVALUATION OF RESULTS
REPLACEMENT POTENTIAL
CONCLUSION

Throughout the known history of medicine, the wrist received fairly limited scientific interest from basic investigators. However, in the past three decades the explosion of interest in the wrist reminds us that the problems have always existed and that the lack of interest was not shared by the patients. The wrist is not vital to life, but it is constantly invoked in a manual lifestyle which is unique and necessary to our constant needs. We would be a different life-form without it. Now that attention is focused on the wrist, thousands of papers have been written about its every aspect. We now know enough to know that we do not know enough; hopefully, the future will bring the knowledge, the insights, and the diagnostic and management methods that we need. Each wrist aficionado can make up a list of what is wanted in the future. Here is ours!

ANTHROPOLOGIC ADAPTATIONS

Perhaps we have passed the point of no return in forcing adaptations on our body parts. Those ways in which the human wrist differs from our anthropoid cousins or from earlier primates seem chiefly to have been concerned with brachiation (withdrawal of the ulna from direct articulation with the carpus) and the use of objects for play or work (strengthening and independence of the thumb ray; locking of the carpal supports of the index ray).[32,34,35] Our development and use of devices serving functional, artistic, and recreational purposes may have delivered us from the need to acquire further adaptations in the wrist, but not necessarily. Robotics and the mechanization of farm, office, and factory help to maintain the present functional design.[2] Manual skills are no longer needed for survival, nor are they a high priority in overcompetitive, industrial societies. However, further adaptive responses could occur in response to the computer age, and manual skills are still highly regarded by our civilization, particularly in the arts, in entertainment, and in sports.

Because we now know that adaptation may take place randomly but be quickly adopted and expanded if it proves useful, it is possible that the hand span of a Paganini, the central carpometacarpal stability useful to a boxer, the added manipulative skills provided by an ulnar thumb, or some useful changes not apparent to our questing spirits may yet take place. The time is near when there will be no need to wait for the random intervention of nature, if a desired adaptation can be clearly formulated. In general, humanity has profited from the lack of specialization of the hand and wrist past a fairly primitive pattern. But that need not be acceptable forever.

Specialty hands and a specialty wrist can be devised and eventually created. Even now one might countenance the breeding of a scapholunate synofibrosis as an alternative to the somewhat weak joint that now occupies that area. There are already various wrist types (the overall lax or loose wrist, the stable wrist, and the carpal coalition wrist). There are also various shapes, sizes, and articulations of the carpal bones; variation of radius to ulnar length proportions; and various carpal accessories. Even some of these may or have become more prevalent in certain population groups. Indeed, it is likely that from the reported high incidence of lunotriquetral coalition in the Bantu and the high incidence of ulna minus variance in the Scandinavian and ulna positive variance in people from the Pacific rim that some preferential wrist constructs are already favored in certain occupational or cultural groups. Investigation of the type of wrist favored by the musician, the artist, the farmer, and the heavy manual worker and whether such types persist in family lines has not been initiated, to our knowledge. Let us end this small detour into the unknown by merely saying that the wrist has developmental multipotential, as it has proved to have functional multipotential.

SOURCES OF WRIST INJURY—PRESENT AND FUTURE

One might think that there is little likelihood of sources of injury other than those already known but, if the past is indication of the future, newer mechanisms of injury and descriptions of damage to wrist structures will certainly appear.[3,4,8] Currently, the known sources of wrist injury are as follows.

Trauma: single episode and sufficient to disrupt normal physiology[3,42,63]

Trauma: repetitive[46,66]

Trauma: single event exacerbated by repetitive damage[46,66]

Energy forms other than direct load or force: vibration, thermal, radiation (x-ray, radioactive), laser

Disease: arthritides, infections, neurologic, vascular, autoimmune

Neoplasia

Congenital and developmental

Metabolic

New entries are constantly appearing in these familiar categories. A simple device such as the skateboard immediately increased the incidence of wrist injuries among its devotees.[3] Similar increases in wrist-related problems have been noted in gymnastics,

snowboarding, in-line roller-blading, and racquet sports.[1,3,18,42] In industry, the repetitive motion of the assembly line; vibration of air guns, air hammers, or staplers; and impact loading of pneumatic wrenches, among others, will bring new or different problems to human physiology and psychology, including the wrist.[66] It is difficult to explain the almost epidemic level of wrist-related complaints during the past few decades without reaching the conclusion that stress involving the wrist increased during that period. Luckily, our knowledge of biomechanics, pathomechanics, and diagnostic methods has also increased.

ASSESSMENT OF STRUCTURE AND FUNCTION

STRUCTURE

The tissues and architecture of the normal wrist and its common and even unique variations are well known and can be specifically determined to a precise degree by one or more of the following.

1) Clinical history and, in particular, physical examination (see Chapter 12)

2) Standard radiographs, routine arthrography,[12,13] and special imaging; new techniques still evolving include three-dimensional and gadolinium-enhanced magnetic resonance imaging, phase-contrast arthrography, positron emission tomography scanning, computer-enhanced spatial tomography, and high-resolution microcomputed tomography[*]

3) Diagnostic arthroscopy,[12,13,63,64] stressed and therapeutic arthroscopy,[14] thermography,[17] phase-contrast ultrasonography,[21] and arthrotomography[7]

4) Specialized ligament, tendon, and vascular nerve studies,[†] including microangiography, vascular magnetic resonance imaging, and quantitative sudomotor autonomic reflex testing

5) Special histologic studies (confocal microscopy)[10,43,69]

6) Comparison of the above findings between different age and population groups[21] and different mechanisms of injury,[61] with eventual outcomes analysis.[28]

In addition to the study of gross malformations, absences, or dysfunctions, many attempts have been made to predict functional characteristics, risk levels, and deterioration potential from such findings.

FUNCTION

Knowledgeable manual examination and testing are still the basis for evaluating the presence and functional status of wrist elements. This can be enhanced by

---

* References 8,15,16,18,20,27,30,48,50,60,67.
† References 15,30,48,49,58,62.

strength, endurance, and specific occupational testing machines, such as the BTE, the Cybex, microtransducer grip, and pinch dynamometers.[22,53,54] Direct pressure measurements within the wrist joint, demonstrated in the laboratory setting, may next be applicable to the human wrist.[22] The same is true for vascular magnetic resonance imaging (time of flight magnetic resonance imaging) and neurologic assessment (e.g., quantitative sudomotor autonomic reflex test). New forms of ultrasonography, vibrometry, electrophysiologic goniometers, laser refraction sarcomere measurements, in vivo force transducers, and joint contact force probes are waiting to augment or replace traditional functional assessment measures.*

FUTURE ANTICIPATIONS

More of the same can be expected in the future. Machines will become more sensitive, reliable, and complex for more precise determinations. For example, it should become possible to view the actions of musculotendinous structures while simultaneously determining strength, coordination, and synergism of muscle groups; vascular alterations; and nerve function.[11,25] Such developments will still require the guidance of a knowledgeable and skilled examiner. In fact, the skills of physical examination should be sharpened by the increased knowledge about performance of the wrist structures. Such increased awareness has already been demonstrated by the development of new "provocative maneuvers" for wrist instability problems, all based on combining clinical and radiologic signs.

Perhaps the best protection of all will be afforded by ergonomic evaluation of manual-use patterns and the development of improved workstations, improved work methods, and improved support devices for the wrist-hand unit.[57]

DIAGNOSTIC METHODS

It will be increasingly tempting to rely on imaging and other test devices to evaluate the wrist or any other part of the body. Compared with the lungs, heart, and other viscera, the wrist is relatively accessible and the clinical examination should not only be preserved but augmented in the future.[9] It should, for instance, be possible to determine the definitive nature of the abnormality that results in pain, tenderness, noises, and unusual motions that accompany each provocative maneuver and to develop others.

Augmenting physical signs could be improved by better tactile response, transillumination, and magnification. Video-screen capture and augmentation are possible now and can be accompanied by audio enhancement of the various creaks, snaps, and pops of the wrist. Force transducers to mark more accurately degrees of carpal instability such as scaphoid shift test may be developed.[68] This may allow a diagnosis at a distance without the added information obtained by palpation.

Although tissue perfusion, turgor, temperature, and internal pressure can be determined by the examining digit, these findings can also be recorded, perhaps more precisely, by sensing devices. The same is true of skin-surface changes, sweat alterations, small masses, anomalous structures, hair distribution, and nail changes. It is more difficult to envision a device that could detect as well as the examining hand(s) the mobility, entrapment, or instability of tendon and nerve; the passive translational ranges of joint motion; simultaneous traction or compression; and luxations of joints or tendons. It is likely that all of these will be developed in time and that a judicious balance will be retained between the clinical senses and the mechanical determinations. Fortunately, there is usually an excess of signs and of findings for wrist problems. Perhaps the most difficult exercise, done by mind or computer, is the weighing of the various findings to select the most important that best fit a pattern typical of a certain diagnosis. Computerized, diagnostic algorithms may assist in this regard.

Such examination methods are either in development or obviously feasible. Near-term needs include the following.
1) Accurate, minimally invasive determinations of pressure in compartments, joints, and bones
2) Quick determination of altered vascular states
3) Rapid assessment of altered neural states, including real-time monitoring
4) Confirmation of occult bone, tendon, ligament, or muscle injury
5) Precise and reliable confirmation of the degree of joint abnormality or instability

MANAGEMENT OF DAMAGE

Central to all damage control is identification of cause and alteration or prevention. For congenital and developmental problems such prevention may come from DNA mapping and genetic sequence engineering, particularly when the wrist deformity accompanies generalized or systemic hereditary abnormalities. However, there are so many extraneous factors that damage the developing embryo that a complete and continually updated list of those factors, means of identifying them, and better methods of control are vital future needs. Current controversies over permissible investigation (e.g., AIDS or hepatitis testing of at-risk patients such as prisoners or drug users) and permissible

---

* References 16,21,22,33,37,40,49,55.

management methods (e.g., chemical toxicity reduction for expectant mothers) demonstrate all too well that knowledge of cause is only the beginning in the process of gaining control and giving treatment.

Infection or disease as causes of wrist damage may relate to exposure to external risks or predisposition to internal risks. Both types of risks can be identified and controlled much better than is currently the case. The Centers for Disease Control and the genome project are already contributing in this area.

Use-related risks have been much discussed and evaluated but the incorporation of such knowledge in prevention is still in its infancy. Selection by both physiologic and psychologic criteria for occupations, sports, and other tasks should be possible with the proviso that training will still be necessary and may upgrade some marginal performers to effective performers.[45,51,70] It is truly astonishing how little selection is permitted by our culture, resulting in nature's deselection by inadequate performance or injury. Training for known tasks or functions and which is continued throughout the course of such performance is another known but poorly utilized method of preventing injury.[2,25,46,55] Even if selection and training were optimal, there would still be a need for work modification, altered recreational techniques, and special equipment to minimize strain on the body parts of humans, who should be programmed as *random-action specialists,* not repetitive-action robots! Luckily, ergonomics has become an accepted discipline and, although insufficiently used or respected, it has made an impact on such problems. *Much more can be expected or demanded of ergonomics in the future.*[46]

Also in their infancy are the development and use of performance protection or enhancement (or both) by internal splinting. A combination of internal devices (surgically placed posts or plates) and splinting (orthotics or prosthetics) could act as static protection-reinforcements or as dynamic devices in tetraplegia, after amputation, and perhaps even in gymnastics to respond to levels of acceleration or force. A hand or wrist mini-airbag, for example, might rest in a wrist support, responding only to excessive impact loads but preventing fracture or ligament damage. The wrist is also a reliable structure for heavy traction or compression use, if supported. It is an augmenting structure for the prehension of digits because of its capability for tenodesis, which can deliver a cascade of digit motion even without the participation of digital motors. Future developments may bring internal reinforcements; internal control elements; and internal devices to release hormones, enzymes, and electrolytes on demand. Exoskeletons, external control devices, and bioprosthetic linkages could benefit the wrist as well as other parts of the body.[36,56,65]

The "healing ray" concept of treatment for wrist problems has not approached Star Trek levels, but

striking modifications and additions to the present armamentarium of electricity, magnetic fields, and ultrasound may aid trauma healing,[24] while various forms of x-rays and lasers become more specific (e.g., tumor destruction). Lasers may be used for resection of cartilage lesions (e.g., triangular fibrocartilage tear) or for spot welding ligament disruptions. The desire for closed or mini-open treatment methods makes anticipation of such therapy particularly susceptible to false hopes and fraud, but there will be continuing developments with promise.[65]

For the moment, open forms of treatment are most used for wrist problems. Endoscopic diagnosis, applied to the interior of the wrist, and endoscopic surgery, principally applied to the release of the transverse carpal ligament, will be further refined in the future. This treatment method has already forced development of other forms of minimally invasive surgery, and this trend is likely to continue and to be applied to other areas.[65] In the wrist area, this means that specific compartments outside the wrist proper, such as the ulnar nerve canal (Guyon's canal or cubital tunnel) radial tunnel, forearm compartments, and tendon compartments (within the palm or digit), will be subjected to "limited access surgery" by endoscopy combined with soft-tissue distension techniques. Even areas that are not natural compartments may be accessed to treat Dupuytren's disease, extensor tendon entrapment or injury, or fascial abnormalities.

Even with standard open surgery, better preliminary or intraoperative guidance to the source(s) of the pathologic condition is a need likely to be fulfilled. Three-dimensional models for reconstruction of the osseous and the soft-tissue structures will become available as surgical guides.[5,20,27,29] Our routine radiographic assessments will include three-dimensional reconstruction, virtual reality surgical procedures, and cybervision.[11,19,65] Improved methods of repair will surely follow. For ligament injuries, varied treatment from spot welding of small tears and avulsions to total replacement with autologous or replicated tissues will be developed. If bones cannot be salvaged by fixation with a bone or cartilage graft, total replacement of cartilage surface or bony stock will be possible.[38] Fixation, when needed, will include the sealing or bonding of tissues with the use of nonbiologic glues, grommets, or cements. Biologic bone and soft-tissue substitutes, augmented or activated by bone morphogenic protein or fibroblastic growth factor (FB6F), will be used and in some cases are already in use clinically and experimentally.[6] A bone substitute (Norion SRS) is currently used in distal radius fractures for bone replacement and immediate fixation because it replaces and bonds. Bone substitutes (collagen) with bone morphogenic protein have been used selectively for scaphoid nonunions.

Nevertheless, these biologic repair and replacement techniques will continue to be rivaled by mechanical replacements for part(s) or all of the wrist area joint systems.[9] This may be true of ligaments as well as replacement tendons, both of which are perfectly feasible. Advanced augmented healing in tendon, nerve, and vessel repair will probably favor the biologic methods for these structures. The use of vascularized flaps, whether free or attached, will continue to be the simplest method for providing needed skin or soft-tissue protection, gliding tissues, and neurovascular support, but tissues made available from tissue banks should become more available. Enhancement of healing by medications, enzymes, and other biochemical support will become commonplace. Use of hyaluronidase substitutes will assist in reducing joint adhesions, improving tendon gliding, and limiting capsular fibroblastic responses, all of which can affect normal joint motion. Will there remain a place for the surgical team or will it be relegated to guiding or overseeing precise, programmable, and sterile machinery? It should be obvious that the evolution of treatment techniques will produce a need for more, not fewer, very "narrow niche" specialists.

FUTURE DIRECTIONS

The wrist has been called the "low back" of the upper limb, the "no man's land" of the upper limb, and similar disparaging terms, because it is well known as a source of diagnostic and treatment problems and associated with indifferent and occasionally unpredictable results of treatment. With or without surgical management, lingering problems are frequent, as is dissatisfaction of patient and physician. All of the methods mentioned in the text to counter these situations are known and practiced currently, but they must be perfected even more for better future results.

EDUCATION

Knowledge of anatomy has long been known to be a key ingredient for any surgeon and this will not change, but the methods of learning anatomy may well change or at least broaden. Fresh amputated specimens are ideal, but infrequently available. Better preservation methods are needed, so that older specimens more nearly resemble the fresh specimen. It is quite likely that much anatomy of the future will be taught via three-dimensional, interactive video or computer simulation, and improvements in these techniques will make them increasingly competitive with fresh specimen dissection.

There is no area of medical knowledge that may not shed light on some wrist problems, but next to anatomy, the most needed knowledge bank for the wrist investigator and clinician will be that of normal and pathologic biomechanics. There are few areas of

the body where the components have so precisely evolved for the mechanical and functional needs of the effector unit—the hand. The simple one degree of motion of a hinge joint has been increased by complex angulatory, translational, and rotatory capabilities that not even a universal joint easily simulates. The wrist provides a functional interdependence on intercalated segment kinetic chains. "Slider-crank" mechanisms, "screw home" movements, and other descriptions emphasize the cooperative coordinated movements. Free-body analysis and finite element models of standard wrist motions and structures have taught us much concerning these mechanisms, but dynamic three-dimensional models of normal and abnormal wrists will teach us much more.

TECHNICAL TRAINING

We have done much with the old "watch, learn, and teach" methods. They will continue to be useful but must be expanded and augmented.[52] Each wrist therapeutic procedure has so many variations that live television or video reproduction should only be the centerpiece for an interactive learning process, in which questions can be asked, anatomy displayed, and alternative methods tried. Although much of this can be done via Internet linkages or CD-ROM programs for the home computer, training centers are needed where actual or simulated upper limbs can be used with the required equipment for the development of the manual coordination essential to good surgery.

Even new procedures will soon be simulated and their likely effects on the kinematics of the system observed well before they are actually performed on the patient. Open surgery, performed to minimize ligament, tendon, and neurovascular damage, will continue to be the major skill requirement of the wrist surgeon for the next few decades. However, increasing benefit from limited surgical approaches, endoscopic procedures, and computer-directed techniques that use laser destructive or patch procedures is likely.[11] All of these treatment methods will benefit from improved imaging methods that will show soft-tissue or bone damage from all positions and in all functional modes before, during, and after the treatment. The future may hold an important role for robotics, virtual reality, and surgical simulators, not greatly different from pilot or astronaut equivalents currently in use.[*]

No matter what the equipment or training level, it will be superseded by ongoing developments. Reviews and retraining will be a constant need, probably recognized at a minimum level by a certification requirement (more than a baseline requirement for the practitioner).[45]

---

[*] References 11,19,36,39,44,47,51,52,59,70.

ATTENTION TO DETAIL

Regardless of advances in training, equipment, and methods, safe and proficient treatment requires great attention to the details of preplanning, periprocedural attentiveness, and postprocedural monitoring. The physician's memory may be matched to a computer checklist that is monitored by another team member. The room, its contents, and the procedure equipment will be monitored by another individual, generally the surgical nurse. Similarly, the equipment and supplies needed for anesthesia will be monitored. A full description of the procedure, including any untoward incidents, will be part of the record, which may include complete video monitoring of the entire procedure. This will permit viewing and reviewing of the entire procedure by the responsible person, the operator, whether present in the operating room or not. Errors or accidents, if noted in time, may be immediately rectified or, if not, compensated to some degree.

The attention to detail continues through the dressing application, postanesthesia positioning and transportation, and the postoperative period. Instructions to nursing attendants, patient, and the patient's attendants should be detailed and should be monitored. This attentiveness should continue throughout the early recovery stage (3-6 weeks in most instances). Future methods will make it possible to initiate guarded function (at least, range of motion) soon, but tissue reactivity will demand some rest and support. Furthermore, excessive reactivity with pain, swelling, stiffness, and other signs of abnormal response will always be the warning signals from the body. Tissue or nerve response monitoring may signal potential complications such as reflex dystrophy, compartment syndromes, or infection. Bone and soft-tissue healing (ligament and tendon) may be assisted by dynamic loading within duo threshold responses to stimulate stress but not produce permanent injury. Other problem signals such as color, temperature, and sweat abnormalities; protective postures; and excessive weakness can also be electrically, thermographically, or chemically quantitated and followed. A monitor of vascular or sudomotor response at the wrist and digits might well become routine in future management. Countermeasures can then be used as soon as the close monitoring picks up these signals.

EVALUATION OF RESULTS

Results of medical management is an area of expertise in transition.[28] The older methods of evaluation such as objective findings often had poor correlation with radiologic parameters, did not correlate with patient expectations, and were often difficult to validate statistically. During the past 5 years, outcomes assessment, wherein quality of life, patient satisfaction, and return to usual functional patterns are paramount, has become the principal focus of results evaluation.[23,28] The two methods of analysis, objective and subjective (outcome), may yield similar results, but not necessarily.[28,31] Because outcomes assessment may determine funding and referrals for the near future, it will probably become the preferred method, but it has weaknesses related to generalities of assessment rather than specifics that may prove fatal in the long run. Problems include a skewing toward short-term rather than long-term results and toward evaluation parameters that are responsive to sociologic and psychologic factors rather than toward physical and physiologic factors.[26] Eventually, an amalgam of the best features of both evaluation methods will be developed. However, the present emphasis on outcomes studies may be a useful trend for a few years in that it will focus attention on the peripheral patient-related factors that affect recovery and rehabilitation as much as the structural and pathologic problems of the original disease or injury.

REPLACEMENT POTENTIAL

Like joints, the wrist is the focus of a search for replacement parts for either part or all of its various joint systems.[41] Replacements can be biologic or prosthetic; the latter is currently favored. For soft-tissue elements about the wrist, the need, and therefore the investigative activity, will more likely be for biologic replacement. Ligament and capsule substitutes will evolve that match the inherent "modulus of elasticity" and strength characteristics of normal materials. Vascularized reconstruction of ligaments, tendons, and fibrocartilage substrates evolves. In fact, we have had preliminary experiences in selected patients.

A new era may emerge of manufacturing of spare parts within the body by means of tissue growth features. For example, a molded scaphoid may be formed subcutaneously or intramuscularly by a combination of bone graft, bone morphogenic protein, an osteoconductive catalyst, and possibly a vascular graft. Soft-tissue attachments (i.e., ligaments or capsule) can be added with fibroblastic growth factor, collagen, and appropriately designed molds attached directly to the bone substitute. In time, the biologic replacements for joint components may well be preferred over the prosthetic offerings, but the latter are already in use and are quite satisfactory for the weaker wrist. Improvements in tissue ingrowth capability for better anchoring of the implants and improved materials for less surface wear are a focus of investigation for all joint implants. Improvement will surely be forthcoming. Allograft replacements for part or all of a carpal bone have had some success and may yet prove useful if vascularization can be accelerated and the immune response can be suppressed. Whole joint transfers of allografts have not yet been attempted in the wrist, but resolution of the above problems and better control of the already weak immunologic response to joint material may make this a feasible venture for wrist reconstruction.

CONCLUSION

After being considered as such a poor relation to other parts of the body that its constituent elements were given no names or just number designations until well into the 19th century, the wrist has exploded onto the stage in the last half of the 20th century. Second to none in intrigue (where is the pain arising and why), complexity (a dynamic composite of joints with multidirectional motion), frequency of direct injury (fall on the outstretched hand is the common form of body instability), and frequency of repetitive injury (median neuritis in the carpal tunnel and wrist complaints rival the back for industrial problems), the wrist is drawing more attention now than ever before. Protection of the wrist will continue to be a high priority in sports, work, and leisure activity. Investigation of the development, anatomy, biomechanics, pathomechanics, trauma patterns, diseases, infections, and neoplasms of the wrist will continue. Treatment methods and techniques, already myriad, will also proliferate until treatment can be matched to the stage of damage. Repair or replacement of the injured structure will be a better option than developing an entirely new pattern of wrist function. Information gathering and peak development of effective diagnostic and treatment methods for the wrist should be well advanced in another 30 to 50 years.

REFERENCES

1. Abu-Laban RB: Snowboarding injuries: an analysis and comparison with alpine skiing injuries, *Can Med Assoc J* 145:1097-1103, 1991.
2. Armstrong TJ, Fine LJ, Goldstein SA, et al.: Ergonomics considerations in hand and wrist tendinitis, *J Hand Surg [Am]* 12:830-837, 1987.
3. Banas MP, Dalldorf PG, Marquardt JD: Skateboard and in-line skate fractures: a report of one summer's experience, *J Orthop Trauma* 6:301-305, 1992.
4. Belsole RJ, Hilbelink DR, Llewellyn JA, et al.: Carpal orientation from computed reference axes, *J Hand Surg [Am]* 16:82-90, 1991.
5. Belsole RJ, Hilbelink DR, Llewellyn JA, et al.: Computed analyses of the pathomechanics of scaphoid waist nonunions, *J Hand Surg [Am]* 16:899-906, 1991.
6. Bentley G, Greer RB III: Homotransplantation of isolated epiphyseal and articular cartilage chondrocytes into joint surfaces of rabbits, *Nature* 230:385-388, 1971.
7. Blair WF, Berger RA, el-Khoury GY: Arthrotomography of the wrist: an experimental and preliminary clinical study, *J Hand Surg [Am]* 10:350-359, 1985.
8. Brahme SK, Resnick D: Magnetic resonance imaging of the wrist, *Rheum Dis Clin North Am* 17:721-739, 1991.
9. Buckwalter J, Rosenberg L, Coutts R, et al.: *Articular cartilage: injury and repair.* In Woo SLY, Buckwalter JA, editors: *Injury and repair of the musculoskeletal soft tissues,* Park Ridge, Illinois, 1988, American Academy of Orthopaedic Surgeons, pp 465-482.
10. Carlsson K, Wallen P, Brodin L: Three-dimensional imaging of neurons by confocal fluorescence microscopy, *J Microsc* 155:15-26, 1989.
11. Coleman J, Nduka CC, Darzi A: Virtual reality and laparoscopic surgery, *Br J Surg* 81:1709-1711, 1994.
12. Cooney WP: Evaluation of chronic wrist pain by arthrography, arthroscopy, and arthrotomy, *J Hand Surg [Am]* 18:815-822, 1993.
13. Cooney WP: The future of arthroscopic surgery in the hand and wrist, *Hand Clin* 11:97-99, 1995.
14. Cooney WP, Berger RA: Treatment of complex fractures of the distal radius. Combined use of internal and external fixation and arthroscopic reduction, *Hand Clin* 9:603-612, 1993.
15. Dalinka MK, Meyer S, Kricun ME, et al.: Magnetic resonance imaging of the wrist, *Hand Clin* 7:87-98, 1991.
16. Engelke K, Graeff W, Meiss L, et al.: High spatial resolution imaging of bone mineral using computed microtomography. Comparison with microradiography and undecalcified histologic sections, *Invest Radiol* 28:341-349, 1993.
17. Feldman F: Thermography of the hand and wrist: practical applications, *Hand Clin* 7:99-112, 1991.
18. Feldman F, Staron R, Zwass A, et al.: MR imaging: its role in detecting occult fractures, *Skeletal Radiol* 23:439-444, 1994.
19. Frohlich B, Grunst G, Kruger W, et al.: The responsive workbench: a virtual working environment for physicians, *Comput Biol Med* 25:301-308, 1995.

20. Gautsch TL, Johnson EE, Seeger LL: True three dimensional stereographic display of 3D reconstructed CT scans of the pelvis and acetabulum, *Clin Orthop* 305:138-151, 1994.

21. Goldenstein C, McCauley R, Troy M, et al.: Ultrasonography in the evaluation of wrist swelling in children, *J Rheumatol* 16:1079-1087, 1989.

22. Hara T, Horii E, An KN, et al.: Force distribution across wrist joint: application of pressure-sensitive conductive rubber, *J Hand Surg [Am]* 17:339-347, 1992.

23. Heck DA, Maar DC, Lowdermilk GA, et al.: Comparative analysis of total knee arthroplasty in two health care delivery systems, *J Arthroplasty* 7:93-100, 1992.

24. Heckman JD, Ryaby JP, McCabe J, et al.: Acceleration of tibial fracture-healing by non-invasive, low-intensity pulsed ultrasound, *J Bone Joint Surg Am* 76:26-34, 1994.

25. Hemami H: Modeling, control, and simulation of human movement, *Crit Rev Biomed Eng* 13:1-34, 1985.

26. Ireland DC: Psychological and physical aspects of occupational arm pain, *J Hand Surg [Br]* 13:5-10, 1988.

27. James SE, Richards R, McGrouther DA: Three-dimensional CT imaging of the wrist. A practical system, *J Hand Surg [Br]* 17:504-506, 1992.

28. Keller RB, Rudicel SA, Liang MH: Outcomes research in orthopaedics, *J Bone Joint Surg Am* 75:1562-1574, 1993.

29. Kirschenbaum D, Sieler S, Solonick D, et al.: Arthrography of the wrist. Assessment of the integrity of the ligaments in young asymptomatic adults, *J Bone Joint Surg Am* 77:1207-1209, 1995.

30. Klug JD: MR diagnosis of tenosynovitis about the wrist, *Magn Reson Imaging Clin N Am* 3:305-312, 1995.

31. Labelle H, Guibert R, Joncas J, et al.: Lack of scientific evidence for the treatment of lateral epicondylitis of the elbow. An attempted meta-analysis, *J Bone Joint Surg Br* 74:646-651, 1992.

32. Linscheid RL: The hand and evolution, *J Hand Surg [Am]* 18:181-194, 1993.

33. Marciello MA, Herbison GJ, Ditunno JF Jr, et al.: Wrist strength measured by myometry as an indicator of functional independence, *J Neurotrauma* 12:99-106, 1995.

34. Marske MV, Shackley MS: Hominid hand use in the pliocene and pleistocene evidence from experimental archaeology and comparative morphology, *J Hum Evolution* 15:439-460, 1986.

35. Marzke MW: Origin of the human hand, *Am J Phys Anthropol* 34:61-84, 1971.

36. Masri BA, McGraw RW, Beauchamp CP: Robotrac in total knee arthroplasty. The silent assistant, *Am J Knee Surg* 8:20-23, 1995.

37. Mizuno M, Secher NH, Quistorff B: 31P-NMR spectroscopy, rsEMG, and histochemical fiber types of human wrist flexor muscles, *J Appl Physiol* 76:531-538, 1994.

38. O'Driscoll SW, Recklies AD, Poole AR: Chondrogenesis in periosteal explants. An organ culture model for in vitro study, *J Bone Joint Surg Am* 76:1042-1051, 1994.

39. Ota D, Loftin B, Saito T, et al.: Virtual reality in surgical education, *Comput Biol Med* 25:127-137, 1995.

40. Paivansalo M, Jalovaara P: Ultrasound findings of ganglions of the wrist, *Eur J Radiol* 13:178-180, 1991.

41. Patterson R, Viegas SF: Biomechanics of the wrist, *J Hand Ther* 8:97-105, 1995.

42. Pino EC, Colville MR: Snowboard injuries, *Am J Sports Med* 17:778-781, 1989.

43. Puck TT, Bartholdi M, Krystosek A, et al.: Confocal microscopy of genome exposure in normal, cancer, and reverse-transformed cells, *Somat Cell Mol Genet* 17:489-503, 1991.

44. Pullin G, Gammie A: Current capabilities of rehabilitation robots, *J Biomed Eng* 13:215-216, 1991.

45. Radwin RG, Lin ML, Yen TY: Exposure assessment of biomechanical stress in repetitive manual work using frequency-weighted filters, *Ergonomics* 37:1984-1998, 1994.

46. Ranney D: Work-related chronic injuries of the forearm and hand: their specific diagnosis and management, *Ergonomics* 36:871-880, 1993.

47. Rau G, Becker K, Kaufmann R, et al.: Fuzzy logic and control: principal approach and potential applications in medicine, *Artif Organs* 19:105-112, 1995.

48. Rettig ME, Raskin KB, Melone CP Jr: Clinical applications of MR imaging in hand and wrist surgery, *Magn Reson Imaging Clin N Am* 3:361-368, 1995.

49. Rofsky NM: MR angiography of the hand and wrist, *Magn Reson Imaging Clin N Am* 3:345-359, 1995.

50. Rominger MB, Bernreuter WK, Kenney PJ, et al.: MR imaging of anatomy and tears of wrist ligaments, *Radiographics* 13:1233-1246, 1993.

51. Satava RM: Virtual reality and telepresence for military medicine, *Comput Biol Med* 25:229-236, 1995.

52. Satava RM, Ellis SR: Human interface technology. An essential tool for the modern surgeon, *Surg Endosc* 8:817-820, 1994.

53. Schuind F, Cooney WP, Linscheid RL, et al.: Force and pressure transmission through the normal wrist. A theoretical two-dimensional study in the posteroanterior plane, *J Biomech* 28:587-601, 1995.

54. Short WH, Werner FW, Fortino MD, et al.: Distribution of pressures and forces on the wrist after simulated intercarpal fusion and Kienbock's disease, *J Hand Surg [Am]* 17:443-449, 1992.

55. Shung KK: Recent developments in diagnostic ultrasound, *Crit Rev Biomed Eng* 15:1-28, 1987.

56. Siddiqi NA, Ide T, Chen MY, et al.: A computer-aided walking rehabilitation robot, *Am J Phys Med Rehabil* 73:212-216, 1994.

57. Skahen JR III, Palmer AK, Levinsohn EM, et al.: Magnetic resonance imaging of the triangular fibrocartilage complex, *J Hand Surg [Am]* 15:552-557, 1990

58. Smith DK: MR imaging of normal and injured wrist ligaments, *Magn Reson Imaging Clin N Am* 3:229-248, 1995.

59. Sternad D, Collins D, Turvey MT: The detuning factor in the dynamics of interlimb rhythmic coordination, *Biol Cybern* 73:27-35, 1995.

60. Stewart NR, Gilula LA: CT of the wrist: a tailored approach, *Radiology* 183:13-20, 1992.

61. Sullivan PP, Berquist TH: Magnetic resonance imaging of the hand, wrist, and forearm: utility in patients with pain and dysfunction as a result of trauma, *Mayo Clin Proc* 66:1217-1221, 1991.

62. Timins ME, Jahnke JP, Krah SF, et al.: MR imaging of the major carpal stabilizing ligaments: normal anatomy and clinical examples, *Radiographics* 15:575-587, 1995.

63. Whipple TL: The role of arthroscopy in the treatment of scapholunate instability, *Hand Clin* 11:37-40, 1995.

64. Whipple TL, Cooney WP III, Osterman AL, et al.: Wrist arthroscopy, *Instruct Course Lect* 44:139-145, 1995.

65. Wickham JE: Minimally invasive surgery. Future developments, *BMJ* 308:193-196, 1994.

66. Williams R, Westmorland M: Occupational cumulative trauma disorders of the upper extremity, *Am J Occup Ther* 48:411-420, 1994.

67. Wills AJ, Jenkins IH, Thompson PD, et al.: A positron emission tomography study of cerebral activation associated with essential and writing tremor, *Arch Neurol* 52:299-305, 1995.

68. Wolfe SW, Crisco JJ: Mechanical evaluation of the scaphoid shift test, *J Hand Surg [Am]* 19:762-768, 1994.

69. Wotton SF, Jeacocke RE, Maciewicz RA, et al.: The application of scanning confocal microscopy in cartilage research, *Histochem J* 23:328-335, 1991.

70. Ziegler R, Fischer G, Muller W, et al.: Virtual reality arthroscopy training simulator, *Comput Biol Med* 25:193-203, 1995.

Carpal bones
  developmental anomalies, 1003-1004
  fetal development, 33-34
  motions; *see* Kinematics
  multiple, comparative morphology, 15, 16f
  ontogenesis, 62
  ossification, 1003t
  pediatric abnormalities, 1017
Carpal boss, 241-242, 242f
  in athletes, 1035, 1037
Carpal dislocations
  in children, 1021
  isolated, 696-708
    dorsal lunate, 700-702
    hamate, 705
    lunate, 696-700
    pisiform, 706
    scaphoid, 702-704
    trapezium, 705
    trapezoid, 704-705
    triquetrum, 704
  Mayo classification, 654
Carpal fractures, isolated, 474-487
  capitate, 482f, 483-484, 485f
  diagnosis and imaging, 474-475
  epidemiology, 474
  hamate, 481, 482-484f
  lunate, 475, 476-478f, 477, 479
  mechanism of injury in fall on outstretched hand, 475f
  physical examination, 243
  pisiform, 480f, 481
  trapezium-trapezoid, 483, 484f
  triquetrum, 479, 479f, 481
Carpal height ratio, 206
Carpal instability; *see also* Instability
  classification, 497, 498t, 499
    classic post-traumatic instability, 496t, 497
    goals, 490-491
    historical perspective, 491
    Lichtman, 491, 491t
    Mayo, 497, 498t, 639t
    McMurtry, 491-492, 493t
    Sennwald, 492, 495t
    Taleisnik, 492, 494t
    terminology, 492-497
    Viegas, 491, 492t
  definition, 493
  distal radius fracture and, 1093, 1095, 1097-1098f
  scaphoid fracture and, 598
Carpal instability combined/complex, 494, 498t, 559
Carpal instability dissociative
  after perilunate dislocation treatment, 648
  carpal instability nondissociative vs., 494, 498t, 550, 551f, 558f
Carpal instability nondissociative, 550-568, 551-552f; *see also*
      Radiocarpal instability and dislocations
  after perilunate dislocation treatment, 648
  carpal instability dissociative vs., 494, 498t, 551f, 558f
  classification, 559, 639t
  diagnosis, 556, 557-558f
  etiology and pathomechanics, 550-551, 553-555, 553-555f, 569
  physical examination, 559f
  radiographic evaluation, 556, 557-560f, 558
  treatment
    authors' recommendations, 561, 563-566f, 563-567
    DISI deformity and repair, 556, 557f, 565-566f
    options and results, 550-551, 560-561, 562f

  ulnar-leveling procedure, 555, 556f
  VISI deformity and repair, 552f, 563-564f, 563-565
Carpal ligaments; *see* Ligament anatomy
Carpal row; *see also* Distal carpal row; Proximal carpal row
Carpal slip, in multiple hereditary osteochondromata, 992f, 996
Carpal stability; *see also* Carpal instability; Instability; Stability
  reintroduction of concept of, 9-10
Carpal tunnel
  anatomy, 1198-1201f, 1199
  compartment syndrome and, 1107, 1108-1109f, 1109
  magnetic resonance imaging, 279f
Carpal tunnel compression test, 1045, 1205, 1206f
Carpal tunnel incision
  in hook of hamate nonunion, 155f, 156, 157f
  for median nerve release, 1082f
  in perilunate dislocations, 640, 642, 645f
Carpal tunnel release; *see also* Transverse carpal ligament release
  endoscopic visualization for, 1218, 1218f
  in ischemic contracture, 1133
  in Kienböck's disease, 460
  palmar tenosynovectomy in, 1159-1160
Carpal tunnel syndrome, 1084, 1197-1233
  anatomy, 1199-1201f
  in athletes, 1045
  bilateral, 1210
  clinical characteristics, 1202
  conservative treatment, 1208-1210
  cortisone injections in, 1207-1209f, 1210
  differential diagnosis and associated conditions, 1207-1208
  in distal radius malunion, 362
  historical perspective, 1197, 1198f
  incidence, 1202
  nerve conduction and electromyographic studies, 1207
  physical examination, 1045, 1202, 1203-1206f, 1204-1205
  physiology, 1201-1202, 1202f
  recurrent, 1228-1230
  rehabilitation, 1045
  surgical treatment, 1210
    author's preferred approach, 1220, 1221-1224f, 1223
    complications, 1227-1228
    endoscopic visualization for carpal tunnel release, 1218, 1218f
    Paine release with transverse limited wrist incision and retinacu-
        latome, 1216f, 1218
    for recurrent carpal tunnel syndrome, 1229-1230
    release through palmar incision, 1214, 1216f
    release through two nonpalmar incisions, 1217f, 1218
    release with incision above wrist, 1210, 1214, 1215f, 12111-1213f
    release with limited-excision techniques, 1214, 1216f, 1217
    reoperations, 1228
    results, 1228
    single-portal technique of endoscopic release, 1223, 1224-1226f,
        1225, 1227, 1227f
    tenosynovectomy alone, 1227
    two-portal technique of endoscopic release, 1219f, 1220
Carpal tunnel view, 265-267, 268f
Carpal-ulnar distance ratio, 582, 582f
Carpectomy; *see* Proximal row carpectomy
Carpometacarpal arthrosis, ulnar, 246
Carpometacarpal bones, comparative morphology, 20f
Carpometacarpal joint(s)
  anatomy, 69
  common, 70
  first
    anatomy, 69
    exposure, 158, 161-162f, 163
    morphology, 20, 21f

Carpometacarpal joint(s)—cont'd
  fractures and fracture dislocations
    in athletes, 1059-1060, 1060f
    classification, 1060, 1061f
  instability, 495, 496t
  physical examination, 241-242, 242f
Carpometacarpal ligament, 47f
Carpus; see also Wrist entries
  axial disruption of; see Axial dislocations and fracture dislocations
  chevron, 967, 968f, 970
    pain from, 975, 975f
    surgical treatment, 972-973
  coalitions, 1004-1006, 1005-1006f, 1017
  fusion, in carpal instability nondissociative, 566
  international terminology/etymology, 2, 3, 5f, 61-62
  omission of, in medieval drawing, 3f
  pediatric anomalies, 1016
    deformities and developmental conditions, 1006-1007, 1017-1018
    ligament laxity, 1016-1017
    skeletal abnormalities, 1017
  pediatric injuries, 1021-1022
  in rheumatoid arthritis
    changes in juvenile rheumatoid arthritis, 949, 950-951f
    collapse deformities, 881
    palmar subluxation/dislocation, 888-889, 889f, 901f
    stabilization, 885
  ulnar translocation of, 582, 583-586f, 586-587
  vulnerable zones of, 652f
Cartilaginous lesions, arthroscopy
  diagnostic, 298, 298f
  therapeutic, 301
Casts; see also Immobilization
  for distal radius fractures, 322f, 324, 330, 338, 347
  for perilunate dislocations, 639-640
  for perilunate fracture dislocations, 669
  for scaphoid fractures, 389f, 390f, 396, 397-398f, 409
  skin complications of, 1076-1077, 1077f
  in total wrist arthroplasty, 937
Catch-up clunk
  in children, 1025
  in midcarpal instability, 247, 250f, 555f, 558
  reverse, 558
Catheters, in compartment pressure measurement, 1119f, 1120
Causalgia; see also Reflex sympathetic dystrophy; Somatic nerve pain
  definition, 1098t
Centralization, in radial aplasia, 1009, 1010f, 1011-1013
Cervical radiculopathy, 1207
Chaput, Henri, 9
Charcot-Marie-Tooth disease, 1117
Charpy, A., 10
Chauffeur fracture, 320, 352
Cheilotomy/cheilectomy, 1064, 1065
Chen compression test, in scaphoid fractures, 1048
Cheselden, William, 3
Chevron carpus, 967, 968f, 970
  pain from, 975, 975f
  surgical treatment, 972-973
Children; see Pediatrics
Chimpanzees, wrist and hand of, 17f, 18t, 21f, 25
Chondrodesis, in radial aplasia, 1011
Chondromalacia, 788, 789
  arthroscopy, 301
  of distal radioulnar joint, 842-843, 845f
  triangular fibrocartilage and, 846
  in ulnar impingement syndrome, 298, 298f
Chondrosarcoma, 1256, 1256f
Chow technique of transverse carpal ligament release, 1219f, 1220
CIND; see Carpal instability nondissociative

Cineradiography, of lunotriquetral sprains, 534-535
Clayton, Ferlic, and Volz total wrist arthroplasty, 941, 942f
Clayton-Ferlic procedure, 1146, 1147-1149f
Closed reduction
  of distal radius fractures, 322f, 328, 329-333f
  Mayfield paradox of, 511
  of perilunate dislocations, 638-640, 641-643f
Club hand, radial, exposures, 163-167f, 164, 166-167
Coalitions, carpal, 1004-1006, 1005-1006f, 1017
Cold therapy, 1263-1265, 1265f
Collagen fascicles, 74-76f
Collapse deformities; see also Scaphoid nonunion advanced collapse;
    Scapholunate advanced collapse wrist
  historical perspective, 9
  in rheumatoid arthritis, 881, 900
Colles fracture, 315, 315f; see also Distal radius fractures
  angulation deformity in, 358
  carpal alignment after, 362
  complications, 321, 1089
  loss of motion in, 361
  malunion after, 356, 1090; see also Distal radius malunion
    arthrodesis for, 373
    osteotomy for, 358t, 361f, 363, 364-365f, 365, 365t
    pressure distribution and, 327, 327f
  pathomechanics, 388f
  reverse; see Smith fracture
  silver fork deformity in, 362
  treatment
    closed reduction, 328, 329-330f
    displaced extra-articular fractures, 347, 350
    extra-articular fractures, 347
    open reduction, 328, 334-335f, 338
  with triangular fibrocartilage tear, 722
  ulnar styloid and triangular fibrocartilage injuries with, 841
Columnar dislocations; see Axial dislocations and fracture dislocations
Columnar instability, 494
Comparative anatomy; see Morphology, comparative
Compartment syndrome, 1107-1135
  anatomy, 1107, 1108-1110f, 1109
  biomechanics, 1109-1110, 1111-1112f
  diagnosis, 1116-1117
  etiology, 1114, 1115-1116f, 1116
  historical perspective, 1111, 1113f, 1113-1114
  measurement of compartment pressure in, 1108-1109f, 1117-1118
    techniques, 1118, 1119f, 1120
  overuse injury, 1299
  signs and symptoms of reported syndromes, 1120t
  surgical treatment, 1122
    forearm, 1122-1124f, 1123, 1125, 1126-1127f
    hand and wrist, 1121f, 1122-1123
  Volkmann's contracture and, 1125-1134
Complex motion tomography, 271
Complications of wrist injury, 1076-1106
  bone and joint, 1089-1095
  pain syndromes, 1095-1104
  soft-tissue injuries, 1076-1089
Compression neuropathy; see also Carpal tunnel syndrome; Nerve
    entrapment syndromes in athletes
  treatment, 1087, 1088f
Compression plate, in ulna recession, 782f, 783, 784f, 850f
Compression test
  lunotriquetral, 531f, 532
  in scaphoid fractures, 1048
Computed tomography, advantages and applications, 277-278, 277-278f
  arthritis deformity, 790f
  degenerative joint disease, 845f
  distal radioulnar joint instability, 755f

distal radioulnar joint subluxation, 762f
growth-plate injuries, 983
hook of hamate fractures, 1058f
rheumatoid arthritis, 889
ulnar head subluxation, 829f, 837f
Concept traction tower for arthroscopy, 181, 184f
Condylar implants, in wrist arthrodesis for rheumatoid arthritis, 913f
Congenital anomalies/disorders
carpal changes in, 1006-1007, 1006-1007f, 1007t
damage control in, 1308-1309
in differential diagnosis, 1024
distal radioulnar joint, 854f, 854-855
distal radius
centralization, 1009, 1010f, 1011-1013
deficient radius, 1007-1008, 1008f
treatment, 1008-1009, 1008-1010f
distal ulna, 1013, 1016
in Kienböck's disease, 441
ulna deficiency, 1013-1016
Continuous passive motion, 1262-1263, 1263-1264f
Contracture
distal radioulnar joint, 843, 845
ischemic; see Volkmann's ischemic contracture
Coronal sectional anatomy, 57-58, 58-59f
Corson, E.R., 5
Cortical bone graft inlay, in wrist arthrodesis for rheumatoid arthritis, 903f
Corticosteroids
in athletic tendon disorders, 1033, 1037
in carpal tunnel syndrome, 1045
in juvenile rheumatoid arthritis, 950, 952
in tendinitis, 1182
de Quervain's disease, 1034, 1185
of extensor pollicis longus, 1187
Linburg's syndrome, 1194
Cortisone injections, in carpal tunnel syndrome, 1207-1209f, 1210
CPM, 1262-1263, 1263-1264f
Crush injury of carpus, 685f, 686-687, 687f, 688f; see also Axial dislocations and fracture dislocations
Cryotherapy, 1263-1265, 1265f
Crystalline deposition disease, in rheumatoid arthritis, 872t
Crystalline-induced synovitis, 1146-1147, 1149-1150f
Cumulative trauma disorder, 1296; see also Overuse syndrome
epidemiology, 1297, 1297f
work hardening in, 1291
Currents, for electrical stimulation, 1268-1269
Cutaneous dysesthetic pain, 122
Cutaneous nerves
dorsal and palmar, 121f
lateral antebrachial cutaneous nerve, 119f, 120, 120f
posterior antebrachial cutaneous nerve, 119f
Cutaneous neuropathy, 1084-1085, 1087
Cyclist's palsy, 1040, 1042f, 1042-1043
Cyriax, E.F., 10
Cysts
bone
aneurysmal, 1252, 1253f, 1256
solitary, 1251f, 1252
epidermoid inclusion, 1240
ganglion; see Ganglion cysts
in lunate, 777f, 779f

D
Dacron silicone ligamentous tether, 833f
Danninger portable continuous passive motion, 1264f
Darrach resection
in arthritis deformity, 789, 791f, 792
technique, 794, 796-799f, 800, 801f

in distal radioulnar joint disorders, 753, 759, 844f
as salvage procedure, 855-858f, 857
in distal radius malunion, 367-368
of distal ulna, 781, 781f
modifications, 856f, 857, 858-859f
in rheumatoid arthritis, 909
for synovitis, 1141, 1141f
fusion-arthroplasty with, 895f
Dart-thrower's motion, 6, 10
de Quervain's disease (tenosynovitis), 1183, 1184f, 1185
in athletes, 1034-1035, 1034-1036f
physical examination, 238, 239f
treatment, 1078-1079
nonoperative, 1184-1185f, 1185
surgical, 1185f, 1185-1186
Débridement
in arthroscopic synovectomy, 1160
for triangular fibrocartilage tears, 1068
Decompression
in de Quervain's tenosynovitis, 1034-1035, 1034-1036f
in flexor carpi radialis tendinitis, 1192, 1193f, 1194
Decoulx classification of Kienböck's disease, 443
Deep heat, 1265, 1266-1267
Deformity
from arthritis; see Arthritis deformity of distal radioulnar joint;
Rheumatoid arthritis
carpus, 1017-1018
in distal radius malunion, 362
distal ulna, congenital, 1016
from multiple hereditary osteochondromata, 991-1001
Degenerative arthritis; see also Arthritis deformity of distal radioulnar
joint; Post-traumatic arthritis
of distal radioulnar joint, 842-843, 843-845f
Degenerative tears of triangular fibrocartilage, 720-722
Denervation
in Kienböck's disease, 453
in scaphoid nonunion advanced collapse, 622
in synovitis, 895
DePalma technique of pin placement, 341, 343
DePuy arthroplasty, 926f
DePuy prosthesis, 928f
Dermatofibroma, 1236
Dermatology; see Skin entries
Dermatomyositis, 884f
Destot, Etienne, 7f, 7-8, 502f, 503f
Development, ossification of carpal bones, 1003t
Developmental disorders
anomalies of wrist skeleton
carpal coalitions, 1004-1006, 1005-1006f
coalitions, accessory carpal bones, and other variations, 1003-1004, 1004f
congenital or developmental syndromes (carpal changes), 1006-1007, 1006-1007f, 1007t
carpal deformities and, 1017-1018
damage control, 1308-1309
in differential diagnosis, 1024
in Kienböck's disease, 441
Dexamethasone, in carpal tunnel syndrome, 1210
Diagnostic methods, future perspective, 1308
Diaphyseal aclasis; see Multiple hereditary osteochondromata
Diathermy, short wave, 1266-1267
Digital arteries, 39f
Digital nerves, 36f, 37f
Digital subtraction arthrography
in scapholunate instability, 509
in ulnocarpal abutment, 780f
Dimple sign, 246f

Direct current, for electrical stimulation, 1268-1269
Disability, accommodation in, 1291-1292
Discus articularis, 65f, 760, 761f
DISI; *see* Dorsal intercalated segment instabilities
Dislocations; *see also specific anatomy and* Fracture dislocations
    axial; *see* Axial dislocations and fracture dislocations
    in carpal instability classification, 496t
    in carpal instability nondissociative, 556, 557f
    isolated carpal; *see* Carpal dislocations, isolated
    ulnar head, 826-839
Dissociation, 493-494
Distal carpal row
    interosseous ligaments, 94-96, 95f, 95t
    normal kinematics, 209-210
Distal radioulnar joint
    anatomy, 66f, 69, 295f, 775f, 820-826, 820-826f
        arthroscopic, 179, 181, 182f, 294f, 295
        transverse section, 51
        variations in shape, 219-222, 220f, 221t
    arthrodesis, 781f; *see also* Sauvé-Kapandji procedure
    arthrography, 275f, 276
    in arthroscopic synovectomy, 1161
    arthroscopy, 297
        examination in sports injuries, 1065t
        inspection, 187
        portals, 291-292
    biomechanics, 819-826, 820-826f
    computed tomography, 277f, 278
    in distal radius fracture, 323
    evolution of, 819
    prosthetic replacement, 789, 792f
    radiographic examination, 264
    rotational injury, 711
    stability, 225-226f, 225-228, 227t, 760-764
    subluxation, 762f, 766-767; *see also* Distal radioulnar joint instability
        in rheumatoid arthritis, 891-892
    torque transfer and, 819, 820f
    ulna recession and, 781, 782f, 786
Distal radioulnar joint dislocations, 227-228, 758-772, 759f
    classification, 764-765
    diagnosis, 766-767f, 766-768
    literature review, 758-759
    pathomechanics, 765-766
    terminology, 760
    treatment and complications
        extra-articular fracture dislocations (type III), 765f, 768-770, 769f
        intra-articular fracture dislocations (type II), 762f, 768
        pure dislocations (type I), 766f, 768
Distal radioulnar joint disorders
    anatomy and physiology, 820-826
    arthritis; *see* Arthritis deformity of distal radioulnar joint
    chrondromalacia and degenerative arthritis, 842-843, 843-845f
    congenital malformations, 854f, 854-855
    contracture, 843, 845
    gymnast's wrist, 853
    miscellaneous, 862
    proximal migration of radius, 849, 852
    rotational injury; *see also* Triangular fibrocartilage tears
    salvage procedures
        radioulnar synostosis with proximal segment excision, 857, 859-860f
        ulnar head excision, 855-859f, 857
    synovitis, 1140f
    tendinitis and tendon subluxation, 859, 861-862, 861-862f
    triangular fibrocartilage injuries and styloid fractures, 839-842, 840t, 840-842f; *see also* Triangular fibrocartilage tears
    ulna minus conditions, 853-854

    ulna variance conditions
        treatment, 849, 850-852f
        ulnar impaction (abutment) syndrome, 846-847, 846-849f
        ulnar styloid impingement and loose bodies, 852-853, 853f
        Vaughan-Jackson lesion, 1138, 1139f
Distal radioulnar joint fractures, 743-757
    adult ulnar fractures, 748f, 749-755
    anatomy, 743-745
    embryology, 743
    pediatric ulnar fractures, 745f, 746-749
Distal radioulnar joint instability, 227-228, 495, 496t; *see also* Distal radioulnar joint dislocations; Distal radioulnar joint mechanics, stability
    associated injuries, 722
    chronic, 826-839
    dorsal subluxation or dislocation of ulna
        pathogenesis, 826-828, 830f
        radiographic examination, 828-829, 829f
        treatment, 829-835, 830-836f
    historical and literature review, 758-759
    palmar subluxation and dislocation
        pathogenesis, 835-836, 836f
        radiographic examination, 836, 837f
        treatment, 836-839, 838f
    physical examination, 244, 245f, 246f
    provocative stress testing, 245f, 260
Distal radioulnar joint mechanics, 219-230
    contacts, 224-225
    force transmission, 228-229t, 228-230, 229f
    kinematics
        basic concepts, 219
        normal range of forearm motion, 222, 224
        pronation-supination, 222-224f
        shape of joint and, 219-222, 220f, 221t
        "ulnocarpal" joint, 224
    stability, 225-226f, 225-227, 760, 763f; *see also* Distal radioulnar joint instability
        axial migration of forearm bones limited by ligaments, 228
        infratendinous extensor retinaculum, 763-764
        interosseous membrane, 227, 764
        musculotendinous stabilizers, 227
        orientation and congruity of articular surfaces, 760, 761f
        pronator quadratus muscle, 764
        soft-tissue constraints, 760-764
        triangular fibrocartilage, 227t, 760, 761f, 762
        ulnocarpal ligamentous complex, 763, 763f
Distal radioulnar ligaments, in joint stability, 226f, 226-227, 228, 760, 761f, 762
Distal radioulnar portal, 172f
Distal radius
    anatomy, 64f, 66-67f, 68, 80f
        fractures and, 310, 311-313f, 312-314
        vascular supply, 38, 40f, 41, 107-108, 111f, 116-118, 117f
    congenital deficiency, 1007-1008
        centralization in, 1009, 1010f, 1011-1013
        classification, 1008f
        treatment, 1008-1009, 1008-1010f, 1013
    gymnastic injuries, 1062f, 1063-1064
    hemiepiphyseal stapling of, in multiple hereditary osteochondromata, 996, 997f
    pedicle grafts, 116-117, 117f
    premature partial fusion of, 983f
Distal radius fractures, 310-355; *see also* Barton fracture; Colles fracture; Distal radius malunion; Smith fracture
    arthritis and, 844f
    arthroscopy, 299, 304-305

associated injuries
    distal radioulnar joint, 323, 323f
    loss of reduction, 321, 322f, 1089-1090, 1089-1092f, 1092
    median neuropathy, 321
    open fractures, 323
carpal instability and, 1093, 1095, 1097-1098f
in children, 1018, 1020, 1020f
classification, 315
    Barton fracture, 315, 316f
    Colles fracture, 315, 315f
    Frykman, 315, 317, 317f, 317t
    Mayo, 319-320, 320f
    Melone, 319, 319f
    Smith fracture, 315, 316f
    universal, 317, 318f, 319, 319t
complications, 356, 1089-1095
degenerative arthritis of distal radioulnar joint after, imaging, 789f
force transmission and, 198, 202
malunion; see Distal radius malunion
mechanisms of injury, 314f, 314-315, 320-321
median neuropathy in, 1082f, 1084
nonunion, 1092, 1093-1094f
presentation, 321
radiographic examination, 266
rehabilitation exercises, 325f
tomography, 272f
treatment
    algorithm, 319t, 337f
    author's preference, 322-325f, 324, 347, 350, 352
    Barton fracture, 352
    bone grafting, 330, 336-337f, 346f
    Chauffeur fracture, 352
    closed reduction, 322f, 328, 329-333f
    complex fractures, 346-347f, 350, 352
    displaced extra-articular Colles-type fractures, 347, 350
    displaced fractures and anatomic reduction, 324, 326-327f, 327-328
    external fixation, 338, 339-340f, 341
    extra-articular fractures, 347
    immobilization, 330, 337f, 338
    intra-articular fractures, 350
    open reduction, 328, 330, 334-337f, 343, 346-350f, 347
    percutaneous pin fixation, 338, 340-342f, 341, 343, 344-345f
    Smith fracture, 352
    undisplaced fractures, 323-324
triangular fibrocartilage avulsion or tear with, 738
Distal radius malunion, 356-384, 1092-1093, 1095-1096f
angulation, 357f, 357-358, 359f
complications
    arthrosis, 361
    carpal instability, 362, 362f
    cosmetic deformity, 362
    loss of motion, 361
    neuropathy, 362
    pain, 360-361
    tendon attrition, 363
    weakness, 361
corrective osteotomy in, 577f
dorsally malangulated, 571, 571f
epidemiology, 356-357
joint incongruity, 360
radiocarpal and midcarpal instability in, 572f, 573f
shortening, 357f, 358-360, 359f
treatment procedures, 363
    authors' preferred method, 373, 374-381f, 376-378
    to eliminate pain, 368-370, 370-373f, 373
    for extra-articular malunions, 376-380f, 378

    to gain functional improvement, 365, 367-368, 369f
    for intra-articular malunions, 374-377f, 376-378
    to restore anatomic relationships, 358t, 361t, 363-365, 364-367f, 365t
Distal ulna
anatomy, 64-66f, 68-69
    muscle attachments, 743-745, 744f
    structural support, 745
caput ulnae syndrome, 874, 874f, 909
congenital deficiency, 1013
congenital deformity, 1016
embryology, 743
fractures; see Distal radioulnar joint fractures; Ulnar fractures
impingement, treatment methods, 781, 781f
multiple hereditary exostoses and, 854
osteotomy, 145f
pediatric injuries, 1020-1021
resection
    Darrach procedure, 794, 796-799f, 800, 801f, 855f
    in distal radius malunion, 367-368
    matched, 808, 810f, 811, 857, 859f
    methods, 781, 781f, 855-856f
    in multiple hereditary osteochondromata, 994-995f, 999
    patient selection, 1090
    in total wrist arthroplasty, 930, 931f, 937
    Tsai technique, 800, 804-807f
soft-tissue stabilization, in rheumatoid arthritis, 884
stabilized by pronator quadratus interposition, 800, 808f
synostosis to radius, 754-755
wafer excision, 1068-1069, 1069f
Distraction, distal radius and ulna physeal injury from, 1063-1064
Distraction frame, in radial aplasia, 1009-1010f, 1011
Distraction resection arthroplasty, in scaphoid nonunion advanced
    collapse, 621-622
Doppler ultrasonography, of ganglions, 1176f
Dorsal approaches, 126-127, 127-132f, 132-133
    dorsal radial approach to scaphoid, 149, 153-154f, 155, 1053
    in lunate dislocations, 698, 699f
    in perilunate dislocations, 640, 644f
    in perilunate fracture dislocations, 663, 670-671f, 677f
    radial, 133, 134-136f
        to scaphoid, 146, 149-152f
    in radial aplasia, 167f
    synovectomy, 952, 954f, 1143f
    in triangular fibrocartilage tears, 723-724f, 724
    ulnar, 140, 141-143f, 144
Dorsal capsulotomy options, 99
Dorsal distal radioulnar ligament, 760, 762, 763
Dorsal extensor tendinitis, in athletes, 1035
Dorsal flap (Nahigian) arthroplasty, in Kienböck's disease, 451, 451f
Dorsal intercalated segment instabilities (DISI)
    carpal instability nondissociative and, 556, 557f, 565-566f
    in carpal tunnel syndrome, 1202f
    definition, 493
    historical perspective, 9, 10
    in rheumatoid arthritis, 881f, 901f
    scaphoid fracture and, 387, 388-389f, 392f, 399f
    in scaphoid nonunion, 598f
Dorsal intercarpal ligament; see also Scaphotriquetral ligament
    anatomy, 67f, 88, 88f, 89f, 656f
    in arthrodesis for scapholunate instability, 521f
    in fracture dislocations, 656f
Dorsal portals, 173f
Dorsal radial wrist examination
    carpal boss, 241-242, 242f
    scapholunate interval, 240-241, 241f
    in soft tissue injuries, 242-243, 244f

Dorsal radiocarpal ligament, 87, 87t, 88f, 89f
Dorsal radiolunate ligament, 656f, 657f
Dorsal radiolunotriquetral ligament, 656f
Dorsal radiotriquetral ligament, 656f, 657f
    in lunotriquetral joint kinematics, 528, 529f
    in radiocarpal rotation and stability, 827f
Dorsal radioulnar joint, 823-825, 824-825f
    kinematic constraints, 824-825, 825f
Dorsal radioulnar ligament
    augmentation or replacement, 830, 832, 832f
    in joint stability, 225-226, 226f
    in kinematic constraint of distal radioulnar joint, 761f, 763f, 824-825,
        825f, 835-836
    mechanical properties, 227t
    in triangular fibrocartilage complex, 97, 98-99, 821f, 821-822
Dorsal rim intra-articular fractures, 576, 578-579f, 581
Dorsal scaphotriquetral ligament, 174f
    in lunotriquetral joint kinematics, 528, 528f
Dorsal superficial ulnar sensory nerve disorders, 862
Dorsal surface anatomy, 34-35
Dorsal synovectomy, 952, 954f
Dorsal transcarpal ligament, 174f
Dorsal translation/translocation, 495
Dorsal triquetral hamate ligament, 656f
Dorsal ulnar sensory nerve, transverse retinacular branch, 1038f
Dorsal ulnar wrist examination, 243
    carpometacarpal arthrosis, 246
    distal radioulnar joint instability, 244, 245f, 246f
    lunotriquetral instability, 245-246, 248-249f
    midcarpal instability, 246-247, 250-251f
    triquetral-hamate impaction, 246
    ulnar impaction syndrome, 244-245, 247f
Dorsal wedge corrective osteotomy, 572, 574-577f, 576
Dorsal wrist synovectomy, 1156-1157, 1157-1158f, 1159
Dorsal-medial approach to ulna, 751, 752f
Dorsiflexion jam syndrome, 1062
Dowel grips in gymnastics, 1063f, 1063-1064
DRUJ; see Distal radioulnar joint
Drummer's wrist, 1037
Dupuytren, Guillaume, 3, 1113-1114
Dynamic splinting, 1279-1280f, 1281, 1282
Dyschondrosteosis, 966, 967, 968-969f; see also Madelung's deformity
Dysplasia
    radial, 973, 975f
    skeletal, 1007t, 1024

E
Edema
    in compartment syndrome, 1115f, 1116
    postoperative, management, 1273-1274
Egg-cup deformity, 879f, 882f
Ehlers-Danlos syndrome, 1016
Elastic semirigid splint, 1280f
Elastic wraps and garments, 1273-1274, 1274f
Electrical stimulation; see also Pulsed electromagnetic stimulation
    for muscle contraction, 1268-1269
    for pain control, 1268, 1269f
    in scaphoid nonunion, 407
    in somatic nerve pain, 1101-1102, 1102-1103f, 1104
    transcutaneous electrical nerve stimulation (TENS), 1104, 1268, 1269t
Electromyography, in carpal tunnel syndrome, 1207
Electrotherapy, 1268
Elevators, in transverse carpal ligament release, 1214, 1216f, 1220,
        1221-1222f
Embryology, 32-34
    radioscapholunate ligament, 81-82, 84f
    ulna, 743
Enchondroma, 1250f, 1252

Enchondromatosis, 1006f
Endoscopic carpal tunnel release, 1218, 1218f
    author's preferred approach, 1220, 1221-1223f, 1223
    single-portal technique, 1223, 1224-1226f, 1225, 1227, 1227f
    topographic landmarks, 1201f
    two-portal technique, 1219f, 1220
Endoscopy; see also Arthroscopy
    diagnostic, in children, 1027
    future of, 1309
Enteropathic arthritis, 872
Entrapment
    of abductor pollicis longus and extensor pollicis brevis, 239f
    nerve; see Carpal tunnel syndrome; Nerve entrapment syndromes in
        athletes
    tendon, 1079, 1079f, 1081, 1081f
Epidermoid inclusion cysts, 1240
Epiligamentum, 74-75, 75f
Epiphysiolysis, 970
Epiphysis, displacement and reduction of, 985
Epithelioid sarcoma, 1245, 1249f
Epithelioma, 1237f
Equipment for arthroscopy, 183-184f, 286-290, 1160
Ergonomics, 1309
Eryops, 16f, 22
Essex-Lopresti fractures, 228, 722, 769
    prosthetic replacement and, 770f
    ulnar styloid and triangular fibrocartilage injuries with, 841
Evolution, 25-27
Ewing's sarcoma, 1257f, 1258
Examination; see Imaging; Physical examination of wrist
Excision arthroplasty
    in Kienböck's disease, 450-451, 450-452f
    in post-traumatic arthritis, 611, 614-615f, 624
Exostoses, multiple hereditary; see also Multiple hereditary osteochondromata
    in distal radioulnar joint disorders, 854, 855
Extension/flexion, axis for, 211f
Extensor carpi radialis, in ligamentous augmentation for scapholunate
        dissociation, 515f
Extensor carpi radialis brevis, 46f
Extensor carpi radialis longus, 46f
    in synovitis treatment, 1141, 1147f, 1149f
Extensor carpi ulnaris
    anatomy, 46f, 47f, 170f, 744f, 1038f
        triangular fibrocartilage complex and, 97-98, 97-98f
    in Bowers hemiresection arthroplasty, 809f
    in distal radioulnar joint salvage, 857, 859, 860f
    distal ulna and, 744f, 744-745
    in distal ulna excision, 794, 796f, 799f, 800
        Tsai technique, 800, 804-807f
    in dorsal dislocation of ulnar head, 828f
    entrapment, 1081f
    in joint stability, 227, 761f
    in modified Darrach procedure, 856f
    in Sauvé-Kapandji procedure, 811, 812f
    stenosing tenosynovitis, in athletes, 1037
    subluxation, 861-862, 862f, 1188-1189
        in athletes, 1038, 1039f, 1040
    subsheath
        in radiocarpal rotation and stability, 827f
        release and reconstruction, in stenosing tenosynovitis, 1037, 1039f
    in synovitis treatment, 1141, 1144f, 1147f
    tendinitis, 859, 1188-1189, 1188-1190f
    in treatment of dorsal subluxation or dislocation of ulna, 832
    in ulnar approaches in arthrotomy, 133, 140
Extensor digiti minimi
    anatomy, 46f, 170f
    tendinitis, 1188
    in ulnar approaches in arthrotomy, 133

Extensor digiti quinti
    anatomy, 98f
    in distal ulna excision, 794, 797f, 800
Extensor digitorum (communis), 46f, 170f, 744f
Extensor indicis proprius
    anatomy, 46f, 170f, 744f
    transfer, 1078, 1080f
Extensor indicis proprius syndrome, 1188
    in athletes, 1037
Extensor insertional tenosynovitis, in athletes, 1035, 1037
Extensor manus brevis, in physical examination, 243
Extensor pollicis brevis
    anatomy, 34f, 46f
    in de Quervain's disease, 1183, 1183f, 1185
    entrapment, 239f
    in intersection syndrome, 1186
Extensor pollicis longus
    anatomy, 34f, 35, 46f, 170f, 237f, 744f
    dorsal wrist synovectomy and, 1159
    injury to, 1077, 1079f
    rupture, treatment, 897, 1080f
    tendinitis, 1187f, 1187-1188
    tenosynovitis, in athletes, 1037
    transposition radial to Lister's tubercle, 1037
Extensor retinaculum
    anatomy, 43-44, 45-47, 46-47f, 98f, 99f
    in dorsal approach in arthrotomy, 128f, 131-132f
    in dorsal ulnar approach in arthrotomy, 141f
    in extensor carpi ulnaris instability treatment, 1189, 1190f
    infratendinous, in distal radioulnar joint stability, 761f, 763-764
    in radiocarpal rotation and stability, 827f
    in recurrent subluxation of extensor carpi ulnaris tendon, 1040
    sling, 1040
    in synovectomy, 1143-1144f, 1146f, 1148-1149f
        dorsal wrist synovectomy, 1157, 1158f, 1159
    in ulnar approach in arthrotomy, 138f
Extensor tendons
    dorsal extensor tendinitis in athletes, 1035
    injuries, 1077, 1079-1080, 1079-1081f
    radial wrist, functional absence in, 927
    ruptures, 243
        treatment of, 896-897
    tenosynovitis, 876f, 890
        treatment of, 892-893
Extensor tenosynovectomy, 1157-1158f
    in juvenile rheumatoid arthritis, 952, 953-955f
External fixation
    complications from pin placement, 1086f
    of distal radius fractures, 331f, 333-334f, 338, 339-340f, 341, 346f, 350, 352, 1086f

F
Fasciitis, nodular, 1243
Fasciotomy, in compartment syndrome, 1118
    technique, 1121-1124f, 1122-1123, 1125
Feldon procedure, 737, 738f, 739, 781f
Fetal development of wrist, 32-34
Fibroma, 1243
Fibromatosis, 1243, 1244f
Fibrosarcoma, 1245, 1248f
Fibrositis syndrome, 1299
Fibrous histiocytoma
    benign, 1243
    malignant, 1247, 1250
Fibrous stratum, 74f, 75f
Fibrous synostosis, in scaphoid nonunion, 407, 409
Fibrous tumors, 1243
Fick, Rudolph, 4, 6f, 6-7

Fingers
    arteries and nerves, 36f, 37f, 39f
    extensor tendon ruptures at wrist, treatment of, 896
    flexor tendon ruptures at wrist, treatment of, 897
    flexor tenosynovitis, 252, 890
Finger-trap traction
    device, 295f, 296
    in distal radius fracture, 322f
Finkelstein's test, 238, 239f, 1034, 1183
First carpometacarpal joint
    anatomy, 69
    exposure, 158, 161-162f, 163
    morphology, 20, 21f
First dorsal compartment anatomy, 1183f
First intermetacarpal nerve, 119f
Fisk, Geoffrey, 9, 9f
"Fist" exercise, 325f
Fixation of fractures; see External fixation; Internal fixation; Pin fixation; Plate fixation; Screw fixation
Fixed unit hypothesis, 206
Flaps
    in Bowers hemiresection arthroplasty, 809f
    in ischemic contracture, 1132
    in modified Darrach procedure, 856f
    in recurrent carpal tunnel syndrome, 1229-1230
    for soft-tissue coverage, 1077, 1078f
    in synovectomy for juvenile rheumatoid arthritis, 952
    vascularized, 1310
Flexion
    comparative morphology, 15, 17-19
    range of, 21
Flexion/extension, axis for, 211f
Flexor carpi radialis
    anatomy, 1191-1192f
    in ligamentous augmentation for scapholunate dissociation, 516f
    tendinitis, 252, 1191-1192, 1193f
        nonoperative treatment, 1192
        operative treatment, 1192, 1193f, 1194
Flexor carpi ulnaris
    advancement from pisiform to dorsum of triquetrum, 832, 836f
    anatomy, 47f
    in compartment syndrome treatment, 1122f
    in distal radioulnar joint salvage, 857, 860f
    in ligamentous augmentation, 834f
    tendinitis, 253, 1189, 1191
    in treatment of palmar subluxation and dislocation of ulnar head, 838f, 839
    in ulnocarpal tendinous tethers, 832, 833-834f
Flexor digitorum profundus, in Linburg's syndrome, 1194
Flexor digitorum superficialis, in compartment syndrome treatment, 1122f
Flexor pollicis longus
    entrapment, 1079f
    in Linburg's syndrome, 1194
    rupture at thumb, treatment of, 897
Flexor retinaculum
    anatomy, 43-45, 45f
    components, 1201f
    in transverse stability of carpus, 687
Flexor slide procedures, in ischemic contracture, 1130f, 1132
Flexor tendons
    anatomy, 35
    injuries, 1077-1078, 1079, 1079f
    tenosynovitis, 252, 877f, 890, 893
Flexor tenosynovectomy, 893, 1142f, 1159-1160, 1161
Fluidotherapy, 1266, 1267f
Football injuries, epidemiology, 1032

Force transmission
  through distal radioulnar joint, 229t, 229-230
  through radiocarpal joint, 190-194
    analytical measurement, 191, 194, 196-197f
    experimental studies, 191, 192-196f
    normal wrist joint, 196-197, 198-199t, 199-200f
    pathologic conditions, 197-198, 200-202f, 201-203
  triangular fibrocartilage degeneration and, 230
  ulnocarpal, 228-229, 228-229f, 229t
Forearm
  compartment syndrome, 1109, 1109f
    signs and symptoms, 1120t
    surgical treatment, 1122-1124f, 1123, 1125, 1126f
  interosseous membrane of, in distal radioulnar joint stability, 227
  ischemic contracture, surgical treatment, 1127, 1130-1133f, 1132-1133
  kinematics, 822-823, 823f
  pronation-supination, in distal radioulnar joint instability, 260
  rotation, normal range of, 222, 224
Forte plate system, 349f
Fossil wrist bones, 22-25
Fracture dislocations
  Barton, 578-580f, 581-582
  in carpal instability classification, 496t
  distal radioulnar joint, 768-770
  perilunate; see Perilunate fracture dislocations
  tomography, 273
Fractures; see also specific anatomy and eponyms
  ancient treatment, 1111, 1113f
  arthroscopy
    diagnostic, 299
    therapeutic, 304-305
  carpal bone, 243; see also Carpal fractures, isolated
  in children, 1022
  dorsal rim intra-articular, 576, 578-579f, 581
  fixation; see specific methods
  malunion, 1094-1095, 1095-1096f
  nonunion, 1092, 1093-1094
  occult, tomography, 272, 272f
  physeal, 983, 984f, 985, 989
  reduction; see also Closed reduction; Open reduction
    loss of, after treatment, 1089-1090, 1089-1092f, 1092
Free body diagrams, in force analyses, 194, 196f
Friction massage, 1275
Frykman classification of distal radius fractures, 315, 317, 317f, 317t
Frykman fractures, 317, 319
Fuji film, in force analyses, 191, 192f
Fulkerson-Watson technique, 833
Functional assessment, 1272-1273, 1307-1308
Functional capacity evaluation, 1292f, 1292-1293
Fusion; see Arthrodesis

G
Galeazzi fracture
  fracture dislocation, 765f, 768-770, 769f
  of radius, 722
  triangular fibrocartilage avulsion with, 738
Galvanic current, for electrical stimulation, 1268-1269
Ganglion cysts, 1166, 1167f; see also Ganglions
  aspiration of, 1169, 1171
  dorsal, 1172
    origin of, 1172, 1173f
    physical examination, 241, 241f, 243
    surgical treatment, 1174-1175f, 1174-1176
    ultrasonography, 276, 276f
  palmar, 1176, 1176f
    origin of, 1177t
    physical examination, 248, 252
    surgical treatment, 1176-1177, 1177f

Ganglions, 1166-1180; see also Ganglion cysts
  aspiration of, diagnostic and therapeutic, 1169, 1171
  diagnosis, 1167-1168
    differential, 1168, 1168t, 1170-1171
    imaging, 1168f, 1169, 1169f
    medical history, 1168
    physical examination, 1168-1169
    tests, 1169-1171
    transillumination, 1169
  in distal radioulnar joint region, 862
  dorsal, 1169, 1170f
    treatment, 305, 1172-1176
  etiology, 1166-1167
  location and incidence, 1166, 1167t
  occult, 1167-1168, 1168f
  palmar, 1169, 1171f
    treatment, 1176-1178
  recurrence, 1178, 1179
  treatment
    algorithm, 1172f
    complications, 1172, 1178-1179
    dorsal wrist ganglion surgery, 1172, 1174-1175f, 1174-1176
    nonoperative, 1171
    operative, 1171-1172
    palmar wrist ganglion surgery, 1176t, 1176-1177f, 1176-1178
    postoperative care and rehabilitation, 1178
Giant cell tumor
  of bone, 1254f, 1256
  of tendon sheath, 1240, 1241f
Gill technique, modified, 919f
Gilula's line, 698
Golf, hook of hamate fractures in, 1055, 1056f
Goniometers, 1272
Gorilla, wrist movements in, 18t
Gout, 872-873, 1146-1147, 1149-1150f
Grafts; see also Bone grafts
  skin, 1237f, 1238f
  vascular pedicle, 117f, 117-118
  vein, 1046f, 1047
Graner procedure, in Kienböck's disease, 451, 452f
Granulomatous inflammatory response to silicone, 1155
Greenstick fracture, 746-747
Grip
  in hominid evolution, 25-27
  repetitive, strength and tolerance testing, 1289f
  strength, in post-traumatic arthritis, 601, 625f, 626
Grips, dowel, in gymnastics, 1063f, 1063-1064
Growth-plate injuries, 982-990
  classification, 982-983
  clinical investigations, 983, 983f
  injuries of physes at wrist, 982
  management, 984-985
    author's experience, 987-989f, 989
  physeal arrest, 983-984
    treatment, 985, 986f, 987
GUEPAR total wrist arthroplasty, 941, 942f
Guyon's canal
  anatomy, 35, 44
  approach, in hook of hamate nonunion, 155, 155f
  ulnar nerve compression and, 1040, 1042-1043
  ulnar neuropathy and, 1084
Gymnastic events, mechanisms of loading end joint positions in, 1033t, 1061
Gymnasts
  dorsal wrist block splint for, 1064f
  dowel grips for, 1063f, 1063-1064
Gymnast's wrist, 853, 1060-1061
  chronic osseous injuries with physeal stress reaction, 1061-1062, 1062f
  diagnosis and treatment, 1062-1063f

distal radius and ulna physeal injury from distraction in, 1063-1064
posterior interosseous nerve palsy, 1043-1044f
scaphoid impaction syndrome, 1064
triquetrolunate impaction syndrome, 1064-1065
ulnocarpal impaction syndrome, 1062-1063, 1063f

H

Hamate
    anatomy, 34f, 41f, 47f, 64-67f, 68, 237f, 238f
    in axial-ulnar disruption, 690f, 693f
    comparative morphology, 17f
    dislocations, 705, 706f
    fractures, 481, 482-484f; see also Hamulus, fractures
    hook of; see Hamulus
    kinematics, 212t, 216
    palmar tenderness, physical examination, 253-254, 256f
    vascular supply, 115-116, 116f
Hamate facet for fifth metacarpal, morphology, 19-20, 20f
Hamate groove, morphology, 17f, 20
Hamate view, 269, 270f, 271
Hamate-triquetral joint, 67f
Hamatolunate abutment, arthroscopy, 302, 304f
Hamatolunate contact, 26, 65f
Hamatometacarpal fracture dislocation, 1060f
Hamilton, Frank Hastings, 1113-1114
Hamulus (hook of hamate)
    anatomy, 34f, 42f, 68, 238f
    comparative morphology, 17f
    exposure, 155-156, 155-158f
    fractures, 115-116, 253-254, 256f, 259f, 481, 482f
        in athletes, 1055, 1056-1057f, 1058
        nonunion, 484f, 1057-1058
        radiologic examination, 268f, 270f, 270-271, 1055, 1057, 1058f
    physical examination, 253-254, 256f, 259f
Hand compartment syndrome, 1109
    signs and symptoms, 1120t
    surgical treatment, 1121f, 1122-1123
Harris growth arrest lines, 983, 983f
Heat therapy, 1265f, 1265-1266
    deep heat, 1266-1267
    fluidotherapy, 1266, 1267f
    hot packs, 1266, 1266f
    hydrotherapy, 1268
    paraffin bath, 1266
    ultrasound, 1267, 1267f
Hemangiomas, 1242, 1242t
Hematomas, lidocaine block and, 1078f
Hemiepiphyseal stapling of distal radius, in multiple hereditary osteo-
        chondromata, 996, 997f
Hemi-interposition transposition, Bowers technique, 781, 781f
Hemimelia, 1017
    radial, 1007-1008, 1008f
        centralization in, 1009, 1010f, 1011-1013
        treatment, 1008-1009, 1008-1010f, 1013
Hemiresection interposition arthroplasty
    in arthritis of distal radioulnar joint, 803, 808, 809f
    in distal radius malunion, 368, 369f, 379f
    as salvage procedure for distal radioulnar joint, 858f
    ulnar stump instability after, 795f
Henke, P.J.W., 4, 10
Henle, F.G.J., 3, 4, 62
    ligamentum subcruentum of Henle, 821, 821f
Herbert classification of scaphoid fractures, 394f, 395t, 1049
Herbert screw osteosynthesis
    of lunate fractures, 438f
    in lunotriquetral arthrodesis, 545-546f, 547
    of perilunate fracture dislocations, 665-666, 667f, 672
    of scaphoid fractures, 401f, 404f

acute unstable scaphoid fractures, 409f, 410, 413f, 415, 415f
    in athletes, 1052, 1053, 1054f
    retrograde screw fixation, 415-416f, 417
in scaphoid nonunion, bone grafting and, 417, 418-419f
Hippocrates, 1111
Histiocytoma, fibrous
    benign, 1243
    malignant, 1247, 1250
Histology, ligament, 74-76, 74-77f
History
    of carpal terminology, 2, 3, 5f, 61-62
    of compartment syndrome, 1111, 1113f, 1113-1114
    patient, in children, 1024
    of total wrist arthroplasty, 924-925
    of wrist joint study, 2-13
        anatomy, 3-4, 3-6t
        Destot, 7-8, 7-8f
        ligament anatomy, 10, 73-74
        physiology after Roentgen, 4-7
        physiology before Roentgen, 4
        reintroduction of concept of carpal stability, 9-10
Hoffmann external fixator, C-series, 1094f
Homo erectus, 24
Homo habilis, 24, 26
Homo sapiens neanderthalensis, 24
Homocystinuria, 1007
Hook of hamate; see Hamulus
Hot packs, 1266, 1266f
Huene jig, in scaphoid fracture repair, 413f, 1052-1053, 1052-1053f
Hui-Linscheid procedure, 732
    ulna stump stability in, 802-803f
Hultén, O., 10
Humpback deformity of scaphoid, 207f, 417, 418f
Humphry, G.M., 5
Hunting reaction, 1264
Hyaluronidase substitutes, 1310
Hydrotherapy, 1268
Hyperextension injury
    lunotriquetral dissociation from, 530, 530f
    radiographic examination, 266-267
Hyperlaxity
    joint, 1006-1007
    ligament, 1016-1017
Hypervitaminosis A, 1024
Hypoplasia of carpal bones, 1017
Hypothenar flap, in recurrent carpal tunnel syndrome, 1229-1230
Hypothenar hammer syndrome, 1046f, 1046-1047

I

Ice therapy, 1263-1265, 1265f
IgM autoantibody, 871
Iliac crest grafts
    in dorsal radiocarpal instability, 572, 574-575f
    in radiolunate arthrodesis, 908f, 909
    in Smith fracture malunion, 581f
    in ulnar translocation, 586f
    in wrist arthrodesis for rheumatoid arthritis, 916, 917-918f
Ilizarov frame, in radial aplasia, 1012f
Imaging, 262-283; see also specific modalities and disorders
    algorithm, 263f
    arthrography, 273-276
    in children, 1025-1027
    computed tomography, 277-278
    magnetic resonance imaging, 278-282
    radiography
        general examination, 262-263
        in kinematic analysis, 206-207, 206-207f, 209-210f
        ligamentous instability series, 271

Imaging—cont'd
  radiography—cont'd
    in radioulna variance measurement, 220f, 220-222, 221t
    routine views, 263-265
    special views, 265-271
  radionuclide imaging, 282
  tomography, 271-273
  ultrasonography, 276
  videofluoroscopy, 273
Immobilization; *see also* Casts; Splints
  after arthroscopic synovectomy, 1161
  after ganglionectomy, 1178
  after wrist arthrodesis for rheumatoid arthritis, 918, 920
  in carpal instability nondissociative, 561
  for distal radius fractures, 322f, 323-324, 330, 337f, 338, 343
    displaced extra-articular Colles-type, 350
    extra-articular Colles-type, 347
  in perilunate dislocation, 639-640
  in perilunate fracture dislocation, 669
  in scaphoid fracture, 389f, 390f, 396, 397-398f
    acute undisplaced scaphoid waist fracture, 409
    in athletes, 1053
  skin complications of, 1076-1077, 1077f
  in total wrist arthroplasty, 937
Immunoglobulin M autoantibody, 871
Impaction
  triquetral-hamate, physical examination, 246
  ulnar impaction syndrome, 846-847, 846-849f
    physical examination, 244-245, 247f
Impingement
  scaphoid, physical examination, 243, 244f
  ulna, 298, 298f
  ulnar styloid, loose bodies and, 852-853, 853f
Implants; *see also* Prostheses; Silicone implants
  in excisional arthroplasty of scaphotrapezial trapezoid joint, 624
  in radioscaphoid arthritis, 600f, 604
  in ulnar head replacement, 789, 792, 793f
  in wrist arthrodesis for rheumatoid arthritis, 913-914f
Incisions; *see* Surgical approaches and joint exposures
Incisura ulnaris radii, 68
Infection
  after carpal tunnel surgery, 1227-1228
  control, 1309
  in rheumatoid arthritis, 871, 872t
  synovitis from, 1152
Inflammation, silicone and, 1155
Infrared heat application, 1265f, 1265-1266
Infratendinous extensor retinaculum, in distal radioulnar joint stability, 761f, 763-764
Injuries to wrist
  complications, 1076-1106
    bone and joint, 1089-1095
    pain syndromes, 1095-1104
    soft tissue, 1076-1089
  immature wrist, 1018, 1020f, 1020-1022, 1023f
  sources of, present and future, 1307
Innervation of wrist, 36-37f, 37-38, 119-120, 119-121f, 122
Insertional tenosynovitis, extensor, in athletes, 1035, 1037
Instability; *see also* Carpal instability
  adaptive carpus or pseudo carpal, 495, 498t
  arthroscopy and, 306
  axial, 494, 496t
  capitolunate instability pattern, 495
  carpometacarpal, 495, 496t
  in children, 1021
  columnar or longitudinal, 494

distal radioulnar joint; *see* Distal radioulnar joint instability
  in distal radius malunion, 362, 362f
  dorsal intercalated segment; *see* Dorsal intercalated segment instabilities
  historical perspective, 9
  lateral view, 265f
  ligamentous, radiographic series, 270f, 271
  lunotriquetral, physical examination, 245-246, 248-249f
  midcarpal, 494, 496t; *see also* Carpal instability nondissociative
    ulnar, physical examination, 246-247, 250-251f
  perilunate, 653, 653f
    stages, 496t, 652f
  provocative stress testing
    distal radioulnar, 245f, 260
    midcarpal, 250-251f, 259
    scaphoid, 254, 256, 258-259f, 259
    ulnocarpal, 248-249f, 259-260
  radiocarpal, 494, 496t
  scaphoid fractures and, 387-388
  scapholunate; *see* Scapholunate instability
  terminology, 492-497
  transverse, 494-495
  transverse spinal, 495
  traumatic, 569
  volar intercalated segment; *see* Volar intercalated segment instabilities
Instruments for arthroscopy, 287-290
Intercalary ulna excision, in distal radius malunion, 368
Intercalated segment, 493
Intercarpal arch, vascular anatomy, 107, 107f, 108f, 110f
Intercarpal arthrodesis
  in distal radius malunion, 373
  in scapholunate advanced collapse, 605-606, 607-610f, 611, 612-613f, 623
  in scapholunate dissociation, 513, 517-519f
Intercarpal ligament
  dorsal, 67f, 88, 88f, 89f, 656f; *see also* Scaphotriquetral ligament
  palmar, 90f
Interfacet prominence, 67f, 68
Interligamentous sulcus, 69, 79
Intermittent pneumatic compression pumps, 1274
Internal fixation; *see also* Open reduction and internal fixation
  for hamate fractures, 482f
  for lunate fractures, 438f, 477f
  for perilunate fracture dislocations, 665f, 665-666, 667, 667f, 669, 673f, 675f
  for scaphoid fractures, 1051-1052, 1053, 1054f
  in wrist arthrodesis for rheumatoid arthritis, 915-916, 916-919f
    pin removal, 920
    with Stanley-Shelley plate in radiolunate arthrodesis, 905, 907f, 909
    two-pin fixation, 917-918
Interosseous ligaments; *see* Ligament anatomy
Interosseous membrane
  in distal radioulnar joint stability, 763f, 764
  of forearm, in joint stability, 227
  radioulnar, 744f, 745
Interposition wedge graft, in scaphoid nonunion, 417, 418f
Intersection syndrome, 1186
  in athletes, 1033-1034
  nonoperative treatment, 1186
  physical examination, 240, 240f
  surgical treatment, 1186f, 1186-1187
Intra-articular ligaments, 75-76, 77f
Intracapsular ligaments, 313f
Intrascaphoid angle
  in scaphoid fracture, 390f, 391f
  in scaphoid malunion, 424f
Iontophoresis, 1268

Iridocyclitis, 948
Irradiation, for soft-tissue tumors, 1240
Irrigation system, for arthroscopy, 287
Ischemia, muscle, in compartment syndrome, 1115f, 1116
Ischemia-edema cycle, traumatic, 1115f
Ischemic contracture; *see* Volkmann's ischemic contracture

J

Jebsen objective standardized test, 1273
Johnson procedure
  in arthritis deformity, 808, 808f
  modified, 859, 860f
Joints
  anatomy, 69-70
  exposures; *see* Surgical approaches and joint exposures
  laxity of
    criteria for, 1006-1007
    provocative maneuvers and, 1025
  mobilization techniques, 1275
Juvenile rheumatoid arthritis, 871, 877-878f, 945-946
  classification, 945-948, 946t, 1147
  diagnostic criteria, 946t
  diagnostic studies, 948-949, 948-951f
  management summary, 952, 955-956
  onset modes, 947t
  pauciarticular, 947t, 947-948
  polyarticular, 947, 947t
  systemic, 947, 947t
  treatment, 950, 1152
    intra-articular steroid injection, 950, 952
    splinting and physiotherapy, 950, 951-952f, 1152
    surgical procedures, 952
    synovectomy, 952, 953-955f, 1152

K

K wires; *see* Kirschner wires
Kapandji, A.I., 10
Kapandji pinning technique, 342f, 343, 344-345f, 347
Kapandji procedure, 857, 859-860f; *see also* Sauvé-Kapandji procedure
  in degenerative joint disease, 843f
  in rheumatoid arthritis, 882f, 884
Kauer, J.M., 10
Keratoacanthoma, 1236, 1236f
Keratosis
  actinic, 1235, 1235f
  seborrheic, 1235
Kessler frame, 1009-1010f, 1011
Keyboard operators
  overuse syndrome in, 1299
  posture for, 1290
Kienböck's disease, 437-465
  classification, 443, 443t, 445-448f
  clinical presentation, 442
  diagnosis, 442-443
  differential diagnosis, 241, 243
  distal radioulnar joint and, 219, 230
  etiology, 438-439
  force distribution across wrist in, 197-198, 201-202
  historical perspective, 10, 437-438
  imaging, 306, 443, 847
    magnetic resonance imaging, 279, 281f, 443t, 444f
    radiographs, 440f, 444f
    stages of disease, 453f, 454f
    tomography, 272f, 272-273, 439f, 445, 848f
  incidence, 442
  lunate in; *see* Lunate, in Kienböck's disease

multiple hereditary osteochondromata and, 1000
  risk factors, 439-442
  treatment, 201-202, 445
    authors' preferred method, 464-465
    biomechanical studies, 449-450
    capitate shortening, 460, 461f
    carpal tunnel release, 460
    excision arthroplasty, 450-451, 450-452f
    limited intercarpal fusions, 458, 460, 460f
    lunate decompression, 453-454
    nonoperative conservative, 449
    proximal row carpectomy, 463-464, 464f
    radial osteotomy, 458, 459f
    radius and ulna shortening, 458
    radius shortening, 444f, 453-456f, 454, 457-458
    revascularization, 460, 462-463, 462-463f
    ulna lengthening, 457, 457f
    wrist denervation, 453
    wrist fusion, 464
  ulna variance in, 432, 853-854
Kinematics; *see also* Motion of wrist
  distal radioulnar joint
    basic concepts, 219
    normal range of forearm motion, 222, 224
    pronation-supination, 222-224f
    "ulnocarpal" joint, 224
    variations in shape of joint, 219-222, 220f, 221t
  forearm, 822-823, 823f
  lunotriquetral joint, 527-528, 528-529f
  proximal carpal row, 551, 553f, 553-554
  radiocarpal joint, 205-218
    abnormal, 216f, 216-217
    analysis, 206-207, 206-211f
    distal carpal row, 209-210
    historical perspective, 205-206
    normal, 208-216, 211f, 212t
    proximal carpal row, 210, 212-214, 213-215f, 216
    reference axes, 211f
Kirschner wires, applications
  arthritis deformity of distal radioulnar joint, 812f, 815
  axial dislocations, 691f, 692, 693f
  distal radius fracture pin fixation, 341-342f, 343, 347, 350
  dorsal wedge corrective osteotomy, 576, 576f, 577f
  lunate fracture repair, 478f
  lunotriquetral arthrodesis, 545-546f, 547
  perilunate dislocations, 640, 642-643f, 646
  perilunate fracture dislocations, 660f, 663-664, 665, 677f, 679f
  radial osteotomy, 363, 364f
  scaphoid fracture repair, 400, 404f
    acute unstable scaphoid fractures, 409f, 410, 413f
    in athletes, 1050, 1052, 1053
    retrograde screw fixation and, 415, 416f
  scaphoid nonunion, bone grafting and, 417, 418-420f, 421
  scapholunate advanced collapse wrist, 523, 608f, 622-623
  scapholunate dissociation, 510f, 511, 514f, 515f
  scaphotrapezial trapezoidal arthrodesis, 623
  triangular fibrocartilage tears, 729f, 732
  wrist arthrodesis for rheumatoid arthritis, 919f
Kleinman technique, 604f
Klippel-Trénaunay syndrome, 1007f
Kuhlmann, J.N., 10

L

Landsmeer, J.M.F., 9
Langenskiöld technique, 985
Lasers, 1309

Lateral antebrachial cutaneous nerve, 119f, 120, 120f
Lateral view, 262, 264-266f, 265
Latex-fixation test, 948
Latissimus dorsi transfer, in ischemic contracture, 1132-1133f
Lauenstein fusion, 914; *see also* Sauvé-Kapandji procedure
Laxity
    joint, 1006-1007, 1025
    ligament, 957, 1016-1017
Lentigo maligna melanoma, 1239
Lewis, O.J., 74
Lichtman classification
    of instability, 491, 491t
    of Kienböck's disease, 443, 445f
LIDO Workset, 1263f
Lidocaine
    in athletic tendon disorders, 1033, 1034, 1037
    in carpal tunnel release, 1212-1213f, 1214
    in carpal tunnel syndrome, 1045
    hematomas and, 1078f
    in triangular fibrocartilage tears, 1067
Ligament anatomy, 73-105
    arthroscopic, 173-179f
        inspection, 185
    carpal ligament organization, 76-78
    distal radius and, 313, 313f
    distal row interosseous ligaments, 95f, 95t
        capitohamate interosseous, 95-96, 95-96f
        trapeziocapitate interosseous, 94-95, 95-96f
        trapezium trapezoid interosseous, 94-95, 95f
    dorsal intercarpal ligament, 88, 89f
    dorsal radiocarpal ligament, 87, 87t, 88f
    histology, 74-76, 74-77f
    history, 10, 73-74
    mechanical function, constraint and material property studies, 96-97
    palmar midcarpal ligaments, 79f, 88-91, 90f
        pisohamate, 79f, 91
        scaphocapitate trapezoid, 79f, 89, 90f, 91
        scaphotrapezium trapezoid, 79f, 89, 90f
        triquetrocapitate, 79f, 90f, 91
        triquetrohamate, 79f, 90f, 91
    palmar radiocarpal ligaments, 78, 79f, 79t, 80f, 81-84, 553f
        long radiolunate, 78-79, 79-81f, 81
        radioscaphocapitate, 78, 79-81f
        radioscapholunate, 79-84f, 81-83
        short radiolunate, 79-81f, 83-84, 85f
    proximal row interosseous ligaments, 92t
        pisotriquetral, 79f, 94
        scapholunate and lunotriquetral interosseous, 81f, 91-93f, 91-94
    suggestions for anatomically based capsulotomies, 99, 100f, 101, 102-103f, 104
    triangular fibrocartilage complex, 97-99, 97-99f
    ulnocarpal ligaments, 79-80f, 84-85, 85t, 85-86f, 87
Ligament of Testut, 79-84f, 81-83
Ligaments
    augmentation, in distal radioulnar joint instability, 830, 832-834f, 838f
    in distal radioulnar joint stability, 760, 761f, 762-763, 763f
    injuries, magnetic resonance imaging, 280, 280f
    instability, radiographic series, 270f, 271
    laxity of, 1016-1017
        in juvenile systemic lupus erythematosus, 957
    in lunotriquetral joint kinematics, 527-528, 528-529f
    in lunotriquetral joint sprains, 529f, 529-530
    in perilunate fracture dislocations, 655-656, 657f
    in proximal carpal row kinematics, 551, 553f, 553-554f
    replacement, 1310, 1311
    sectioning, 202f

sports injuries, arthroscopic management
        diagnostic, 299
        therapeutic, 305, 1065
    tears, ulna positive variance with, 779f
Ligamentum subcruentum of Henle, 821, 821f
Linburg test, 1194, 1194f
Linburg's syndrome, 1194
Linear tomography, 271
Lipoma, 1240, 1242
Lister's tubercle
    anatomy, 34, 34f, 41f, 46f, 68, 170f, 172f, 237f
    distal radius and, 311f, 314
    dorsal skin incision centered over, 127f
    in physical examination, 240-241
    in soft-tissue reconstruction in rheumatoid arthritis, 893, 897
LMB splint, 1281f, 1282
Load cells, in force analyses, 191, 196f
Long radiolunate ligament
    anatomy, 78-79, 79-81f, 81, 553f
        arthroscopic, 173, 174f, 176f, 178f
        in sagittal section, 48
    in carpal instability nondissociative treatment, 561, 562f
    dorsal, 656f
    in perilunate fracture dislocations, 657f
    in scaphoid fracture repair, 1050-1051f
Longitudinal disruption; *see* Axial dislocations and fracture dislocations
Longitudinal instability, 494
Loose bodies
    arthroscopy
        diagnostic, 299
        therapeutic, 305
    ulnar styloid impingement and, 853
Lunate
    anatomy, 64-65, 64-65f, 175f, 181f, 432-434f
        dorsal perspective, 41f
        palmar perspective, 42f
    cysts, 777f, 779f
    dorsal pole of, 34f, 237f
    fragmentation and collapse, 446-448f
    historical perspective, 10
    in Kienböck's disease
        decompression of, 453-454
        etiology/pathogenesis, 64, 108, 111, 201, 432, 434, 437-439, 441, 442f, 479, 1017
        excision arthroplasty for, 450-451, 450-452f
    kinematics, 212t, 213-214, 214-215f
    multiple ossification centers, 1017
    multisegment, 1003
    ontogenesis, 62
    shape of, 570f, 571
    vascular supply, 108, 110-111, 114f
Lunate dislocations, 633f, 635f, 696, 697f, 698; *see also* Perilunate dislocations
    diagnosis, 698, 698f
    dorsal, 700, 701f, 702, 702f
    treatment, 698-700, 699-700f, 704f
        closed reduction and cast immobilization, 638-640, 641f
        closed reduction and pin fixation, 640, 642-643f
        open reduction and direct repair, 640, 642, 644-647f, 646
Lunate fossa
    anatomy, 67f, 68
    displaced fractures, 323
    distal radius fractures and, 310, 311f, 312
Lunate fractures, 434-435, 437; *see also* Kienböck's disease
    classification, 436, 436f
    clinical presentation, 435-436
    imaging, 435f, 439f, 475, 476-478f

isolated, 475, 476-478f, 477, 479
    mechanism, 476f
    treatment, 436, 438f, 477
Lunatomalacia; *see* Kienböck's disease
Lunocapitate joint, perilunate dissociation at, 633f
Lunotriquetral ballottement and compression test, 248-249f
Lunotriquetral dissociation, 527, 535, 537, 545f
    and triangular fibrocartilage instability, ulna recession in, 852f
    kinematics, 208-209f, 217
Lunotriquetral interosseous ligament, 81f, 91-93f, 91-94, 657f
Lunotriquetral joint
    anatomy and kinematics, 35, 527-528, 528-529f
    arthrodesis, 536f, 543-546f, 544-545, 547
        in distal radius malunion, 373
    coalitions, 1004, 1005f
    instability, physical examination, 245-246, 248-249f, 259
    perilunate dissociation at, 633f
Lunotriquetral ligament, arthroscopy of
    anatomy, 176f, 177, 179f
    inspection, 185
    therapeutic, 305
Lunotriquetral shear tests, 249f, 259-260; *see also* Lunotriquetral stress tests
Lunotriquetral sprains, 527-549
    clinical findings
        arthroscopy, 535, 535f
        bone scans, 535, 543f
        examination, 531f, 532-533
        radiography, 532-534f, 533-535, 543-544f
        symptoms, 532
    mechanism of injury, 530, 530f, 532
    pathomechanics, 529f, 529-530
    treatment
        lunotriquetral arthrodesis, 536f, 543-546f, 544-545, 547
        lunotriquetral reconstruction, 536f, 539-542f, 542
        lunotriquetral repair, 537, 537f, 538f, 539
        methods and considerations, 535, 536f, 537
Lunotriquetral stress tests, 531f, 532
Lunotriquetral tears, 527, 535f, 536f, 841f
    treatment, 535, 536f
        reconstruction, 539-541f, 542
        repair, 537, 537f
Lupus erythematosus, systemic, 872, 956
    classification criteria, 958t
    diagnostic studies, 956-957, 956-957f
    management summary, 957, 959
Lyme disease, 873
Lymphangiomatosis, 1242, 1243f
Lyser, Michael, 3, 61

M
Madelung's deformity, 244, 966-981
    clinical manifestations, 967, 969-970, 1021
    discussion and clinical examples, 973, 974-977f
    in distal radioulnar joint disorders, 854f, 854-855
    etiology and clinical appearance, 966, 967f
    management, 970, 1021
        author's preferred treatment, 970
        in established late Madelung's deformity, 977-978, 978-979f, 980
        surgical technique, 970-973, 971-972f
    multiple hereditary osteochondromata and, 1000, 1000f
    pathology and natural history, 966-967, 968-969f
    reverse, 966, 967-969f
        surgical treatment, 972-973
    ulnocarpal abutment and, 773, 781
Maffucci's syndrome, 1006f

Magnetic resonance imaging
    advantages and applications, 278-281, 279-281f
        chrondromalacia, 845f
        ganglions, 1169f, 1170, 1171f
        gout, 1150f
        growth-plate injuries, 983
        Madelung's deformity, 969f, 977
        overuse syndrome, 1299
        rheumatoid arthritis, 880
        scapholunate instability, 509, 509f
        styloid erosion and tenosynovitis, 861f
        triangular fibrocartilage tears, 716, 718, 719f
    physics and technique, 281-282
Malignant fibrous histiocytoma, 1247, 1250
Malignant melanoma, 1237, 1238-1239f, 1239
Malignant schwannoma, 1250
Malunion of fractures, 1094-1095, 1095-1096f; *see also* Distal radius malunion; Scaphoid malunion
Marfan's syndrome, 1007, 1016
Massage, friction, 1275
Matched arthroplasty, 857, 859f
Mayfield, J.K., 10
Mayfield paradox of closed reduction, 511
Mayo classification
    of carpal dislocations, 654
    of carpal instability, 497, 498t, 639t
    of distal radius fractures, 319-320, 320f
    of scaphoid fractures, 394f, 395t
    of triangular fibrocartilage tears, 720, 722f
Mayo Foundation Forearm Holder, 184f
McMurrich, 3
McMurty classification of instability, 491-492, 493t
Mechanics; *see specific anatomy and* Biomechanics
Median nerve, 1041f
    anatomy, 37f, 38
    in carpal tunnel syndrome, 1202, 1203f, 1204, 1205f, 1207f
    classification of motor nerve distribution, 1203f
    distance to radius and ulna from, 1081, 1084, 1084t
    injuries, 1081, 1082f, 1084
        in carpal tunnel surgery, 1228
        treatment, 1087, 1088f
    in ischemic contracture treatment, 1129-1130f, 1133, 1134
    palmar cutaneous branch, 119f, 121f
Median neuropathy, 1084, 1085f
    in distal radius fracture, 321
    in distal radius malunion, 362
    in perilunate dislocation, 648
Medications; *see also* Corticosteroids
    in carpal tunnel syndrome, 1209
    narcotics in pain syndromes, 1104
    in overuse syndrome, 1301
Melanoma, 1237, 1238-1239f, 1239
Melone classification of distal radius fractures, 319, 319f
Melorheostoses, 1007
Meniscus homologue, 70
Menon technique of transverse carpal ligament release, 1227f
Menon total wrist arthroplasty, 941, 942f, 943
Metacarpal bones
    bases of, 69
    comparative morphology, 19-21, 21f
    metacarpal V, 47f
    palmar perspective, 41f
Metacarpal styloid process, 69
Metacarpophalangeal joints, in juvenile rheumatoid arthritis, 949f
Methyl methacrylate cement, in total wrist arthroplasty, 934-935f, 936

Meuli prosthesis, 927f, 940
    design development, 928
    in distal radius malunion, 369
    initial design, 925f
Meyer, R., 4
Midcarpal joint
    anatomy, 35, 36, 43, 44f, 64f, 65f, 70
    arthrodesis
        in rheumatoid arthritis, 902f
        in scaphoid nonunion advanced collapse, 621f
        in scapholunate advanced collapse, 611, 612-613f
    arthrography, 274, 274f, 276
    arthroplasty
        radiocarpal arthrodesis and, 894, 894f
        radioscapholunate arthrodesis and, 912, 913-914f, 914
    arthroscopy, 297
        anatomy, 293, 294f, 295, 295f
        examination in sports injuries, 1065t
        inspection, 185, 187
        portals, 177, 180f
    capsulotomy, 101
    force transmission through, 196, 199t
    instability, 496t, 572, 572f; see also Carpal instability nondissociative
        definition, 494
        provocative stress testing, 250-251f, 259
        ulnar, physical examination, 246-247, 250-251f
    subluxation, in rheumatoid arthritis, 891
Midcarpal ligaments, palmar, 79f, 88-91, 90f
Midcarpal portal, 172f
Minnesota Rate of Manipulation Test, 1292f
Mitek anchor, 733f
Moberg objective method, 1273
Mobility, comparative morphology, 15, 17f, 17-19, 18t, 19f
Monro, Alexander, 3, 61-62
Morphologic evolution, prehistoric tools and, 25-27
Morphology, comparative, 14-29
    classification of animals, 15
    features shared by humans and other animals
        midcarpal stabilizing features, 16-17f, 19
        multiple carpal bones, 15, 16f
        wrist mobility: supination, ulnar deviation, and flexion, 15, 17f, 17-19, 18t, 19f
    features unique to human wrist
        broad and moderately contoured first carpometacarpal joint, 20, 21f
        broad capitate with distally oriented facet for second metacarpal, 20, 21f
        hamate groove between hook and metacarpal articular surfaces, 17f, 20
        large hamate facet for fifth metacarpal, 19-20, 20f
        proportionately large scaphotrapezial and small scaphotrapezoid joints, 21
        proximally to coronally oriented facet on second metacarpal for trapezium, 19f, 20-21
        restricted range of flexion, 21
        short pisiform bone, 17f, 19
    fossil wrist bones, 22-25
Motion of wrist; see also Kinematics
    after total wrist arthroplasty, 937
    after wrist arthrodesis for rheumatoid arthritis, 904t, 915t
    continuous passive, 1262-1263, 1263-1264f
    imaging, 270f, 271, 273
    loss of, in distal radius malunion, 361
    studies
        in rheumatoid arthritis, 876
        in scapholunate instability, 507-508f

Multiple hereditary osteochondromata, 991-1001
    background and problem, 991, 992-995f
    incidence, 992f
    incidence of deformity in, 993f
    Kienböck's disease and, 1000
    Madelung's deformity and, 1000, 1000f
    proximal radial dislocation and, 996f, 999-1000
    treatment of deformities and problems in
        distal ulna excision, 999
        excision of osteochondromata, 992-993, 996, 996f
        hemiepiphyseal stapling of distal radius, 996, 997f
        osteotomy and shortening of radius, 999
        ulna lengthening, 996, 997-998f, 999
        ulna straightening, surgical, 998f, 999
Muscle(s)
    biofeedback and, 1269f, 1269-1279
    contraction, electrical stimulation for, 1268-1269
    delayed-onset soreness, 1299
    in distal ulna fractures, 743-745
    intrinsic to hand, 1110f
        in ischemic contracture, 1121f
    spasticity, 1264
    testing, 1273
    transfer, in ischemic contracture, 1132-1133f
Musculotendinous stabilizers, in joint stability, 227
Musicians, overuse syndrome in, 1297, 1299
Mycobacterium marinum, 1152

N

Narcotics, in pain syndromes, 1104
Navarro, A., 8, 9
Naviculocapitate syndrome, 635, 669
Neanderthals, 24, 26
Necrosis, avascular
    of lunate; see Kienböck's disease
    in perilunate dislocations, 648
    in perilunate fracture dislocations, 681
Needle manometer technique of compartment pressure measurement, 1118, 1119f, 1120
Neoplasms; see Tumors
Nerve blocks, 120, 1088
    in pain syndromes, 1100, 1103, 1104
Nerve conduction studies, in carpal tunnel syndrome, 1207
Nerve entrapment syndromes in athletes, 1040
    carpal tunnel syndrome, 1045
    cyclist's palsy, 1040, 1042f, 1042-1043
    etiology, 1040, 1041f
    gymnast's palsy, 1043-1044f
    Wartenberg's syndrome, 1044-1045
Nerve injuries, 1081, 1084
    cutaneous neuropathy, 1084-1085, 1087
    median nerve, 1081, 1082f, 1084
    radial sensory nerve, 1083f, 1084-1085
    treatment, 1087-1089, 1088f
    ulnar nerve, 1084
Nerve pain; see Reflex sympathetic dystrophy; Somatic nerve pain
Nerves
    compression, in rheumatoid arthritis, 884
    distance to radius and ulna from, 1081, 1084, 1084t
    innervation of wrist, 119-120, 119-121f, 122
Neurectomy, posterior interosseous, 1043-1044f
Neurilemoma, 1243, 1245
Neuritis
    after wrist injury, 1088
    posterior interosseous, physical examination, 243
    radial, physical examination, 238, 240

Neurofibrolipoma, 1245, 1246f
Neurofibroma, 1245, 1245f
Neurologic disorders and injuries; *see* Nerve *entries;* Neuropathy
Neurolysis
    in carpal tunnel syndrome, 1229
    in ischemic contracture, 1129-1130f, 1130, 1132-1133
Neuromas, 122
    after ganglionectomy, 1178
    posterior interosseous nerve, 243
Neuromuscular deficits, in children, 1024
Neuropathy, in distal radius malunion, 362
Nevi, 1236-1237
Nightstick fracture, 749
Nodular fasciitis, 1243
Nodular melanoma, 1239
Nonunion of fractures, 1092, 1093-1094
Nutritional disorders, in children, 1024

O

Oarsman's wrist; *see* Intersection syndrome
Occult fractures, tomography, 272, 272f
Occupational therapy, 1272
    postoperative management, 1273-1275
    preoperative evaluation, 1272-1273
    splinting in, 1276-1283
One-bone forearm procedures, 1013, 1014-1015f, 1016
Ontogenesis of carpus, 62
Open reduction
    of distal radius fractures, 328, 330, 334-337f, 343, 346-350f, 347
    of growth-plate injuries, 985
    of perilunate dislocations, 640, 642, 644-647f, 646
    of perilunate fracture dislocations, 660f, 663-667, 664-679f
Open reduction and internal fixation
    of hamate fractures, 482f
    of lunate dislocations, 698, 699
    of scaphoid fractures, 399-400, 400-401f, 404f
        acute unstable scaphoid fractures, 409f, 410, 413-414f
        retrograde screw fixation, 415-416f, 417
    of trans-radial-styloid fracture dislocations, 664-665f, 673-674
    of transscaphoid fracture dislocations, 666-667f, 669, 672, 673-674, 677f
    of trapezium-trapezoid fractures, 483, 484f
Open wedge osteotomy, in Madelung's deformity, 970, 972, 972f
Openheimer spring splint, 1282
Opponens muscle, in carpal tunnel syndrome, 1204, 1204f
Orangutans, feeding and climbing postures of, 19f
Orthoplast splint, 324f, 1161
Orthoses; *see also* Splints
    for gymnasts, 1064f
Os centrale, 1003, 1004f
    anatomy, 62, 62f
    comparative morphology, 19
Os Daubentonni, 853
Os metacarpale I to V; *see* Metacarpal bones
Os secondarium, 853
Os styloideum, 1004, 1017
Os triangulare, 743, 1003
Os ulna; *see* Distal ulna
Ossification of carpal bones, 62, 1003t
    multiple ossification centers, 1017
Osteoarthritis
    chronic scapholunate dissociation with, treatment, 521-523, 522f
    evolution and, 26
    synovitis in, 1146
Osteochondroma, 1251f, 1252; *see also* Multiple hereditary osteochon-dromata

Osteochondromatosis, synovial, of distal radioulnar joint, 862
Osteogenesis imperfecta, 1007
Osteogenic sarcoma, 1255f, 1256
Osteoid osteoma, 1252, 1252f
Osteolysis, carpal row, 1007t
Osteopenia, in rheumatoid arthritis, 878f, 879f, 883f
Osteosynthesis; *see also specific methods*
    in scaphoid nonunion, 406-407, 407f, 408f
Osteotomy
    in Barton dorsal fracture dislocation, 580f, 581-582
    in Darrach resection, 800, 801f
    in distal radius malunion, 1096f
    distal ulna, 145f
    in dorsal radiocarpal instability, 572, 574-577f, 576
    in Kienböck's disease, 455-457f, 457-458, 459f, 461f
        biomechanical studies, 449-450
    in Madelung's deformity, 854, 970, 971-972f, 972
        established late deformity, 978-979f, 980
        physiolysis and, 973, 976f
    in multiple hereditary osteochondromata deformity, 996, 997-998f, 999
    radial; *see* Radial osteotomy; Radial recession osteotomy
    in radial aplasia, 1012f
    scaphoid, 424-425
        motion changes after, 207f
    in Smith fracture malunion, 581f
    in ulna deficiency, 1015f, 1016
    ulnar, radioulnar fusion and, 811, 812-814f, 813, 815
    in ulnar impaction (abutment) syndrome, 849, 850-851f
    ulnar recession, 780f, 781, 782-784f
Overuse syndrome, 1295-1303
    epidemiology, 1297-1298f, 1297-1299
    historical background, 1295
    investigations, 1299-1300
    terminology, 1296-1297
    treatment, 1300f, 1300-1301

P

Pain in wrist
    in carpal tunnel syndrome, 1229
    in chevron carpus, 975, 975f
    in compartment syndrome, 1117
    cutaneous dysesthetic, 122
    in de Quervain's disease, 1183
    deep and superficial nerves in, 120
    in distal radius malunion, 360-361
        procedures to eliminate, 368-370, 370-373f, 373
    dysfunction classification, 1098t
    in Madelung's deformity, 969-970
    in overuse syndrome, 1296
    palmar ulnar, 253-254, 254-256f
    TENS treatment, 1268
Pain syndromes, 1095
    somatic nerve pain, 1101-1102
    sympathetic dystrophy, 1095, 1098-1101
    treatment alternatives, 1104
    treatment plan, 1103-1104
Paine release with transverse limited wrist incision and retinaculatome, 1216f, 1218
Palmar approaches, 146, 147-148f
    in carpal tunnel syndrome, 1210, 1211f, 1214, 1217f, 1220, 1221f
    in first carpometacarpal joint exposure, 162f
    in hook of hamate exposure, 155f
    in lunate dislocations, 698, 700f
    in perilunate dislocations, 640, 642, 645-646f
    in perilunate fracture dislocations, 655-656, 664-665, 666f, 667, 668f, 669, 672-673f, 675f, 680f

Palmar approaches—cont'd
    to scaphoid, 146, 149-152f, 1050-1051f, 1052
    tenosynovectomy, 1159
    to ulna, 750f, 751
Palmar arch, 238f
Palmar beak (tubercle), 69
Palmar capsule imbrication and tendinous augmentation, 837-838f, 839
Palmar capsulotomy options, 101, 103
Palmar carpal ligaments
    anatomy, 77, 77f, 78f
    extrinsic, 551, 553f, 553-554
    in perilunate fracture dislocations, 655-656
Palmar distal radioulnar ligament, 760, 762
Palmar intercalated segment instabilities; see Volar intercalated segment
        instabilities
Palmar intercarpal ligaments, 90f
Palmar ligament repair, with radial recession osteotomy, 560f
Palmar metaphyseal artery, 40f
Palmar midcarpal ligaments, 79f, 88-91, 90f
Palmar radiocarpal ligaments, 78-84, 79f, 79t, 80-81f, 84-85f
    in perilunate fracture dislocations, 669
Palmar radioscaphoid ligament, 657f
Palmar radioulnar ligament, 86f
    in joint stability, 225-226, 226f, 763f
    in kinematic constraint of distal radioulnar joint, 824-825, 825f,
        835-836
    mechanical properties, 227t
    in transverse section, 52
    in triangular fibrocartilage complex, 97, 98, 821f, 821-822
Palmar surface anatomy, 35
Palmar tenosynovectomy, 1141, 1142f
    in carpal tunnel release, 1159-1160
Palmar tilt, 570f
Palmar translation/translocation, 495
Palmar wrist examination
    ganglion cysts, 248, 252
    radial-side pain, 247-248
    scaphotrapezial arthritis, 248, 252f
    tendinitis, 252-253, 253f
Palmaris longus muscle, 35
Palmer classification, of triangular fibrocartilage complex injuries, 720,
        721f, 839-840, 840t
    arthroscopic treatment based on, 1068
Pan, wrist movements in, 18t
Pan troglodytes, wrist and hand in, 17
Paraffin bath, 1266
Paranthropus robustus, 24
Particulate arthritis, 873
Particulate synovitis; see Silicone synovitis
Pauciarticular juvenile rheumatoid arthritis, 947t, 947-948
Pediatrics
    diagnostic and treatment problems, 1002-1030
        carpal disorders, 1016-1018
        congenital anomalies, 1007-1013
        deformed distal ulna, surgical procedures, 1016
        developmental anomalies, 1003-1007
        diagnostic methodology, 1024-1027
        differential diagnosis, 1022, 1024
        injuries to immature wrist, 1018-1022
        treatment guide, 1026t
        ulnar deficiency, surgical procedures, 1013-1016
    distal radioulnar joint fractures, 745f, 746-749
    growth-plate injuries, 982-990
    juvenile rheumatoid arthritis, 945-956
    Madelung's deformity, 966-981
    multiple hereditary osteochondromata, 991-1001

Percutaneous pin fixation
    complications, 1085, 1086f
    for distal radius fractures, 324, 338, 340-342f, 341, 343, 344-345f
    for perilunate dislocations, 640, 642-643f, 647f
    for perilunate fracture dislocations, 659, 660f, 661-663
Perifascicular spaces, 74-76f
Perihamate peripisiform axial-ulnar disruption, 690f, 693f
Perilunate dislocations, 632-650; see also Lunate dislocations
    axial dislocations vs., 691
    chronic, 648-649
    classification, 638, 638f, 639t, 640, 659f
    complications, 648, 1085f
    diagnosis, 634
        radiographic studies, 634, 635-636f, 636-638
    etiology, 632-634
    palmar, 700, 701f, 702
    pathways of ligamentous and bone cleavage in, 635f
    stages, 632-633, 633-634f
    treatment
        closed reduction and cast immobilization, 638-640, 641f
        closed reduction and pin fixation, 640, 642-643f
        open reduction and direct repair, 640, 642, 644-647f, 646
        open reduction and pin fixation, 647f
        of variants, 646
Perilunate fracture dislocations, 651-683
    classification, 654, 656-658, 658t
    complications, 674, 680f, 681
    diagnosis, 658
        delayed, 658
        imaging, 658, 660-661f
    epidemiology, 651
    etiology, 634
    historical perspective, 651
    Mayo classification, 639t
    mechanism of injury, 652f
        pathology, 654-656, 655-657f
        pathophysiology, 653-654
    stages, 635f
    treatment, 651, 653
        algorithm, 661f
        clinical scoring chart, 663t
        management principles, 659, 662f
        open reduction, 663-666, 664-679f
        percutaneous pin fixation, 659, 660f, 661-663
        transscaphoid perilunate fracture dislocations, 666-667, 668-669f,
            669, 670-674f, 677-678f, 680f
        transscaphoid transcapitate fracture dislocations, 669, 672,
            675-676f
Perilunate instability, 496t, 652f
    stages, 653, 653f
Perineurioma, 1245, 1247f
Peripheral nerve blocks, 1088
Peripheral nerve injuries; see Nerve injuries
Peritendinitis crepitans, 240; see also Intersection syndrome
Peritrapezium axial-radial dislocation, 689f, 690, 690f
Peritrapezoid peritrapezium axial-radial dislocation, 689f, 690, 691f
Phalen's test, in carpal tunnel syndrome, 1045, 1204-1205, 1205-1206f,
        1229
Phonophoresis, 1267
Physeal arrest, 983-984
    treatment, 985, 986f, 987
Physeal fractures, 983, 984f, 985, 989
Physeal injuries, 982-983; see also Growth-plate injuries
    in gymnasts, 1061-1062, 1062-1063f, 1063-1064
    to ulna, 747f, 747-748
Physeal surgery technique, 970-973, 971-972f

Physical examination of wrist, 236-261
  in children, 1025
  dorsal radial, 240-243
  dorsal ulnar, 243-247
  palmar, 247-253
  in palmar ulnar wrist pain, 253-254
  principles, 236-237
  provocative stress testing, 254-260
  radial, 237-240
Physical therapy
  in juvenile rheumatoid arthritis, 950
  modalities, 1262-1271
    biofeedback, 1269f, 1269-1270
    continuous passive motion, 1262-1263, 1263-1264f
    cryotherapy, 1263-1265, 1265f
    deep heat, 1266-1267
    electrical stimulation for pain control, 1268, 1269t
    electrotherapy, 1268
    fluidotherapy, 1266, 1267f
    hot packs, 1266, 1266f
    hydrotherapy, 1268
    muscle stimulation, 1268-1269
    in overuse syndrome, 1301
    paraffin bath, 1266
    phonophoresis, 1267
    therapeutic heat, 1265f, 1265-1266
    ultrasound, 1267, 1267f
Physiolysis, 970, 973, 974-976f
  in growth-plate injuries, 984, 985, 986-987f, 987, 989
  physeal surgery technique, 970-973, 971-972f
Piano key sign, 245f, 260, 713, 715f, 827, 830f, 844f
Pigmented villonodular synovitis, 1155
Pin fixation; see also Kirschner wires, applications
  complications, 1085, 1086f
  for distal radius fractures, 324, 338, 340-342f, 341, 343, 344-345f
  in growth-plate injuries, 985
  for perilunate dislocations, 640, 642-643f, 647f
  for perilunate fracture dislocations, 659, 660f, 661-663
  in wrist arthrodesis for rheumatoid arthritis, 915-916, 917f, 917-918
Pisiform
  anatomy, 34f, 66, 66f, 238f
    dorsal perspective, 41f
    in extensor retinaculum system, 47f
    palmar perspective, 42f
  in axial-ulnar disruption, 690f, 693f
  dislocations, 706f, 707
  excision, 480f
  exposure, 156, 158, 159f
  fractures, 480f, 481
    radiographic examination, 267f
  morphology, 17f, 19
Pisohamate ligament, 47f, 79f, 91
Pisometacarpal ligament, 20
Pisotriquetral grind test, 255f
Pisotriquetral joint, 70, 862
  arthritis
    evolution and, 26
    physical examination, 253, 254f
Pisotriquetral ligament, 79f, 94
Plate fixation
  for displaced ulnar fractures, 749, 751, 751f, 752f
  for distal radius fractures, 348-351f
  for intra-articular malunions, 375f
  in osteotomy for Madelung's deformity, 972f
  radial osteotomy and, 363, 366f
  in radiolunate arthrodesis, 905, 907f, 909

Pneumatic compression pumps, 1274
Poirier, P., 10
  space of Poirier, 10, 79
    in palmar capsulotomy, 104
Polinsky Advantage, 1292, 1293
Polyarthritis, 946
Polyarticular juvenile rheumatoid arthritis, 947, 947t
Polytomography, 271
  of perilunate fracture dislocation, 658, 661f
  of solitary bone cyst, 1251f
Pongo, wrist movements in, 18t
Portals for arthroscopy, 169, 171-173f, 173, 291f
  distal radioulnar joint, 291-292
  midcarpal joint, 177, 180f
  radiocarpal joint, 186f, 291
Posterior antebrachial cutaneous nerve, 119f
Posterior interosseous nerve, 36f, 38, 119f, 120, 121f
  palsy, 1043-1044f
Post-traumatic arthritis, 588-629
  classification, 601-602
  diagnosis, 598-601, 599-601f
  etiology, 593, 594f
    scaphoid fracture and secondary arthritis, 597-598, 597-599f
    scapholunate instability and secondary degenerative arthritis, 593, 595f, 596
    scaphotrapezial trapezoidal arthritis, 596f, 596-597
  incidence, 592-593
  patterns, 588, 589f, 591-592
  stages, 590f, 592-593f, 601-602
  treatment
    conservative, 602
    excisional arthroplasty, 611, 614-615f, 624
    general considerations, 602
    limited arthrodesis for scaphoid nonunion, 620-621f, 620-622
    proximal row carpectomy, 616, 617-619f, 620
    results, 624, 624t, 625f, 626
    for scapholunate advanced collapse and scaphotrapezial trapezoid pattern, 624
    scapholunate advanced collapse wrist surgery, 603-610f, 603-611, 612-613f, 622-613, 622-623
    scaphotrapezial trapezoidal arthrodesis, 604f, 623-624
    surgical, 602t, 602-603
Pouteau, Claude, 3
Preiser's disease (avascular ischemia of scaphoid), 1003, 1017, 1022
  magnetic resonance imaging, 278-279
Pressure testing; see Provocative stress testing
Pressure-sensitive conductive rubber, in force analyses, 191, 193-194f, 229
Pressure-sensitive film, in force analyses, 191, 192f, 229, 229f
Prestyloid recess, 69, 86f, 87
Proconsul africanus, 22
ProFlex splint, 1280f
Pronation-supination
  axis for, 211f
  distal radioulnar joint, 219, 222-224f, 226f
Pronator fat stripe, 265, 266f
Pronator quadratus
  advancement, in dorsal subluxation or dislocation of ulna, 832, 835f
  in distal radioulnar joint stability, 763f, 764
  distal ulna and, 744f
  interposition, 1080f
    in arthritis deformity, 800, 808f
  in joint stability, 227
  in modified Johnson procedure, 859, 860f
Pronator teres syndrome, 1207

Prostheses; *see also* Total wrist arthroplasty
    in arthritis deformity, 789, 792f
    future of, 1309-1310, 1311
    in Kienböck's disease, 450f, 450-451
    radial head, 770, 770f
    in scaphoid nonunion, 408f, 409
Provocative stress testing
    in children, 1025
    in distal radioulnar joint instability, 245f, 260
    in lunotriquetral sprains, 531f, 532
    in midcarpal instability, 250-251f, 259
    in scaphoid instability, 254, 256, 258-259f, 259
    in ulnocarpal instability, 248-249f, 259-260
Proximal carpal row; *see also* Proximal row carpectomy
    developmental wrist synovitis and, 891
    instability; *see* Carpal instability nondissociative; Radiocarpal instability
        and dislocations
    interosseous ligaments, 91-93f, 91-94, 92t
    kinematics, 551, 553f, 553-554
        normal, 210, 212-214, 213-215f, 216
    pediatric anomalies, 1016
    in radiocarpal rotation and stability, 826f, 827f
    radiographic examination, 270f
Proximal pole fracture of scaphoid, 395, 400, 402-404f, 403
Proximal radius dislocation, multiple hereditary osteochondromata and,
        996f, 999-1000
Proximal row carpectomy
    in arthrogryposis multiplex congenita, 1018
    complications, 620
    indications, 616
    in Kienböck's disease, 463-464, 464f
    limited wrist arthrodesis vs., 626
    in perilunate dislocations, 648, 648f
    in perilunate fracture dislocations, 669f, 674, 680f
    in post-traumatic arthritis, 616-620, 624t, 625f, 626
    technique, 616, 617-619f
Pseudarthrosis
    of distal ulna, 781f
    in total wrist arthroplasty, 939, 939f
Pseudo carpal instability, 495
Pseudogout, 873, 1147, 1151f
Psoriasis, 872
Psoriatic arthritis, 884f, 959
    diagnostic studies, 959f, 960-961
    etiology, 959-960
    management summary, 962
    surgical treatment, 960-961f, 961-962
Pterygium syndromes, 1007
Pulsed electromagnetic stimulation
    in scaphoid fracture, 400, 402f
    in scaphoid nonunion, 407
Pyridoxine, in carpal tunnel syndrome, 1209

Q
Quervain's disease; *see* de Quervain's disease

R
Radial aplasia, 1007-1008, 1008f
    centralization in, 1009, 1010f, 1011-1013
    surgical approaches in, 163-167f, 164, 166-167
    treatment, 1008-1009, 1008-1010f
Radial approach in arthrotomy, dorsal, 133, 134-136f
    to scaphoid, 149, 153-154f, 155
Radial artery
    anatomy, 34f, 35, 38, 39-40f, 107f, 108, 109f, 110, 110f, 238f
    occlusion, 282
Radial articular angle, 992f
    in multiple hereditary osteochondromata deformity, 992f, 996, 999

Radial avulsion triangular fibrocartilage tears, open repair of, 732, 733f
Radial club hand, exposures for, 163-167f, 164, 166-167
Radial collateral ligament, 174f
Radial dysplasia, 973, 975f
Radial epiphysis, teardrop shape of, 973, 977f
Radial forearm flap, in recurrent carpal tunnel syndrome, 1229, 1230
Radial head, prosthetic replacement, 770, 770f
Radial inclination, 570f
Radial nerve
    anatomy, 38, 119f, 120, 120f, 121f
        dorsal cutaneous branches, 170f
        superficial branch, 36f
    dorsal sensory branch, traction neuropathy of, 1044-1045
    sensory nerve injury, 1083f, 1084-1085
Radial neuritis, physical examination, 238, 240
Radial osteotomy
    biomechanical studies, 450
    in carpal instability nondissociative, 566
    for distal radius malunions
        extra-articular, 378-379f
        intra-articular, 375f, 376, 376f
        palmar approach, 380-381f
    for Kienböck's disease, 458, 459f
    for malunion of Colles fracture
        anatomic results, 358t
        in dorsal angulation fractures, 363, 364-366f
        indications, goals, and preoperative planning, 363
        in intra-articular malunions, 365, 367f
        in palmar angulation fractures, 365
        postoperative care, 365
        series results, 365t
        strength and motion results, 361t
Radial palmar carpal artery, 40f
Radial palmar carpal ligaments, arthroscopic inspection, 185
Radial recession osteotomy
    for carpal instability nondissociative, 560f
    for lunate fracture, 438f
Radial rim tear of triangular fibrocartilage, treatment of, 726, 727-730f
Radial styloid
    anatomy, 34f, 35, 172f, 237f, 238f
        dorsal perspective, 41f
        palmar perspective, 42f
    fractures, 352
        perilunate instability and, 635f, 653f, 657f, 660f
    physical examination, 237-238, 239-240f
    trans-radial-styloid fracture dislocations, 664f, 672-674
Radial styloid process, 67f
    ontogenesis, 62
Radial styloidectomy
    for post-traumatic arthritis, 605, 611
        technique, 611, 614-615f
    in scaphoid malunion, 425
Radial translation/translocation, 495
Radial wrist examination, 237-238, 239-240f
    in de Quervain's tenosynovitis, 238, 239f
    dorsal; *see* Dorsal radial wrist examination
    in intersection syndrome, 240, 240f
    in palmar wrist pain, 247-248
    in snuffbox tenderness, 240
    in Wartenberg's cheiralgia, 238, 240
Radial wrist extensors, functional absence in, 927
Radialization procedure, in radial aplasia, 1011
Radial/ulnar deviation, axis for, 211f
Radian method, 1110, 1112f
Radiation therapy, for soft-tissue tumors, 1240
Radiocapitate ligament; *see* Radioscaphocapitate ligament
Radiocapitate subluxation index, 559f, 561
Radiocarpal arch, vascular anatomy, 107, 107f, 109f, 118f

Radiocarpal instability and dislocations, 496t, 569-587
  Barton dorsal fracture dislocation, 578-580f, 581-582
  definition, 494
  dorsal radiocarpal instability
    author's corrective osteotomy technique, 576-577f
    evaluation, 570-573f, 571-572
    treatment, 572, 574-576f
  dorsal rim intra-articular fractures, 576, 578-579f, 581
  Mayo classification, 639t
  palmar radiocarpal instability, 581f, 582
  pathomechanics, 569
  ulnar translocation, 582, 583-586f, 586-587
Radiocarpal joint
  anatomy, 43f, 64f, 69-70
  arthrodesis
    in distal radius malunion, 370
    in psoriatic arthritis, 960f, 962
    in synovitis, 894-896f
  arthrography, 93f, 274, 275, 275f
  arthroscopy, 296f, 296-297
    anatomy, 173, 175-178f, 177, 292-293, 292-293f
    examination in sports injuries, 1065t
    inspection, 185, 186f
    portals, 186f, 291
  capsulotomy, 99, 100f, 101
  dorsal wrist examination of, 244f
  fetal development, 33, 33f
  force transmission through, 190-194
    analytical measurement, 191, 194, 196-197f
    experimental studies, 191, 192-196f
    normal wrist joint, 196-197, 198-199t, 199-200f
    pathologic conditions, 197-198, 200-202f, 201-203
  normal alignment, 571f
  pressure distribution, 327f
  rotation and stability, 825-826, 826-827f
  subluxation, in rheumatoid arthritis, 891
Radiocarpal joint kinematics, 205-218
  abnormal, 216f, 216-217
  analysis, 206-207, 206-211f
  historical perspective, 205-206
  normal, 208, 211f, 212t
    distal carpal row, 209-210
    proximal carpal row, 210, 212-214, 213-215f, 216
  reference axes, 211f
Radiocarpal ligaments
  dorsal, 87, 87t, 88f, 89f
  palmar, 78-84, 79f, 79t, 80-81f, 84-85f
    repair in perilunate fracture dislocations, 669
Radiocarpal portal, 172f
Radiocarpal-to-carpometacarpal approach to capsulotomy, 101, 103f
Radiography; see also specific disorders and Imaging
  general examination, 262-263
  in kinematic analysis, 206-207, 206-207f, 209-210f
  in radioulna variance measurement, 220f, 220-222, 221t
  in rheumatoid arthritis, 878-879f, 879-880, 889, 890-891f, 900, 901f
  routine views, 263
    lateral, 264-266f, 265
    oblique, 265, 267f
    posteroanterior, 263-265, 264f
  special views
    carpal tunnel, 265-267, 268f
    hamate, 269, 270f, 271
    scaphoid, 267-269, 269f
  in ulna variance assessment, 432, 434f, 440, 440f, 777, 778f
Radiology; see Imaging; Radiography
Radiolunate arthrodesis
  in distal radius malunion, 373
  in rheumatoid arthritis, 902f

postoperative protection, 909
range of motion after, 904t
results, 909
spontaneous, 882f, 903-904
surgical, 904-905, 905-908f, 909, 910f
  in ulnar translocation, 586
Radiolunate ligament; see also Long radiolunate ligament; Short radio-
    lunate ligament
  chevron carpus and, 972-973, 975, 975f
  dorsal, 656f, 657f
  in Madelung's deformity, 967, 968-969f, 972-973
Radiolunotriquetral (long radiolunate) ligament
  anatomy, 78-79, 79-81f, 81, 553f
    arthroscopic, 173, 174f, 176f, 178f
    in sagittal section, 48
  in carpal instability nondissociative treatment, 561, 562f
  dorsal, 656f
  in perilunate fracture dislocations, 657f
  in scaphoid fracture repair, 1050-1051f
Radionuclide imaging, 282
Radioscaphocapitate ligament
  anatomy, 78, 79-81f, 553f
    arthroscopic, 173, 174f, 176f
    in sagittal section, 48
  in carpal instability nondissociative treatment, 561, 562f
  magnetic resonance imaging, 280f
  in perilunate fracture dislocations, 657f
  in scaphoid fracture repair, 1050-1051f
  wrist motion and, 215f
Radioscaphoid joint
  arthritis, 591f, 600f; see also Scapholunate advanced collapse wrist
    arthrodesis
      in post-traumatic arthritis, 624t, 625f
      in scaphoid nonunion, 409
  early changes on tomography, 519f
Radioscaphoid ligament, 175f, 178f, 657f
Radioscapholunate arthrodesis
  in distal radius malunion, 372-373f, 373
  in Kienböck's disease, 460
  in post-traumatic arthritis, 624t, 625f
  in rheumatoid arthritis, 902f, 909, 911-912f, 912
    with midcarpal arthroplasty, 912, 913-914f, 914
    range of motion after, 915t
  in synovitis, 896f
  in ulnar translocation, 586f
Radioscapholunate ligament, 79-84f, 81-83
  arthroscopic anatomy, 173, 174f
Radiotriquetral ligament, dorsal, 656f, 657f
  in lunotriquetral joint kinematics, 528, 529f
Radioulna variance, measurement of, 220f, 220-222, 222t
Radioulnar carpal joint; see also Distal radioulnar joint
  force transmission and pressure distribution in, 196, 199f, 199t
Radioulnar fusion
  and ulnar osteotomy, in arthritis deformity, 811, 812-813f, 813
    technique, 813, 814f, 815
  in rheumatoid arthritis, 884
Radioulnar interosseous membrane, 744f, 745
Radioulnar joint, dorsal, 823-825, 824-825f
Radioulnar ligaments; see also Dorsal radioulnar ligament; Palmar radio-
    ulnar ligament
  in joint stability, 225-227, 226f, 227t, 228
  in kinematic constraint of distal radioulnar joint, 761f, 763f, 824-825,
    825f, 835-836
  in triangular fibrocartilage complex, 97, 98-99, 821f, 821-822
Radioulnar synostosis, with proximal segment excision, 857, 859-860f
Radius
  distal; see Distal radius
  distance of nerves to, 1084t

Radius—cont'd
  normal carpal bone motions with respect to, 208, 212t
  osteotomy; *see* Radial osteotomy; Radial recession osteotomy
  palmar perspective, 41f
  premature fusion of, 983f, 984
  proximal dislocation, multiple hereditary osteochondromata and, 996f, 999-1000
  proximal migration of, 849, 852
  resection in total wrist arthroplasty, 930
  synostosis of distal ulna to, 754-755
Radius shortening
  biomechanical studies, 449
  in carpal instability nondissociative, 566
  in distal radius malunion, 357f, 358-360, 359f
  for Kienböck's disease, 201, 444f, 453-456f, 454, 457-458
    dorsal approach, 455f, 458
    palmar approach, 456f, 458
    ulna shortening and, 458
  in multiple hereditary osteochondromata, 999
  radioulnar joint articular pressure and, 229t
Ramamorphs, 23
Range of motion
  after wrist arthrodesis for rheumatoid arthritis, 904t, 915t
  passive, 1274-1275
  postoperative exercises, 1274
Rayan dorsal "bone" plate technique, 918f
Rayhack technique
    of percutaneous pin fixation, 341, 341f, 343, 347
    of ulna recession, 783, 784f, 850f
Raynaud's phenomenon, 282
RBSM, 194, 229
Recessus preradialis, 64f, 69
Recessus prescaphoideus, 69
Recessus prestyloideus, 69, 87
Recessus pretriquetralis, 69-70
Reduction of fractures and dislocations; *see* Closed reduction; Open reduction
Reflex sympathetic dystrophy, 1095
  clinical presentation, 1098, 1099f, 1100
  clinical stages, 1099t
  definition, 1098t
  diagnosis, 282, 1100, 1100f, 1100t
  somatic nerve pain vs., 1101t, 1102
  treatment, 1100-1101, 1103-1104
Rehabilitation, 1262, 1272
  occupational therapy and splinting, 1272-1286
  physical therapy modalities, 1262-1271
  work, 1287-1294
Reiter's syndrome, 872
Repetitive strain injury, 1296; *see also* Overuse syndrome
  epidemiology, 1297-1299, 1298f
Replacement of wrist; *see also* Prostheses; Total wrist arthroplasty
  potential for, 1311-1312
Resection arthroplasty, in synovitis, 895
Resorption, in rheumatoid arthritis, 881
Restrictive thumb-index tenosynovitis, 1194, 1194f
Retinacular anatomy, 43-47, 45-46f; *see also* Extensor retinaculum; Flexor retinaculum
Retinaculatome, Paine, 1216f, 1218
Reuleaux, Franz, 4
Revascularization, for Kienböck's disease, 460, 462-463, 462-463f
Reverse Phalen's test, in carpal tunnel syndrome, 1205, 1205f
Rhabdomyosarcoma, 1247
Rheumatic fever, acute, 872
Rheumatoid arthritis
  classification of conditions in
    tendon ruptures, 892
    tenosynovitis, 890

  wrist synovitis, 890-892
  clinical guides to treatment decisions
    balancing priorities of person, disease, and treatment, 884-885
    confirming diagnosis, 881-882
    evaluating pathologic features, 882, 884
  diagnosis, 888-889, 888-890f
  differential diagnosis, 870
    diseases affecting linings of joints and tendons, 871
    rheumatoid (seropositive) and seronegative arthritis, 871-873
  epidemiology, 870-871
  etiology, 888
  historical perspective, 870
  imaging findings, 878-884f, 879-881, 900, 901f
  juvenile; *see* Juvenile rheumatoid arthritis
  laboratory findings, 879
  management, 887-888
  nonsurgical treatment, 900
  palpation and manual testing, 876-877f, 879
  pathogenesis, 871, 880-881
  pathophysiology, 899-900
  signs, symptoms, and findings, 872t, 873-875f, 873-876
  soft-tissue reconstruction in, 887-898
    etiology and, 888
    principles, 887
    problems and complications, 897
    in tendon rupture, 895-897
    in tenosynovitis, 892-893
    in wrist synovitis, 893-895, 894-896f
  surgical treatment, 884-885; *see also* Total wrist arthroplasty; Wrist arthrodesis for rheumatoid arthritis
    midline ulnar approach, 144-145f, 146
    Sauvé-Kapandji procedure, 812f
    synovectomy, 900
  Wrightington classification, 1139, 1141
Rheumatoid synovitis, 888, 890-891, 899, 1137
  with articular cartilage destruction, 892, 894-895
  etiology and pathogenesis, 1137-1138
  isolated, with preserved joint congruity, 891, 891f, 893-894
  with joint subluxation but preserved articular surfaces, 891f, 891-892, 894
  juvenile, 1147, 1152
  pathomechanics, 1138, 1139-1140f
  recurrent, 897
  synovectomy for, 1139, 1141-1142, 1141-1142f
  treatment, 893-895, 893-896f
    authors' preferred method, 1142, 1143-1149f, 1146
  wrist synovitis, 1138
Rigid body spring modeling, 194, 229
Ring sign
  cortical, in scapholunate instability, 505
  in perilunate instability, 636, 636f, 637f, 643f, 698f
Roentgen, Wilhelm Conrad, physiology before and after, 4-7
Rongeur, for synovectomy, 893f
Rosette strain gauge, in force analyses, 195f
Rotation, forearm, normal range of, 222, 224
Rotational axes, 208, 211f, 212t, 223f
Rotatory subluxation of scaphoid; *see* Scaphoid subluxation, rotatory
Rubber, pressure-sensitive conductive, in force analyses, 191, 193-194f
Rush pinning, of displaced ulnar fractures, 751, 753, 753f
Rüsse bone grafting
  in scaphoid fracture in immature wrist, 1023f
  in scaphoid nonunion, 406, 407f, 408f, 417
Rüsse classification of scaphoid fractures, 394f, 395t, 1049, 1049f
Rüsse incision, 146, 149, 149f

S

Sagittal sectional anatomy, 47-49, 48-50f
Salter type I fractures, 748
Salter type II fractures, 747f

Salter-Harris classification, of growth-plate injuries, 982

Saphenous vein bypass graft, 1046f, 1047

Sarcomas
    chondrosarcoma, 1256, 1256f
    epithelioid, 1245, 1249f
    Ewing's, 1257f, 1258
    fibrosarcoma, 1245, 1248f
    incidence, 1254f
    osteogenic, 1255f, 1256
    rhabdomyosarcoma, 1247
    synovial, 1247
    work-up for, 150t, 1241f

Sauvé-Kapandji procedure, 781, 781f; see also Kapandji procedure
    in arthritis deformity, 789, 791f, 811, 812-813f, 813
        technique, 813, 814f, 815
    in distal radioulnar joint fractures, 753
    in distal radius malunion, 368
    in rheumatoid arthritis, 914-915
        radiolunate arthrodesis and, 909, 910f

Scaphocapitate arthrodesis, 217
    biomechanical studies, 449
    in Kienböck's disease, 202, 460
    kinematics and, 217
    for scapholunate advanced collapse wrist, 605-606f

Scaphocapitate ligament, 174f

Scaphocapitate syndrome, 483-484, 635

Scaphocapitate trapezoid ligament, 79f, 89, 90f, 91

Scaphoid
    anatomy, 34f, 41f, 63, 64f, 181f, 237f, 385-386, 387f
        vascular supply, 385-386, 387f
    avascular necrosis, in perilunate injury, 648
    dislocations, 702-704, 703-704f
        axial dislocations vs., 692
    distal pole of, 35
    excision, in post-traumatic arthritis, 606, 607-610f, 611, 624t, 625f
    fracture dislocations
        transscaphoid perilunate, 666-667, 668-669f, 669, 670-674f
        transscaphoid transcapitate, 669, 672, 675-676f
    humpback deformity, 207f
    impingement, physical examination, 243, 244f
    implants, in radioscaphoid arthritis, 600f, 604
    instability
        historical perspective, 9
        provocative stress testing, 254, 256, 258-259f, 259
    kinematics, 212t, 213, 214-215f
    multiple ossification centers, 1017
    ontogenesis, 62
    osteotomy, motion changes after, 207f
    proximal, 34f
    surgical approaches
        dorsal radial, 149, 153-154f, 155
        palmar, 146, 149-152f
    tubercle of, 42f

Scaphoid displacement test, 506f

Scaphoid fat stripe, 263, 264f, 395

Scaphoid fossa, 67f, 68, 310, 311f, 312

Scaphoid fractures, 385-403; see also Scaphoid malunion; Scaphoid nonunion
    anatomy and vascularity, 385-386, 387f
    arthritis after, 597-598
    in athletes, 1047
        classification, 1048-1050, 1049f
        diagnosis, 1047-1048
        misdiagnosis, 1049f
        nonoperative treatment, 1050
        operative treatment, 1050-1054f, 1052-1053
        return to competition for, 1053-1054
    carpal instability and, 598
    carpal kinematics after, 207f, 217

in children, 386f, 1022, 1023f
clinical presentations, 388, 393
diagnosis and assessment, 393, 395
    arthroscopy, 299
    magnetic resonance imaging, 278, 281f
    radiographic examination, 267-269
    tomography, 272, 272f
distal articular, 395, 403, 405f
epidemiology, 385
morphology, 394f, 395, 395t
pathomechanics, 386-388, 388-392f
perilunate instability and, 635f, 653f, 654-655, 655f, 657f, 660f
proximal pole, 395, 400, 402-404f, 403
radiographs, 389-393f, 395-398f, 401-403f
snuffbox tenderness and, 240
treatment, 395-396, 395-396f
    acute undisplaced scaphoid waist fractures, 409
    acute unstable scaphoid fractures, 409-410, 409-414f, 414
    cast immobilization, 396, 397-398f
    complications, 421, 421f
    failed, salvage of, 422, 423f
    open reduction and internal fixation, 399-400, 400-401f
    retrograde screw fixation, 415-416f, 417
    surgical approach, 410-414f

Scaphoid impaction syndrome, in athletes, 1064

Scaphoid lift test, 256, 260f, 504

Scaphoid ligament, 175f

Scaphoid malunion, 422, 599f
    clinical findings, 422
    etiology, 387-388
    pathomechanics, 422
    radiographic findings, 422, 424
    treatment, 424-425

Scaphoid nonunion, 403, 405, 599f
    arthritis in, 598, 598f
    in children, 1023f
    degenerative changes in, 599f
    dorsal intercalated segment instability in, 598f
    etiology, 387-388
    imaging, 405, 406f
    treatment, 405
        electrical stimulation, 407
        excision and prosthetic replacement, 408f, 409
        fibrous synostosis, 407, 409
        humpback deformity, 417, 418f
        interpositional wedge grafts, 410-414f, 417, 418f, 421
        limited arthrodesis, 620-621, 620-621f, 620-622
        osteosynthesis, 406-407, 407f, 408f, 417, 419f
        proximal row carpectomy, 616
        radioscaphoid arthrodesis, 409
        Rüsse bone grafting, 407f, 408f, 417
        salvage procedures, 409
        surgical approach, 410-414f

Scaphoid nonunion advanced collapse (SNAC), 591-592, 597f
    clinical examples, 594f
    stages, 592-593f, 601-602
    treatment
        algorithm, 602t
        conservative, 602
        denervation of wrist joint, 622
        distraction resection arthroplasty, 621-622
        limited arthrodesis, 620-621f, 620-622
        total wrist arthroplasty, 622

Scaphoid shift test, 254, 256, 258f, 259, 504, 506

Scaphoid subluxation
    dorsal, 259f
    rotatory, 198, 492, 501-502; see also Scapholunate instability
        isolated, treatment, 510f, 511, 512f

Scaphoid subluxation—cont'd
rotatory—cont'd
radiography, 504-506
secondary, treatment, 511-512, 614f
Scaphoid thrust test, 256
Scaphoid tuberosity, 238f
Scaphoid view, 267-269, 269f
Scapholunate advanced collapse (SLAC) wrist, 591, 591f
degenerative process, 589f, 596
diagnosis, 601
scaphotrapezial trapezoidal arthritis in, 596f
stages, 590f, 601
synovitis and, 1146
treatment, 522-523
algorithm, 602t
conservative, 602
intercarpal fusion, 605-606, 607-610f, 611, 612-613f
limited wrist arthrodesis, 603-605, 604-610f
reconstruction technique, 607-610f, 613f, 622-623
results, 626
wrist arthrodesis, 603, 603f
Scapholunate angle, 214f
Scapholunate ballottement, 504, 504f
Scapholunate complex, anatomy, 80f, 82f, 93f
Scapholunate dissociation, 202-203, 501, 502; *see also* Scapholunate
instability
in children, 1025
in Destot's work, 8, 8f
diagnosis, 503-504, 505f, 509f
kinematics, 216f, 217
physical examination, 241, 241f
in rheumatoid arthritis, 881f
schematic appearance, 510f
Scapholunate dissociation treatment
acute scapholunate dissociation
isolated rotatory subluxation of scaphoid, 510f, 511, 512f
secondary rotatory subluxation of scaphoid, 511-512, 514f
after acute stage (without osteoarthritis)
capsulodesis, 517-518
intercarpal arthrodesis, 513, 517-519f
ligament repair-reconstruction, 512-513, 515-516f
ligamentous repair and dorsal capsulodesis, 512f, 518, 520-521f
scaphotrapezium-trapezoid fusion, 520-521
chronic scapholunate dissociation with osteoarthritis, 521-523,
522f
Scapholunate gap, on frontal radiograph, 504-505, 505f
Scapholunate instability, 501-526
after ganglionectomy, 1178
clinical examination, 504, 504f
arthrography, 507-509
arthroscopy, 511
bone scintigraphy, 507
frontal radiograph, 504-505, 505f
lateral radiograph, 505-506
magnetic resonance imaging, 509, 509f, 511
scaphoid displacement test, 506f
degenerative arthritis and, 593, 595f, 596
diagnosis, 503-504
historical perspective, 501
mechanism of injury, 502-503
stages, 502
terminology, 501-502
treatment
acute scapholunate dissociation, 510f, 511-512, 512f, 514f
chronic scapholunate dissociation with osteoarthritis, 521-523,
522f

scapholunate dissociation after acute stage (without osteoarthritis),
512-513, 515-519f, 517-518, 520-521, 520-521f
SLAC wrist, 522-523
video fluoroscopy, 507-508f
Scapholunate interosseous ligament, 81f, 91-93f, 91-94
Scapholunate joint
anatomy, 35
arthrodesis, 513
arthroscopic inspection, 187
perilunate dissociation at, 633f
Scapholunate ligament
arthroscopy
anatomy, 175, 176f, 177, 178f
inspection, 185
therapeutic, 305
ganglions originating in, 1166, 1173-1175f
repair-reconstruction, in scapholunate dissociation, 512f, 512-513,
515-516f, 518, 520
Scaphotrapezial capitate joint, arthroscopic appearance, 180f
Scaphotrapezial joint
arthritis, physical examination, 248, 252f
morphology, 21
Scaphotrapezial ligament, 174f
Scaphotrapezial trapezoid arthrodesis, 216f
biomechanical studies, 449
in Kienböck's disease, 201, 458, 460, 460f
kinematics and, 216f, 217
in post-traumatic arthritis, 604f, 623-624
for scapholunate advanced collapse wrist, 604, 604f
in scapholunate dissociation, 513, 517
results and complications, 513, 517, 519f
successful, radiographs, 517-518f
technique, 520-521
technique, 604f, 623-624
Scaphotrapezial trapezoid joint
arthritis, 591, 591f, 596f
diagnosis, 601
arthroscopic anatomy, 294f
exposure, 158, 160f
Scaphotrapezium trapezoid ligament, 79f, 89, 90f
Scaphotrapezoid joint, morphology, 21
Scaphotriquetral interosseous ligaments, 94
Scaphotriquetral ligament; *see also* Dorsal intercarpal ligament
dorsal, 174f, 656f
in lunotriquetral joint kinematics, 528, 528f
Schwannoma
benign, 1243, 1245
malignant, 1250
Scintigraphy, skeletal; *see* Bone scans
Scleroderma, 883f
Sclerosis of distal articular surface of ulna, 777f
Scopes for arthroscopy, 287, 288f
Screw fixation; *see also* Herbert screw osteosynthesis
for hamate fractures, 483f
for lunate fractures, 438f
for perilunate fracture dislocations, 665-666, 667f, 672, 673f
for scaphoid fractures, 1052, 1053, 1054f
Seborrheic keratosis, 1235
Sectional anatomy
coronal, 57-58, 58-59f
sagittal, 47-49, 48-50f
transverse, 50-57, 51-56f
Segmuller, G., 10
Sennwald, G., 10, 74
Sennwald classification of instability, 492, 495t
Sensory recovery, 1291

Sensory testing, in carpal tunnel syndrome, 1204, 1207

Sepsis, fusion from, 989, 989f

Shear tests, lunotriquetral, 249f, 259-260, 531f, 532

"Shepherd's crook" wrist splints, 1278f, 1281

Short radiolunate ligament, 79-81f, 83-84, 85f, 553f, 657f
    anatomy, 79-81f, 83-84, 85f, 553f
        arthroscopic, 175, 178f
    magnetic resonance imaging, 280f
    in perilunate fracture dislocations, 657f
    in scaphoid fracture repair, 1050-1051f

Short stature, 1024

Short wave diathermy, 1266-1267

Sigmoid notch, 68, 311f, 312, 851f

Silastic implants, in radioscaphoid arthritis, 600f, 604

Silicone implants
    in excisional arthroplasty of scaphotrapezial trapezoid joint, 624
    in Kienböck's disease, 450f, 450-451
    in psoriatic arthritis, 961f, 962
    radiocarpal arthrodesis with, 895f
    in radioscaphoid arthritis, 600f, 604
    synovitis from, 1153, 1155-1156, 1156f; see also Silicone synovitis
    in ulnar head replacement, 789, 792, 793f

Silicone ligamentous tether, 833f

Silicone replacement arthroplasty of lunocapitate joint, radioscapholunate arthrodesis and, 912, 913-914f, 914

Silicone rubber, 1152-1153

Silicone rubber interpositional arthroplasty, 925

Silicone synovitis, 450f, 451, 1152-1156, 1153-1154f, 1156f
    dorsal wrist synovectomy in, 1159

Silicone wrist arthroplasty, 925; see also Total wrist arthroplasty

Silver fork deformity, of Colles fractures, 362

Sixth dorsal compartment anatomy, 1188, 1188f

Skeletal dysplasia, 1007t, 1024

Skin anatomy and innervation, 36-37

Skin complications of wrist injury, 1076-1077, 1077-1078f

Skin grafts, 1237f, 1238f

Skin tumors
    benign, 1235t, 1235-1236f, 1235-1237
    evaluation and treatment principles, 1235
    malignant, 1235t, 1236-1237f, 1237, 1238-1239f, 1239

SLAC; see Scapholunate advanced collapse wrist

Smilodectes gracilis, 22

Smith fracture, 315, 316f
    angulation deformity in, 358
    loss of motion in, 361
    malunion in, surgical correction, 365, 378, 581f, 582
    treatment, 328, 330, 332-333f, 350-351f, 352

Smith-Petersen approach, 915

SNAC; see Scaphoid nonunion advanced collapse

Snuffbox
    anatomic, 35
    tenderness, physical examination, 240
    ulnar, 36

Soft-tissue constraints, in distal radioulnar joint stability, 760-764

Soft-tissue injuries of dorsal wrist, physical examination, 242-243

Soft-tissue injury complications
    nerves, 1081-1089
    skin, 1076-1077
    tendons, 1077-1081

Soft-tissue reconstruction; see Rheumatoid arthritis, soft-tissue reconstruction in

Soft-tissue tumors
    benign, 1240, 1240t, 1241f, 1242t, 1242-1243, 1243-1245f, 1245
    evaluation and treatment principles, 1239-1240
    malignant, 1240t, 1245, 1246-1249f, 1247, 1250
    management algorithm, 1241f

Solitary bone cyst, 1251f, 1252

Somatic nerve pain
    clinical presentation, 1101
    sympathetic dystrophy vs., 1101t, 1102
    treatment, 1101-1104, 1102-1103f

Space of Poirier, 10, 79
    in palmar capsulotomy, 104

Spilled teacup sign, 637, 637f

Splints; see also Immobilization
    commercially available, 1280-1282f, 1282, 1283
    internal, 1309
    practice of splinting, 1276, 1282
        dynamic splinting, 1279-1280f, 1281, 1282
        principles, 1276-1277
        static splinting, 1276-1278f, 1277-1279, 1281, 1282
    in specific situations
        after arthroscopic synovectomy, 1161
        carpal instability nondissociative, 561
        carpal tunnel syndrome, 1209-1210
        distal radius fractures, 324, 324f
        dorsal wrist block splint for gymnasts, 1064f
        intersection syndrome, 1033
        juvenile rheumatoid arthritis, 950, 951-952f
        overuse syndrome, 1301
        radial aplasia, 1009, 1011
        rheumatoid arthritis, 888
        total wrist arthroplasty, 937
        work hardening programs, 1290
    synovitis and, 1139f

Sports injuries; see Athletic injuries

Sprains
    carpometacarpal, 241, 242
    lunotriquetral; see Lunotriquetral sprains
    scaphoid fracture and, 388, 389f

Squamous cell carcinoma, 1237, 1237f

Stability; see specific anatomy and Instability

Ståhl classification of Kienböck's disease, 443

Stanley-Shelley plate, 905, 907f, 909

Stapling, hemiepiphyseal, of distal radius, in multiple hereditary osteochondromata, 996, 997f

Stark, W.A., 9

Static splinting, 1276-1278f, 1277-1279, 1281, 1282

Steinmann pins
    in psoriatic arthritis treatment, 960f, 961f
    in wrist arthrodesis for rheumatoid arthritis, 915-916, 917f
        removal of, 920

Stenosing tenosynovitis
    of extensor carpi ulnaris, in athletes, 1037
    of first extensor compartment; see de Quervain's disease
    of sixth extensor compartment, 1189f

Steroids; see Corticosteroids

Still's disease, 945

Strain gauges, in force analyses, 191, 195f

Strengthening, in work hardening program, 1291f

Stress fracture of ulna, 753-754

Stress loading; see also Stress testing
    of carpometacarpal joint, 242f
    of distal radioulnar joint, 245f, 260
    of flexor tendons, 259f
    of midcarpal joint, 251f

Stress testing, provocative
    in children, 1025
    in distal radioulnar joint instability, 245f, 260
    in lunotriquetral sprains, 531f, 532
    in midcarpal instability, 250-251f, 259
    in scaphoid instability, 254, 256, 258-259f, 259
    in ulnocarpal instability, 248-249f, 259-260

Stretching, postoperative, 1274, 1275
Subluxation; see also specific anatomy
    in carpal instability classification, 496t
    in carpal instability nondissociative, 556, 557f, 559f
    in rheumatoid arthritis, 888-889, 889f, 891-892, 901f
Superficial heat, 1265
Superficial spreading melanoma, 1239
Supertrauma, 983, 985
Supination
    comparative morphology, 15, 17-19
    distal radioulnar joint dislocation and, 228
Supination-pronation
    axis for, 211f
    distal radioulnar joint, 219, 222-224f, 226f
Surface anatomy, 34f, 34-36; see also Topographic anatomy
Surgery
    as diagnostic method in children, 1027
    future of, 1309-1310, 1311
Surgical approaches and joint exposures, 126-168
    general approaches, 126
        dorsal, 126-127, 127-132f, 132-133
        dorsal radial, 133, 134-136f
        dorsal ulnar, 140, 141-143f, 144
        midline ulnar, 144-145f, 146
        palmar, 146, 147-148f
        ulnar, 133, 137-140f, 140
    specific approaches
        in arthritis deformity of distal radioulnar joint, 814f
        carpal tunnel incision for median nerve release, 1082f
        in carpal tunnel syndrome; see Carpal tunnel release; Transverse
            carpal ligament release
        in compartment syndrome, 1121-1124f, 1122-1123, 1125
        in complete arthrodesis for rheumatoid arthritis, 905f, 915
        Darrach resection technique, 796f
        dorsal radial approach to scaphoid, 149, 153-154f, 155, 1053
        dorsal synovectomy, 952, 954f, 1143f
        first carpometacarpal joint exposure, 158, 161-162f, 163
        in first extensor compartment release, 1035-1036f
        hook of hamate exposure, 155-156, 155-158f
        in ischemic contracture, 1129f
        in lunate dislocations, 698, 699-700f
        lunotriquetral joint exposure, 537, 538f
        osteotomy in Madelung's deformity, 978, 978f
        palmar approach to scaphoid, 146, 149-152f, 1050-1051f, 1052
        palmar tenosynovectomy, 1159
        in perilunate dislocations, 640, 642, 644-646f
        in perilunate fracture dislocations, 655-656, 663-669, 666f, 670-673f,
            675f, 677f, 680f
        pisiform exposure, 156, 158, 159f
        radial club hand exposures, 163-167f, 164, 166-167
        in radiolunate arthrodesis, 904, 905f
        in scapholunate instability, 510f, 511
        scaphotrapezial trapezoid joints exposure, 158, 160f
        total wrist arthroplasty, 930, 931f
        in triangular fibrocartilage tears, 723-724f, 724
        to ulna, 750f, 751, 752f
Sutro, C.J., 10
Swanson implants, in distal radius malunion, 369
Swanson technique of prosthetic replacement of distal head of ulna, 789,
    792, 793f
Swanson wrist arthroplasty, 920, 922f, 925
Sympathetic dystrophy; see Reflex sympathetic dystrophy
Synostosis of distal ulna to radius, 754-755
Synovectomy, 893, 1139, 1140-1142f, 1141-1142
    arthroscopic, 301, 1160-1161
    dorsal wrist, 1156-1157, 1157-1158f, 1159
    in juvenile rheumatoid arthritis, 952, 953-955f, 1152

    palmar tenosynovectomy in carpal tunnel release, 1159-1160
    in rheumatoid arthritis, 884, 900
    rongeur for, 893f
Synovial hypertrophy, in carpal tunnel syndrome, 1201-1202
Synovial osteochondromatosis, of distal radioulnar joint, 862
Synovial sarcoma, 1247
Synovial stratum, 74f
Synovitis, 1137-1164; see also Tenosynovitis
    arthroscopy, diagnostic, 299
    crystalline-induced, 1146-1147, 1149-1150f
    evaluation, 882
    historical perspective, 1137
    miscellaneous forms, 1152
    in osteoarthritis, 1146
    pigmented villonodular, 1155
    in rheumatoid arthritis; see Rheumatoid synovitis
    silicone, 450f, 451, 1152-1156, 1153-1154f, 1156f
    surgical treatment; see Synovectomy
Synovium, 1137
Systemic juvenile rheumatoid arthritis, 947, 947t
Systemic lupus erythematosus, 872, 956
    classification criteria, 958t
    diagnostic studies, 956-957, 956-957f
    management summary, 957, 959

T
"Tabletop" exercise, 325f
Taleisnik, J., 7, 9, 10, 74
Taleisnik classification of instability, 492, 494t
Taleisnik procedure, in rheumatoid arthritis, 912, 913-914f, 914
Tears, triangular fibrocartilage; see Triangular fibrocartilage tears
Technetium-99 scans, of ulnar impaction (abutment) syndrome, 849f
Teisen and Hjarbaek classification of lunate fractures, 436, 436f
Telegraphists' cramp, 1295
Tendinitis, 1181-1196
    abductor pollicis longus, 252
    in athletes, 1032-1033, 1035
    diagnosis, general considerations, 1182
    etiology, 1181-1182
    of extensor compartments
        de Quervain's disease, 1183-1185f, 1185-1186
        extensor carpi ulnaris, 859, 1188-1189, 1188-1190f
        extensor digiti minimi, 1188
        extensor indicis proprius syndrome, 1188
        extensor pollicis longus, 1187-1188
        intersection syndrome, 1186f, 1186-1187
    of flexor compartments
        flexor carpi radialis, 252, 1191-1192, 1191-1193f, 1194
        flexor carpi ulnaris, 253, 1189, 1191
        restrictive thumb-index tenosynovitis, 1194, 1194f
    palmar, physical examination, 252-253, 253f
    treatment, general considerations, 1182
Tendon grafts, 1078
    in carpal instability nondissociative, 564, 564f
    in lunotriquetral joint reconstruction, 539-541f, 542
Tendon surgery, in rheumatoid arthritis, 884
Tendon transfer, 1078, 1080f
    in ischemic contracture, 1129f, 1132, 1134
    in radial aplasia, 1011
    in synovitis, 1141, 1147f
Tendons
    athletic disorders
        de Quervain's tenosynovitis, 1034-1035, 1034-1036f
        extensor insertional tenosynovitis, 1035, 1037
        intersection syndrome, 1033-1034
        recurrent subluxation of extensor carpi ulnaris tendon, 1038, 1039f,
            1040

stenosing tenosynovitis of extensor carpi ulnaris, 1037
    tendinitis, 1032-1033
historical perspective, 10
injuries, 1077-1079, 1079-1081f, 1081
retinacular anatomy, 43-47, 45-46f
ruptures
    in distal radius malunion, 363
    physical examination, 243
    in rheumatoid arthritis, 892, 895-897
    from synovitis, 1141-1142
ulnocarpal tendinous tethers, 832, 833-834f, 837-838f, 839
Tennis, hook of hamate fractures in, 1055, 1056f
Tenodesis, synovectomy and, 1159
Tenosynovectomy, 892, 893
in carpal tunnel syndrome, 1214, 1215f, 1227
dorsal, 1157-1158f
extensor, 1157-1158f
    in juvenile rheumatoid arthritis, 952, 953-955f
flexor, 893, 1142f, 1159-1160, 1161
palmar, 1141, 1142f
    in carpal tunnel release, 1159-1160
Tenosynovial thickening, in carpal tunnel syndrome, 1201-1202
Tenosynovitis
de Quervain's; see de Quervain's disease
in dorsal compartments of wrist, 859, 861f
etiology, 1181
extensor, 876f, 890
    insertional, in athletes, 1035, 1037
    sixth extensor compartment, 1189f
extensor carpi ulnaris, 1188-1189
    in athletes, 1037
extensor pollicis longus, 1187-1188
    in athletes, 1037
flexor, 252, 877f, 890
physical examination, 242-243
restrictive thumb-index, 1194, 1194f
in rheumatoid arthritis, 888, 890
    recurrent or untreated, 897
    treatment, 892-893
surgical treatment; see Tenosynovectomy
villonodular, 1240, 1241f
TENS
for pain control, 1268, 1269t
in somatic nerve pain, 1104
Tension band wires
in dorsal wedge corrective osteotomy, 576, 576f
in ulnar styloid reattachment, 732, 733f
Terminology
historical, 2, 3, 5f, 61-62
instability, 492-497
Terry-Thomas sign, 504, 636
Testut, L.L., 10
ligament of Testut, 79-84f, 81-83
Testut and Kuenz, ligament of, 173f
TFC(C); see Triangular fibrocartilage (complex)
Thomas suspension splint, 1282
Thoracic outlet syndrome, 1207
Thrombosis, ulnar artery, 1046f, 1046-1047
Thumb shell splint, 1277f, 1278
Thumb spica splint, in intersection syndrome, 1033
"Thumb to tip" exercise, 325f
Tinel's sign, in carpal tunnel syndrome, 1045, 1204, 1229
Tomography, advantages and applications, 270-271f, 271-273; see also
    Computed tomography
Barton dorsal fracture dislocation, 578f
carpal instability nondissociative, 556, 557f
dorsal subluxation of ulnar head, 829f

gout, 1150f
growth-plate injuries, 983-984f
Madelung's deformity, 969f
perilunate fracture dislocation, 658, 661f
radioscaphoid joint, 519f
rheumatoid arthritis, 880
scaphotrapezium-trapezoid arthrodesis, 519f
ulnar impaction (abutment) syndrome, 849f, 851f
Tools, prehistoric, in morphologic evolution, 25-27
Topographic anatomy, 34f, 169, 170-174f, 173, 237-238f; see also Surface
    anatomy
Torus fracture, 745-746
Total wrist arthroplasty, 924-944
alternative devices, 927f, 940-941, 941-942f, 943
design development, 925f, 928-929f
in distal radius malunion, 368-370, 370-371f
history, 924-925
indications and contraindications, 925, 927
postoperative care, 937, 939
revision surgery and salvage after, 938-940f, 939-940
in scaphoid nonunion advanced collapse, 622
surgical technique, 930, 931-936f, 936-937
T-plate fixation
for intra-articular malunions, 375f
radial osteotomy and, 363, 366f
Traction, for distal radius fractures, 322f, 329f, 343
Traction tower for arthroscopy, 181-182, 184f
Trampoline effect/test, 730, 734, 734f
Transcapitate fractures, 657f
Transcarpal ligament, dorsal, 174f
Transcutaneous electrical nerve stimulation; see also TENS
for pain control, 1268, 1269t
in somatic nerve pain, 1104
Trans-radial-styloid fracture dislocations, treatment, 664-665f
Trans-radial-styloid fractures, 657f
Transscaphoid fracture dislocations, 662f
tomography, 660, 661f
treatment, 666-667f
    perilunate fracture dislocations, 666-667, 668-669f, 669, 670-674f,
        677-678f, 680f
    transcapitate fracture dislocations, 669, 672, 675-676f
Transscaphoid fractures, 657f
Transtriquetral fractures, 657f
Transulnar fractures, 657f
Transverse carpal ligament, 67f
Transverse carpal ligament release; see also Carpal tunnel release
author's preferred approach, 1220, 1221-1223f, 1223
endoscopic visualization in, 1201f, 1218, 1218f
with incision above wrist, 1210, 1211-1213f, 1214, 1215f
incomplete, 1228
with limited-excision techniques, 1214, 1216f, 1217
Paine release with transverse limited wrist incision and retinaculatome,
    1216f, 1218
single-portal technique, 1223, 1224-1226f, 1225, 1227, 1227f
by tenosynovectomy alone, 1227
through palmar incision, 1214, 1216f
through two nonpalmar incisions, 1217f, 1218
two-portal technique, 1219f, 1220
Transverse instability, 494-495
Transverse sectional anatomy, 50-57, 51-56f
Trapezial tuberosity, 238f
Trapeziocapitate interosseous ligament, 94-95, 95-96f
Trapeziometacarpal joint, 70
Trapezium
anatomy, 41f, 64f, 66, 66f, 67f
in axial-radial dislocation, 689f, 690, 690f, 691f
dislocations, 705, 706f

Trapezium—cont'd
 fractures, 483, 484f
 morphology, 20-21
 tubercle of, 42f
Trapezium trapezoid interosseous ligament, 94-95, 95f
Trapezoid
 anatomy, 64f, 65f, 66-67, 67f
  dorsal perspective, 41f
  palmar perspective, 42f
 dislocations, 704-705
 fractures, 483
Trapezoidal bone graft, in distal radius malunion, 375f, 377f
Trauma
 in children, 1024
 ischemia-edema cycle in, 1115f
 in rheumatoid arthritis, 871, 872t
 supertrauma, 983, 985
Traumatic instability, 569
 classification, 496t, 497
Traumatic tears of triangular fibrocartilage, 720, 721, 723; see also
    Triangular fibrocartilage tears, treatment
Triamcinolone, in juvenile rheumatoid arthritis, 950, 952
Triangular fibrocartilage
 abnormalities, 775
 anatomy, 224, 225, 225f, 711, 712f, 821-822, 821-822f
  arthroscopic, 175f, 176f, 177, 178-179f, 181, 182f
  microstructure, 713-714f
  vascular supply, 118f, 118-119, 714f
  zones, 713f
 arthrography, 274
 arthroscopic inspection, 185, 187, 718, 720
 compression, 247f
 degeneration, 230
 in distal radioulnar joint stability, 224-225f, 226, 227t, 244, 760, 761f, 762
 distal radius and, 312, 314
 distal ulna and, 745
 in dorsal dislocation of ulnar head, 828f
 exposure, 133
 in force transmission through wrist, 198, 200-201f, 201
 injuries, 839-842, 840t, 840-842f; see also Triangular fibrocartilage tears
  in distal radius fracture, 323
 magnetic resonance imaging, 280f
 mechanical properties, 227t
 physical examination, 713, 715f, 716
 repair or reconstruction, 830-831f
 in ulnar impaction (abutment) syndrome, 774, 846
Triangular fibrocartilage complex
 anatomy, 67f, 97-99, 97-99f, 175, 822, 1066
 arthroscopy
  diagnostic, 290f, 298-299, 300f
  therapeutic, 301-302, 303f
 excision, force transmission and, 228t
 in Kienböck's disease, 441
 lunate and, 432
 Palmer classification of injuries to, 720, 721f, 839-840, 840t, 1068
Triangular fibrocartilage tears, 710-742
 anatomy and biomechanics, 711, 712-714f
 arthroscopy (diagnostic), 300f, 718, 720, 1067-1068
 classification, 720-722, 721-722f, 1068
 clinical presentation, 711, 713, 715f, 716, 840
 diagnostic examinations, 244, 245, 716-719f, 718, 840
 mechanism of injury, 1067
 trampoline effect/test in, 730, 734, 734f
 treatment
  acute traumatic tears, 722
  arthroscopic repair, 301-302, 303f, 732, 734-736f, 737, 1066-1067f,
    1068-1070, 1069f

 author's preference, 737-739, 738f
 isolated tears, acute repair, 723-724f, 724
 open repair, 724, 725f, 726
 palmar tears, open repair, 731f, 732
 radial avulsion tears, open repair, 732
 radial repair technique, 726, 727-730f
 reattachment of ulnar styloid (bone avulsion injury), 731-732,
   733f
 type IA tears (radial lesions), open repair, 726
 ulnar tears (avulsions), open repair, 723-724f, 726, 730-731
Tricyclic antidepressants, in overuse syndrome, 1301
Triple-injection arthrography, in scapholunate instability, 507-508
Triquetral-hamate impaction, physical examination, 246
Triquetral-hamate ligament, anatomy, 47f, 79f, 90f, 91, 174f, 553f
 dorsal, 656f
Triquetrocapitate ligament, 79f, 90f, 91
Triquetrolunate impaction syndrome, in athletes, 1064-1065
Triquetrum
 anatomy, 34f, 65-66, 65-67f, 237f
  arthroscopic, 175f, 181f
  dorsal perspective, 41f
  in extensor retinaculum system, 47f
  palmar perspective, 42f
 dislocations, 704, 705f
 dorsal displacement, 697f
 fractures, 115, 479, 479f, 481
  in athletes, 1058-1059, 1059f
  perilunate instability and, 635f, 653f, 657f
 kinematics, 212t, 214, 216
 vascular supply, 115, 116f
Trispherical total wrist arthroplasty, 941, 941f
Trochlea, 42f
Tsai technique, 800, 804-807f
Tubercles, anatomy, 42f
Tulipan modification of Darrach procedure, 856f
Tumors, 1234-1259; see also Ganglions
 bone; see also Multiple hereditary osteochondromata
  benign, 1250t, 1251-1254f, 1252, 1256
  evaluation and treatment principles, 1250, 1250t, 1252
  malignant, 1250t, 1254-1257f, 1256, 1258
 in children, 1024
 in distal radioulnar joint region, 862
 skin
  benign, 1235t, 1235-1236f, 1235-1237
  evaluation and treatment principles, 1235
  malignant, 1235t, 1236-1237f, 1237, 1238-1239f, 1239
 soft-tissue
  benign, 1240, 1240t, 1241f, 1241t, 1242-1243, 1243-1245f, 1245
  evaluation and treatment principles, 1239-1240
  malignant, 1240t, 1245, 1246-1249f, 1247, 1250
  management algorithm, 1241f
Tuohy needle, in triangular fibrocartilage tear repair, 736f, 737, 1066-1067f,
   1068

U
Ulna
 caput ulnae syndrome, 874, 874f, 909, 1139-1140f, 1142f
 congenital deficiency
  treatment, 1013, 1014-1015f, 1016
  types, 1013, 1014f
 distal; see Distal ulna
 distance of nerves to, 1084t
 dorsal subluxation or dislocation
  pathogenesis, 826-828, 830f
  radiographic examination, 828-829, 829f
  treatment, 829-835, 830-836f
 embryology, 743

injuries in children, 1020-1021
intercalary excision, in distal radius malunion, 368
midshaft fracture, 1092f
palmar dislocation, 754-755f
palmar perspective, 41f
plastic deformation, 748-749
surface anatomy, 36
surgical approaches to, 750f, 751, 752f
surgical straightening, in multiple hereditary osteochondromata, 998f, 999
translocation/translation, 495, 570f, 582-584f, 586-587
    pathomechanics, 585f
    treatment, 586, 586f
vascular supply, 38, 40f, 41, 107-108, 116-118
Ulna lengthening
    biomechanical studies, 449
    in children, 1020-1021
    in Kienböck's disease, 201, 457, 457f
    in multiple hereditary osteochondromata, 996, 997-998f, 999
    in radial aplasia, 1011, 1012f
Ulna minus conditions, 853-854
Ulna physeal injury, from distraction, 1063-1064
Ulna plus/minus, 69
Ulna recession, 780f, 785f; see also Ulna shortening
    in lunotriquetral dissociation and triangular fibrocartilage instability, 852f
    Madelung's deformity and, 854f
    methods, 781, 781f
    procedure, 781, 782-785f, 783, 786
    Rayhack technique, 783, 784f
    in ulnar impaction (abutment) syndrome, 849, 850-851f
Ulna shortening; see also Ulna recession
    in children, 1020-1021
    in distal radius malunion, 368
    in Kienböck's disease, 368
Ulna variance
    biomechanics, 774, 821, 821f
    in gymnasts, 1062, 1063
    in Kienböck's disease, 432, 434f, 439-441, 440f
    measurement, 777, 778f, 846
    positive, negative, and neutral, 43
    radiographic examination, 264-265, 266f
    in rheumatoid arthritis, 879f
    treatment, 849, 850-852f
    in ulnocarpal abutment, 779f, 785f, 846-847, 846-849f
Ulnar anlage excision, 1013, 1015f, 1016
Ulnar approaches in arthrotomy, 133, 137-140f, 140
    dorsal, 140, 141-143f, 144
    in hook of hamate nonunion, 155f, 156, 158f
    midline, 144-145f, 146
    in radial aplasia, 163-166f
Ulnar artery
    anatomy, 34f, 38, 39-40f, 107f, 110f, 238f
    occlusion, 282
    reconstruction with saphenous vein bypass graft, 1046f, 1047
    thrombosis, 1046f, 1046-1047
    triangular fibrocartilage and, 118f, 118-119
Ulnar compression test, 260
Ulnar deviation
    comparative morphology, 15, 17-19
    in juvenile rheumatoid arthritis, 948f
    lunate in, 571f
Ulnar fractures; see also Ulnar styloid, fractures
    in adults, 749, 751, 753
        articular fractures, 753, 753f
        complications, 754
        displaced fractures, 749-753f, 751, 753
        nightstick fracture, 749

pathologic, 754
        stress fractures, 753-754
        synostosis of distal ulna to radius, 754-755
        treatment, 749, 750-753f, 751, 753
        treatment algorithm, 748f
    in children
        complete fractures, 746f, 747
        complications of physeal injuries to ulna, 748
        greenstick fracture, 746-747
        physeal injury, 747-748
        plastic deformation of ulna, 748-749
        torus fracture, 745-746
        treatment, 746-747
        treatment algorithm, 745f
Ulnar gutter splint, 1278f
Ulnar head
    anatomy and kinematics, 34f, 68-69, 237f, 823-824, 824f, 826f
    chondromalacia and degenerative arthritis of, 842-843, 843-845f
    dorsal subluxation or dislocation
        pathogenesis, 826-828, 830f
        radiographic examination, 828-829, 829f
        treatment, 829-835, 830-836f
    palmar subluxation and dislocation
        pathogenesis, 835-836, 836f
        radiographic examination, 836, 837f
        treatment, 836-839, 838f
    replacement, in arthritis deformity, 789, 792, 793-794f
    resection/excision, 855-859f, 857; see also Darrach resection
        in arthritis deformity, 789, 792, 794, 795f
        complications, 792, 794, 795f
Ulnar impaction (abutment) syndrome, 846-847, 846-849f; see also
        Ulnocarpal abutment
    physical examination, 244-245, 247f
Ulnar impingement syndrome, 298, 298f; see also Ulnar impaction
        (abutment) syndrome; Ulnocarpal abutment
Ulnar nerve
    anatomy, 34f, 38, 119f, 120, 121f, 238f
        deep branch, 37f
        dorsal branch, 36f
        dorsal cutaneous branches, 170f
        transverse retinacular branch of dorsal sensory branch, 1038f
    compression, in cyclist's palsy, 1040, 1042-1043
    distance to radius and ulna from, 1084, 1084t
    injuries, 1084
        treatment, 1087, 1088f
Ulnar osteotomy, radioulnar fusion and, in arthritis deformity, 811, 812-814f, 813, 815
Ulnar palmar carpal artery, 40f
Ulnar recession osteotomy, 780f, 781, 782-784f
Ulnar styloid
    anatomy, 34f, 36, 175f, 237f, 238f
        dorsal perspective, 41f
        palmar perspective, 42f
    fractures, 839-842, 843f
        fixation, 323, 323f, 324
        in gymnasts, 1062f
        treatment, 722
        triangular fibrocartilage tears and, 716f
    impingement, loose bodies and, 852-853, 853f
    peripheral tears from, treatment, 723-724f, 726, 730-731
    reattachment of, in bone avulsion injury, 731-732, 733f
Ulnar styloid process, 67f
    ontogenesis, 62
Ulnar styloid prominence, 69
Ulnar tunnel syndrome, in distal radius malunion, 362
Ulnar wrist examination, dorsal; see Dorsal ulnar wrist examination
Ulnar/radial deviation, axis for, 211f

Ulnocapitate ligament, 79f, 80f, 86f, 87, 174f
Ulnocarpal abutment, 773-787, 840t; *see also* Ulnar impaction (abutment)
    syndrome
  biomechanics, 773-774, 774f
    force distribution across wrist, 197-198
  classification, 774-775
  diagnosis, 775-777, 776-780f
  etiology, 773
  in gymnasts, 1062-1063, 1063f
  treatment, 777, 781, 781f
    ulna recession procedure, 782-785f, 783, 786
Ulnocarpal force transmission, 228-229, 228-229t
Ulnocarpal instability, provocative stress testing in, 248-249f, 259-260
Ulnocarpal joint
  capsulotomy, 101, 102f
  kinematics, 224
Ulnocarpal ligaments
  anatomy, 79-80f, 84-85, 85t, 85-86f, 87, 175f
    arthroscopic, 175f
  arthroscopic inspection, 185
  triangular fibrocartilage and, 822, 822f
Ulnocarpal tendinous tethers, 832
Ulnolunate ligament
  anatomy, 79f, 80f, 84, 85f, 86f
    arthroscopic, 174f, 175, 179f
  in distal radioulnar joint stability, 763
  in perilunate fracture dislocations, 657f
Ulnotriquetral ligament
  anatomy, 79f, 80f, 84-85, 86f, 87
    arthroscopic, 174f, 179f
  in distal radioulnar joint stability, 763
  in perilunate fracture dislocations, 657f
Ultrasonography, 276, 276f
  of ganglions, 1167-1168, 1168-1169f, 1169-1170, 1172, 1176f
  in phonophoresis, 1267
  in rheumatoid arthritis, 880
Ultrasound therapy, 1267, 1267f
Unciform process; *see* Hamulus
Uni-Cut system of endoscopic release, 1227f
Universal Classification of distal radius fractures, 317, 318f, 319, 319t

V

Vaillant, Sebastian, 9
Valpar 9, 1292f
Vascular anatomy (blood supply), 38, 41, 106-119
  capitate, 111, 115f
  distal radius and ulna, 38, 40f, 107-108, 111f, 116-118, 117f
  dorsal and palmar surfaces, 39f
  extrinsic and intrinsic systems, 106-108, 109f, 110
  hamate, 115-116, 116f
  intercarpal arches and anastomoses on dorsal side of wrist, 108f
  lateral aspect of carpus, 109f
  lunate, 108, 110-111, 114f, 432, 434f
  palmar aspect of carpus, 110f
  palmar extrinsic, 109f
  scaphoid, 108, 110, 112-113f, 386
  triangular fibrocartilage, 118f, 118-119, 714f
  triquetral, 115, 116f
Vascular disorders in athletes, 1046f, 1046-1047
Vascular pedicle grafts, 117f, 117-118
Vascular tumors, 1242t, 1242-1243, 1243f
Vascularized bone grafts, in scaphoid nonunion, 422, 423f
Vascularized flaps, 1310
VATER (VACTERL) syndromes, 1008
Vaughan-Jackson, O.J., 10
Vaughan-Jackson lesion, 1138, 1139f
Vein grafts, 1046f, 1047

Vesalius, Andreas, 3, 4f, 61
Vibration, tendinitis and, 1182
Videofluoroscopy, 273, 273f
  in carpal instability nondissociative, 558, 559, 560f
  in scapholunate instability, 507-508f
Viegas classification of instability, 491, 492t
Villonodular tenosynovitis, 1240, 1241f
Viral arthritis, 872
VISI; *see* Volar intercalated segment instabilities
Vitamin A, overdosage, 1024
Vitamin B_6, in carpal tunnel syndrome, 1209
Volar intercalated segment instabilities (VISI), 493
  carpal instability nondissociative and, 552f, 563-564f, 563-565
  historical perspective, 9, 10
  in lunotriquetral sprains, 529f, 529-530, 533f, 535, 547
  in rheumatoid arthritis, 878f
  scaphoid fracture and, 387
Volkmann's ischemic contracture, 1107, 1126f
  biomechanics, 1109, 1110
  digital and wrist extension in, 1111f
  historical perspective, 1113-1114
  surgical treatment, 1121f, 1125-1127, 1128-1133f, 1130, 1132-1133
    author's preferred approach, 1133-1134
Volz prosthesis
  design development, 928
  initial design, 925f

W

Wafer procedure, 302, 304, 781, 783, 786, 1069f
Wartenberg's cheiralgia, physical examination, 238, 240
Wartenberg's syndrome, 1044-1045
Water therapy, 1268
Watson matched arthroplasty, 857, 859f
Watson resection of distal ulna, 781, 781f
Watson scaphoid shift/stress test, 254, 256, 258f, 259
Watson-Jones closed manipulation, 659
Whipple compression screw (Herbert-Whipple screw), 1052
Whitesides technique of compartment pressure measurement, 1118, 1119f, 1120
Whitlow, acral melanotic, 1239f
Wick catheter technique of compartment pressure measurement, 1119f, 1120
Wolff's law, 1262
Wood's bursa, 240; *see also* Intersection syndrome
Work, overuse syndrome and, 1297
Work hardening programs, 1287
  concepts and design, 1287-1288
  in cumulative trauma disorder, 1291
  disability accommodation and, 1291-1292
  elements of, 1289-1290f, 1289-1291
  initial evaluation in, 1289
  in overuse syndrome, 1301
  referral to, 1288
  in specific injuries, 1291
  therapy team in, 1288-1289
Work rehabilitation, 1287; *see also* Work hardening programs
  functional capacity evaluation, 1292f, 1292-1293
Work simulation tasks, 1290-1291
Wrestling injuries, epidemiology, 1032
Wrightington classification of rheumatoid arthritis, 1139, 1141
Wrist; *see also* Carpal *entries;* Carpus
  discomfort, diagnosis, 775; *see also* Pain in wrist
  international terminology/etymology, 2, 3, 5f, 61-62
  morphology; *see* Morphology, comparative
Wrist arthrodesis
  advantages and disadvantages, 924
  for Kienböck's disease, 464

for perilunate dislocations, 648, 649
for scapholunate advanced collapse, 603, 603f
    limited, 603-605, 604-610f
Wrist arthrodesis for rheumatoid arthritis, 899-923
    after failed arthroplasty, 922, 922f
    bilateral, 920
    complete
        immobilization after, 918, 920
        indications, 915
        internal fixation in, 915-916, 916-919f
        pin removal after, 920
        position of fusion, 916-917
        surgical approach, 906f, 915
        surgical closure, 918
        two-pin fixation in, 917-918
    complications, 920
    limited, 900-901, 902-903f, 903
    midcarpal, 902f
    radiolunate
        range of motion after, 904t

spontaneous, 903-904
surgical, 902f, 904-905, 905-908f, 909, 910f
radioscapholunate, 902f, 909, 911-912f, 912
    with midcarpal arthroplasty, 912, 913-914f, 914
    range of motion after, 915t
Sauvé-Kapandji fusion, 914-915
WristJack frame, 339f
Writer's cramp, 1295

X
Xanthoma, 1240, 1241f

Z
Zaidemberg vascular bone graft, 117
    in scaphoid nonunion, 422, 423f
Zolpidem, in overuse syndrome, 1301
Z-plasty
    in arthrogryposis multiplex congenita, 1018, 1019f
    in radial aplasia, 1010f
    in radial club hand, 165f, 166